Nutrition and Integr Medicine for Clinicians

Mystery illness can be helped, and this book lays the groundwork for it!

Can a water-damaged building ruin your health and cause debilitating exhaustion, chronic pain, insomnia, anxiety, obesity and "brain fog?" Could a flood or wet basement make you sick even if it has long dried out? Building on its predecessor, *Nutrition and Integrative Medicine for Clinicians: Volume Two* is an essential, peer-reviewed resource for practitioners to help patients with various illnesses found in society, including those contracted from water-damaged structures, that can lay the groundwork for a healthy road to recovery.

Written by authors at the forefront of their respective fields, this book presents information for people "written off" as having a "mystery illness," fibromyalgia or chronic fatigue. Chronic inflammatory response syndrome (CIRS) is ubiquitous and affects many body systems, yet it is largely unrecognized by doctors, who misdiagnose CIRS patients daily. This book is a comprehensive guide on evaluating illnesses that are difficult to diagnose, including CIRS.

This volume contains information on various subjects, including:

- Illnesses resulting from water-damaged buildings and subsequent change in the microbiome of the building.
- Steps to heal from mold/mycotoxin illnesses.
- Legal and ethical considerations in health issues from exposure to a water-damaged building as well as introducing the "building science" to clinicians.
- Effects of CIRS on metabolism and insulin resistance.
- Environmental hormone disruptors.
- Myalgic encephalitis/chronic fatigue syndrome.
- Regenerative agriculture.
- Pediatric sleep-related breathing disorders and their effects on growth and development.
- Circadian effects of artificial light and their effects on mitochondria.
- Nutritional support in Covid.
- The design nature of sound and its relationship to neural networks.
- The human body as a biological sound healing instrument.
- The use of color in clinical application.
- Art in medicine.
- Living life with intentionality and mindfulness.
- Making childbirth a positive experience.

Nutrition and Integrative Medicine for Clinicians

Volume Two

Edited by

Aruna Bakhru

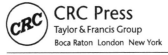

CRC Press is an imprint of the
Taylor & Francis Group, an **informa** business

Designed cover image: © Shutterstock

First edition published 2023
by CRC Press
6000 Broken Sound Parkway NW, Suite 300, Boca Raton, FL 33487-2742

and by CRC Press
4 Park Square, Milton Park, Abingdon, Oxon, OX14 4RN

CRC Press is an imprint of Taylor & Francis Group, LLC

© 2023 Taylor & Francis Group, LLC

ISBN: 978-0-367-42895-2 (hbk)
ISBN: 978-1-032-11012-7 (pbk)
ISBN: 978-1-003-36583-9 (ebk)

DOI: 10.1201/b23304

Typeset in Times
by Deanta Global Publishing Services, Chennai, India

Access the Support Material: www.routledge.com/9781032110127

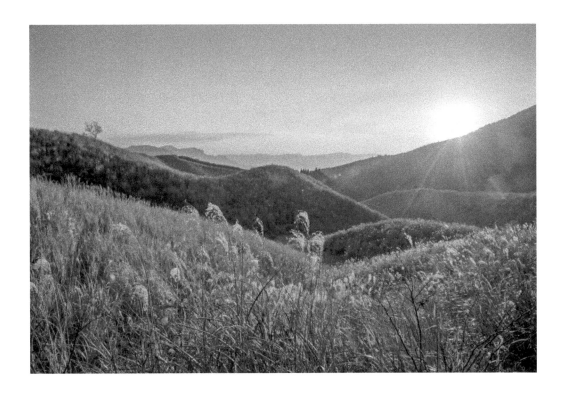

The sun is a daily reminder that we too can rise again from the darkness, that we, too, can shine our light.
S. Ajna

Contents

SECTION I Environmental Medicine, Chronic Illness and Innovations in Standard of Care

SECTION II Functional and Integrative Medicine: Perspectives in Deep Healing

Editor

Aruna Bakhru is Board Certified in Internal Medicine and a Fellow of The American College of Physicians. She graduated in Medicine and Surgery from Lady Hardinge Medical College, New Delhi, India and did her Residency in Internal Medicine at Prince George's Hospital and Medical Center affiliated with The University of Maryland. She also conducted research with Valerie Johnson at New York Medical College, Lincoln Hospital and Medical Center. Currently, she is affiliated with Vassar Brothers Medical Center, Poughkeepsie, New York.

A respected and long-standing figure in her field, Dr. Bakhru currently serves as a physician with a focus on integrative and internal medicine in her private practice, which she has maintained for over 25 years. Dr. Bakhru has held numerous appointments over the course of her career: She acted as the Young Physician Section Representative of The Dutchess County Medical Society and also as the Chair of the Integrative Medicine Subcommittee of The Dutchess County Medical Society. She has also served in the past on the Ambulatory and Emergency Services Committee at Vassar Brothers Medical Center, the Medical Audit Committee of Vassar Brothers Medical Center and the Complementary Care Committee at Vassar Brothers Medical Center. She has also served on the Utilization Review and Quality Assurance Committee of Mohawk Valley Plan Health Plan.

She has over 20 years of experience and training in many other modalities, such as Nutrition, Intravenous Nutrient Therapy, Functional Medicine, Ayurvedic Medicine, Herbal Medicine as well as Bioenergetic Medicine, Sound and Light as healing modalities. She trained with The American Academy of Environmental Medicine, learning to treat 21st-century problems caused by our lifestyle and environmental issues, including Building Biology, heating, ventilation and air conditioning systems, and mold.

She has also been involved with numerous community service activities such as the medical clinic for the indigent at Vassar Hospital and volunteer physician for the summer camp run by SVSC, a nonprofit group. She has also written for numerous publications and appeared on radio and television as well as lecturing on medically related topics. Dr. Bakhru has been endorsed by Marquis Who's Who as a leader in the healthcare industry. She recently was named a Lifetime Achiever by Marquis Who's Who, the world's premier publisher of biographical profiles. As in all Marquis Who's Who biographical volumes, individuals profiled are selected on the basis of current reference value. Factors such as position, noteworthy accomplishments, visibility and prominence in a field are all taken into account during the selection process. In addition to her status as Lifetime Achiever, Dr. Bakhru has previously received the Excellence in Integrative Medicine Award from Emord and Associates and has also been honored by The Holistic Doctors Recognition Board as one of the Top Ten doctors in New York State. Additionally, she received Awards in Pathology and Forensic Medicine from the University of Delhi as well as the Certificate of Excellence from many insurance groups. Furthermore, Dr. Bakhru has been a featured listee in Who's Who in America, Who's Who in Medicine and Healthcare, Who's Who in the World and Who's Who in Science and Engineering. She also volunteers at Cyber safety India International Board of Advisors and is an Executive Committee member of the Dutchess County Regional Science Fair. She has also published various articles in her local newspapers as well as appearing on public television in White Plains and radio talk shows for WKIP and WVKR 91.3 FM out of Vassar College. Her website is www.centerforenergymedicine.com. She currently practices in New York and believes that treating the patient as a whole leads to better outcomes and satisfaction for both the physician and the patient.

Contributors

Arden Andersen, DO, MSPH, PhD
Family and Occupational Medicine Physician
Kansas, USA

Kristina Baehr, JD
Owner, Just Well Law
Austin, TX

John Beaulieu, ND, PhD
Professor of Integrative Health Studies
California Institute of Integral Studies
and
Owner, BioSonic Enterprises
Stone Ridge, New York

Kathleen Keats Beaulieu
BioSonic Enterprises
Stone Ridge, New York

Dona Biswas, MD, FRANZCP
Integrative Psychiatrist
Fellow of the Royal Australian and
    New Zealand College of Psychiatrists
Blacktown, New South Wales, Australia

Payal Chaudhary, MD
Senior Consultant
Madhukar Rainbow Children's Hospital
New Delhi, India

Kenneth J. Friedman, PhD
Adjunct Associate Professor of Medicine
School of Osteopathic Medicine
Rowan University

Michael J. Gonzalez, NMD, DSc, PhD
Professor (Full)
University of Puerto Rico
Medical Sciences Campus
School of Public Health

Jerry L. Hatfield, PhD
Affiliate Professor
Iowa State University
and
Laboratory Director
United States Department of Agriculture

Andrew Heyman, MD, MHSA
Medical Director of Integrative Medicine
Department of Clinical Research and
    Leadership
School of Medicine and Health Sciences
George Washington University
Washington D.C., USA
and
Director of Academic Affairs
Metabolic Medical Institute and American
    Academy of Anti-Aging Medicine

Shawn Marie Higgins, DO, NMM
Osteopathic Physician
Board Certified in Neuromuscular Medicine
Owner and Founder of Osteopathic Wellness
Faculty and Board of Directors of the
    Osteopathic Cranial Academy
Raymond, Maine, USA

Susan Imholz, PhD
Scholar, Program Designer, Clinician, and
    Educator
New Bern, NC

David Lark, B. App. Sci., CIEC, CMC
Principal Mycologist and Director
NSJ EnviroSciences Pty Ltd
Newcastle, Australia

Marsha L. Luginbuehi, PhD, NCSP
President and CEO
Child Uplift
Fairview, WY, USA

Nisha J. Manek, MD, FACP, FRCP (UK)
Integrative Rheumatologist and Independent
    Consultant
Aptos, CA

David Perez Martinez, MD
Integrative Psychiatrist
New York, New York

Scott W. McMahon, MD
Clinical Associate Professor
Burrell College of Osteopathic Medicine
New Mexico State University

Jorge R. Miranda-Massari, BS Biol, RPh, PharmD
University of Puerto Rico
Medical Sciences Campus
School of Pharmacy
and
EDP University
Naturopathic Sciences Program
San Juan, Puerto Rico

Jeffrey Moss, DDS, CNS, DACBN
Owner, Moss Nutrition

Chris Newton, PhD
Research Director
Center for Immuno-Metabolism
Microbiome and Bio- Energetic Research
East Yorkshire, UK

Peter O'Brien, PhD
Research Agronomist
USDA Agricultural Research Service
United States Department of Agriculture

Manju Puri, MD
Director Professor
Department of Obstetrics and Gynecology
Lady Hardinge Medical College
University of Delhi, India

Joshua Rosenthal, MD
Holistic Sleep and Regenerative Medicine
    Specialist
Huntington, NY

Judy Sachter, MA, PhD
Artist and Media Technologist
Los Angeles, CA

Larry Schwartz, BSME, MBA, CIEC
CEO
Safestart Environmental and Safestart Building
    Consulting
USA

Stephanie Seneff, PhD
Senior Research Scientist
Computer Science and Artificial Intelligence
    Laboratory

Massachusetts Institute of Technology
Cambridge, MA, USA

Alyse Shockey, RDH, CHHP, CSOM
Certified Holistic Healthcare Practitioner
Highlands Ranch, CO, USA

Ritchie Shoemaker, MD
Director
Center for Research on Biotoxin-Associated
    Illness
Pocomoke City, MD, USA

Martha Stark, MD
Faculty
Harvard Medical School
Cambridge, MA
Co-Founder/Co-Director, Center for
    Psychoanalytic Studies

Maria A. Vera-Nunez, MD, MS
Staff Physician
Center for Functional Medicine
Cleveland Clinic, Ohio

April Vukelic, DO
Shoemaker Certified Physician
Institute of Functional Medicine Certified
    Physician (IFMCP)
and
ReCODE 2.0 Certified Physician, Wahls
    Certified Physician
American Academy of Osteopathy
Osteopathic Cranial Academy
and
Table Trainer with Indiana Academy of
    Osteopathy
Biodynamic Osteopath

Kenneth M. Wacha, PhD
Agricultural Engineer Research Scientist
USDA Agricultural Research Service
United States Department of Agriculture)

Jerry Wintrob, OD
Optometrist
Colored Light as a Healing Modality
Accord, New York

Preface

The first volume was a mighty undertaking; luckily, each chapter was "stand alone," and the reader could choose to begin the book at any chapter. My aim was to bring an understanding of the different aspects of integrative medicine and nutrition to the clinician interested in healing the whole patient.

This volume was "unintended." An unintended consequence of a negligent ductless heating, ventilation and air conditioning (HVAC) installation in my own home. At first, the water was seeping inside the walls and the attic, and we were unaware until a major water leak occurred that brought attention to the situation. Then, the nightmare began. The box store that recommended the installers, the installers, and the insurance company that insured them all knew what had happened; they knew exactly what the problem was and what needed to be done, and instead of taking swift action, they instituted a gaslighting campaign. Since the installer had been putting these in homes up and down the east coast, negligently I am sure, ruining the health of the occupants, who were likely unaware, it was of prime importance to the insurance company to stifle my voice. Not to do the right thing; rather, to shove it under the rug.

We had to tear our house down to the studs and rebuild it. Every wall where the ductless air conditioning was installed had to be torn down. Our lives were upended and our health affected due to mycotoxins and mold. I turned to a Shoemaker Protocol physician for help. I also joined a Facebook group for people whose lives had been affected by water damage and mold. The stories were heart rending, and eventually, I could not take the suffering. I had to stop reading their stories, but I realized that I could help by creating a Volume Two for clinicians that dealt with mold as a big part of the book. There are people who have their own ideas about treating mold-related health problems, but Dr. Ritchie Shoemaker gets credit for being the forerunner in this field.

You will read a short commentary by Kristina Baehr JD in this book, relating what happened to her. My hope is to provide a book, even if it is a starting point, for doctors, regulators, lawyers, judges and regular people, maybe even some decent ones who work for the insurance industry and the home building and HVAC industry and who have not sold their soul for money, to gain an understanding of water-damaged homes and health issues caused by mold and mycotoxins and the change in the microbiome of the water-damaged building.

Dr. Scott McMahon is a top expert witness for mold legal cases, and he told me that it is his calling. Dr Stephanie Seneff's chapter brings attention to the complex biological issues relating to Euthyroid Sick Syndrome, caused again by – you guessed it – chronic inflammatory response syndrome (CIRS) due to mold/mycotoxin toxicity and the interaction between mycotoxins and the ubiquitous glyphosate.

Larry Schwartz lends his expertise to Building Science. He is an expert witness in water-damaged homes litigation. There are many people who take a short course, call themselves remediators and exploit those who are already suffering.

Dr. April Vukelic is passionate about treating mold patients and is also an expert osteopathic physician. Her standalone chapter on central nervous system injuries from mold is a classic. So of course, are all the chapters that she coauthored.

Mold- and mycotoxin-related illness is a serious public health issue. It is responsible for many diverse medical conditions, as it causes multisystem illnesses that have not yet been properly recognized by the medical, legal, building or regulatory agencies. Original research published in the *Frontiers of Immunology* shows that "[l]ong-term exposure to dampness microbiota induces multi-organ morbidity."[1]

Harding et al. in their article in *Brain, Behavior and Immunity*, titled "Mold inhalation causes innate immune activation, neural, cognitive and emotional dysfunction," state:

> Individuals living or working in moldy buildings complain of a variety of health problems including pain, fatigue, increased anxiety, depression, and cognitive deficits. Mold inhalation causes innate immune activation, neural, cognitive and emotional dysfunction.[2]

Exposure to water-damaged buildings can damage the mitochondria. "In trying to understand the mechanism of injury to the mitochondria that triggers an autoimmune response, researchers have learned that pyruvate carboxylase is a major site of antigenicity for antimitochondrial antibodies (AMA)."[3]

A study by Dennis et al. published in *Toxicology and Industrial Health*, titled "Fungal exposure endocrinopathy in sinusitis with growth hormone deficiency: Dennis-Robertson syndrome,"[4]found that patients with a significant history of indoor mold exposure and chronic rhinosinusitis, determined by computed tomography scan or endoscopy, had deficiency of human growth hormone, primary or secondary hypothyroidism, and deficiency of adrenocorticotropic hormone.

In another original article, "Neural autoantibodies and neurophysiologic abnormalities in patients exposed to molds in water-damaged buildings,"[5] the authors state:

> Recently, it has been suggested that mold exposure causes neurological injury. The authors investigated neurological antibodies and neurophysiological abnormalities in patients exposed to molds at home who developed symptoms of peripheral neuropathy (i.e., numbness, tingling, tremors, and muscle weakness in the extremities).

Daschner in *Frontiers in Immunology*[6] describes "Dampness and mold hypersensitivity syndrome" that results in multi-organ symptoms. He states:

> Even chronic fatigue syndrome or clinical features similar to this entity have been connected not only to relevant environmental histories of exposure to water-damaged buildings but also to the detection of mycotoxins.

An article by Brewer et al. published in the journal *Toxins*, titled "Chronic illness associated with mold and mycotoxins: Is naso-sinus fungal biofilm the culprit?"[7] came to the following conclusions, among others (for the full list, see the article):

CONCLUSIONS[7]

> Indoor water-damaged environments contain a variety of mold and bacterial species that produce mycotoxins, volatile organic compounds, exotoxins and other metabolites that are present in the dust, furnishings and air.
>
> The occupants of these environments experience chronic adverse health effects that range from upper and lower respiratory disease, central and peripheral neurological deficits, chronic fatigue type illness, among others.
>
> Prior exposure to toxic mold and mycotoxins may represent an important feature of chronically ill patients such as CFS as well as those with CRS. An internal reservoir of toxin producing mold (e.g., sinuses) that persists in biofilms could produce and release mycotoxins. This model of fungal persistence may help explain these chronic illnesses and represent a potential new understanding of mechanisms of disease that can be treated and/or lessened.

In another article titled "Mold exposure and respiratory health in damp indoor environments," published in the journal *Frontiers in Bioscience*, the authors, Park and Cox-Ganser,[8] make the following point regarding respiratory outcomes with mold exposure in indoor damp environments:

> In this article we have presented abundant evidence of associations of various respiratory health outcomes with mold exposure and some potential disease mechanisms. Thus, even if we do not fully understand specific causal agents or mechanisms for mold-related illnesses yet, it is very sensible for physicians, environmental professionals, and building managers to recognize potential risk of exposure to mold and support proactive measures for remediation of water damage and mold contamination to protect occupants' health. The major driving force for mold and other microbial growth in indoor environments is moisture. Thus, identification and repair of the sources of excess moisture such as humid

air, or water intrusion or leaks, prompt and complete repair or replacement of water-damaged materials, and thorough cleaning of all indoor surfaces after remediation are essential to minimize mold exposure and decrease mold exposure-related respiratory illnesses. The problem of water damage and mold contamination in indoor environments and related health effects is now a global issue, as is evident from reports from several countries, and thus, needs to be taken much more seriously.[8]

Lynch and Teitelbaum of the Illinois College of Optometry report an adult woman with exposure to black mold who developed atopic dermatitis with anterior subcapsular cataracts:[9] "Anterior subcapsular cataracts are pathognomonic for atopic illness."[9]

Chapter 6 of this book, titled "Chronic Inflammatory Response Syndrome (CIRS) and Metabolism: Proliferative Physiology and Insulin Resistance" by Ritchie C. Shoemaker and April Vukelic, explains how exposure to water-damaged buildings can cause, among other issues, heart failure, insulin resistance and dementia. CIRS causes metabolic acidosis and grey matter nuclear atrophy, which in turn, results in pulmonary hypertension and heart failure.

The relationship of suppression of production of ribosomal mRNA and nuclear-encoded mitochondrial genes to multiple facets of glucose metabolism, especially aerobic glycolysis, resulting in neuronal injury, including cognitive impairment, and pulmonary hypertension.

Specifically,

The combination of the development of hypoxemia (from fatty acid oxidation [FAO]) and aerobic glycolysis is the development of pulmonary hypertension.

And you will read more, as here:

In CIRS, we worry about the Warburg Effect, because it underlies the pathologic development of clinically significant metabolic acidosis and pulmonary hypertension; it underlies abnormalities, including metabolism in branched chain glycans, that will lead to insulin resistance. Further, we also see multiple examples of injury to neuronal tissue associated with the Warburg Effect, both peripherally, creating peripheral neuropathy, and centrally, possibly contributing to dementing illnesses.

The innate immune system activation caused by CIRS does not get better on its own, does not self-heal, even after the patient has been removed from the source of exposure.

There is not an intrinsic issue with the mitochondria. The problem is the failure to effectively use the electron transport chain and the inability to use acetyl CoA, only producing maybe 5% of ATP and reduced oxygen delivery to the cells. That is why CIRS patients are so tired. Lactic acidosis and closure of voltage-dependent anion channels cause fatigue and pain.

Mold and CIRS is the great equalizer because it affects both the wealthy and the poor. Yet there is so little knowledge, so little understanding, so little sympathy and close to zero responsibility taken by those who are actually responsible, whether it is the home building industry, the HVAC industry, the landlords, the insurance industry and so on.

On average, most patients have spent around $50,000 and seen approximately a dozen doctors before they are diagnosed with CIRS. People are wasting precious time and money while getting sicker!

If you are a physician, then you are probably already taking care of CIRS patients every single day and don't know it! It is ubiquitous. CIRS patients are high users of the medical system because people are missing the diagnosis. Instead of calling these people chronically or mysteriously ill, you can help them.

Drs. Maria Vera-Nunez and Ken Friedman are experts in myalgic encephalitis (chronic fatigue syndrome), and their chapter deals with the latest advances in the field. A must-read chapter in my opinion.

Our environment is literally under attack by endocrine-disrupting plastics, and Dr. Arden Anderson's chapter, another classic chapter, highlights this.

Dr. Moss talks about a commonsense approach to dealing with chronic fatigue syndrome/ME by dealing with allostatic overload and avoiding overwhelm.

When talking about chronic illness, it is important to understand that we humans are not separate from the earth. Those in the environmental field know of Dr. Jerry Hatfield, and his chapter on soil and regenerative agriculture is a masterpiece.

The Health of Our Cells Is Shaped by the Soil

Dr. Vandana Shiva

Regarding the science of light, I consider myself lucky to have found Dr. Joshua Rosenthal, an expert on the circadian and mitochondrial effects of artificial light, an emerging public health problem.

Again, this volume is all about highlighting the new medicine, new illnesses that those trained in traditional allopathic medicine are not educated on unless they seek out the knowledge sources. I have attempted to corral many of these diverse topics in two books. Perhaps there will be a Volume Three, as the knowledge and information that needs to be known by the healer-clinician is endless. Humanity is suffering, and the need is great.

I had thought that I had covered the oro-facial and dental correlations with the entire human organism in detail in the first volume; however, there was more! The correlation between pediatric sleep-related breathing disorders and behavior and their systemic connections are masterfully covered by Marsha Luginbuehl and Alyse Shockey. Anyone wanting to fill out a survey, whether parent or clinician, can go to Child Uplift's website and fill out the questionnaire for a detailed report.

A deeper understanding of metabolic and physiologic correction using nutrition is covered in Dr. Michael Gonzalez's chapter, while nutritional support for Covid in the different stages is covered by Chris Newton. This is not to be considered an alternative to standard medical care for Covid but rather, an adjunct as nutritional support.

Dr. Martha Stark described this book as follows: I would read her words whenever I felt down, and they gave me the courage to keep going.

Your line up of authors is absolutely spectacular!!

You have somehow managed to gather together – probably as challenging as trying to "herd cats into a box"!! – such an impressive, broad-ranging, and in-depth collection of chapters spanning everything from Environmental to Functional to Complementary and Alternative to Integrative to Holistic to Energetic to Nutritional to Innovative to Spiritual …

… all of which are approaches that will benefit both those who have long been suffering from complex chronic conditions and those who are deeply invested in optimizing the overall well-being of their mind, body, and soul!!

Aruna, this second volume of yours (replete with its pearls of theoretical and clinical wisdom) promises to constitute a landmark contribution to the many fields it embraces!!

Her chapter, another groundbreaking one on "Living Life Forward: The Neuroplastic Synergy of Mindfulness and Intentionality," changes the way we look at healing to one in which the patient has the power, using the power of intention and mindfulness to change their circumstances.

My dear friends, Dr. John Beaulieu and Thea Beaulieu, are gifted healers, and Dr. Beaulieu is a master of sound healing and author of the chapters on "Mind, Consciousness and the Design Nature of Sound" and "Syntonic Phototherapy." Both chapters are outstanding contributions to the field of medicine. Indeed, it is about time that sound healing with all its splendor became mainstream. Music, for instance, can change your mood, and songs can give voice to your feelings when you don't have the words to express yourself. It has been established that there is a relationship between sound and form. The world emerged from "unstruck sound;" why can we not heal using sound? That brings me to the chapter by Dr. Shawn Marie Higgins, which suggests that the human body itself is a biological sound healing instrument. I am proud to say that Dr. Higgins teaches a CME course on sound healing. Those of you who are lucky enough to travel to see Dr. Beaulieu would find it life-changing to learn from him.

In the course of my being a doctor, as well as studying and learning with many teachers, it was quite self-evident that art and creativity had a special place in healing. Children can draw before they write. If we drew and used our imagination to find our way out of illness and many other life situations, I am confident that it would be a powerful self-help tool. I am proud to present Susan Imholz and Judy Sachter as the authors of "Art in Medicine."

My first volume had a chapter on sunlight as information; this volume takes it a step further with Dr. Nisha Manek's chapter on Information Medicine for the 21st Century.

I studied medicine at Lady Hardinge Medical School, New Delhi, in India, and one of the affili-ated hospitals had a major Ob/Gyn service for New Delhi and surrounding areas. As an intern, rotating through that department, I must have either assisted or single-handedly delivered at least a hundred babies. My experience as a young intern and later, my own experience at the other end, giving birth to my two sons in the United States, were the impetus to my imperative that there needs to be a shift in the understanding of childbirth. I had great difficulty in finding the right author(s), as Ob/Gyns either have no time or did not have the understanding, as perhaps a doula might have, of the patient's mental state, or even the newborn, who cannot "speak" in our vocabulary but does feel and sense. Where did this little one come from? Yes, it might be a spiritual question, but we must not lose our sense of wonder and amazement. I was honored to secure the Head of the Ob/Gyn department in my *Alma Mater*, Dr. Manju Puri, and also Dr. Payal Chaudhary as authors of the chapter on "Birthing the Light."

Evidence that matter can be generated directly from light comes from the Brookhaven National Laboratory, a multipurpose research institution funded by the U.S. Department of Energy. Their study demonstrates a long-predicted process for generating matter directly from light. This study came from scientists studying particle collisions at the Relativistic Heavy Ion Collider (RHIC):[10]

> The primary finding is that pairs of electrons and positrons—particles of matter and antimatter—can be created directly by colliding very energetic photons, which are quantum "packets" of light. This conversion of energetic light into matter is a direct consequence of Einstein's famous E=mc2 equation, which states that energy and matter (or mass) are interchangeable. Nuclear reactions in the sun and at nuclear power plants regularly convert matter into energy. Now scientists have converted light energy directly into matter in a single step.[10]

Last but not least is Dr. Dona Biswas' chapter on "Hidden Societal Enigmas That Have Significant Impact on Mental, Physical and Spiritual Health." This chapter was born out of her, and to a lesser extent my, forays in the hidden world of psychiatry, where shamans of Asia, Europe, and North and South America tap into nonlocal information for healing. I am not talking about charlatans here but real healers of a bygone era who could obtain information from "the field" that assisted the sick.

A jaded and stressed physician is not good for society. Doctors need to rediscover their love for medicine. Patients need to appreciate their doctors, and insurance companies need to be done away with in their present form, with the emphasis on profits and more well-paid administrators than doctors.

It is my sincere wish that the reader will take what helps and forgive anything that "triggers" a reaction, because there may come a time, just around the bend, when the sun will shine again and society will be ready for the information presented in this book. So, with great love and great respect, this book is offered to clinicians and anyone with an interest in a different kind of medicine.

Aruna Bakhru M.D., F.A.C.P.

REFERENCES

1. Somppi, T. L. (2017). Non-thyroidal illness syndrome in patients exposed to indoor air dampness micro-biota treated successfully with triiodothyronine. *Frontiers in Immunology*, 8. https://doi.org/10.3389/fimmu.2017.00919

2. Harding, C. F., Pytte, C. L., Page, K. G., Ryberg, K. J., Normand, E., Remigio, G. J., DeStefano, R. A., Morris, D. B., Voronina, J., Lopez, A., Stalbow, L. A., Williams, E. P., & Abreu, N. (2020). Mold inhalation causes innate immune activation, neural, cognitive and emotional dysfunction. *Brain, Behavior, and Immunity*, 87:218–228. https://doi.org/10.1016/j.bbi.2019.11.006

3. Lieberman. (2020). Mold exposure and mitochondrial antibodies. *Alternative Therapies in Health and Medicine*, 26(6):44–47.

4. Dennis, D., Robertson, D., Curtis, L., & Black, J. (2009). Fungal exposure endocrinopathy in sinusitis with growth hormone deficiency: Dennis-Robertson syndrome. *Toxicology and Industrial Health*, 25(9–10):669–680. https://doi.org/10.1177/0748233709348266

5. Campbell, A. W., Thrasher, J. D., Madison, R. A., Vojdani, A., Gray, M. R., & Al Johnson (2003). Neural autoantibodies and neurophysiologic abnormalities in patients exposed to molds in water-damaged buildings. *Archives of Environmental Health: An International Journal*, 58(8):464–474. https://doi.org/10.3200/AEOH.58.8.464-474

6. Daschner, A. (2017). An evolutionary-based framework for analyzing mold and dampness-associated symptoms in DMHS. *Frontiers in Immunology*, 7. https://doi.org/10.3389/fimmu.2016.00672

7. Brewer, J. H., Thrasher, J. D., & Hooper, D. (2014). Chronic illness associated with mold and mycotoxins: Is naso-sinus fungal biofilm the culprit? *Toxins*, 6(1):66–80. https://doi.org/10.3390/toxins6010066

8. Park, J. H., & Cox-Ganser, J. M. (2011 January 1). Mold exposure and respiratory health in damp indoor environments. *Frontiers in Bioscience*, 3(2):757–71. https://doi.org/10.2741/e284. PMID: 21196349.

9. Lynch, K. B., & Teitelbaum, B. A. (2019). Anterior subcapsular cataract secondary to black mold exposure. *Optometric Clinical Practice*, 1(1):7.

10. *Collisions of Light Produce Matter/Antimatter from Pure Energy*. Brookhaven National Laboratory. (2021, July 28). Retrieved June 25, 2022, from https://www.bnl.gov/newsroom/news.php?a=119023

Acknowledgments

This book would not have been possible without the expertise of each of the contributing authors. It is their dedication to research and study in their chosen field, as well as their generous willingness to share with the readers of this book, that has brought this volume into existence.

Special thanks to Dr. April Vukelic for her assistance with most of the chapters on mold illness, CIRS and Building Science. She credits her writing skills to the help of her husband Mihailo Vukelic.

I would like to thank all the people at Taylor and Francis (Routledge Press) for their hard work behind the scenes during production.

My Senior Editor, Ms. Randy Brehm, who helped me navigate the editing process and has been my rock during my editing career. Without her helpful advice and expedient replies to my queries, I would not have been able to take this project to completion.

Thanks also to Tom Connelly, Editorial Assistant at Taylor and Francis Group, who has been a pleasure to work with throughout this process. I would like to thank Vijay Bose and his team at Deanta for their outstanding and detail oriented work in copy editing the manuscript.

My husband, Sushil Dhawan M.D., and my sons, Nikhil and Rahul Dhawan, have helped me in more ways than I can count. My brothers, Umesh and Dinesh Bakhru, for their never-ending support, and my mother, Gita Bakhru, who is a gift of God in my life. My late father, Govind Bakhru, who always wanted me to be a writer.

Section I

Environmental Medicine, Chronic Illness and Innovations in Standard of Care

1 Introduction to Chronic Inflammatory Response Syndrome (CIRS)

Andrew Heyman and April Vukelic

CONTENTS

1.1 PREFACE

Chronic inflammatory response syndrome (CIRS) represents a common clinical condition. CIRS is a progressive, multi-system, multi-symptom illness characterized by exposure to biotoxins. The ongoing inflammation can affect virtually any organ system of the body and if left untreated, become debilitating.

For patients with CIRS, the innate immune system fails to communicate with the adaptive immune system due to a defect in antigen presentation. The result is inflammation that remains "stuck" in the early phases of the innate immune response. The body cannot transition to the more mature and specific actions coordinated by T cells and B cells in the adaptive immune system.

DOI: 10.1201/b23304-2

1.2   WHAT IS A BIOTOXIN?

Any living organism or fragment of an organism that triggers an innate immune response can function as a biotoxin. This can result from mold and mycotoxins from water-damaged buildings (WDBs), endotoxins, actinobacteria, pathogens as seen in tick-borne illnesses, viruses, dinoflagellates, apicomplexans, cyanobacteria, Mediterranean spider bites, babesia and about 30 other identified pathogens (Table 1.1).

There are many known triggers for CIRS, and more are likely to be discovered. Ciguatera fish poisoning results from eating fish contaminated with the marine toxin ciguatoxin. A single exposure to this toxin may result in CIRS-ciguatera. Airborne or contact exposure to cyanobacteria in freshwater ponds, lagoons and lakes can also cause CIRS-cyanobacteria. Many who suffer from chronic illness seen after antibiotic therapy of acute Lyme disease present with post-Lyme syndrome (CIRS-PLS). Another form of CIRS is caused by Pfiesteria, a dinoflagellate responsible for fish kills along the Eastern seaboard.

Eighty percent of biotoxin illness cases are due to WDBs. About 24% of the population is genetically susceptible, and over 50% of buildings in the United States are water damaged. CIRS-WDB is CIRS that develops after chronic exposure to the interior of WDB typified by resident microbial growth, including bacteria, filamentous fungi (molds), mycobacteria and actinobacteria. Symptoms may be triggered or exacerbated by biologically produced toxins and inflammagens, including mannans, beta-glucans, hemolysins, proteinases, spirocyclic drimanes and volatile organic compounds (VOCs).

Regardless of the initial trigger, each form of CIRS shows similar characteristics in its final manifestations. Doctors may diagnose patients with CIRS as having depression, anxiety, post-traumatic stress disorder (PTSD), somatization, Alzheimer's disease, Parkinsonism, allergy, fibromyalgia and chronic fatigue syndrome (CFS). Treating the symptoms of these patients does not improve their underlying condition.

1.3   PERTINENT NEGATIVES: AN ELUSIVE DISEASE HIDING IN PLAIN SIGHT

CIRS activates the innate immune system, making a proper diagnosis difficult since common inflammation parameters are generally negative upon laboratory evaluation. Normal results may include white blood count, complete metabolic panels, immunoglobulins, autoimmune markers, sedimentation rate, C-reactive protein and interleukin (IL)-6.

Much of modern clinical immunology has focused on diseases associated with cardiometabolic risk, autoimmune diseases, allergies and cancer. In other words, these inflammatory processes can

---

TABLE 1.1

Common Biotoxins (Indoor Environmental Professionals Panel of Surviving Mold, Consensus Statement)

• Beta-glucans	• Microbial volatile organic compounds
• Mannans	• Mycotoxins
• Spirocyclic drimanes	• Mycolactones
• Lipopolysaccharides	• Hemolysins
• Actinobacteria	• Proteinases
• Hyphal fragments	• Gram (+) and G (−) bacteria
• Cell wall fragments	• Particulates (small, fine, ultra)
• Bioaerosols	• Conidia
• Endotoxins	• Protozoa

occur outside the innate immune system. Inflammation increases visceral fat (adipokines), loss of immune tolerance or defects in *adaptive* immunity.

Identifying a patient with CIRS requires collecting subjective and objective information to demonstrate activation of innate immunity while ruling out other causes of symptoms. The evaluation process includes the assessment of proteomics, neuroinflammation, transcriptomics, immune dysregulation and hormonal imbalances. Additional assessments include cardiopulmonary exercise testing, autonomic testing and biliary tree testing.

Despite 25 research papers and 2 clinical trials having been published on the subject of CIRS across 4000 subjects, the evaluation process remains unfamiliar to the general practitioner. The testing for CIRS is specific, and the biomarkers should be done in concert, as no one biomarker can identify CIRS.

1.4 GENETIC SUSCEPTIBILITY: HUMAN LEUKOCYTE ANTIGEN

If CIRS is "difficult to diagnose," how common is it? Who is vulnerable to CIRS? The answer is found on chromosome 6, containing the Human Leukocyte Antigen (HLA) alleles. HLA-DR underlies the mechanism by which antigen-presenting cells identify antigens as "foreign."

When foreign antigens are presented to T lymphocytes by antigen-presenting cells (APCs), the complex process that leads to antibody production begins. If the antigen presentation process is defective, as seen in CIRS, there will be a limited production of protective antibodies and therefore, nothing to stop the expanding inflammatory cascade. As a result, the normally protective innate immune response becomes destructive.

For 95% of patients with known CIRS-WDB, increased relative risk (>1.9) for the acquisition of illness is associated with just 6 of 54 major HLA haplotypes. These six haplotypes exist in roughly 24% of the population (see Table 1.2). Similarly, only four HLA haplotypes are associated with roughly 95% of patients with chronic symptoms following antibiotic treatment for Lyme disease or PLS. Twenty-two percent of patients initially infected by Lyme have these four haplotypes.

TABLE 1.2
HLA Alleles Associated with Poor Antigen Presentation

	DRB1	DQ	DRB3	DRB4	DRB5
Multisusceptible	4	3		53	
	11/12	3	52B		
	14	5	52B		
Mold	7	2/3		53	
	13	6	52A, B, C		
	17	2	52A		
	*18	4	52A		
Borrelia, post-Lyme syndrome	15	6			51
	16	5			51
Dinoflagellates	4	7/8		53	
Multi antibiotic resistant *Staphylococcus epidermidis* (MARCoNS)	11	7	52B		
Low MSH	1	5			
No recognized significance	8	3,4,6			
Low-risk mold	7	9		53	
	12	7	52B		
	9	3/9		53	

Up to 40 million people in the United States are vulnerable to CIRS, given how common these HLA alleles are in the general population. HLA typing becomes important for epidemiologic risk assessment. However, it is also important to consider who else in a family may be susceptible to heightened inflammatory responses following exposure to biotoxins.

1.5   VISUAL CONTRAST SENSITIVITY

The visual contrast sensitivity (VCS) test has been used clinically for over 50 years by the Air Force and remains the most accurate assessment for functional vision. Contrast is one of the seven main functions of the optic nerve that provide the neurologic basis of vision. When testing for contrast, control of the other elements of vision must occur: near vision, far vision, static, motion, peripheral, and night vision.

Contrast is the ability to see an edge. Contrast sensitivity looks at the graded change of contrast at a different light frequency (cycles per degree of visual arc) used to make a grid of five separate frequencies. This grid begins at 1.5 cycles per degree of a visual arc extending in discrete intervals (3, 6, 12, 18) up to 18 cycles per degree of visual arc. Remember, we test visual acuity at 24 cycles per degree of visual arc.

Dr. Ken Hudnell, neurotoxicologist for the United States Environmental Protection Agency (US EPA) National Health and Environmental Effect Research Laboratory (NHEERL) in Research Triangle Park, NC, was the first to use VCS testing in biotoxin illnesses. His landmark work in 1997 paved the way for others to follow. Dr. Shoemaker and Dr. Hudnell noted abnormal VCS in Pfiesteria patients. Visual contrast abnormalities reversed with Dr. Shoemaker's treatment. However, visual contrast deficits, identical to the initial deficits, reappeared with re-exposure, usually within 36 hours.

The VCS test can be completed in person or online under the correct conditions in about 10 minutes and offers an immediate score of a pass or fail. Some patients may pass one eye but not the other, a result still classified as a failure. When combined with positive symptoms (8 of 13 clusters), the diagnosis of CIRS reaches 98.5% sensitivity.

The VCS test also verifies therapeutic progress and detects when re-exposure has occurred. As patients become acquainted with this test, they rely on its accuracy to track clinical progress. Once passed, VCS is a necessary threshold to the next therapeutic step: Multiple Antibiotic Resistant Coagulase-Negative Staphylococci (MARCoNS) treatment. About 8% of CIRS patients can pass the VCS test. Therefore, a pass does not rule out CIRS.

1.6   THE BIOTOXIN PATHWAY IN ACTION

In the HLA-susceptible population, a cascade of events can occur, leading to chronic activation of the innate immune system due to poor antigen presentation. Without the ability to fully upregulate the adaptive immune response with proper antigen disposal, biotoxins are left free to bind to certain cell surface receptors such as Toll, mannose and L-type lectin. Recognition and binding of the biotoxin at these receptors leads to specific upregulation of inflammatory pathways, resulting in an abnormal rise in inflammatory markers such as matrix metalloproteinase (MMP)-9, cytokines, transforming growth factor (TGF)β-1, and split products of complement.

Leptin also plays a key role in the biotoxin illness pathway. Leptin is primarily produced in adipocytes and acts as both a hormone and a cytokine, and it links the neuroendocrine and immune systems. Cytokines compete at the leptin hypothalamic receptor due to their structural similarity to induce leptin resistance, which in turn causes upregulation of leptin production.

In normal physiology, leptin binds receptors located within the arcuate nucleus of the hypothalamus, signaling enzymatic cleavage of the preformed prohormone proopiomelanocortin (POMC) into the following hormones: Alpha melanocyte stimulating hormone (MSH), adrenocorticotropic hormone (ACTH), and endorphins. Disruption of the POMC pathway will decrease levels of the hypothalamic hormones and lead to a decreased ability to mobilize fat stores for energy, resulting in recalcitrant weight gain in some patients that does not respond to typical measures of diet and exercise.

MSH acts as an important neuroregulatory peptide hormone with anti-inflammatory actions by inducing cyclic adenosine monophosphate (cAMP) and inhibiting nuclear factor κ β (NF-κ β). MSH can also downregulate the expression of pro-inflammatory cytokines seen in intracerebral inflammation. MSH deficiency leads to unchecked cytokine effects, manifesting as numerous symptoms such as muscle aches, temperature instability, headaches and decreased concentration ability.

Low MSH levels lead to other immune system dysfunction, sleep issues and gut malabsorption. The MSH-driven conversion of T helper cells into CD4+CD25+ regulatory T cells (Treg cells) prevents hypersensitivity and autoimmune diseases. MSH deficiency diminishes this protective mechanism. With the loss of leukocyte regulation over cytokine responses, patients may succumb to opportunistic infections, such as MARCoNS, and have a slower recovery from infections.

MSH tightens junctions in the gut lining and has anti-inflammatory effects on the colon. MSH deficiency leads to increased intestinal permeability (aka leaky gut), allowing foreign material such as toxins, bacteria and food antigens into the body. Leaky gut and predisposition to autoimmunity have a link, as evidenced by the following antibodies: AGA (gluten sensitivity), anti-cardiolipin antibodies (ACLA), antineutrophil cytoplasmic antibodies (ANCA) and more. Leptin resistance also causes low endorphin levels, resulting in loss of modulation of pain perception, leading to chronic pain and unusual pain.

Fifty percent of CIRS patients with low MSH will experience a loss of cortisol regulation. During the beginning stages of CIRS, simultaneous measurements of ACTH and morning cortisol are often high with minimal symptoms. However, as CIRS progresses, ACTH and morning cortisol levels fall, resulting in a marked increase in symptoms.

Androgen production is downregulated in 40–50% of CIRS patients. Additionally, in patients deficient in vasoactive intestinal polypeptide (VIP), estradiol levels may be elevated due to an over-active aromatase enzyme that converts androgens (i.e., dehydroepiandrosterone [DHEA], androstenedione, testosterone) into estrogens (i.e., estrone, estradiol).

VIP is a neuroregulatory peptide hormone produced in the hypothalamus that often diminishes in CIRS. VIP deficiency can lead to shortness of breath with exercise and pulmonary hypertension (increased pulmonary artery systolic pressure or PASP) reversible with exogenous VIP administration. Lastly, VIP can downregulate cytokines, making it invaluable to the CIRS treatment protocol.

Additionally, cytokines can cause elevated levels of plasminogen activator inhibitor-1 (PAI-1) and abnormal levels of von Willebrand's factor (vWF) and Factor VIII, leading to coagulopathies in some CIRS patients. Cytokines also induce macrophages to release MMP-9, which enzymatically degrades the proteins found in the protective extracellular matrix of blood vessel walls, allowing other inflammatory markers originating in the bloodstream to penetrate sensitive tissues such as the brain. Elevated MMP-9 has a link with an increased risk of atherosclerotic plaque formation, progression and rupture. Additionally, high MMP-9 adversely affects joints, muscles and nerves. Capillary hypoperfusion can also occur due to cytokine effects, including those produced by tumor necrosis factor (TNF)-α. There is a suggestion that this decrease in microvascular perfusion could be caused by vasoconstriction due to direct cytokine effects or recruitment of leukocytes obstructing vessels.

Upregulation of hypoxia inducible factor (HIF) genes occurs in response to cytokine-induced hypoxia, which in turn, promotes the increased production of vascular endothelial growth factor (VEGF) and TGFβ-1. VEGF is known for vasodilation, angiogenesis and neuroprotection. VEGF can be conspicuously high or low in patients with CIRS. A deficiency results in loss of neuroprotection with noted increased permeability of the blood–brain barrier and capillary hypoperfusion. Symptoms associated with low VEGF include shortness of breath, cognitive dysfunction, fatigue and muscle cramps.

TGFβ-1 promotes stiffening of soft, pliable epithelial cells, leading to remodeling in the lung tissue, resulting in a restrictive airway pattern and fibrosis. Like VEGF, TGFβ-1 can increase blood–brain barrier permeability.

CIRS can also involve derangements in the complement cascade, indicated by elevated C4a levels. C4a elevations occur through activation of the classical and mannose-binding lectin pathways and trigger an amplified release of downstream-signaling proteins, promoting a swift inflammatory response. Additionally, some patients may experience auto-activation of the C4a protease enzyme mannose-binding protein-2 (MASP-2), leading to markedly elevated C4a levels. The MASP-2 auto-activation results in a "sicker quicker phenomenon" upon re-exposure. Symptoms of elevated C4a include fatigue, musculoskeletal issues, capillary hypoperfusion and cognitive impairment.

1.7 REGULATORY NEUROPEPTIDES: CHANGES IN BRAIN FUNCTION

The neuroinflammation of CIRS also affects the production of regulatory neuropeptide hormones, especially VIP and alpha MSH. Direct measurement of VIP is possible but misleading, as the crucial problem with VIP physiology is the variable production of one of its two receptors. VIP is available as a therapeutic agent, and exogenous administration has greatly benefited CIRS patients and those with grey matter nuclear atrophy.

Regulatory neuropeptide hormones affect (i) hypothalamic hormone function, (ii) pituitary hormone production, (iii) peripheral hormone regulation by pituitary hormones, (iv) immune cell and innate immune functions, (v) cytokine physiology, (vi) limbic system activity, (vii) genomic activity and (viii) pulmonary artery pressure.

1.7.1 MSH – Melanocyte Stimulating Hormone

Normal Range: 35–81 pg/mL

MSH deficiency is important in CIRS. The hormone is made in the hypothalamus and to a lesser extent, in part of the pituitary. It is a neuropeptide that regulates inflammation and immunity. MSH influences other hormone functions, especially the pituitary and peripheral hormones, and has important regulatory features in the limbic system, circadian rhythm, pain perception, mood, mucus membrane defenses, pulmonary response, appetite and weight. MSH "patrols" the periphery of the skin, respiratory system, gastrointestinal tract and blood. MSH is invested in just about every cell in the gut, including tight junctions. The deficiency of MSH will result in what others call a leaky gut.

Low MSH causes a variety of hormonal dysregulation. Approximately 67% of CIRS patients lack normal regulation in ACTH/cortisol, and 80% lack antidiuretic hormone (ADH)/osmolality regulation. Symptoms of ADH dysregulation include static electrical shocks, migraine-like headaches, excessive thirst with frequent urination, and dehydration. Androgen abnormalities, particularly including upregulation of aromatase, are found in 50% of CIRS cases. Understanding the impact of hormone dysregulation requires looking at feedback loops involving central and peripheral hormones.

Another correlation of MSH deficiency in CIRS is the presence of biofilm-forming, multiple-resistant coagulase-negative staphylococci in deep aerobic nasopharyngeal cultures, essentially found exclusively in those with low MSH.

1.7.2 Additional Innate Immune Markers

MMP-9, TGFβ-1 and split product of complement 4 (C4a) are some of the diagnostic and prognostic variables to assess for inflammation in CIRS. The complement system can be activated to the point that some people with elevated C4a are suffering from auto-activation of MASP-2, the enzyme that cleaves C4a. Removal from exposure does not stop the production of C4a. This so-called "sicker, quicker" process is recognizable with persistent elevation of C4a.

1.7.3 MMP-9

Normal Range: 85–332 ng/mL

MMP-9 is an enzyme that in humans is encoded by the MMP9 gene. Proteins of the MMP9 family are involved in the breakdown of extracellular matrix in normal physiological processes such as embryonic development, reproduction, tissue remodeling and disease processes.

It has been implicated in the pathogenesis of rheumatoid arthritis, atherosclerosis, cardiomyopathy, abdominal aortic aneurysm and chronic obstructive pulmonary disease (COPD) by the destruction of lung elastin. MMP-9 delivers inflammatory elements in the blood into subintimal spaces, where further delivery into solid organs (brain, lung, muscle, peripheral nerve and joint) begins.

1.7.4 TGFβ-1 – TRANSFORMING GROWTH FACTOR β-1

Normal Range: <2380 pg/mL

TGFβ-1 is a protein with important regulatory effects throughout innate immune pathways. This protein helps control the growth and division (proliferation) of cells, the process by which cells mature to carry out specific functions (differentiation), cell movement (motility) and the self-destruction of cells (apoptosis). The TGFβ-1 protein exists throughout the body. It plays a role in development before birth, the formation of blood vessels, the regulation of muscle tissue, body fat development, wound healing and immune system function (especially regulatory T cells).

TGFβ-1 can impair T regulatory cell function, which in turn, contributes to the activation of autoimmunity. However, TGFβ-1 also plays a role in suppressing autoimmunity. TGFβ-1 has become important in the exploding incidence of childhood asthma, raising the issue of pulmonary remodeling due to biotoxin exposure. The EPA says that 21% of all new cases of asthma are due to exposure to WDBs. If an individual develops wheezing after exposure to a WDB, look for remodeling to be a cause. Measuring a PASP is also *critical*. Neurologic, autoimmune, and other systemic problems occur with high TGFβ-1. Individuals with HLA 11-3-52B tend to have higher TGFβ-1.

1.7.5 C4A

Normal Range: 0-2830 ng/mL

C4a has become an inflammatory marker of great significance in immune responses in patients with CIRS. The complement system is a group of proteins that move freely through the bloodstream. Only National Jewish Laboratories® and Sunrise Laboratories can process C4a.

These short-lived products are re-manufactured rapidly, so that an initial rise of plasma levels occurs within 12 hours of exposure to biotoxins. The sustained elevation occurs until definitive therapy begins.

1.7.6 VEGF

Normal Range: 31–86 pg/mL

VEGF is a polypeptide that stimulates new blood vessel formation and increases blood flow in the capillary beds. VEGF deficiency is quite common and is a serious problem in biotoxin illness patients that must be corrected.

Delivery of oxygen in capillary beds is reduced in CIRS. This reduced delivery sets off alarm signals in the body through the activity of a nuclear transcription factor called hypoxia inducible factor (HIF). Low oxygen in tissue means HIF will be produced in high amounts to stimulate VEGF production, which increases new blood vessel growth. VEGF affects TGFβ-1, which in turn, is linked to countless genomic pathways that lead to fibrosis, differential gene activation, the "leakiness" of the blood–brain barrier, and a host of effects on the normally beneficial T regulatory cells.

1.7.7 ACTH/Cortisol

Normal Range: ACTH 8–37 pg/mL; Cortisol a.m. 4.3–22.4 / p.m. 3.1–16.7 µg/dL

ACTH is a hormone released from the anterior pituitary gland in the brain. Cortisol is a steroid hormone produced by the adrenal cortex, which is the outer part of the adrenal gland. As MSH begins to fall, high ACTH is associated with few symptoms early in the illness. As ACTH falls, patients experience more symptoms. Using steroids with low MSH worsens clinical outcomes. Finding simultaneous high cortisol and high ACTH may prompt consideration of screening tumors, but the reality is that the dysregulation is usually corrected with therapy.

1.7.8 ACLA IgA/IgG/IgM

Normal Range: IgA 0–12; IgG 0–10; IgM 0–9

Anti-cardiolipins (ACLA) are autoantibodies produced in response to the accumulation of abnormal lipid content in the double lipid bilayer of the mitochondria. IgA, IgM and IgG are autoantibodies often identified in collagen vascular diseases such as lupus and scleroderma and are often called anti-phospholipids.

An increased risk of spontaneous fetal loss in the first trimester of pregnancy often occurs in women with the presence of these autoantibodies. They occur in over 33% of children with biotoxin-associated illnesses.

1.7.9 Anti-Gliadin Antibodies (AGA)

Normal Range 0–19

Anti-gliadin antibodies form in response to a protein in gluten. Eating gluten can cause an inflammatory response that appears to be similar to attention deficit disorder in children. Elevated AGA requires a trial of a gluten-free diet. Prolonged elevation and symptoms can necessitate a gluten-free diet for life.

1.7.10 ADH/Osmolality

Normal Range: ADH 1.0–13.3 pg/mL; Osmolality 280–300 mOsm/kg

Antidiuretic hormone (ADH), or vasopressin, is a substance produced naturally by the hypothalamus and released by the pituitary gland. The hormone controls the amount of water the body removes. ADH stimulates cells in renal tubules to reabsorb free water in response to rising osmolality in blood. Intravascular dehydration occurs in 80% of patients with low MSH.

Symptoms associated with dysregulation of ADH include dehydration, frequent urination (with urine showing low specific gravity), excessive thirst, and sensitivity to static electrical shocks. Edema and rapid weight gain can occur due to fluid retention during the initial correction of ADH deficits.

1.7.11 Leptin

Normal Range: Male 0.5–13.8 ng/mL; Female 1.1–27.5 ng/mL

Leptin regulates fat metabolism. High leptin promotes fat storage and weight gain. Standard approaches to weight loss, like calorie reduction and exercising more, will fail. The inflammatory responses cause leptin levels to rise, leading to patients who are chronically tired, in chronic pain and forever overweight.

1.8   SECONDARY SOURCE OF BRAIN INFLAMMATION: MARCoNS

MARCoNS bacteria colonize in mucosal membrane surfaces due to MSH deficiency in CIRS patients. MARCoNS evade host defenses through biofilm formation and secrete exotoxins A and B, which split MSH molecules apart, causing further reduction in MSH levels. Coagulase-negative *Staphylococcus* secretes hemolysins, which can increase inflammation in the host and even alter the genomic expression of host genes.

MARCoNS in deep nasal passages release small neurotoxins through the olfactory bulb into the central nervous system, worsening the patients' clinical condition. The infection must be eliminated for symptom improvement because it interferes with the efficacy of VIP nasal spray, the last step of therapy used to correct brain-related changes and aberrant genomic responses.

1.9   THE NEW LANGUAGE OF GENES: TRANSCRIPTOMICS

We now know that the static genome is actively manipulated, constantly increasing the production of some gene transcripts and decreasing others in response to its environment. Regulation is complex: Nuclear transcription factors and newly discovered long non-coding RNAs, together with microRNAs and circular RNAs, methylation and acetylation (also demethylation and deacetylation), can turn on and shut off gene function.

Research into the interacting complexities of so many layers of regulation has progressed beyond its infancy. This shift from measuring the presence of genes to assessing every level of activity along the molecular pathway is called Genomics.

1. Genomics is the branch of molecular biology concerned with the structure, function, evolution and mapping of genomes.
2. Transcriptomics is the study of the transcriptome, the complete set of RNA transcripts produced by the genome, under specific circumstances or in a specific cell.
3. Proteomics is the large-scale study of proteomes. A proteome is a set of proteins produced in an organism, system or biological context.
4. Metabolomics is the large-scale study of small molecules, commonly known as metabolites, within cells, biofluids, tissues or organisms. These small molecules and their interactions within a biological system are collectively known as the metabolome.

1.10   THE FUTURE OF CIRS

The future is coming into focus. Our understanding of CIRS science has grown exponentially due to transcriptomics. These advances reflect the landmark work of Dr. Jimmy Ryan and Dr. Ritchie Shoemaker. The sarcin/ricin loop is a preserved genetic sequence that creates permanent vulnerability to biotoxins in all living creatures. Because of their universal nature, doctors can never fully eliminate susceptibility to biotoxins. In fact, from an evolutionary perspective, CIRS can be seen as an adaptation to cellular threats, albeit ultimately a debilitating one for a large minority of the population.

Many well-trained doctors are unfamiliar with CIRS and cannot fully address common complaints like fatigue, chronic pain, mood issues, functional bowel disorders and weight gain. Every doctor should have the ability to recognize CIRS in order to best address these common complaints. Specialists may diagnose an isolated condition in the CIRS patient but may not recognize it as part of the greater constellation of CIRS.

Dr. Shoemaker has almost single-handedly defined, described and formulated treatment for an incredibly common and devastating illness that has eluded the rest of the medical community. Most practicing doctors see these patients every day and have no idea how to alleviate their symptoms. One cannot overstate Dr. Shoemaker's contribution to medicine, and his combination of genius and grit is without parallel.

We must recognize this disease as squarely in the domain of primary care. Primary care doctors should have command of this topic. Additionally, the vital signs of every patient must include the health of our indoor spaces. There is just no way around these ideas. Furthermore, the science that underpins CIRS has matured to the point where it seems almost malpractice to offer "medication management" to patients in lieu of proper treatment that is actually curative.

1.10.1　Science

Every new piece of data will reinforce, expand or refine our understanding of CIRS. *New findings will never fundamentally undermine the science that came before them.* Transcriptomics appears to be the true breakthrough in diagnosing CIRS. Gene expression has revealed the disease's hallmarks: molecular hypometabolism, altered immune efficiency, defective apoptosis and aerobic glycolysis. Dr. Shoemaker and Dr. Ryan have linked these molecular abnormalities to several risk factors like vascular dementia, diabetes, thrombotic events and pulmonary hypertension.

Additionally, applying new metabolomics techniques to measure mitochondrial production of downstream small molecule patterns may also help identify subsets of CIRS. Metabolomics is a means to unlock issues around those resistant to standard therapy and chemically sensitive individuals and elucidate the impact of the exposome on cellular health. Genomics helps fine-tune therapies and improve patient outcomes.

Where we lag is a broad array of treatments that reliably cure the illness. Certain molecular and genomic features of CIRS respond to earlier steps in the Shoemaker Protocol before the administration of VIP. VIP is a miraculous but single arrow in our therapeutic quiver that restores the individual to health, heals the brain and corrects gene response. Maybe, new treatments will be discovered in emerging regenerative techniques such as peptides, exosomes, stem cells, phage therapy, CRISPR, nutrients or even high extract natural compounds. Maybe, as was the case with cholestyramine, an old drug will be identified that demonstrates unique characteristics well suited for CIRS.

As we dive deeper into the condition's pathophysiology, a key finding is the mitochondria's profound orchestration of cell behavior and the shift toward a pathologic but permanently altered gene expression state. While downstream consequences of this molecular activity show measurable changes in levels of signaling molecules, nutrients, amino acids, lipids, inflammatory markers, the microbiome and more, these are merely the leaves on the tree.

Without casting aspersions, "Functional Medicine" has been overly focused on assessing and treating these abnormal small molecule findings while ignoring the key insight transcriptomics offers. To cure these patients, we have to find therapies that shift the genomic expression of the mitochondria back to a healthy state of oxidative phosphorylation and normal cellular energetics. Merely treating the leaves on the tree will not achieve this end. We have to fix the roots of this disease instead.

Overall, the clinical imperative should be to heal patients more quickly, build resiliency to future exposures, and ensure complete resolution in all tissues and organs. Unfortunately, there is currently little to no outside funding for CIRS.

1.10.2　Professionals

Dr. Shoemaker and the author are committed to offering a graduate-level learning experience on the subject of CIRS. This community of excellent providers will grow, and they will treat hundreds of thousands of CIRS patients over the coming years.

This expanding network of trained professionals offers a larger opportunity to conduct patient-centered outcomes research. There is power in numbers. If we cannot obtain funding for formal investigations, we can draw upon the collective contributions of many providers to aggregate properly sized data sets to assess outcomes.

Technology, especially cloud-based, has been revolutionary in this regard. New "point of care" platforms, wearables, apps and devices can be the nexus between practitioner and patient while funneling data across large populations to centralized research hubs.

Family Medicine in the 1990s was the first medical specialty to assemble practice-based research networks (PBRN) to achieve just this goal. Electronic medical records were still new, if not uncommon, and accessing data at the clinic level required superhuman efforts to mine paper charts. Now, technology efficiencies have reduced these barriers to entry on large-scale research.

CIRS providers will need to commit to participating in the PBRN model to accelerate research findings. While the early and ongoing work of Dr. Shoemaker and Dr. Ryan has been singular and heroic, an opportunity has arisen for the current generation of CIRS providers to give back to them, to their patients and to medicine overall by engaging in the research effort. An organized network of trained and certified providers, unified by their education and connected within a technological ecosystem, will allow an acceleration of discoveries in CIRS.

A centralized data network requires a participatory spirit, the adoption of unified technology platforms and a commitment to expand the practitioner identity to include researchers. The goal is to usher in a shared spirit of collaborative research in the coming years to accelerate our understanding of CIRS.

1.10.3 POLICY

Everyone deserves an opportunity for health. It is a social good that should not serve only those who can afford it. People cannot reach their potential, compete in the marketplace or participate effectively in society if they are sickened by their living environment. Likewise, people deserve the right to work and receive education in healthy environments. It does not take much thought to see the financial, social and cultural implications of CIRS. This may be the largest, and most expensive, unrecognized public health crisis of the modern era.

It has particular implications for the underserved who lack access to medical care, proper nutrition and social opportunities. We already struggle with managing their obesity, diabetes and heart disease, mental health disorders, substance abuse, violence and neglect.

Additionally, we do not have nearly enough properly trained doctors and primary care practitioners to manage the millions of CIRS patients currently living in the United States. The amount of resources required to match health services to this particular population is underfunded and grossly under-recognized by medical institutions. Health advocacy that leads to meaningful policy changes will need to occur on the state and federal levels to support formal education, inclusion in clinical guidelines, and recognition as a distinct disease category that impacts vulnerable populations.

Large-scale clinical outcomes data will likely lead the way as the basis for policy-related changes. Public health advocacy work may be occurring soon, but it is not imminent. In the meantime, patient groups can act as a vehicle for meaningful dialogue as a starting point beyond the support groups used by individuals only seeking medical advice.

Awareness-raising activities, recognizing healthy environments as a human right, and lobbying for protections against landlords, building owners, construction companies and employers will need to be energized by effective advocates for change. This is an uphill battle at best, but pressure from the public on politicians, the medical community and social institutions has a track record of success in other movements for change.

At some point, public awareness will reach a critical mass. Doctors need to take their role as cultural leaders seriously. Doctors giving local talks on CIRS is an important step. Raise awareness, advocate for change, encourage community-based groups to take the issue seriously as a public health problem while continuing to treat patients, and help collect data to change medicine. There is much to be done.

However, we have approached the point of no return. CIRS is real. CIRS is common. It has enormous socioeconomic and health services implications and deserves its own social movement for change. Otherwise, practitioners remain vulnerable to state medical boards. Patients remain underdiagnosed and untreated. Those responsible for ensuring clean interior environments do not bear responsibility. Moreover, the crisis continues on a grand scale.

1.10.4 FINAL THOUGHTS

Who knew a person's home could make them fat, depressed and demented? Who knew that water damage leads to amplified microbial growth of bacteria more impactfully than fungal elements? Who knew that this is as much a proliferative disorder as inflammatory? Now, we know.

We have a roadmap for the clinical aspects of CIRS. The scientific foundation is now relatively firm and offers a framework to expand our data sets overall, seek additional effective therapies and apply new research methods to a very old disease. Medicine, and society, need to catch up. Dr. Shoemaker gave us a gift through his insights and almost 30 years of work on the subject.

It is time for the next generation of providers, in partnership with the public, to raise awareness of CIRS, conduct high-quality outcomes research, establish reliable clinical guidelines and ensure people have access to clean interior environments. No one is coming to save us. CIRS doctors must build on the current momentum to create a better future for ourselves, our patients and the general population.

BIBLIOGRAPHY

Bagnis, R., T. Kuberski, and S. Laugier. "Clinical Observations on 3,009 Cases of Ciguatera (Fish Poisoning) in the South Pacific." *The American Journal of Tropical Medicine and Hygiene*, vol. 28, no. 6, 1979, pp. 1067–1073. https://doi.org/10.4269/ajtmh.1979.28.1067.

Bartram, J., and I. Chorus. *Toxic Cyanobacteria in Water.* Geneva: World Health Organization, 1999. https://doi.org/10.1201/9781482295061.

Campbell, Andrew W., Jack D. Thrasher, Michael R. Gray, and Aristo Vojdani. "Mold and Mycotoxins: Effects on the Neurological and Immune Systems in Humans." *Advances in Applied Microbiology*, vol. 55, 2004, pp. 375–406. https://doi.org/10.1016/s0065-2164(04)55015-3.

Charlton, Bruce G., and I. Nicol Ferrier. "Hypothalamo-Pituitary-Adrenal Axis Abnormalities in Depression: A Review and a Model." *Psychological Medicine*, vol. 19, no. 2, 1989, pp. 331–336. https://doi.org/10.1017/s003329170001237x.

Delgado, M. "Vasoactive Intestinal Peptide: The Dendritic Cell -> Regulatory T Cell Axis." *Annals of the New York Academy of Sciences*, vol. 1070, no. 1, 2006, pp. 233–238. https://doi.org/10.1196/annals.1317.020.

Ehrhart-Bornstein, Monika, Joy P. Hinson, Stefan R. Bornstein, Werner A. Scherbaum, and Gavin P. Vinson. "Intraadrenal Interactions in the Regulation of Adrenocortical Steroidogenesis." *Endocrine Reviews*, vol. 19, no. 2, 1998, pp. 101–143. https://doi.org/10.1210/edrv.19.2.0326.

Gennaro, Renato, Tatjana Simonic, Armando Negri, Cristina Mottola, Camillo Secchi, Severino Ronchi, and Domenico Romeo. "C5a Fragment of Bovine Complement. Purification, Bioassays, Amino-Acid Sequence and Other Structural Studies." *European Journal of Biochemistry*, vol. 155, no. 1, 1986, pp. 77–86. https://doi.org/10.1111/j.1432-1033.1986.tb09460.x.

Habashi, J. P. "Losartan, an AT1 Antagonist, Prevents Aortic Aneurysm in a Mouse Model of Marfan Syndrome." *Science*, vol. 312, no. 5770, 2006, pp. 117–121. https://doi.org/10.1126/science.1124287.

Jessop, D. S. "Review: Central Non-Glucocorticoid Inhibitors of the Hypothalamo-Pituitary-Adrenal Axis." *Journal of Endocrinology*, vol. 160, no. 2, 1999, pp. 169–180. https://doi.org/10.1677/joe.0.1600169.

Kuhn, D. M., and M. A. Ghannoum. "Indoor Mold, Toxigenic Fungi, and Stachybotrys Chartarum: Infectious Disease Perspective." *Clinical Microbiology Reviews*, vol. 16, no. 1, 2003, pp. 144–172. https://doi.org/10.1128/cmr.16.1.144-172.2003.

Lin, K., and R. Shoemaker. "Inside Indoor Air Quality: Environmental Relative Moldiness Index (ERMI)." *Filtration News*, March 2007.

Metcalf, Lee N., Neil R. McGregor, and Timothy K. Roberts. "Membrane Damaging Toxins From Coagulase-Negative Staphylococcus Are Associated With Self-Reported Temporomandibular Disorder (TMD) in Patients With Chronic Fatigue Syndrome." *Journal of Chronic Fatigue Syndrome*, vol. 12, no. 3, 2004, pp. 25–43. https://doi.org/10.1300/j092v12n03_03.

Morris, J. Glenn. "Human Health Effects and Pfiesteria Exposure: A Synthesis of Available Clinical Data." *Environmental Health Perspectives*, vol. 109, suppl. 5, 2001, p. 787. https://doi.org/10.2307/3454928.

Nagase, Hideaki, and J. Frederick Woessner. "Matrix Metalloproteinases." *Journal of Biological Chemistry*, vol. 274, no. 31, 1999, pp. 21491–21494. https://doi.org/10.1074/jbc.274.31.21491.

Nigrovic, L. E., Amy D. Thompson, Andrew M. Fine, and Amir Kimia. "Clinical Predictors of Lyme Disease Among Children With a Peripheral Facial Palsy at an Emergency Department in a Lyme Disease-Endemic Area." *Pediatrics*, vol. 122, no. 5, 2008, pp. e1080–e1085. https://doi.org/10.1542/peds.2008-1273.

Ogata, R. T., P. A. Rosa, and N. E. Zepf. "Sequence of the Gene for Murine Complement Component C4." *Journal of Biological Chemistry*, vol. 264, no. 28, 1989, pp. 16565–16572. https://doi.org/10.1016/s0021-9258(19)84744-0.

Opdenakker. "MMP9 Functions as Regulator and Effector in Leukocyte Biology." *Journal of Leukocyte Biology*, June 2001.

Ross, David E., A. L. Ochs, J. M. Seabaugh, C. R. Shrader, and Alzheimer's Disease Neuroimaging Initiative. "Man Versus Machine: Comparison of Radiologists' Interpretations and NeuroQuant® Volumetric Analyses of Brain MRIs in Patients With Traumatic Brain Injury." *The Journal of Neuropsychiatry and Clinical Neurosciences*, vol. 25, no. 1, 2013, pp. 32–39. https://doi.org/10.1176/appi.neuropsych.11120377.

Ryan, James C., Qingzhong Wu, and Ritchie C. Shoemaker. "Transcriptomic Signatures in Whole Blood of Patients Who Acquire a Chronic Inflammatory Response Syndrome (CIRS) Following an Exposure to the Marine Toxin Ciguatoxin." *BMC Medical Genomics*, vol. 8, no. 1, 2015, pp. 1–12. https://doi.org/10.1186/s12920-015-0089-x.

Schwartz, Larry, Greg Weatherman, Michael Schrantz, Will Spates, Jeff Charlton, Keith Berndtson, and Ritchie Shoemaker. "Indoor Environmental Professionals Panel of Surviving Mold Consensus Statement." 12 April 2016.

Shoemaker, R. "Differential Association of HLADR Genotypes With Chronic Neurotoxin Mediated Illness: Possible Genetic Basis for Susceptibility." *American Journal of Tropical Medicine*, vol. 67, 2002, p. 160.

Shoemaker, R. "Posure." *5th International Conference on Bioaerosols*, September 2003.

Shoemaker, R. "Presentation to the Indoor Air Quality Association." *Sequential Upregulation of Innate Immune Responses During Acute Acquisition of Illness in Patients Exposed to Water-Damaged Buildings*, October 2007.

Shoemaker, R., and H. Hudnell. "5th International Conference on Bioaerosols." *Sick Building Syndrome in Water Damaged Buildings: Generalizations of the Chronic Biotoxin-Associated Illness Paradigm to Indoor Toxigenic-Fungi Exposure*, September 2003.

Shoemaker, R., and S. McMahon. "Policyholders of America Research Milani Committee Report on Diagnosis and Treatment of Chronic Inflammatory Response Syndrome Caused by Exposure to the Internal Environment of Water-Damaged Buildings." July 2010.

Shoemaker, R. C. "Defining Sick Building Syndrome in Adults and Children in a Case-Control Series as a Biotoxin-Associated Illness: Diagnosis, Treatment and Disorders of Innate Immune Response, MSH, Split Products of Complement IL-1B,IL-10, MMP-9, VEGF, Autoimmunity and HLADR." *American Journal of Tropical Hygiene and Health*, June 2005.

Shoemaker, Ritchie C. "Residential and Recreational Acquisition of Possible Estuary-Associated Syndrome: A New Approach to Successful Diagnosis and Treatment." *Environmental Health Perspectives*, vol. 109, suppl 5, 2001, p. 791. https://doi.org/10.2307/3454929.

Shoemaker, Ritchie C. *Surviving Mold: Life in the Era of Dangerous Buildings*. Baltimore, MD: Otter Bay Books, LLC, 2010.

Shoemaker, Ritchie C., and Dennis E. House. "A Time-Series Study of Sick Building Syndrome: Chronic, Biotoxin-Associated Illness From Exposure to Water-Damaged Buildings." *Neurotoxicology and Teratology*, vol. 27, no. 1, 2005, pp. 29–46. https://doi.org/10.1016/j.ntt.2004.07.005.

Shoemaker, Ritchie C., and Dennis E. House. "Sick Building Syndrome (SBS) and Exposure to Water-Damaged Buildings: Time Series Study, Clinical Trial and Mechanisms." *Neurotoxicology and Teratology*, vol. 28, no. 5, 2006, pp. 573–588. https://doi.org/10.1016/j.ntt.2006.07.003.

Shoemaker, Ritchie C., Dennis House, and James C. Ryan. "Vasoactive Intestinal Polypeptide (VIP) Corrects Chronic Inflammatory Response Syndrome (CIRS) Acquired Following Exposure to Water-Damaged Buildings." *Health*, vol. 5, no. 3, 2013, pp. 396–401. https://doi.org/10.4236/health.2013.53053.

Shoemaker, Ritchie C., Patricia C. Giclas, Chris Crowder, Dennis House, and M. Michael Glovsky. "Complement Split Products C3a and C4a Are Early Markers of Acute Lyme Disease in Tick Bite Patients in the United States." *International Archives of Allergy and Immunology*, vol. 146, no. 3, 2008, pp. 255–261. https://doi.org/10.1159/000116362.

Shoemaker, Ritchie C., and Patti Schmidt. *Mold Warriors: Fighting Americas Hidden Health Threat.* Baltimore, MD: Gateway Press, 2007.

Shoemaker, Ritchie W., et al. *The Art and Science of CIRS Medicine.* 2020.

Swanson, David L., and Richard S. Vetter. "Bites of Brown Recluse Spiders and Suspected Necrotic Arachnidism." *New England Journal of Medicine*, vol. 352, no. 7, 2005, pp. 700–707. https://doi.org/10.1056/nejmra041184.

Tibbles, Carrie D., and Jonathan A. Edlow. "Does This Patient Have Erythema Migrans?" *JAMA*, vol. 297, no. 23, 2007, p. 2617. https://doi.org/10.1001/jama.297.23.2617.

Vesper, Stephen, Craig McKinstry, Richard Haugland, Larry Wymer, Karen Bradham, Peter Ashley, David Cox, Gary Dewalt, and Warren Friedman. "Development of an Environmental Relative Moldiness Index for US Homes." *Journal of Occupational & Environmental Medicine*, vol. 49, no. 8, 2007, pp. 829–833. https://doi.org/10.1097/jom.0b013e3181255e98.

2 The Evolution of Chronic Inflammatory Response Syndrome (CIRS) and the Biotoxin Pathway

Ritchie Shoemaker and April Vukelic

CONTENTS

2.1 HISTORY OF CIRS

Chronic inflammatory response syndrome (CIRS) is a multisystem, multi-symptom illness acquired following exposure to environmentally produced biotoxins. CIRS has gone through an evolution of names over the years. In the 1990s, CIRS was called a neurotoxin-mediated illness. The term changed to chronic biotoxin-associated illness (CBAI) with more information. The third and current change to CIRS nomenclature occurred following the development of a commercial assay for transforming growth factor β-1 (TGFβ-1) in 2008 and then a commercial assay for acquired T regulatory cells in 2009.

CIRS involves many arms of the immune response systems acting simultaneously and in combination. CIRS follows the acute systemic inflammatory response syndrome (SIRS) model, most commonly sepsis. In patients with sepsis, there is simultaneous activation of Th1, Th2 and Th17 immunity, coagulation factors and complement in response to an overwhelming stimulus of infection and endotoxin presence in the bloodstream. In this regard, the illness is the host response. Survivors of sepsis have a heightened level of innate immune activation post-sepsis, show a significant increase in interleukin (IL)-10, and suffer a greater incidence of chronic fatiguing illnesses. By adding one inflammatory feature of an illness on top of another, much like bricks laid on a foundation, we begin to recognize that our attempts to define diseases by organ system will fail. Physicians recognize, however, that infectious diseases often set off systemic inflammation that can persist beyond the clearance of infectious agents.

2.2 EVOLUTION OF CASE DEFINITION OF CIRS

In some instances, the initial sources of illness could not be identified reliably. The case definition in 2003 simply included:

1. The potential for exposure.
2. Presence of a multisystem, multi-symptom illness.
3. Absence of confounding exposures or diagnosis.
4. There must be the potential for exposure to a damp indoor space.
5. There must be a multisystem, multi-symptom illness present with symptoms similar to those seen in peer-reviewed publications.
6. There must be laboratory testing results similar to those seen in peer-reviewed, published studies.
7. There must be documentation of response to therapy.

With the addition of objective laboratory studies, including visual contrast sensitivity (VCS), HLA DR by polymerase chain reaction (PCR), and melanocyte stimulating hormone (MSH), there was a commonality of inflammatory abnormalities and the similarity of symptom groups within subsets of this neurotoxin-mediated illness.

In 2008, the US General Accountability Office (GAO) published an overview of publications from US agencies working on the problem of damp indoor buildings.[24] Fifty-four studies were noted, showing no coordination of efforts across agency lines. But for the first time, a Federal case definition for what has become CIRS-WDB was proposed.

2.3 EVOLUTION OF THE PARADIGM OF CIRS

Initially, CIRS seemed to be simply an inflammatory response to exposure to environmentally produced neurotoxins. Dinoflagellate illnesses, such as Pfiesteria and ciguatera, were used to develop the case definition in the late 1990s. Later, additional findings, first from exposure to cyanobacteria (1997) and then to the interior environment of water-damaged buildings (WDBs, 1998), showed an uncanny similarity of symptoms shared by each of these diverse sources of inflammatory illness. In 2008, followed by a publication in 2010,[24] members of the "mold" medical community began using the term CIRS-WDB to describe illness seen with the same activation of Th1, Th2 and Th17, coagulation and complement activation. Physicians who treat CIRS have noted little variation in symptoms recorded from patients living around the globe. WDBs are the most significant source that results in CIRS.

A treatment protocol employed removal from exposure, initiation of cholestyramine (CSM) together with clearance of multiple antibiotic resistant coagulase negative staphylococci (MARCoNS) resident in deep nasopharyngeal space. In rapid-fire order, in the early 2000s, physicians were able to see the following:

1. Low levels of vascular endothelial growth factor (VEGF).
2. Elevated levels of split products of complement activation, especially C4a, which would become additional targets for sequential treatment.

MSH was the first regulatory neuropeptide identified as deficient in the early CIRS cases. Because MSH exerts a regulatory role on the production of other hormones, especially gonadotropins, it was not a surprise to find that androgens, together with estrogens, were affected by MSH deficiency. To this day, physicians are attempting to "balance" androgens and estrogens. Correcting MSH deficiency is the true method to address the "root cause." Correction of MSH is mandatory for correcting androgens and estrogens. Researchers also saw that MSH interacted with antidiuretic hormone (ADH) in the hypothalamus to regulate other hormone activities in addition to salt and water balance. MSH controls tight junctions in the gut, a fact often overlooked by those who diagnose "leaky gut."

The discovery that vasoactive intestinal polypeptide (VIP), another regulatory neuropeptide, was deficient in >90% of patients with the syndrome set off another avenue of inquiry into the physiology of the illness. Providers now know that measurements of VIP receptors 1 and 2 are also essential to understand VIP's efficacy fully. Transcriptomics shows us how VIP receptors intimately tie to the activities of a family of nuclear transcription factors, Ikaros.

As objective laboratory parameters became associated loosely with some specific grouping of symptoms, the sequential treatment method enabled providers to approach symptom reduction in a disciplined manner. By correcting one objective parameter at a time, patients could identify improved symptoms, implying that objective parameters correlated with specific laboratory abnormalities.

The concept of the "final common pathway" began to emerge following the 2010 Physician Consensus Statement[27] and the naming of this inflammatory illness as chronic inflammatory response syndrome (CIRS). In other words, CIRS caused by chronic exposure to WDB was nearly indistinguishable from CIRS caused by post-Lyme syndrome, ciguatera, Pfiesteria or cyanobacteria. The initial inciting triggers might differ in each case, but the end clinical presentation was similar. Since providers could not rely on VCS deficits, laboratory abnormalities or symptoms alone to adequately distinguish one illness from another, all physicians had to support a diagnosis was the potential for exposure. Even this reliable method of history taking became confounded when someone who had a dinoflagellate illness then moved into a moldy apartment, creating two sources of biotoxin exposure. Even worse, some individuals lived next to freshwater areas, lakes or ponds, for example, in which there would be cyanobacteria blooms in addition to moldy buildings and sick fish.

Physicians needed a diagnostic method that would specify individual illnesses and provide the basis for monitoring treatment results. With the addition of transcriptomics to CIRS case management, based on case-controlled studies and prospective intervention trials, there is a molecular basis for the final common pathway suggested by the commonality of symptoms in sources of CIRS. This final common pathway is like a spiderweb. Genomics is at the core of the spiderweb. Here, we find the source of all the objective laboratory abnormalities, the confusing complexities of symptoms and their groupings (called clusters), and the basis for CIRS illness.

To quote a current Primer in Transcriptomics[25]:

> Transcriptomics has now crossed from research to application. It not only serves as a diagnostic aid, but it also provides precision in monitoring the complexities found in many immune-based illnesses, such as chronic inflammatory responses acquired following environmental exposures. We see transcriptomics as an ideal mechanism to fine-tune therapies to correct inflammatory abnormalities.
>
> The initial finding by Ryan et al.[33] showed that intranasal use of VIP in CIRS patients, partway through their treatment protocols, modulated expression of both nuclear-encoded mitochondrial genes and ribosomal genes. We later confirmed that patients naïve to treatment had profound suppression of these same genes. These genes usually recover with the first ten steps of the Shoemaker Protocol; they often become higher than normal controls. A tantalizing possibility for the overshoot lies with genes important in glycolysis (breakdown of glucose into two 3-carbon fragments). One of these genes, glyceraldehyde-3-phosphate dehydrogenase (GAPDH), also regulates inflammatory gene suppression after initial activation in the presence of interferon-gamma.
>
> What we think is happening is an attack on the basic cellular metabolic elements. It is well documented that microbial toxins (i) attack protein production at the level of the ribosome and (ii) energy production in the mitochondria. Patients with CIRS will not recover unless exposure to these microbes and their cellular toxins ceases. Further, it is well documented that in the face of infectious diseases, especially from viruses, cells become "hypometabolic" to prevent viral "takeover" of cellular function.

This idea is relevant for the abnormal immune responses we see in CIRS. Hypometabolic immune cells activate primordial mechanisms: innate immunity, complement, defensins. These protective inflammatory elements do not require the participation of cells. When cells begin to recover from the illness-induced hypometabolic state, the protective mechanisms of innate immunity begin to wane. Cells then upregulate protein production, energy production and begin to use sugar properly. Call it a "synchronized reboot" of cellular systems. Re-exposure simply means a recall of innate immunity and all its protective mechanisms.

Changes in transcriptomics show the sequence of hypometabolism and recovery. Certainly, the CIRS protocol could prime ribosomal and mitochondrial gene expression. Then VIP could upregulate GAPDH gene expression. Could increased pyruvate from glycolysis fire up the mitochondrial furnace for energy production and then protein expression? Or will it stay suppressed as not to increase lactate production?

With a genomics basis established for CIRS, physicians began to see the application of the principles of CIRS to other illnesses that involve inflammation but did not have all the elements of CIRS. For example, in a small number of patients with impending heart transplants for dilated cardiomyopathy, gene expression of adrenoceptors and "contractility receptors" found in peripheral blood cells respond to CIRS protocols. If there is confirmation that cardiac myocytes improve as white blood cells do, perhaps providers will prevent further myocardial injury from genomic abnormalities.

Growing evidence shows atherosclerosis to be an inflammatory illness. Oxidized low-density lipoprotein (LDL) is a potent nuclear transcription factor. Insulin and insulin resistance are the inflammatory bases of diabetes and obesity. Alzheimer's, specifically Type III, is shown to be an inflammatory illness. Inflammation is the underlying mechanism, not just a source of the symptoms and not just the cause of laboratory abnormalities. As the next decade of CIRS approaches, the expansion of the application of the principles of CIRS to other illnesses, possibly including pediatric acute-onset neuropsychiatric syndrome (PANS), is becoming clear.

2.4   OFFICE VISIT

Based on the experience of thousands of initial office visits with CIRS providers, most patients have seen at least ten doctors and are still ill. Fibromyalgia and psychosomatic disorders are common misdiagnoses. Review of past medical records remains the most critical initial duty of the CIRS provider to the patient. The initial visit should take place only after a thorough review of all relevant documents. In the example of 5,000 pages of records, there may only be several pages of pertinent data. Symptoms of CIRS vary from day to day and are subject to unnoticed environmental exposures. Patients should also log symptoms to correlate with exposures. The patients should stop nasal oral, and intravenous antifungals, as they are creating resistant mutant MARCoNS.

2.5   SPECIFIC SYMPTOMS

From a list of 37 different symptoms, 8 main categories (general, musculoskeletal, eye, respiratory, gastrointestinal, cognitive, hypothalamic and neurologic) were formed to classify symptoms. Cluster analysis provides a mechanism to take subjective symptoms, pass them through a skilled medical history, and convert them to objective elements using abstruse statistical methods, including cluster analysis. Clusters can take the seemingly endless roster of symptoms to make their use amenable to a scoring system. Statistically, these 13 clusters of symptoms yield a diagnostic capability to separate CIRS from essentially all diseases. If an adult patient has eight or more clusters of symptoms, the likelihood of CIRS exceeds 95%. When combined with VCS deficits, symptom clusters can yield an accuracy in the diagnosis of 98.5% (the sum of false positives and false negatives is less than 2%).

CIRS providers have looked at symptoms described by character, including fatigue, weakness and executive cognitive dysfunction. Does a patient have muscle cramps? Are there unusual, sharp stabbing pains that seemingly come unexpectedly and lancinate in one area of the body only to disappear and reappear elsewhere the next day? This type of pain description is typical of what CIRS patients experience. It is not confabulated but will sound bizarre to the unaware physician. Patients will recognize a physician as an insightful historian when he knows to ask unusual questions about "odd" symptoms.

During the appointment with a CIRS patient, ask about unusual posturing of fingers or toes, sometimes called "clawing." These involuntary spasms in small muscles of fingers and toes can be painful and are certainly distinctive elements of history. Some patients will have their long and fourth fingers split apart, making a sign of a V, as we often saw from Mr. Spock in Star Trek. Sometimes, there will be arching of the metacarpophalangeal and metatarsophalangeal joints as well. These spasms are far more commonly brought on by lying down in bed or arising from sleep. CIRS patients quickly learn that the spasm experienced in the middle of the night can be severe, especially if they sleep with their ankles extended. Simple dorsiflexion of the ankles can create spasms and sometimes cramping of the gastrocnemius.

Joint stiffness occurs in CIRS patients with *cessation* of activity, called "gelling." If a patient says that he would prefer to stay standing after activity rather than sit down and rest, that may be an indication of his awareness of his rate of gelling.

CIRS patients will often describe fatigue and aching by saying they feel like they ran a marathon, yet they have hardly moved. Aching is perhaps the most common CIRS pain. Muscle aches are largely unrelated to activity and can recur with little exertion. Aches from CIRS will not respond to most meds, including non-steroidal anti-inflammatory drugs. The aching often comes from muscle insertion areas on tendons, raising the concern regarding enthesopathies. A healthy enthesium has a limited blood supply and reduced capillary perfusion. Inflammatory responses in CIRS worsen capillary hypoperfusion of the enthesium, which increases pain. If one sees an enthesopathy (extensor epicondylitis, patellar tendinitis, Achilles tendinitis and more) but does not find a convincing history of overuse, spend a few minutes exploring the rest of the CIRS symptom roster with the patient.

Instead of postulating *intrinsic* mitochondrial disorders leading to abnormal mitochondrial metabolism of glucose, resulting in lactic acid accumulation, a better approach is recognizing that nuclear transcription factors directly affect mitochondrial function. The physician can understand reduced energy delivery as abnormal due to aberrant genomic control by transcriptomics recording nuclear-encoded mitochondrial gene activation. Still, whatever causes lactic acid accumulation, excessive lactic acid in capillary beds is a source of muscle pain, including aching.

Headaches are not necessarily a musculoskeletal problem but can overlap with any pain syndrome. With CIRS, look for intravascular volume depletion and reduced ADH levels for a given osmolality. If patients are troubled with headaches, especially when told that they have a "migraine that lasts for more than 24 hours," think of ADH/osmolality and not an actual migraine.

A special case in CIRS patients is the unexplained, sudden weight gain just after the onset of CIRS illness. Ask the question, "Was there a time that you gained 20 or more pounds unexpectedly that you just cannot lose?" The physician asks about leptin resistance, a feared complication of inflammatory changes that abnormally alters the responsiveness of the primordial gp130 cytokine receptor that responds to leptin. A great month of weight loss for a leptin-resistant patient is usually 0.5 pounds per month. When the patient is a young female, and this is often the case, societal values of thinness add to her pain from CIRS.

The overwhelming majority of CIRS patients know all about the symptom of "push/crash." Years ago, doctors believed the push/crash phenomenon was diagnostic for chronic fatigue syndrome (CFS). Now, CIRS providers are confident CFS is just a subset of CIRS. Once thought to be simply due to capillary hypoperfusion and anaerobic metabolism, the final common pathway of CIRS involves abnormalities in glycolysis and ribosomal and nuclear-encoded mitochondrial genes that reduce energy availability.

Be sure to ask about abdominal pain. Bile acid reflux occurs in over 66% of CIRS patients. The reflux sounds typical of acid reflux but never responds to acid blockers. Bile acid reflux will not be a problem when a gastroenterologist performs an endoscopy while the patient is fasting. The chances are high that the abdominal pain after meals will be called "functional." Functional, by definition, means there is no discernible pathology: the problem is psychiatric in origin. Objective data, not "functional ideation," define the illness and define the effectiveness of treatments in CIRS patients. Gastroparesis rarely occurs in anyone except older diabetics with poor blood sugar control history, except for CIRS patients in whom delayed gastric emptying occurs. Nuclear emptying studies are abnormal in 5–10% of cases. Do not guess, do the study.

2.6   ENVIRONMENTAL HISTORY

The history must include location and type of exposure as well as mechanism of exposure, with duration less important than intensity. Some exposures are simple: "I swam in a lake later confirmed to have bloom conditions of Microcystis." Some are not: "I walk by a retention pond every day. I never heard of any problems with any algae there." Be careful with Public Health pronouncements regarding cyanobacteria, especially Microcystis in Lake Erie. Since the source of most illness from cyanobacteria comes from inhalation of droplets of water, when one hears that the water from Lake Erie in Toledo is unsafe to drink but safe to use for showering, do not believe it. Every state in the United States gets deliveries of reef fish. Every state has had problems with Harmful Algal Blooms at some time.

Over 80% of reported CIRS cases stem from exposure to the interior environment of WDB. What is not known is the effect microbial toxins have on pathophysiology compared with microbial particles. Studies have shown that for every whole spore found, over 500 fragments are present.[6] Fragments of amplified molds, bacteria, actinobacteria and mycobacteria may possess toxins and certainly contain inflammagenic material. After inhalation of fragments, the innate immune system detects them and starts the CIRS process in those who are genetically predisposed.

It may seem odd that until recently, only fungal DNA measurements assessed human health risks. The Environmental Protection Agency adopted the research advances coming from Vesper and colleagues, selling a license to use Vesper's methods commercially, beginning in 1996. This test, called the Environmental Relative Moldiness Index (ERMI), was cumbersome in interpretation, as fungi counts from benign species added to the supposed risk assessment. A follow-up test, HERTSMI-2, also based on spore equivalents/mg of dust, is more specific and sensitive.[22, 24] Now that advanced testing for endotoxins and actinobacteria is available (EnviroBiomics), the future of accurate microbial assessments is improving.

A distinctive molecular pattern marking gene activation by trichothecenes and actinobacteria,[25] together with clusters of differentiation for endotoxin exposure[25] and beta-glucans,[25] further defines CIRS. The era of reliance on urinary mycotoxin testing, uncompromisingly exposed as unreliable by the Centers for Disease Control, has passed.[15]

2.7   POST-LYME SYNDROME (CIRS-PLS)

In 1998, Lyme researchers Donta and Cartwright patented the identification of a biotoxin made by *Borrelia burgdorferi* (Publication number CA2365424 A1), the causative agent in Lyme disease. Since CSM worked well to treat other biotoxins, its use in Lyme patients followed. The unexpected and precipitous negative reactions of patients with post-Lyme syndrome to CSM caused a stunning rethinking of concepts of biotoxin illnesses. Patients with negative reactions to CSM consisted of people with confirmed Lyme disease, as shown either by physician-witnessed erythema migrans rash associated with a recent tick bite or clear evidence of a significant antibody response shown by western blot testing. When given CSM after a reasonable course of antibiotics, these patients with Lyme did not improve as dinoflagellate, cyanobacteria and WDB patients did. They got worse.

This never-before-seen adverse reaction, labeled "intensification," was quickly shown to be due to a massive pro-inflammatory cytokine response, as manifested by significant elevation of matrix metalloproteinase-9 (MMP-9). This syndrome was recognized initially as showing a fall in VCS scores beginning in row E, followed by a fall in row D. This was not a "Herxheimer" reaction; it had nothing to do with antibiotics or a "die-off."

Chronic inflammatory response syndrome-post-Lyme syndrome (CIRS-PLS) occurs after the acute phase of Lyme disease, marked by the end of antibiotic use. Lyme disease is the most common vector-borne disease in the United States and Europe.[35] In the acute phase of Lyme disease, symptoms reported in older literature include arthritis, meningitis, facial palsy and myocarditis.[2] More recently, however, acute Lyme creates systemic inflammatory illness, with transcriptomic and proteomic markers seen within 48 hours of a tick bite.[32] The erythema migrans (EM) rash is a target lesion seen in fewer than 70% of acute cases.[38] In the acute phase, patients develop increased complement split products of the third and fourth complement elements.[31] These elevations are present in both EM-positive and EM-negative acute Lyme patients, making C4a and C3a useful biomarkers for Lyme disease.

A post-treatment Lyme disease syndrome develops for an estimated 20% of patients treated with antibiotics for acute Lyme disease.[1] This post-treatment Lyme disease is a chronic inflammatory response syndrome because of its parallels to other varieties of CIRS subtypes.[4] These similarities include a strong genetic predisposition based on HLA haplotypes (15-6-51, 16-5-51, 4-3-53, 11-3-52B). Additional proteomic parallels to other chronic inflammatory syndromes are lower levels of regulatory peptides, especially MSH, higher than normal levels of TGFβ-1, split products of activation of the third and fourth element of complement, and disrupted regulation of feedback control of osmolality by ADH and cortisol by adrenocorticotropic hormone (ACTH). Various other diagnostic modalities are disrupted, including deficits in VCS testing; stress echocardiograms revealing acquired pulmonary hypertension; pulmonary function tests demonstrating restrictive lung disease; and brain volumetric (NeuroQuant® [NQ]) findings of excessive atrophy of grey matter nuclear material in the bilateral putamen and right thalamic swelling. The notable proteomic and diagnostic differences between CIRS-PLS and CIRS-WDB, the predominant chronic inflammatory response syndrome, are some of the HLA genetic haplotypes particular to increased Lyme but not WDB sensitivity and an elevation of C3a. C3a is a complement pathway specific to bacterial sources of innate immune system perturbation and brain volumetric findings.

The use of transcriptomics using RNA-seq most strongly affirms the existence and pathophysiology of CIRS-PLS.[4] While the clinical complaints of post-Lyme patients might seem subjective and the proteomic changes considered non-specific, RNA-seq detects unique patterns of differential gene activation. These patterns form a "transcriptomic signature." It demonstrates changes in Lyme disease's acute, post-treatment and chronic phases. Bouquet et al.[4] assessed transcriptomics at three time points: At the initial date seen and diagnosed with Lyme disease, after 3 weeks of antibiotics treatment, and 6 months post-treatment. His study found marked differences in gene activation and suppression between cases and controls in 1,235 genes in the initial period. After 3 weeks of antibiotic treatment, 1,060 genes remained abnormal. The persistence of perturbed differential gene activation after antibiotic treatment offers genomic validation of persistent illness and the concept of CIRS-PLS. After 6 months, 636 genes remained abnormal. Notably, there were no differences in abnormal gene activation between subjects who reported they were "fully recovered" and those who remained persistently symptomatic. The symptoms were not predictive of the persistence of perturbed differential gene activation. This finding advances the notion of the persistence of post-Lyme disease: Patients presumably thought to have recovered from antibiotic treatment are experiencing objective subclinical pathology at the transcriptomic level.

The transcriptomic signature of post-treatment Lyme disease is unique compared with other inflammatory and immune-mediated conditions.[4] There are two disturbed gene pathways specific to Lyme: Glutathione-mediated detoxification and IL-6 signaling pathways. Pathway analysis in the 6-month post-treatment group with publicly available transcriptome data sets from patients with chronic illnesses shows a varying overlap of differentially expressed genes, up to 60%. These other chronic illnesses include CFS, systemic lupus erythematosus (SLE) and rheumatoid arthritis

(RA). A notable gene, eIF2, shows suppression at all three time points. eIF2 is a gene pathway that modulates ribosome-transfer binding, the process underlying the start of translation. Disruption of translation interrupts the vital function of protein synthesis from messenger RNA. Down-regulation of eIF2 is not specific to Lyme disease. This suppression also occurs in patients colonized with MARCoNS, SLE and RA. After adding exogenous VIP as part of the CIRS protocol, eIF2 can normalize.[33]

Consistent with the theory that post-Lyme syndrome is a chronic inflammatory syndrome is the detection of upregulated pro-inflammatory cytokines. There are eight notable upregulated inflammatory genes: Interferon-gamma, IL-1 β, tumor necrosis factor-alpha (TNF-alpha), IL-6, transforming growth factor β-1, anti-inflammatory cytokine IL-4, colony-stimulating factor 2, cell surface, and marker ligand CD40L. Genes upregulated after antibiotics treatment include Toll-like adapter molecule 1(TICAM1) and nuclear factor kappa-B.

Ryan and colleagues have found disruptions in microRNA (unpublished) not covered in the Bouquet study. The significance of perturbed microRNA is the implication that post-Lyme syndrome involves disruptions of the mechanisms of regulation of DNA expression. This finding extends the model for understanding PLS beyond the simplistic model of varying upregulated and downregulated gene pathways. These transcriptomic deficits suggest the need for therapeutic approaches that eventually correct the abnormal gene expression. Prior data has demonstrated the ability of the CIRS protocol to normalize the proteomic disturbances that remain post treatment with antibiotics.

At baseline, patients with Lyme disease have perturbations in TGFβ-1, C4a, C3a, i-Treg and t-Treg biomarkers. The proteomic abnormalities persist after antibiotic treatment except for C3a, which decreases to normal levels. One biomarker (TGFβ-1) worsens after antibiotics. Only after CIRS treatment do all five of these biomarkers approximate the levels found in controls. This finding has three significant implications:

1. Post-treatment Lyme syndrome is a demonstrable disease entity.
2. Post-treatment Lyme syndrome is a chronic inflammatory syndrome with elevated innate immune system biomarkers consistent with inflammation.
3. The use of antibiotics followed by the CIRS protocol can restore patients with this condition, leading to clinical and objective metabolic improvement. Transmission of *B. burgdorferi* from person to person or by nursing has been suggested but never confirmed.
4. Vectors other than ticks, including flies and mosquitoes, have been suggested to be vectors of *Borrelia*.

As of the writing of this statement, there is no confirmation of this speculation.

2.8   DIFFERENTIAL DIAGNOSIS

The first question in the differential diagnosis is: Is there exposure to a WDB? Is there exposure to a source of biotoxins? Is there *potential for exposure*? It is tough to remember in a 20-year illness what building one might have been in 20 years ago. In cases of chronic ciguatera, people will often forget what they ate and when they ate it in relation to illness. With Lyme disease, some people will not remember a tick bite but still have Lyme. Other people will have a tick bite but no Lyme rash (EM). In Lyme, we end up relying on an inherently flawed antibody test instead of a physiologic test to assist us in diagnosis.

If the potential for exposure can be satisfied, the following requirement is that we have a multi-system, multi-symptom illness. In turn, the symptoms must meet the criteria from cluster analysis. The sorting process is becoming more evident, because if one does not have a multisystem, multi-symptom illness, they do not have CIRS. If they do not have eight symptom clusters as an adult or six as a child, they likely do not have CIRS. They may have something similar, but not CIRS.

Furthermore, the case definition includes not just symptoms alone but laboratory abnormalities seen in published peer-reviewed literature. We will see a reduction in levels of the normal regulatory neuropeptides, especially MSH. We will see an elevation of at least one of three inflammatory markers: TGFβ-1, C4a, and MMP-9. We will see dysregulation of ACTH and cortisol. We will also see abnormalities in gliadin antibodies and VEGF. The issue we faced in the past with CIRS is that we did not know the transcriptomic signatures that these illnesses have. We hope to distinguish CIRS-PLS from CIRS-WDB readily with transcriptomics. We have published on transcriptomics of ciguatera and also transcriptomics of mold. We add NQ findings to the differential diagnosis to quickly make things easier. Lyme has distinctive abnormalities, as does CIRS-WDB. Other illnesses do not have those findings.

The differential diagnosis process never stops in the sense that as we continue with therapy, there will be a resolution of individual physiological abnormalities, *one by one*, as we institute sequential treatments that fix physiological abnormalities. We make no effort to do two things simultaneously; such "shotgun" medicine has no role in CIRS.

Differential diagnosis only ends when there is near-100% exclusion of all possible causes of a given patient's illness or we have a resolution of symptom abnormalities, including VCS, laboratory, nasal culture and transcriptomic abnormalities. Keeping an open mind to other diagnoses is vital.

2.9 PHYSICAL EXAM

A carefully performed physical exam remains a second fundamental basis of medical diagnosis beyond history. Perform vital signs on all new patients. Careful respiration assessment is critical. It only takes 30 seconds to count breaths and look for Cheyne–Stokes respirations in individuals with cognitive effects. Orthostatic blood pressures help identify postural orthostatic tachycardia syndrome and problems with adrenoceptors if there is blood pressure suppression. The character of the pulse provides clues to ectopic beats.

There are multiple possible tip-offs to the presence of CIRS. Look for a resting tremor of the outstretched fingers, spread wide apart. Place a piece of paper on top of the fingers to make a resting tremor evident to the examiner and patient alike. Look for evidence of abnormal skin turgor, rashes and venous stasis changes. Look especially for evidence of enlargement of turbinates and polyps upon nasal exam. Transillumination of sinuses is usually not helpful. Look for evidence of gingivitis. One of the most critical indicators of dental biofilm formers is refractory gingival abnormalities. HEENT evaluation includes determining the presence or absence of pallor, erythema of the cheeks approximating a butterfly rash but sparing the nasal bridge ("mold facies" often misdiagnosed as rosacea), the presence of scleral injection and acne. The exam should also note the presence of goiter (thyroid illness frequently accompanies CIRS), the size of cervical lymph nodes and the presence of any cranial nerve dysfunctions (often with CN VII weakness). Carotid upstroke should be full without any bruit. Look for jugular venous distention, especially in someone who has evidence of right ventricular hypertrophy on electrocardiography (EKG).

During the pulmonary exam, listen for symmetry and evidence of mucous plugging with change after cough. Crackling rales and evidence of dullness, usually at the right base, possibly indicate a pleural effusion. Evaluate for wheeze, rhonchi, decreased diaphragm excursion and post-tussic rales. Ask for three maximal inspirations, and then listen for inspiratory rales.

It seems straightforward, but we know that individuals with a wingspan greater than height are at an increased risk of developing abnormalities in the thoracic and abdominal aorta that can lead to aneurysm formation. Listen carefully for the wide splitting of S1 versus a gallop rhythm. Listen for an S3 or an S4. Look for a reason for cardiovascular compromise of either volume overload or pressure overload, both from the right ventricle and pulmonary artery or systemically.

An abdominal exam is rarely helpful unless there is an enlargement of the liver and spleen. Trained observers can feel kidneys reliably, but this skill diminishes with extra patient weight (a problem commonly seen in leptin-resistant patients with CIRS). The CIRS physical rarely requires rectal, pelvic or breast exams except as history indicates. Extremity exam demands looking for evidence of true arthritis together with evidence of peripheral edema (pitting or not, unilateral or not) and venous thrombosis. Capillary refill may diminish in fingers and toes with decreases in end-organ perfusion. Evaluate hands and feet for coolness, discoloration and perfusion. Record proximal (shoulder shrug) and distal arm strength (grip). Note handedness, and dominant arm strength in anti-gravity muscles, compared with the non-dominant arm, should be tested three times (for initial strength and fatiguing). Evaluate joints for pain, erythema, swelling and heat. Look for sensory deficits.

Mental status is usually normal, but there is often a lack of specific abilities. Most notably, math functions, performed without paper and pen, are frequently diminished. Asking questions such as "What is 91 divided by 7" or "What is 65 plus 17" will frequently elicit delayed and incorrect answers.

A few tricks go along with physical exams that CIRS docs will perform but other docs rarely do. Performance of measurement of wingspan compared with height takes 5 seconds but is associated with a more common finding of HLA 11-3-52B and elevated TGFβ-1. Similarly, gently scratching the skin, as if making a tic tac toe board on a patient's back, is an easy way to look for dermatographia. While some providers think this shows evidence of mast cell activation, a positive finding simply reflects increased levels of C4a.

Pulse oximetry, 12-lead EKG, and pulmonary functions with spirometry are vital. If, for example, there is a discrepancy between the counted pulse and the recorded pulse with pulse-ox, the physician must explain the difference. Any oxygen saturation under 92% should raise red flags immediately. Look on an EKG for evidence of abnormal rhythm, prior myocardial injury, and voltage suggesting overload of either the right or left ventricle or both. Spirometry gives us two essential recordings at the bedside for primary care and CIRS. Low forced vital capacity (FVC) tells us about restrictive lung disease, and low forced expiratory volume in 1 second (FEV-1) tells us about obstructive lung disease. If a patient has given their best effort and can only blow out for 3 seconds, look for restrictive lung disease.

2.10   ANCILLARIES – VCS

VCS testing has been used clinically for years and remains the most accurate test for functional vision.[20] It is best to do a VCS test in person at each office visit. Contrast is one of the seven main functions of vision facilitated by the optic nerve, which provides the neurologic basis of vision. If new symptoms appear during therapy or prior symptoms recur, VCS can point the way to re-exposure (scores in columns C and D will fall). Do not use VCS to make nutrition-related diagnoses.

2.11   ANCILLARIES – PULMONARY ARTERY PRESSURE

"Echos" are usually done resting, most often performed to assess the function of the left ventricle as well as to assess the pumping function of the heart. Each echo will assess the function of multiple cardiac structures; we are interested in the velocity of the tricuspid regurgitant flow, also called the tricuspid jet. Blood can go backward from the right ventricle to the right atrium passing "the wrong way" across the tricuspid valve. The measurement of the rate of backward flow is in meters/second. The machine records the velocity on at least four views during a routine echocardiogram. Curiously, cardiac sonographers are trained to label the tricuspid jet qualitatively as either absent, trace, mild or moderate. The CIRS physician needs to know about a quantified pulmonary artery pressure elevation. The echo machine generates numbers for each of the four ways the jet is measured. Use these measurements to calculate an average.

We use the tricuspid jet velocity to calculate the pulmonary artery pressure indirectly. We square the tricuspid jet number and then multiply that number by 4. To that product, we add the right atrial pressure (usually between 5 and 10 mm) to give us a calculated pulmonary artery pressure. Any resting pulmonary artery pressure (PASP) greater or equal to 30 mm Hg is consistent with pulmonary hypertension. *Any tricuspid jet greater than 2.5 meters per second will raise concerns about pulmonary artery systolic pressure in people with CIRS.*

For individuals with normal PASP at baseline or patients with health symptoms such as unexplained cough, shortness of breath or chest pain, it can be helpful to perform stress echocardiography. In this modification of the basic echo technique, an individual has two sonograms done. The first is at baseline, as discussed. The second is done after maximal exercise, requiring a target heart rate of 90% of predicted. Stress testing typically looks for problems with the performance of the left ventricle. *Exercise stress testing* is a fundamental diagnostic aid that can help identify coronary artery disease. In our example, we are not looking for left ventricular problems; we want to know the PASP change with exercise. Any rise in PASP pressure over 8 mm Hg is abnormal.

The mechanics of performing a stress echo can become difficult. Here is someone following possibly 11 minutes of maximal exercise, for example, exhausted, breathing heavily and leaning forward after the stress portion of this stress echo. Now, the echo sonographer will insist that the patient lie down within 30 seconds. The out-of-breath patient lies down on the exam table for a repeat measurement of the tricuspid jet.

Most sonographers do not examine the tricuspid valve after exercise. It helps to talk to the cardiopulmonary staff to make sure they know exactly where they will place their transducer before the exercise begins. We use PASP as an inclusion criterion for VIP treatment. If PA pressure rises more than 8 mm, the indication for VIP use becomes stronger.

2.12   ANCILLARIES – VO$_2$ MAX AND ANAEROBIC THRESHOLD

Another important cardiovascular diagnostic test is a cardiopulmonary exercise test (CPET). While the name of this test sounds like a stress echo, it is different. This test measures oxygen usage and carbon dioxide production in exercise performance, usually on a bicycle. The test is somewhat cumbersome in that a patient is strapped to EKG monitors and pedaling maximally on a bike while breathing with hoses, tubes and a mask used to record oxygen consumption.

In 2015, the Institute of Medicine (IOM)[26] emphasized the importance of cardiopulmonary exercise testing in their redefinition of CFS as Systemic Exercise Intolerance Disorder (SEID). However, this effort fell short of making CPET a biomarker necessary to diagnose SEID. The IOM simply returned to an updated, but still inadequate, non-specific symptom-only definition, one that essentially applies to 100% of all CIRS cases.

Much is known about the importance of VO$_2$ max (milliliters of oxygen consumed per kilogram per minute), as this is an important mechanism used to classify possible disabilities. We know that there is a difference between the VO$_2$ max of women and men. We also know that age has a role in normal ranges for VO$_2$ max. Based on our practice data (unpublished), it is not unusual in the face of chronic fatiguing illness for a 50-year-old woman to have a VO$_2$ max of approximately 20 ml per kilogram per minute (with slightly higher values for men), raising the diagnosis of chronic fatiguing illness. The tables for Cardiovascular Fitness Classification are in the American Medical Association Guides to Evaluation Disability and Impairment; Social Security uses VO$_2$ max as one of the key elements in assessing disability.

More important than VO$_2$ max is delineating the anaerobic threshold (AT). The maximum activity level occurs through available oxygen (aerobic metabolism). Mitochondria need oxygen to break down glucose fragments, releasing water, carbon dioxide and energy (ATP). For those with low AT, even walking slowly up a flight of stairs reduces oxygen delivery, diminishing aerobic energy production. When AT is exceeded, as in the stairs example, oxygen is not available as needed for mitochondria to produce the full complement of 38 ATP from a single molecule of glucose. Without oxygen to supply the electron transport chain, a single glucose molecule will now just provide two molecules of ATP, or a 5% efficiency in the face of oxygen depletion. In turn, as glucose and glycogen stores are quickly exhausted, the energy-depleted cell looks for additional fuel sources. In the face of low MSH, leptin resistance is often present, preventing normal use (through direct beta-oxidation) of fatty acids for fuel (the "second wind" most runners have experienced). Under compromised conditions, lean body mass, our protein reserves, is broken down into amino acids, which are converted (especially alanine and glutamine) into glucose. The demand for ATP may create protein-wasting syndromes that conserve fat reserves. Patients will often complain about weight gain and an inability to gain muscle.

If AT is depressed, even trying to do a few things extra when a patient has a day with a bit more energy than most results in glycogen depletion. Do not forget glycogen replenishment is a slow process: Patients will feel exhausted until the repletion of glycogen stores. Terms for this commonly observed phenomenon include "push/crash," "delayed recovery from normal activity" and "post-exertional malaise." Simply stated: "The patient did too much."

However, contrary to the IOM opinion, low AT is common in conditions other than just SEID. In CIRS, the oxygen delivery problem is complicated by a lack of normal blood flow into capillary beds, not to mention nuclear-encoded mitochondrial gene problems. Still, capillary hypoperfusion is the mechanism that underlies deficits in VCS, which is a hallmark of CIRS.

Performing CPET twice, 24 hours apart, can objectively document the push/crash syndrome. Maximal effort on Day 1 often demonstrates low VO_2 max and impaired AT. With maximal effort (push) the first day, at-risk CIRS patients will often perform even more poorly (crash) on Day 2. VO_2 max and AT are commonly lower on the second day, highlighting the push/crash phenomenon. CPET performed over two consecutive days can provide objective evidence of physical disability.

2.13   ANCILLARIES – VON WILLEBRAND'S FACTORS

Additional problems in CIRS paradoxically include both excessive clotting and bleeding. Just like in sepsis, where multiple inflammatory mediators are activated, including complement, Th1, Th2 and Th17, coagulation defects also appear. Likewise, two-thirds of CIRS patients will have abnormalities in a comprehensive von Willebrand's profile.

Over 80% of CIRS patients will report shortness of breath. Asthma may occur, but restrictive lung disease, interstitial lung disease and pulmonary emboli are all primary features of the differential diagnosis. Similarly, when exposure to a building results in unexplained nosebleeds and hemoptysis, immediately think of acquired von Willebrand's disease (AvWD), a condition that is easily treated using a medication (desmopressin) that costs about a nickel. If the differential diagnosis did not include AvWD, uncontrolled hemorrhage might follow. Conversely, elevated levels of vWF raise the risk of intravascular clotting, with deep vein thrombosis and pulmonary emboli possible. Whenever, for example, a patient suffers clotting around an intravenous catheter (especially PICC lines), make sure that elevated vWF factors are not the underlying problem.

2.14   ANCILLARIES – NEUROQUANT®

NQ has made identification and separation of CIRS-WDB, CIRS-PLS, traumatic brain injury, post-traumatic stress disorder (PTSD), ciguatera and multi-nuclear atrophy straightforward. When added to magnetic resonance imaging of the brain, NQ is an illness-specific indicator. The use of sequential NQ testing has shown there is much more plasticity for an injured brain to heal than was once thought.[6] With low cost, rapid turnaround times and no need for contrast dyes, NQ adds powerful weight to assessing cognitive dysfunction, including evaluation of possible risk for development of dementia.

We can look at a General Morphometry Report (GMR) produced by NQ and rapidly identify microscopic interstitial edema, atrophy and patterns of brain injury accurately. Many unsupported ideas about PTSD being purely a psychiatric condition need re-evaluation now that we have indications of a unique volumetric measure that correlates with symptoms. We hope a new era will arrive in treating neurodegenerative illnesses now that we can use NQ to identify and correct grey matter nuclear atrophy (Figure 2.1).

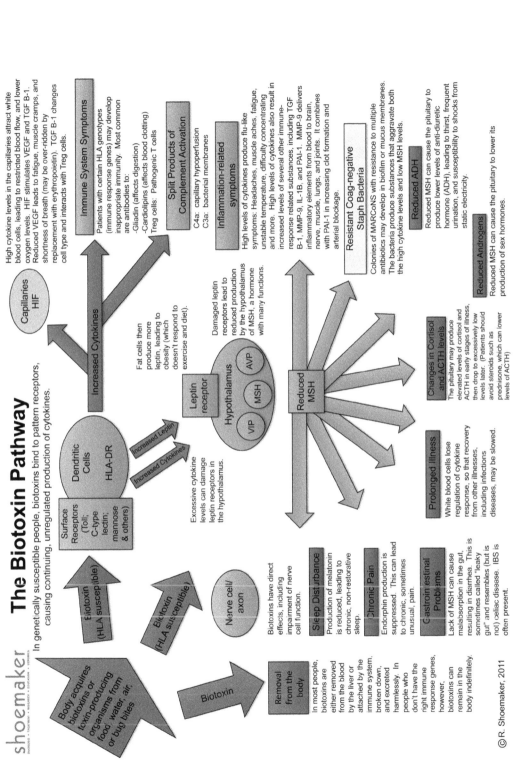

FIGURE 2.1 Biotoxin illness pathway: A description of the progressive stages of CIRS pathophysiology. (Reprinted with permission from Dr. Ritchie Shoemaker, "2018 Diagnostic Process for Chronic Inflammatory Response Syndrome (CIRS): A Consensus Statement Report of the Consensus Committee of Surviving Mold." Internal Medicine Review, May 2018.)

2.15   BIOTOXIN PATHWAY

We are looking at multisystem dysfunction with genetic susceptibility and deficiency of neuroregulatory peptides. The schematic called the Biotoxin Pathway summarizes the basics of the role of innate immune inflammatory pathways.

Within normal hosts, exposure to biotoxins will result in an innate immune response via the production and release of innate inflammatory markers.[3] Biotoxin exposure signals an adaptive immune response with specific antibody formation to the offending agent.[23] The antibody tags the biotoxin, signaling it for destruction and subsequent removal from the body.[19] With the activation of the adaptive immune system, inhibitory signals downregulate the innate immune response, preventing chronic innate immune activation.[18]

In contrast, hosts predisposed to CIRS exhibit disruptions in their adaptive and innate immune mechanisms when exposed to biotoxins,[21] precluding the removal of the offending agents. The resultant, persistent biotoxicity creates an upregulation of the innate immune system,[1, 4] which if left unchecked, will manifest as CIRS.[33] Specific HLA immune response genes (HLA-DR genes) link to an increased risk for CIRS.[26, 23]

In addition to triggering systemic inflammation, biotoxins can also have a direct neurotoxic effect.[26] In most patients, VCS testing can detect deficits caused by biotoxicity affecting the neurologic function in the visual system.[13]

The upregulation of the innate immune system results in increased cytokine levels, which bind to receptors on certain white blood cells,[17] signaling the release of MMP-9 into the bloodstream.[8] Leptin's cytokine action acts upon macrophages, resulting in the synthesis of additional pro-inflammatory cytokines[29], such as TNF-α, IL-1 and IL-6.[14] These cytokines can, in turn, stimulate further production of leptin from adipocytes, creating a positive feedback loop that perpetuates the innate inflammation and weight gain.[14]

As opposed to leptin's driving force on the innate immune system during CIRS, leptin's normal physiologic hypothalamic influence wanes due to competing cytokines that block the leptin hypothalamic receptor.[29] Certain cytokines, such as IL-6, IL-11, IL-12 and oncostatin M, are capable of such a feat due to their structural similarity to leptin.[14] The leptin receptor blockage creates leptin resistance,[20] which causes upregulation of leptin production.[29] In normal physiology, leptin binds receptors located within the arcuate nucleus of the hypothalamus.[9] Inevitably, the leptin receptor blockade in CIRS leads to loss of hormonal regulatory control due to disruption of the pro-opiomelanocortin (POMC) pathway with decreased hypothalamic hormones.[29]

With the release of cytokines, leukocytes marginalize to the venule's endothelial cell (EC) wall. A weak adhesion occurs between the leukocyte and the EC wall via a tethering and rolling process. The adhesion through leukocyte activation results in a stationary attachment.[11]

Persistent innate inflammation leads to abnormal T cell responses[40] and dysregulated complement cascade.[21, 30, 31] In a normal host, there is tight regulation over the production of mature effector helper T (Th) cells and regulatory T (Treg) cells.[40] These mature T cells have specific functions in the immune system: Th1 and Th17 increase in autoimmune diseases; Th2 are involved in allergies; Tregs modulate inflammatory responses through regulation of Th cells.[5] Cytokines play a role in dictating the maturation of naïve CD4+ T cells into the various functional subtypes: IL-12 and interferon-gamma induce TH1 cells; IL-4 induces Th2 cells; IL-6, IL-23 and elevated TGFβ-1 induce Th17 cells; IL-2 and normal levels of TGFβ-1 induce Treg cells.[40] Additionally, specific intracellular proteins known as "suppressors of cytokine signaling" (SOCS) 1 and (SOCS) 3 influence cytokine effects on both maturing effector helper T cells and Tregs.[40]

The forkhead box P3 (FOXP3) gene is the "master of gene control" for Tregs.[7] In SOCS1 deficient Tregs, there is a loss of FOXP3 expression, leading to the production of pathogenic Tregs.[40] Although CD4+CD25+ Treg cells normally suppress autoimmunity,[7] once they become pathogenic T cells in the face of ongoing inflammation, they can induce autoimmunity[40] and create tissue inflammation.[34] In CIRS patients, levels of circulating CD4+CD25+ Tregs decrease on Day 1 upon re-exposure to a WDB without spontaneous return to normalcy.[37] This finding supports the notion that the innate inflammation incited by inhalation of particulates from the WDB exposure induces conversion of CD4+CD25+ Tregs into pathogenic Tregs, thereby decreasing measurable levels of the CD4+CD25+ Tregs.[37] Additionally, TGFβ-1 regulates pathways that initiate and maintain the expression of FOXP3, thereby manipulating the production of Treg cells.[10] CIRS patients can develop autoimmunity, as evidenced by the following antibodies: Anti-gliadin antibodies (gluten sensitivity), anti-cardiolipin antibodies (ACLA),[16] antineutrophil cytoplasmic antibodies (ANCA)[28] and more.

CIRS can also involve derangements in the complement cascade, indicated by elevated C4a levels.[21, 30, 31] As the chronic inflammation continues, further hormonal dysregulation ensues.

Released in response to stress, cortisol is typically tightly regulated by ACTH through the hypothalamic-pituitary-adrenal (HPA) axis and is a good reflection of neuroendocrine wellbeing.[36] Unfortunately, 50% of CIRS patients with low MSH will experience loss of cortisol regulation.[28] During the beginning stages of CIRS, simultaneous ACTH and morning cortisol measurements are often high with minimal symptoms.[28] However, as CIRS progresses, ACTH and morning cortisol levels fall, resulting in a marked increase in symptoms.[28] Decreased ACTH production due to hypothalamic leptin resistance results in altered sleep regulation.[12] Chronic leptin resistance limits the production of MSH.

The posterior pituitary secretes ADH, regulating sodium and water balance.[39] The hypothalamus responds to the solute concentration (i.e., serum osmolality) in the blood through osmoreceptors.[39] When the serum osmolality is too high, the hypothalamus signals to the pituitary to secrete ADH into the bloodstream.[39] ADH subsequently induces the kidneys to reabsorb free water, thus diluting the blood.[39] Approximately 60% of CIRS patients will have dysregulation of ADH/serum osmolality levels.[28]

2.16 SUMMARY

The science behind CIRS has evolved rapidly and expansively. Recent transcriptomics knowledge is advancing the foundation of CIRS proteomics. Implications for metabolic disorders are a staggering and exciting frontier. With the additions of endotoxin knowledge and actinobacteria, the intersection between environment and chronic illness continues to crystallize.

REFERENCES

1. Aucott, John N., Lauren A. Crowder, and Kathleen B. Kortte. "Development of a Foundation for a Case Definition of Post-Treatment Lyme Disease Syndrome." *International Journal of Infectious Diseases* 17, no. 6 (2013): e443–9. https://doi.org/10.1016/j.ijid.2013.01.008.
2. Aucott, John, Candis Morrison, Beatriz Munoz, Peter C Rowe, Alison Schwarzwalder, and Sheila K West. "Diagnostic Challenges of Early Lyme Disease: Lessons From a Community Case Series." *BMC Infectious Diseases* 9, no. 1 (2009): 1–8. https://doi.org/10.1186/1471-2334-9-79.
3. Berndtson, K., S. McMahon, M. Ackerley, S. Rappaport, and R. Shoemaker. "Medically Sound Investigation and Remediation of Water-Damaged Buildings in Cases of CIRS-WDB." www.survivingmold.com, October 2015. https://www.survivingmold.com/MEDICAL_CONSENSUS_STATEMENT_10_30_15.PDF.
4. Bouquet, Jerome, Mark J. Soloski, Andrea Swei, Chris Cheadle, Scot Federman, Jean-Noel Billaud, Alison W. Rebman, B. Kabre, R. Halpert, M. Boorgula, and J. N. Aucott. "Longitudinal Transcriptome Analysis Reveals a Sustained Differential Gene Expression Signature in Patients Treated for Acute Lyme Disease." *mBio* 7, no. 1 (2016): e00100. https://doi.org/10.1128/mbio.00100-16.
5. Chapoval, Svetlana, Preeta Dasgupta, Nicolas J. Dorsey, and Achsah D. Keegan. "Regulation of the T Helper Cell Type 2 (th2)/t Regulatory Cell (Treg) Balance by Il-4 and STAT6." *Journal of Leukocyte Biology* 87, no. 6 (2010): 1011–18. https://doi.org/10.1189/jlb.1209772.
6. Cho, Seung-Hyun, Sung-Chul Seo, Detlef Schmechel, Sergey A. Grinshpun, and Tiina Reponen. "Aerodynamic Characteristics and Respiratory Deposition of Fungal Fragments." *Atmospheric Environment* 39, no. 30 (2005): 5454–65. https://doi.org/10.1016/j.atmosenv.2005.05.042.

7. Dejaco, Christian, Christina Duftner, Beatrix Grubeck-Loebenstein, and Michael Schirmer. "Imbalance of Regulatory T Cells in Human Autoimmune Diseases." *Immunology* 117, no. 3 (2006): 289–300. https://doi.org/10.1111/j.1365-2567.2005.02317.x.

8. Di Girolamo, Nick, Ikuko Indoh, Nicole Jackson, Denis Wakefield, H. Patrick McNeil, Weixing Yan, Carolyn Geczy, Jonathan P. Arm, and Nicodemus Tedla. "Human Mast Cell-Derived Gelatinase B (Matrix Metalloproteinase-9) is Regulated by Inflammatory Cytokines: Role in Cell Migration." *The Journal of Immunology* 177, no. 4 (2006): 2638–50. https://doi.org/10.4049/jimmunol.177.4.2638.

9. D'Agostino, Giuseppe, and Sabrina Diano. "Alpha-Melanocyte Stimulating Hormone: Production and Degradation." *Journal of Molecular Medicine* 88, no. 12 (2010): 1195–201. https://doi.org/10.1007/s00109-010-0651-0.

10. Fu, Shuang, Nan Zhang, Adam C. Yopp, Dongmei Chen, Minwei Mao, Dan Chen, Haojiang Zhang, Yaozhong Ding, and Jonathan S. Bromberg. "TGF-Beta Induces foxp3 + T-Regulatory Cells from CD4 + CD25 - Precursors." *American Journal of Transplantation* 4, no. 10 (2004): 1614–27. https://doi.org/10.1111/j.1600-6143.2004.00566.x.

11. Granger, D. Neil, and Elena Senchenkova. *Inflammation and the Microcirculation*. San Rafael, CA: Morgan & Claypool, 2010.

12. Han, Kuem Sun, Lin Kim, and Insop Shim. "Stress and Sleep Disorder." *Experimental Neurobiology* 21, no. 4 (2012): 141–50. https://doi.org/10.5607/en.2012.21.4.141.

13. Hudnell, H. Kenneth, Quay Dortch, and Harold Zenick. "An Overview of the Interagency, International Symposium on Cyanobacterial Harmful Algal Blooms (ISOC-HAB): Advancing the Scientific Understanding of Freshwater Harmful Algal Blooms." *Advances in Experimental Medicine and Biology*: 1–16. https://doi.org/10.1007/978-0-387-75865-7_1.

14. Iikuni, Noriko, Queenie Kwan Lam, Liwei Lu, Giuseppe Matarese, and Antonio Cava. "Leptin and Inflammation." *Current Immunology Reviews* 4, no. 2 (2008): 70–79. https://doi.org/10.2174/157339508784325046.

15. Kawamoto, M. "Notes From the Field: Use of Unvalidated Urine Mycotoxin Tests for the Clinical Diagnosis of Illness-US 2014." *M MWR*, 2015: 157–58.

16. McMahon, Scott. "An Evaluation of Alternate Means to Diagnose Chronic Inflammatory Response Syndrome and Determine Prevalence." *Medical Research Archives* 5, no. 3 (2017). https://doi.org/10.18103/mra.v5i3.1125.

17. Melamed, D. "Modulation of Matrix Metalloproteinase-9 (MMP-9) Secretion in B Lymphopoiesis." *International Immunology* 18, no. 9 (2006): 1355–62. https://doi.org/10.1093/intimm/dxl068.

18. Mogensen, Trine H. "Pathogen Recognition and Inflammatory Signaling in Innate Immune Defenses." *Clinical Microbiology Reviews* 22, no. 2 (2009): 240–73. https://doi.org/10.1128/cmr.00046-08.

19. Murphy, K. *Janeway's Immunology*. 9th ed. New York, NY: Garland Science Publisher, 2017.

20. Park, Hyeong-Kyu, and Rexford S. Ahima. "Leptin Signaling." *F1000Prime Reports* 6 (2014). https://doi.org/10.12703/p6-73.

21. Ryan, James C., Qingzhong Wu, and Ritchie C. Shoemaker. "Transcriptomic Signatures in Whole Blood of Patients Who Acquire a Chronic Inflammatory Response Syndrome (CIRS) Following an Exposure to the Marine Toxin Ciguatoxin." *BMC Medical Genomics* 8, no. 1 (2015): 1–12. https://doi.org/10.1186/s12920-015-0089-x.

22. Shoemaker, R. "#658 In Proceedings of the 14th International Conference on Indoor Air Quality and Climate, International Society for Indoor Air Quality and Climate." *Healthy Buildings Europe*, 2017.

23. Shoemaker, R. "Exposure to Interior Environments of Water-Damaged Buildings Causes a CFS-like Illness in Pediatric Patients: A Case/Control Study." *Bulletin of the IACFS/ME* 17, no. 2 (2009): 69–81.

24. Shoemaker, R., and D. Lark. "HERTSMI-2 and ERMI: Correlating Human Health Risk With Mold Specific QPCR in Water-Damaged Buildings." *#658 in Proceedings of the 14th International Conference on Indoor Air Quality and Climate*. Ghent, Belgium: International Society for Indoor Air Quality and Climate, 2016.

25. Shoemaker, R., and J. Ryan. *A Gene Primer for Health Care Providers: The Genomics of CIRS and Associated Molecular Pathways: Interpreting the Transcriptomics Results*. Ebook, 2018.

26. Shoemaker, R., J. Rash, and E. Simon. "Sick Building Syndrome in Water Damaged Buildings: Generalization of the Chronic Biotoxin Associated Illness Paradigm to Indoor Toxigenic Fungi. Bioaerosols, Fungi, Bacteria, Mycotoxins and Human Health." In *Bioaerosols, Fungi, Bacteria, Mycotoxins and Human Health: Pathophysiology, Clinical Effects, Exposure Assessment, Prevention and Control in Indoor Environments and Work*, edited by E. Johanning, 52–63. Fungal Research Group Foundation, 2006.

27. Shoemaker, R., S. McMahon, and C. Grimes. "Research Committee Report on Diagnosis and Treatment of Chronic Inflammatory Response Syndrome Caused by Exposure to the Interior Environment of Water-Damaged Buildings." *Policyholders of America*, 2010.
28. Shoemaker, Ritchie C. *Surviving Mold: Life in the Era of Dangerous Buildings*. Baltimore, MD: Otter Bay Books, LLC, 2010.
29. Shoemaker, Ritchie C., and Dennis E. House. "Sick Building Syndrome (SBS) and Exposure to Water-Damaged Buildings: Time Series Study, Clinical Trial and Mechanisms." *Neurotoxicology and Teratology* 28, no. 5 (2006): 573–88. https://doi.org/10.1016/j.ntt.2006.07.003.
30. Shoemaker, Ritchie C., Dennis House, and James C. Ryan. "Vasoactive Intestinal Polypeptide (VIP) Corrects Chronic Inflammatory Response Syndrome (CIRS) Acquired Following Exposure to Water-Damaged Buildings." *Health* 5, no. 3 (2013): 396–401. https://doi.org/10.4236/health.2013.53053.
31. Shoemaker, Ritchie C., Patricia C. Giclas, Chris Crowder, Dennis House, and M. Michael Glovsky. "Complement Split Products C3A and C4A Are Early Markers of Acute Lyme Disease in Tick Bite Patients in the United States." *International Archives of Allergy and Immunology* 146, no. 3 (2008): 255–61. https://doi.org/10.1159/000116362.
32. Shoemaker, Ritchie, Andrew Heyman, Annalaura Mancia, and James Ryan. "Chronic Fatiguing Illnesses: Entering the Era of New Biomarkers and Therapies." *Internal Medicine Review* 3, no. 10 (2017): 1–29. https://doi.org/10.18103/imr.v3i10.585.
33. Shoemaker, Ryan. "RNA-Seq on Patients With Chronic Inflammatory Response Syndrome (CIRS) Treated With Vasoactive Intestinal Peptide (VIP) Shows a Shift in Metabolic State and Innate Immune Functions That Coincide With Healing." *Medical Research Archives* 4, no. 7 (2016). https://doi.org/10.18103/mra.v4i7.862.
34. Shu, Ye, Qinghua Hu, Hai Long, Christopher Chang, Qianjin Lu, and Rong Xiao. "Epigenetic Variability of CD4+CD25+ Tregs Contributes to the Pathogenesis of Autoimmune Diseases." *Clinical Reviews in Allergy & Immunology* 52, no. 2 (2016): 260–72. https://doi.org/10.1007/s12016-016-8590-3.
35. Stanek, Gerold, Gary P. Wormser, Jeremy Gray, and Franc Strle. "Lyme Borreliosis." *The Lancet* 379, no. 9814 (2012): 461–73. https://doi.org/10.1016/s0140-6736(11)60103-7.
36. Stawski, R. S., D. M. Almeida, M. E. Lachman, P. A. Tun, C. B. Rosnick, and T. Seeman. "Associations Between Cognitive Function and Naturally Occurring Daily Cortisol During Middle Adulthood: Timing is Everything." *The Journals of Gerontology Series B: Psychological Sciences and Social Sciences* 66B, suppl. 1 (2011): i71–i81. https://doi.org/10.1093/geronb/gbq094.
37. "T Regulatory Cells in Chronic Inflammatory Response Syndrome From Water-Damaged Buildings (CIRS-WDB)." http://Www.survivingmold.com/Physician-Section/Members%20only%20downloads/Johanning_T%20regs_9_5_2011_MSM.Ppt. 2011.
38. Tibbles, Carrie D., and Jonathan A. Edlow. "Does This Patient Have Erythema Migrans?" *JAMA* 297, no. 23 (2007): 2617. https://doi.org/10.1001/jama.297.23.2617.
39. Unnikrishnan, Ambika Gopalakrishnan, Binu P. Pillai, and Praveen V. Pavithran. "Syndrome of Inappropriate Antidiuretic Hormone Secretion: Revisiting a Classical Endocrine Disorder." *Indian Journal of Endocrinology and Metabolism* 15, no. 7, suppl. 3 (2011): 208. https://doi.org/10.4103/2230-8210.84870.
40. Yoshimura, Akihiko, Mayu Suzuki, Ryota Sakaguchi, Toshikatsu Hanada, and Hideo Yasukawa. "SOCs, Inflammation, and Autoimmunity." *Frontiers in Immunology* 3 (2012): 20. https://doi.org/10.3389/fimmu.2012.00020.

3 The Shoemaker Protocol

Andrew Heyman and April Vukelic

CONTENTS

3.1 THE SHOEMAKER PROTOCOL

The Shoemaker Protocol is an evidence-based, peer-reviewed approach to biotoxin illness. It is a structured, step-by-step method that relies on well-designed studies. The Shoemaker Protocol identifies those sickened from biotoxin illness and uses rigorously tested interventions to help them recover. The implications for the prevention and treatment of Chronic Inflammatory Response Syndrome are profound for individuals and public health. If the lessons learned from the Shoemaker Protocol were put into practice universally, we could prevent the suffering of millions of people.

One should perform a very detailed history of all possible exposures, starting from the childhood home. Interview the patient regarding 37 symptoms in 13 clusters. Formulate a differential diagnosis by taking a thorough history, including a review of past medical history and labs.

These are the 13 clusters of symptoms seen in Chronic Inflammatory Response Syndrome (CIRS):

1. Fatigue.
2. Weakness, assimilation of new information, aches, headache, light sensitivity.
3. Memory impairment, word-finding difficulties.
4. Difficulty with concentration.
5. Joint pain, morning stiffness, cramps.
6. Unusual skin sensations, tingling.
7. Shortness of breath, sinus congestion.
8. Cough, excessive thirst, confusion.
9. Appetite swings, body temperature dysregulation, urinary frequency.
10. Red eyes, blurred vision, night sweats, mood swings, ice-pick pain.
11. Abdominal pain, diarrhea, numbness.

DOI: 10.1201/b23304-4

12. Tearing, disorientation, metallic taste.
13. Static shocks, vertigo.

Adult CIRS patients need to meet 8 symptoms out of 13 different clusters, and children 6 symptoms out of 13 different clusters, to be diagnosed with CIRS. A physical exam may demonstrate dehydration with hypotension and tachycardia, red eyes, muscle fatigue, rales, S3 or S4 upon cardiac auscultation, edema, tremor, dermatographia/rashes, increased body mass index, evidence of brain fog (which may include word-finding difficulties), difficulty following directions, and frequent patient interruptions due to difficulty with executive functions.

Ninety-five percent of patients with CIRS will have susceptible human leukocyte antigens (HLAs). Only about 5% of CIRS patients have non-susceptible HLAs. About 24% of the population is susceptible to illness from water-damaged buildings, and 21% is vulnerable to unresolved illness from Lyme disease after antibiotic treatment. The susceptible HLA signifies a flaw in antigen presentation. The body recognizes a threat exists but cannot properly form antibodies to remove it. Therefore, the innate immune system amplifies inflammation without clearing the biotoxin. There is ever-increasing inflammation and vigilance with no resolution.

A screening visual contrast sensitivity (VCS) test can detect capillary hypoperfusion in the retina and optic nerve by testing the patient's ability to differentiate shades of gray. VCS is a highly effective test that identifies 92% of sick patients and has a false positive rate of only 1%. Individuals who have a false negative test tend to be young women, people trained in art and photography, or people who have vision-intensive careers, like pilots. Exposure to hydrocarbons or solvents may cause a small population to have a false positive VCS. The test is non-invasive, fast, inexpensive, accurate and can be performed at home by the patient. The VCS test should be performed during the protocol period to measure both progress and re-exposure. The test can be performed at home on a computer and verified with a hand-held VCS in the doctor's office. Initiating vasoactive intestinal polypeptide (VIP) treatment requires a negative VCS. Occasionally, the VCS may not completely normalize, but it should stabilize. Passing the VCS means both eyes (if testable) see correctly seven or more patterns in row C and six or more in row D. Failure in one eye means the patient has failed the VCS. When someone has only one eye or limited acuity, the test is valid if the one eye can see 20:50 or better.

A stress echocardiogram can identify elevated pulmonary artery systolic pressures (PASP). An elevation of PASP of >8 mm Hg during exercise is abnormal and requires treatment. These patients can experience heart palpitations and exercise intolerance, and may be short of breath. It is important to ask specifically for the PASP to be quantified by the cardiologist. This objective marker helps confirm the diagnosis and can be measured afterward to demonstrate the response to the protocol.

A cardiopulmonary exercise test can measure VO_2 max. A normal value is >35 ml of oxygen consumed per kilogram per minute. A CIRS patient may have a VO_2 max of <20 ml of oxygen consumed per kilogram per minute. To put this into context, a VO_2 max of 15 ml of oxygen consumed per kilogram per minute is consistent with Stage IV cardiac failure.

All patients should receive pulmonary function tests (PFTs), especially those experiencing shortness of breath. These patients may appear to have asthma, but PFTs often show restrictive lung disease instead of obstructive lung disease. Restrictive lung disease happens in conjunction with abnormalities in transforming growth factor (TGF)β-1, matrix metalloproteinase (MMP)-9, vascular endothelial growth factor (VEGF) and T regulatory cells in the form of remodeling.

In 2006, the Food and Drug Administration (FDA) approved the NeuroQuant® software program by CorTechs. It is a volumetric study of 11 brain areas that only takes about 10 minutes to perform. NeuroQuant® is a vital test added to a traditional magnetic resonance imaging (MRI) without contrast, which shows small variances in volume in select areas of the brain. NeuroQuant® can differentiate the type of exposure based on patterns. An enlargement of the forebrain parenchyma and cortical gray and atrophy of the caudate are characteristic of CIRS-WDB. The thalamus and putamen are normal. In CIRS–post-Lyme syndrome, the putamen shows atrophy and the right thalamus enlargement.

These patterns provide excellent evidence of biotoxin illness and can be repeated after treatment to demonstrate the protocol's efficacy. GENIE (Genomic Expression: Information Explained) testing can track genetic expression associated with illness from CIRS, help tailor treatment and demonstrate resolution of illness. This test is useful in demonstrating hypometabolism through transcriptomics by the mRNA of white blood cells.

Hypometabolism includes pathologic suppression of both ribosomal and nuclear-encoded mitochondrial genes. Hypometabolism shows the dominant role of differential gene activation in the pathogenesis and perpetuation of chronic illnesses. Treatment of hypometabolism with the Shoemaker Protocol shows sequential resolution of gene suppression/activation. We can now track the pathologic basis of chronic fatigue and critical inflammatory elements throughout treatment for the first time. GENIE has advanced our knowledge of CIRS and demonstrated the importance of endotoxins and actinomycetes.

Adrenocorticotropic hormone (ACTH) and cortisol levels may initially rise and then fall as the patient's illness progresses. It is crucial to avoid systemic corticosteroids, such as prednisone, unless absolutely required. Topical and inhaled corticosteroids are safe to use. This dysregulation occurs in about 65% of patients with low melanocyte stimulating hormone (MSH) levels.

3.2   STEP 1: REMOVAL FROM EXPOSURE

Action: Polymerase chain reaction (PCR) test with Environmental Relative Moldiness Index (ERMI) or Health Effects Roster of Type-Specific Formers of Mycotoxins and Inflammagens – 2nd Version (HERTSMI). Leave and avoid all environments with unacceptable levels.

Goal: All environments should be ERMI <2 and/or HERTSMI <11. Low ERMI and HERTSMI scores are one of the requirements before VIP treatment.

This simple-sounding step is deceptively difficult. It starts with identifying the sources of exposure. Each area where the patient spends time requires a PCR test such as an ERMI or a HERTSMI. Mycometrics Lab performs these reliably. Testing is essential for home, school and work. All locations where the patient regularly spends time should undergo testing: A family member's house, church and other buildings they might frequent routinely. If the patient is renting a water-damaged apartment or house, it is best and easiest to move into a new home with an acceptable ERMI (<2 if MSH is less than 35 and C4a <20,000) or HERTSMI (<11) and remediate all belongings. If an individual has an MSH of <35 and a C4 >20,000, the ERMI must be −1 or less. Actinomycetes should be less than 15.

In 2008, the US General Accountability Office (GAO) published a Federal case definition for CIRS-WDB:

- There must be the potential for exposure to a damp indoor space.
- There must be a multi-system, multi-symptom illness present with symptoms similar to those seen in peer-reviewed publications.
- There must be laboratory-tested abnormal results similar to those seen in peer-reviewed, published studies.
- There must be documentation of improvement with therapy.

The US Environmental Protection Agency developed and validated ERMI as a form of Mold Specific Quantitative Polymerase Chain Reaction (MSQPR) from house dust. The method employs MSQPCR to detect and quantify species of fungi found in water-damaged buildings (WDB) compared with buildings without a history of water damage. HERTSMI-2 values provide an inexpensive, objective measure of organisms routinely found in WDB, known to be associated with adverse human health effects. A HERTSMI can be done by itself or derived from an ERMI. The five species measured are *Wallemia sebi, Aspergillus versicolor, Aspergillus penicillioides, Stachybotrys chartarum*, and *Chaetomium globosum*. Recent genomic research has identified actinobacteria as a common microbe in WDB and potentially responsible for CIRS six times more frequently than mycotoxins.

Environmental history includes questions about past and present living conditions, buildings the patient has occupied at school or work, HERTSMI/ERMI tests of the buildings, travel history, rashes, tick or spider bites, consumption of fish, yellow-jacket stings, exposure to freshwater with fish kills, and algae blooms. The history should include medications taken, such as fluoroquinolones, corticosteroids and gadolinium contrast.

If the patient owns a WDB, the home may have to undergo remediation by an expert who regards improvement in human health over an arbitrary spore count. Once the patient has the results of their ERMI, HERTSMI, endotoxin and actinobacteria report, an Indoor Environmental Professional should locate the source of damage. Then, a remediation company will remove the mold properly. Look at www.acac.org to find certified agencies. Indoor Environmental Professionals will carry the CIEC or CMC certification. Remediators will carry CMRS or CIES certification.

There are three phases to making the environment safe:

Phase 1. Inspect and investigate to detect water intrusions, leaks and condensation problems. Also, investigate the HVAC system for potential cross-contamination issues. A plan for correcting problems and preventing recurrences follows, including a plan for remediation of water-damaged structures. In cases of CIRS-WDB, detection, correction and prevention should begin with an interview of the occupant(s) that includes a symptom-based assessment of risk for CIRS-WDB.

Phase 2. Perform the planned corrections required to achieve moisture control and remediate water-damaged building materials. In cases where occupants suffer from CIRS-WDB or other medical conditions affected by WDB contaminants, remediation should include in-depth cleaning of all reservoirs of bioactive particulates inside the affected building.

Phase 3. Perform maintenance procedures to sustain high-quality indoor air over the long term. In cases of CIRS-WDB, maintenance protocols should involve more frequent and intensive monitoring of water damage risks. In addition, proactive measures can be considered for the structure to help improve the overall indoor environmental quality in the home. Some examples of this are optimal air filtration, ventilation, and pressurization of the structure. The Surviving Mold Professional Panel (SMPP) can help provide support/direction regarding this recommendation.

Once remediated, repeat ERMI, HERTSMI-2, endotoxin and actinomycetes testing and continue to use the high-efficiency particulate air (HEPA) filter made by Air Oasis. Move machines around twice a day. Use a HEPA filter vacuum cleaner on floors twice a week and on ceilings and walls every 2 weeks.

The patient may need to temporarily vacate the environment during remediation, though sometimes moving out and selling is the best option. The items in the WDB must receive a careful evaluation. Porous items need to be disposed of or placed in air-tight containers. It is possible to clean non-porous items like glass, metal, finished wood and leather with HEPA vacuums and quaternary solutions such as Windex, Fantastic, 409 or Clorox Clean-up (this is *not* the same as bleach). For the very sensitive, it is better to use paper towels and disposable dusting cloths (e.g., Swiffers) than rags to permanently remove contaminated material from the home. Reusable rags and mop-heads can spread the biotoxins. It may be necessary to wear HEPA respirators and protective gear while cleaning. Some of the most sensitive patients may need to abandon possessions altogether. Failure to remediate the old belongings before bringing them into a new environment will bring the patient back to square one.

It is vital to discard all reservoirs for inflammagens, like rugs, curtains, thick bedding and upholstered furniture. Mattresses may potentially be salvageable with impermeable covers. Wash clothes with detergent, borax and quaternary cleaners. In general, the thicker the fabric, the more difficult it is to clean. Sometimes, cleaning fabric is ineffective, depending on the person's sensitivities, and it is better to buy new items. The patient may reduce the number of items in a home, as a sparse aesthetic translates into a healthier environment with fewer reservoirs and less cleaning. Car interiors should also receive attention. If a vehicle sustained flooding or a longstanding leak from the window, this could cause illness, and the upholstery and carpet can act as a reservoir. Under these conditions, performing a HERTSMI may be advisable. HEPA vacuuming and quaternary fluids are effective cleaners in a car. Use Air Oasis purifiers to improve air quality in the car.

The patient must not attend school or work in a WDB. In most cases, after someone has been sickened, it is best to find another school or workplace. It is impossible to regain health if the patient remains exposed to WDBs. When a school or workplace cleans the environment, the remedial action is often insufficient or much too late for an already ill patient. Unfortunately, the patient is unlikely to find organizations that take full or appropriate responsibility for their compromised buildings and the resulting damage to health. The patient should perform an ERMI or HERTSMI at a prospective school or job before beginning. Spore sampling is inherently flawed and has no bearing on human health per the World Health Organization's stance (2009). Intact mold spores account for about 0.2% of the problem, and for this reason, PCR is the only valid method to ensure safety. Studies of human health and re-exposure trials have validated the ERMI/HERTSMI PCR.

According to the National Institute for Occupational Safety and Health (NIOSH), more than half the buildings in America are water damaged. Once the patient has determined that none of the buildings in question are water damaged, they must remain cautious and vigilant when entering any other untested building. That means grocery stores, banks, pharmacies, movie theaters, big box stores and restaurants must be safe if the patient stands to regain health. If a local post office or shipping distribution center is moldy, online shopping can be a source of exposure. It is impractical to test each building one enters, so here are some general guidelines: If the building has a stucco facade and a flat roof, the odds of water intrusion are higher. Buildings at the bottoms of hills or in a known flood zone are likely to be unsafe. A glance at the roof and fascia can give a clue about the condition of the building. Water-stained ceiling tiles, standing water, musty smells, visible mold, stained carpet and active leaks are red flags to leave quickly. Some people have reported benefits from using a peak-flow meter to identify WDBs. Others have a "gut feeling" about a building. Learning to recognize signs of exposure is critical in avoiding WDBs. The symptoms can vary from person to person, but recognizing the first signs of feeling unwell is critical.

As the living/working environment becomes progressively cleaner, one may notice adverse symptoms occurring more quickly in unclean environments. This increased sensitivity is the "sicker, quicker" pattern associated with mannose-binding lectin serine protease 2 (MASP-2). In time, smaller exposures make the patient sicker and for longer periods. The cascading "sicker, quicker" phenomenon often confuses patients and their loved ones who have not studied CIRS. It baffles many people why they could work somewhere for years, but eventually, they can no longer spend a few minutes in the same building. Some people may get headaches, feel dizzy, become hoarse, feel short of breath, have nausea, and experience ringing or fullness in the ears. People have different ways of describing WDBs. They may characterize them as "stuffy, dark, stale, dank, musty, run-down, cheap" or "dirty." Sometimes the way someone describes a building provides information that they are not consciously processing.

After remediation and when the home has an acceptable ERMI or HERTSMI, HEPA filters can remove particles down to 0.3 microns. For smaller fragments, Air Oasis filters are a good choice. There is also an exciting product called AeroSolver. It employs a fogging solution to remove the smallest fragments and inflammagens from the air. Wipe up particulates once the fog settles.

Dehumidifiers can also discourage mold growth. These are helpful adjuncts but *do not replace proper remediation.*

Pets can also become sick from WDBs, and veterinarians are unlikely to know about mold exposure. A case study from 2007 describes two Himalayan cats that died from pulmonary hemorrhage after Stachybotrys exposure. Doggy daycare, groomers and pet sitters are all potential sources of exposure. If a basement has water damage, it is not suitable for pets or humans to spend time there. Having litter boxes in basements or relegating animals to water-damaged areas is bad for the pets and ultimately, their humans. Basements typically have worse ERMIs and HERTSMIs.

In animals, symptoms to consider are cough, lethargy, vomiting, diarrhea, vocalized pain, unexplained weight loss/anorexia, neurologic issues like dizziness, ataxia or confusion, unexplained behavioral changes, and paw-shaking when no other sources of injury are apparent.

Children may spend time at daycare, in extra-curricular lessons or with family members outside of school. Each of these places can be a source of exposure and contamination. Ensure each of these places is safe by using PCR testing such as ERMI or HERTSMI.

Other sources of biotoxin illness include ciguatera from fish, Lyme and Babesia from ticks, algae blooms and cyanobacteria, Pfiesteria from waterways, Mediterranean spider bites and lionfish. Even if WDB exposure was not the event that made a person sick, anyone with a low MSH (who has had the same final common pathway of inflammation triggered) could be made sicker with mold exposure. People who have had a chronic illness from Lyme disease can become increasingly sensitive to mold. They are frequently made ill from moldy buildings and may not know it. Instead, they can find themselves on unnecessary courses of antibiotics when in fact, their home is causing continued inflammation.

3.3   STEP 2: CHOLESTYRAMINE AND WELCHOL

Action: Cholestyramine 4 grams QID or Welchol 625 mg two pills TID with food.
Goal: Reduce biotoxin load to pass VCS.
Pediatric Considerations: Cholestyramine 60 mg/kg/dose TID, 60–120-lb children 4 mg TID.
     Welchol 20 kg = 1 tab, BID.

Biotoxins are small, negatively charged compounds that continuously cycle through the bile in a process called enterohepatic circulation. The bile is conserved in this process, and because the biotoxins remain in the bile, they do not leave the body by normal physiologic processes. Cholestyramine (CSM) has long polystyrene chains with side groups of positively charged nitrogen (quaternary ammonium). The electrostatic interaction holds toxins in the gut and therefore prevents enterohepatic recirculation. The shape and size of the positive charge interact with a net negative charge found in parts of biotoxins. Treat Lyme with 30 days of antibiotics before administering CSM. Omega 3s and the non-amylose diet should be used at least 10 days before starting CSM.

The biotoxin and CSM can then leave via the digestive system. Each dose of CSM will reduce the amount of biotoxins in the body. Pre-medicating with a week's worth of high-dose fish oil (eicosapentaenoic acid [EPA] 2.4 grams and docosahexaenoic acid [DHA] 1.8 grams) and for the first 5 days after initiation of CSM can reduce the intensification reaction that occurs as these biotoxins leave the body. Patients are dosed with 4 grams of CSM four times a day.

CSM can cause nausea, reflux and constipation. Use magnesium citrate to reduce constipation, the most common side effect. CSM is a very safe medication, as it does not enter the bloodstream. Mix CSM with water. One may eat 30 minutes after taking CSM. It is also important to fast for at least 60 minutes after eating before taking a dose of CSM. If the patient has difficulty tolerating the pharmaceutical formulation, use a compounded version of CSM without sugar, aspartame or additives. Sensitive patients can start slowly with a tweezer full of CSM and titrate as tolerated. The VIP protocol outlined in *The Art and Science of CIRS Medicine* prepares the most sensitive patients for binder.

CSM is a cholesterol binder called a bile acid sequestrant. It should be dosed 4 hours after medications like Synthroid, digitalis, beta-blockers, valproic acid, warfarin and antibiotics. It can also bind to fat-soluble vitamins A, C, D and E. The use of this medication to remove biotoxins is off-label, and the physician should have the patient sign a consent.

Welchol is an alternative for those who cannot tolerate CSM but is only about a quarter as effective because it has fewer positive charges to bind the biotoxin. Patients with multiple chemical sensitivity may be able to tolerate Welchol. It can be dosed with food and comes in pill form, which is more convenient than CSM.

Ultimately, the goal is to remove as much of the biotoxin load as possible and pass the VCS. Repeat the VCS monthly. If there is no improvement, look for another source of biotoxin exposure and check for patient compliance. Then, eliminate MARCoNS for continued improvement of symptoms.

Before entering a new and unknown building, pre-medicating with CSM is advisable. Dosing with full-strength CSM for several days afterward, as described earlier, may be needed if the building is water damaged. Look for resolution of symptoms and improvement of the VCS.

It should be clear that the inflammatory proteins, lipid-soluble anions 1.4 angstroms in size, are not amenable to charcoal, clay, chlorella, zeolite or other common "natural" binders. Only okra and beets have shown pre-clinical promise. The goal is not binding mycotoxins (in fact, most people are sick from actinomycetes); instead, the goal is to remove the inflammatory compounds that traffic through the liver and saponify in the bile. Each time the gall bladder contracts, a load of inflammatory proteins finds its way into the gut, which can be removed by a proper anion binder or remixed through enterohepatic circulation back into the body.

Okra (*Abelmoschus esculentus*) possesses several important biological activities, including antioxidant, anti-inflammatory and immunomodulatory, antibacterial, anticancer, antidiabetic, organ protective and neuroprotective action. Okra effectively binds to bile acids (34% compared with CSM 100%).

Because of its high mucilage, okra is also used in traditional medicine as a dietary meal to treat gastric irritation. A 2014 laboratory study reported a non-specific interaction between high–molecular weight polysaccharides from okra fruits and *Helicobacter pylori* surface. Okra prevented *H. pylori* from adhering to stomach tissue. Okra polysaccharides are antioxidants, and clinical effects, including blood glucose and insulin regulation, are attributed to this property. Okra's antioxidant effects in diabetes models may be from PI3K/AKT mTOR pathway–medicated Nrf2 transport.

In the last decade, beet juice has become a highly studied supplement to improve nitric oxide (NO) production in the laboratory and in human studies. Beets bind to bile acids (54% binding vs. CSM 100%). CSM (Questran) is a potent toxin/mycotoxin binder.

At this stage, the practitioner can consider adding Rg3/Nicotinamide nasal spray to reduce further neuroinflammation. Rg3 is one of several triterpene saponins (ginsenosides) found in the plant genus Panax (including Asian or *Panax ginseng* and American ginseng or *Panax quinquefolius*). Rg3 is produced by steaming the ginseng root and then, extracting and isolating the Rg3 constituent. Laboratory studies report that Rg3 extracted from *Panax ginseng* is neuroprotective, helping to decrease microglial activation and neuroinflammatory processes. Rg3 may have anti-inflammatory activity via cyclooxygenase-2 (COX-2) inhibition and reduction of inducible nitric oxide synthase (iNOS) and pro-inflammatory cytokine expression, including tumor necrosis factor (TNF)-alpha and interleukin (IL)-1B.

Nicotinamide riboside (NR) is a form of vitamin B3 found in cow's milk. Laboratory studies report that administration of NR increases nicotinamide adenine dinucleotide (NAD+) levels in yeast and cultured human and mammalian cells. NR may be incorporated into the cellular NAD+ pool via the action of the Nrk pathway or nicotinamide (NAM) salvage after conversion to NAM by phosphorolysis. Laboratory studies have reported a neuroprotective role for NAD+. NR is a unique precursor to nervous system health when de novo synthesis of NAD+ from tryptophan is insufficient. In laboratory studies, NR supports neuronal NAD+ synthesis without inhibiting sirtuins, which are essential regulators of metabolism and longevity. Stimulation of NAD+ production may decrease axonal degeneration in laboratory studies. Axonal degeneration occurs after physical damage to axons upon traumatic injury. Axonal injury is involved in various neuropathological conditions, including diabetic neuropathies, demyelinating diseases and neurodegenerative diseases, including Alzheimer's disease, amyotrophic lateral sclerosis (ALS) and Parkinson's disease. NAD+ is a rate-limiting co-substrate for the sirtuin enzymes and helps regulate sirtuin function and subsequent regulation of oxidative metabolism.

Aberrant, very long-chain fatty acids (VLCFAs) accumulate in cell membranes in a dysfunctional pattern that affects cell metabolism. These VLCFAs form "lipid rafts" and ceramides, which augment inflammation and destabilize membrane structure. These abnormal folds are an epigenetic insult and can normalize with butyrate and phospholipid supplementation. Specialized testing from Johns Hopkins shows increases in trans isomers, saturated odd fats, VLCFAs, and renegade fats.

Use phosphatidylcholine 1.8 mg BID to repair the outer membrane and double lipid bilayer of mitochondria. Omega 6/3 at a ratio of 4:1 improves membrane fluidity. Butyrate uses short-chain fatty acids (SCFA) to cause beta-oxidation of abnormal long-chain fats and "burn off" of VLCFA from the membrane. If tolerated, wheat germ oil helps strengthen structural lipids in the membrane. Lipid supplementation can be initiated right after the first appointment. Butyrate use comes afterward.

Dr. Patricia Kane wrote about how Lyme spirochetes will preferentially use these aberrant VLCFAs to travel and feed. The VLCFA provides a rigid structure for the flagellum to move and thus feed on the sphingomyelin, oxidized cholesterol and lipid rafts themselves.

3.4   STEP 3: ELIMINATE MARCoNS

Action: 0.25% EDTA two sprays each nostril TID for 6 months, at least a month after binders.

Goal: Eradicate MARCoNS with EDTA and confirm the absence of MARCoNs with culture from MicrobiologyDX after 2 weeks off the spray. Eradication of MARCoNS must precede VIP treatment.

Pediatric Concerns: Test after 15 years of age, 0.25% EDTA one spray BID–TID per day.

MARCoNS are multiple antibiotic-resistant coagulase-negative staphylococci that reside in the deep nasopharynx. Perform a nasal swab to determine colonization. The bacteria form a self-protective biofilm, which can encourage differential gene activation. The biofilm creates hemolysin proteins, which trigger continual cytokine production. MARCoNS then cleave MSH and form exotoxins. MARCoNS are very common in CIRS patients with low MSH. The presence of MARCoNS will reduce MSH and prevent the patient from healing. Children will usually not have MARCoNS before the age of 15. Test younger children who are not improving.

Use 0.2% EDTA, with or without MucoLox as a first-line medication. Some patients may need to stay on EDTA spray for the remainder of treatment for 1 to 2 years. Avoid anti-fungal medications, especially itraconazole, since these close the VDAC receptor, worsen aerobic glycolysis and further injure the brain. Indiscriminate anti-fungal use also increases MARCoNS resistance.

Re-acquisition of MARCoNS can occur if patients have close contact with dogs or individuals with low MSH and MARCoNS. Patients should wash their hands after petting their dogs and avoid sharing a bed with dogs. If needed, a veterinarian can culture for MARCoNS through MicrobiologyDX and treat them with EDTA spray. Cats rarely harbor MARCoNS.

If the patient feels worse during treatment, use high-dose fish oils in the manner we use during CSM treatment (7 days prior and 5 days after with EPA 2.4 grams and DHA 1.8 grams). After treatment, repeat culture and VCS test. A negative MARCoNS test is needed to proceed with VIP.

3.5   STEP 4: CORRECT ANTI-GLIADIN ANTIBODIES

Action: Eliminate gluten and retest anti-gliadin antibodies (AGA).

Goal: Negative AGA or continued avoidance of gluten.

CIRS patients can have positive AGAs and not be able to tolerate gluten well. This sensitivity is more common in children than adults. If the patient has a positive AGA, the patient should avoid gluten for at least 3 months and retest. If the AGA is normal, reintroduce gluten if desired. Many people will not feel as well on gluten, and for these individuals, permanently eliminating gluten is wise. A positive tissue transglutaminase antibody (tTG) signifies celiac disease and the need to eliminate gluten for life. After ruling out celiac, the physician can opt for a full food sensitivity panel at this point for a complete dietary review. Do this step concurrently while using CSM and EDTA.

3.6   STEP 5: CORRECT ANDROGENS

Action: Use VIP or dehydroepiandrosterone (DHEA) 25 mg TID for 30 days and monitor estradiol.
Goal: Normalize androgens and aromatase.
Pediatric concerns: 20 kg = 1/4 adult dose.

Problems with androgens are seen in somewhere between 40% and 50% of CIRS patients. Check aromatase along with DHEA, testosterone and estradiol. Because aromatase converts testosterone to estradiol, replacing testosterone in a high-aromatase patient will increase estradiol in men. For these reasons, testosterone replacement can be counterproductive and may exacerbate symptoms. VIP can normalize androgens. If VIP does not optimize androgens, use DHEA cautiously while closely monitoring estradiol.

3.7   STEP 6: CORRECT ADH/OSMOLALITY

Action: Desmopressin 0.2 mg every other night for a total of five doses. Monitor electrolytes and ADH/osmolality closely (at least once every 10 days).
Goal: Normalize ADH/Osmolality.
Pediatric Concerns: DDAVP one to four sprays per day *only* if absolutely needed (for example, a patient has postural orthostatic tachycardia syndrome or acquired von Willebrand's disease).

ADH and osmolality dysregulation is common in CIRS and affects about 60–80% of patients. The most common manifestation of this is low ADH accompanied by increased thirst, headaches that mimic migraines, static shocks, frequent urination and dehydration. Some individuals with low ADH can exceed the sweat chloride of people with cystic fibrosis. Desmopressin is the treatment of choice. Monitor ADH/osmolality, electrolytes, daily weights and ankle swelling. Watch for low sodium and low osmolality. Symptoms of nocturia and polyuria should stabilize in 1 week.

Acquired von Willebrand's factor (vWF) can also be normalized with this step. Acquired von Willebrand's deficiency can cause a patient to bleed profusely and have an inability to clot normally. Patients with acquired vWF bleeding need to carry DDAVP with them when they travel. Acquired von Willebrand's deficiency is the loss of the ability to form clots via the formation of von Willebrand's multimers (low ristocetin associated cofactor, low multimer formation and low von Willebrand's antigen are common in labs). The multimers are polymers of monomers that cannot form in some individuals with elevated C4a and patients with hematologic cancers.

3.8   STEP 7: CORRECT ELEVATED MMP-9

Action: Use EPA 2.4 grams/DHA 1.8 grams. VIP, when indicated in the protocol, will improve MMP-9.

Goal: Decrease MMP-9 and increase peroxisome proliferator-activated receptor.
Pediatric Concerns: 20 kg = 1/4 adult dose of EPA/DHA.

The next step is normalizing MMP-9. MMP-9 causes inflammation of the nervous system, lungs, muscles, blood vessels and joints. Safely reduce high MMP-9 with high-dose fish oil (EPA 2.4 grams/DHA 1.8 grams). The dose of fish oil is the same dosage discussed earlier in pre-medication for the CSM and MARCoN steps. Initiate a no-amylose diet, which excludes gluten, rice, bananas and all vegetables grown underground (except garlic and onions). TNF, PAI-1, leptin and VEGF may also normalize in this step.

Actos has been used along with an amylose-free diet to reduce MMP-9 in individuals with leptin over 7. There is concern over long-term Actos use regarding bladder cancer, making its use less appealing.

3.9 STEP 8: CORRECT VEGF

Action: Use high-dose fish oil (EPA 2.4 grams/DHA 1.8 grams) to increase low VEGF. VIP, when indicated in the protocol, will improve VEGF.
Goal: Normalize VEGF by raising a low VEGF or lowering a high VEGF.
Pediatric Concerns: 20 kg = 1/4 adult dose of EPA/DHA.

Correlate low VEGF with VO_2 max on pulmonary function testing. Abnormal VEGF frequently normalizes by the same means as MMP-9. Correcting VEGF will improve breathing, fatigue and cognition and reduce muscle cramping. Patients with low VEGF will have capillary hypoperfusion, which must be corrected. Use a program of daily graded exercise to optimize capillary perfusion.

3.10 STEP 9 CORRECT HIGH C3a

Action: Use a high-dose statin (like atorvastatin 80 mg) and pre-medicate with 10 days of Coenzyme Q10, 200 mg per day, and monitor patients on warfarin.
Goal: Reduce high C3a.

It is essential to do a complete metabolic panel with fasting glucose to monitor liver function and detect hyperglycemia. C3a rises within 12 hours of a tick bite with a bacterial membrane in those who develop Lyme disease. Look for infections and correlate with GENIE.

Proper antibiotic treatment for Lyme must take place for a month before addressing the reduction of C3a. Repeat labs after antibiotic treatment. Non-HLA-susceptible patients may obtain a resolution of C3a, C4a and VCS after antibiotics alone. No change in C3a and a rise in C4a 1 week after treatment indicates ongoing exposure to WDBs. A rise in C3a and C4a 1 month after treatment signifies active Lyme disease and the need for additional antibiotic treatment. The patient must be pre-medicated with Coenzyme Q10 for 10 days and then given a high-dose statin such as atorvastatin 80 mg to reduce C3a afterward. Alternatively, use red yeast rice 600 mg BID. Monitor liver enzymes after 1 month.

3.11 STEP 10: CORRECT HIGH C4a

Action: Use VIP to reduce high C4a.
Goal: Reduce high C4a.

One of the many things VIP corrects is high C4a. C4a tends to self-resolve as a patient completes the previous treatment steps and avoids re-exposure. The use of VIP is safe, fast-acting, and effective. If a patient meets the criteria and tolerates VIP, it is a great way to lower C4a.

3.12   STEP 11: REDUCE HIGH TGFβ-1

Action: Use VIP or losartan 25 mg BID to reduce TGFβ-1 and monitor blood pressure. Hypotension is a contraindication for losartan.
Goal: Reduce high TGFβ-1.
Pediatric Considerations: Losartan 0.6–0.7 mg/kg/day divided BID.

High TGFβ-1 causes several pathologic conditions. High TGFβ-1 and MMP-9 cause tissue remodeling by epithelial to mesenchymal transformation (EMT), including restrictive lung disease. EMT transforms a normal cell into one that is fibrotic and ineffective. Increased TGFβ-1 may occur in conditions like multiple sclerosis, tics, tremor and even a Parkinson-like illness. Autoimmune disorders like Crohn's disease and rheumatoid arthritis can respond favorably to reducing TGFβ-1. Nasal and vocal cord polyps may develop, but gastrointestinal polyps are not associated with high TGFβ-1. Either VIP or losartan can lower TGFβ-1. Before the advent of VIP, Procrit was used to correct C4a levels, but it is no longer the treatment of choice.

3.13   STEP 12: REPLACE LOW VIP

Action: Use VIP 50 µg QID supplementation after meeting all requirements. Higher or lower doses may be appropriate.
Goal: Normalize transcriptomics and NeuroQuant® and improve the patient's symptoms.

This 28–amino acid peptide is produced in the body and binds to 2 different VIP receptors. When given in the form of a nasal spray, VIP dilates blood vessels to improve circulation, reduces inflammation, heals the brain and corrects underlying gene expression abnormalities. We do not know of any other treatment that achieves the same results. Titrate VIP nasal spray for maximum clinical benefit.

Although we do not check VIP levels with labs, this is the last step of the protocol. Start VIP after the patient no longer experiences mold exposure, registers an ERMI of less than 2 and a HERTSMI of less than 11, Actinomycetes <15, has a negative VCS test, a negative MARCoNS test and a normal lipase, and signs a waiver to start.

Give the first dose of VIP in the office after a baseline TGFβ-1. Then, one spray of VIP is given, followed by a second TGFβ-1 test performed 15 minutes later. The TGFβ-1 should not rise.

If lipase rises at 30 days, the patient could develop pancreatitis. High lipase is a contraindication for VIP. Rising TGFβ-1 is associated with ongoing mold exposure. The doctor must check for rashes, changes in blood pressure, and improvements in breathing and cognition, which can occur within minutes. Consult with the patient every month to see progress, check lipase level and watch for side effects of headache, dizziness, syncope or abdominal pain. While patients are using VIP nasal spray, they must monitor their blood pressure and pulse daily. Monthly laboratory testing is required and should include at a minimum a complete blood count with differential, comprehensive metabolic panel, amylase and lipase.

VIP corrects many of the protocol steps and can normalize NeuroQuant® studies and transcriptomics. VIP can correct vitamin D, T regulatory cells, androgens, aromatase, MMP-9, VEGF, C4a, TGFβ-1 and of course, VIP levels. Treatment with VIP should also normalize PASP. It can also reduce extreme hypersensitivity to the inflammagens found in WDBs by normalizing MASP2. VIP can increase endorphin production and reduce symptoms of multiple chemical sensitivities (MCS) and chronic fatigue syndrome (CFS).

Hopkinton Drug ships VIP with an icepack, but VIP should not be frozen. The medication should be refrigerated and stored upright (placing it in a mug that will not tip over is a good idea). It can be stored for 90 days and diluted for those who need to titrate to the recommended dose. One full-strength bottle of 24 ml typically provides eight × 50 µg/spray per day for 1 month. Dose VIP

TABLE 3.1
Day and Dosing

Day	Dosing
1–2	1 spray AM
3–4	1 spray AM, PM
5–6	1 spray AM, late morning, pm
7–8	1 spray AM, late morning, late afternoon, PM
9–10	2 sprays AM, 1 spray late morning, late afternoon, and PM
11–12	2 sprays AM, 1 spray late morning and late afternoon, 2 sprays PM
13–14	2 sprays AM, and late morning, 1 spray late afternoon, 2 sprays PM
15–16	2 sprays AM, late morning, late afternoon, and PM

for 6 to 12 months, then taper down to low maintenance doses. Maintenance dose requirements can be less than once per day.

Dr. Scott McMahon has aptly outlined how VIP can help a variety of CIRS patients. VIP can help with unresolved fatigue, cognitive issues, multi-nuclear atrophy (including caudate atrophy), exercise intolerance, multiple chemical sensitivity, those not responding well, and those looking for maximal recovery. VIP is a potent anti-inflammatory peptide and neuroimmunoregulatory peptide, which can correct MARCoNS, PASP, capillary hypoperfusion (may even include helping ED), androgens, exercise tolerance, polyuria/nocturia, MMP-9, VEGF, C4a and TGF β-1. However, VIP must be done in the proper sequence to achieve maximum benefit.

For the sensitive patient, start VIP at 1:10 dilution (50 µg/ml = 5 µg/spray). Build to *eight sprays per day.* Perform two sprays in one nostril. Upon reaching day 16, if tolerated, switch to full-strength VIP 1:1 (500 µg/ml = 50 µg/spray). Then, titrate to *12 doses per day* in the form of three sprays QID.

Very sensitive patients may need to start with a 1:100 dilution (5 µg/ml and 0.5 µg/spray) (Table 3.1).

VIP treatment is the phase that induces the most profound corrections to the brain and the genome. Twelve doses daily × 6 months is the studied dose that demonstrates effectiveness in resolving CIRS. Repeat NeuroQuant® 6 months after beginning the full-dose regimen. Final check to verify stability off medications includes all labs and MRI with NeuroQuant®. Monitor patients''symptoms.

3.14   GRADED EXERCISE

Start an exercise regimen to increase the anaerobic threshold. The patient should work up to 15 minutes of cardiovascular exercise, 15 minutes of weights and 15 minutes of abdominal exercise performed daily. Slowly titrate as tolerated, and perform every day without exception.

3.15   RE-EXPOSURE TRIALS

A re-exposure trial can prove that the building in question caused the clinical symptoms. A requirement is that the patient has undergone adequate treatment. At that point, the medications are stopped for 3 days while baseline VCS and labs (C4a, MMP-9, TGF β-1, VEGF and factor VIII) are measured. The patient is re-exposed to the building for 8 hours at a time for three consecutive days. Labs are performed the morning of the first day before exposure and the next three mornings following exposure. C4a and TGF β-1 will increase on Day 1. VEGF will increase on Day 1 and fall by Day 3. Factor VIII decreases on Day 1 and normalizes by Day 3. Leptin increases, and VCS becomes abnormal on Day 2. By Day 3, vW antigen and ristocetin cofactor may drop, and bleeding can begin. On Day 3, MMP-9 increases as well. The patient should also record their symptoms. These labs follow a predictable pattern and can prove that a particular building is the cause of illness. The patient is then re-treated using the protocol to restore health.

BIBLIOGRAPHY

Bagnis, R., T. Kuberski, and S. Laugier. "Clinical Observations on 3,009 Cases of Ciguatera (Fish Poisoning) in the South Pacific." *The American Journal of Tropical Medicine and Hygiene*, vol. 28, no. 6, 1979, pp. 1067–1073. https://doi.org/10.4269/ajtmh.1979.28.1067.

Bartram, J., and I. Chorus. *Toxic Cyanobacteria in Water*. Geneva: World Health Organization, 1999. https://doi.org/10.1201/9781482295061.

Campbell, Andrew W., Jack D. Thrasher, Michael R. Gray, and Aristo Vojdani. "Mold and Mycotoxins: Effects on the Neurological and Immune Systems in Humans." *Advances in Applied Microbiology*, vol. 55, 2004, pp. 375–406. https://doi.org/10.1016/s0065-2164(04)55015-3.

Charlton, Bruce G., and I. Nicol Ferrier. "Hypothalamo-Pituitary-Adrenal Axis Abnormalities in Depression: A Review and a Model." *Psychological Medicine*, vol. 19, no. 2, 1989, pp. 331–336. https://doi.org/10.1017/s003329170001237x.

Delgado, M. "Vasoactive Intestinal Peptide: The Dendritic Cell -> Regulatory T Cell Axis." *Annals of the New York Academy of Sciences*, vol. 1070, no. 1, 2006, pp. 233–238. https://doi.org/10.1196/annals.1317.020.

Ehrhart-Bornstein, Monika, Joy P. Hinson, Stefan R. Bornstein, Werner A. Scherbaum, and Gavin P. Vinson. "Intraadrenal Interactions in the Regulation of Adrenocortical Steroidogenesis." *Endocrine Reviews*, vol. 19, no. 2, 1998, pp. 101–143. https://doi.org/10.1210/edrv.19.2.0326.

Gennaro, Renato, Tatjana Simonic, Armando Negri, Cristina Mottola, Camillo Secchi, Severino Ronchi, and Domenico Romeo. "C5a Fragment of Bovine Complement. Purification, Bioassays, Amino-Acid Sequence and Other Structural Studies." *European Journal of Biochemistry*, vol. 155, no. 1, 1986, pp. 77–86. https://doi.org/10.1111/j.1432-1033.1986.tb09460.x.

Habashi, J. P. "Losartan, an AT1 Antagonist, Prevents Aortic Aneurysm in a Mouse Model of Marfan Syndrome." *Science*, vol. 312, no. 5770, 2006, pp. 117–121. https://doi.org/10.1126/science.1124287.

Jessop, D. S. "Review: Central Non-Glucocorticoid Inhibitors of the Hypothalamo-Pituitary-Adrenal Axis." *Journal of Endocrinology*, vol. 160, no. 2, 1999, pp. 169–180. https://doi.org/10.1677/joe.0.1600169.

Kuhn, D. M., and M. A. Ghannoum. "Indoor Mold, Toxigenic Fungi, and Stachybotrys Chartarum: Infectious Disease Perspective." *Clinical Microbiology Reviews*, vol. 16, no. 1, 2003, pp. 144–172. https://doi.org/10.1128/cmr.16.1.144-172.2003.

Lin, K., and R. Shoemaker. "Inside Indoor Air Quality: Environmental Relative Moldiness Index (ERMI)." *Filtration News*, March 2007.

McMahon, Scott. "Implementing the Shoemaker Protocol." *Proceedings of When Data Matters*, 2020.

Metcalf, Lee N., Neil R. McGregor, and Timothy K. Roberts. "Membrane Damaging Toxins From Coagulase-Negative Staphylococcus Are Associated With Self-Reported Temporomandibular Disorder (TMD) in Patients With Chronic Fatigue Syndrome." *Journal of Chronic Fatigue Syndrome*, vol. 12, no. 3, 2004, pp. 25–43. https://doi.org/10.1300/j092v12n03_03.

Morris, J. Glenn. "Human Health Effects and Pfiesteria Exposure: A Synthesis of Available Clinical Data." *Environmental Health Perspectives*, vol. 109, suppl. 5, 2001, p. 787. https://doi.org/10.2307/3454928.

Nagase, Hideaki, and J. Frederick Woessner. "Matrix Metalloproteinases." *Journal of Biological Chemistry*, vol. 274, no. 31, 1999, pp. 21491–21494. https://doi.org/10.1074/jbc.274.31.21491.

Nigrovic, L. E., Amy D. Thompson, Andrew M. Fine, and Amir Kimia. "Clinical Predictors of Lyme Disease Among Children With a Peripheral Facial Palsy at an Emergency Department in a Lyme Disease-Endemic Area." *Pediatrics*, vol. 122, no. 5, 2008, pp. e1080–e1085. https://doi.org/10.1542/peds.2008-1273.

Ogata, R. T., P. A. Rosa, and N. E. Zepf. "Sequence of the Gene for Murine Complement Component C4." *Journal of Biological Chemistry*, vol. 264, no. 28, 1989, pp. 16565–16572. https://doi.org/10.1016/s0021-9258(19)84744-0.

Opdenakker. "MMP9 Functions as Regulator and Effector in Leukocyte Biology." *Journal of Leukocyte Biology*, June 2001.

Ross, David E., A. L. Ochs, J. M. Seabaugh, C. R. Shrader, and Alzheimer's Disease Neuroimaging Initiative. "Man Versus Machine: Comparison of Radiologists' Interpretations and NeuroQuant® Volumetric Analyses of Brain MRIs in Patients With Traumatic Brain Injury." *The Journal of Neuropsychiatry and Clinical Neurosciences*, vol. 25, no. 1, 2013, pp. 32–39. https://doi.org/10.1176/appi.neuropsych.11120377.

Ryan, James C., Qingzhong Wu, and Ritchie C. Shoemaker. "Transcriptomic Signatures in Whole Blood of Patients Who Acquire a Chronic Inflammatory Response Syndrome (CIRS) Following an Exposure to the Marine Toxin Ciguatoxin." *BMC Medical Genomics*, vol. 8, no. 1, 2015, pp. 1–12. https://doi.org/10.1186/s12920-015-0089-x.

Shoemaker, R. "Differential Association of HLADR Genotypes With Chronic Neurotoxin Mediated Illness: Possible Genetic Basis for Susceptibility." *American Journal of Tropical Medicine*, vol. 67, 2002, p. 160.

Shoemaker, R. "Presentation to the Indoor Air Quality Association." *Sequential Upregulation of Innate Immune Responses During Acute Acquisition of Illness in Patients Exposed to Water-Damaged Buildings*, October 2007.

Shoemaker, R. "Posure." *5th International Conference on Bioaerosols,* September 2003.

Shoemaker, R., and H. Hudnell. "5th International Conference on Bioaerosols." *Sick Building Syndrome in Water Damaged Buildings: Generalizations of the Chronic Biotoxin-Associated Illness Paradigm to Indoor Toxigenic-Fungi Exposure*, September 2003.

Shoemaker, R., and S. McMahon. "Policyholders of America Research Milani Committee Report on Diagnosis and Treatment of Chronic Inflammatory Response Syndrome Caused by Exposure to the Internal Environment of Water-Damaged Buildings." July 2010.

Shoemaker, R. C. "Defining Sick Building Syndrome in Adults and Children in a Case-Control Series as a Biotoxin-Associated Illness: Diagnosis, Treatment and Disorders of Innate Immune Response, MSH, Split Products of Complement IL-1B,IL-10, MMP-9, VEGF, Autoimmunity and HLADR." *American Journal of Tropical Hygiene and Health*, June 2005.

Shoemaker, Ritchie C. "Residential and Recreational Acquisition of Possible Estuary-Associated Syndrome: A New Approach to Successful Diagnosis and Treatment." *Environmental Health Perspectives*, vol. 109, suppl. 5, 2001, p. 791. https://doi.org/10.2307/3454929.

Shoemaker, Ritchie C. *Surviving Mold: Life in the Era of Dangerous Buildings*. Baltimore, MD: Otter Bay Books, LLC, 2010.

Shoemaker, Ritchie C., and Dennis E. House. "A Time-Series Study of Sick Building Syndrome: Chronic, Biotoxin-Associated Illness From Exposure to Water-Damaged Buildings." *Neurotoxicology and Teratology*, vol. 27, no. 1, 2005, pp. 29–46. https://doi.org/10.1016/j.ntt.2004.07.005.

Shoemaker, Ritchie C., and Dennis E. House. "Sick Building Syndrome (SBS) and Exposure to Water-Damaged Buildings: Time Series Study, Clinical Trial and Mechanisms." *Neurotoxicology and Teratology*, vol. 28, no. 5, 2006, pp. 573–588. https://doi.org/10.1016/j.ntt.2006.07.003.

Shoemaker, Ritchie C., Dennis House, and James C. Ryan. "Vasoactive Intestinal Polypeptide (VIP) Corrects Chronic Inflammatory Response Syndrome (CIRS) Acquired Following Exposure to Water-Damaged Buildings." *Health*, vol. 5, no. 3, 2013, pp. 396–401. https://doi.org/10.4236/health.2013.53053.

Shoemaker, Ritchie C., Patricia C. Giclas, Chris Crowder, Dennis House, and M. Michael Glovsky. "Complement Split Products C3a and C4a Are Early Markers of Acute Lyme Disease in Tick Bite Patients in the United States." *International Archives of Allergy and Immunology*, vol. 146, no. 3, 2008, pp. 255–261. https://doi.org/10.1159/000116362.

Shoemaker, Ritchie C., and Patti Schmidt. *Mold Warriors: Fighting Americas Hidden Health Threat*. Baltimore, MD: Gateway Press, 2007.

Swanson, David L., and Richard S. Vetter. "Bites of Brown Recluse Spiders and Suspected Necrotic Arachnidism." *New England Journal of Medicine*, vol. 352, no. 7, 2005, pp. 700–707. https://doi.org/10.1056/nejmra041184.

Tibbles, Carrie D., and Jonathan A. Edlow. "Does This Patient Have Erythema Migrans?" *JAMA*, vol. 297, no. 23, 2007, p. 2617. https://doi.org/10.1001/jama.297.23.2617.

Vesper, Stephen, Craig McKinstry, Richard Haugland, Larry Wymer, Karen Bradham, Peter Ashley, David Cox, Gary Dewalt, and Warren Friedman. "Development of an Environmental Relative Moldiness Index for US Homes." *Journal of Occupational & Environmental Medicine*, vol. 49, no. 8, 2007, pp. 829–833. https://doi.org/10.1097/jom.0b013e3181255e98.

4 Pediatric Chronic Inflammatory Response Syndrome

Scott W. McMahon

CONTENTS

4.1   INTRODUCTION

Pediatric medical care is terrifying to some practitioners. It is well known that children are not "small adults." Their physiology is different. Their medication dosing and side effect profiles can differ. Their compensatory mechanisms vary from those of their elders. Even within pediatrics, differing age groups show dissimilarities to each other.

All these and other diversities are true of pediatric CIRS (chronic inflammatory response syndrome). Perhaps the biggest difference is in the amount and type of medical research. While many mold-based illness studies have been performed on children, most have looked at allergy and asthma, and considerably fewer at CIRS specifically. There are far more CIRS studies published in adults. Fortunately, this author has evaluated roughly 900 children for CIRS and maintained a searchable database on each. As such, some of the data presented in this chapter is pending publication. Almost all of the unpublished data herein has been presented at international and peer-reviewed CIRS conferences.[1-4]

4.2   HISTORY

The same 37 diagnostic CIRS symptoms are used in children as in adults, but there are caveats. For instance, how does one elicit a history of unusual (neuropathic) pains or metallic taste from a 5-year-old? How would one detect easy confusability in a child just celebrating their third birthday? Can a 6-year-old distinguish vertigo from dizziness? Many adults cannot! Even if small children could, would they be able to articulate that distinction?

These questions point out two important differences between children and adults when reviewing the diagnostic symptom roster. First, some questions have to be reworded to allow a parent

DOI: 10.1201/b23304-5   **49** a reasonable opportunity to answer correctly. For an adult, regarding generalized weakness, one might ask if physical strength and/or endurance have changed over the previous few years. For a small child, asking if the patient has the same amount of strength and endurance as their playmates is more likely to generate a useful response. Questions about fatigue could be asked directly to those who are ten or older. Younger pediatric patients might display fatigue by "being a couch potato" or avoiding play in active games with their peers.

Secondly, some of the symptoms simply cannot be discerned, no matter how attuned the guardian is to their child's behaviors. It just is not possible to determine whether a 2-year-old has a metallic taste, ice pick pains or vertigo, for example. A CIRS diagnostic roster of symptoms specific for pediatrics could be established, but left untreated, children will develop all the same symptoms adults do. As such, no new scale has been created; rather, expectations have been adjusted.

Another observation is that even children with enough self-awareness to answer all symptom questions by themselves (usually by 10 years) have fewer symptoms, fewer symptom clusters and not as many body systems involved as teenagers and adults. Lower standards are set for youngsters for both consideration of possible CIRS and CIRS diagnostic criteria. Manifesting fewer symptoms presumably is related to less time with and less exposure to toxins, inflammagens and microbes found in water-damaged buildings (WDB), but no specific study has documented this in the literature. CIRS youths possessing one (or two) predisposing HLA haplotype(s) are born with such susceptibility. There is potential exposure even in utero, but it is also possible a child may not get their first WDB exposure until starting school, their first job or when they leave home for life in a college dormitory. Without exposure, CIRS will not develop. Patients with fewer exposures and less time in those exposures may be more difficult to diagnose as they are earlier in the continuum of disease and less likely to have a startling number of symptoms and accumulation of abnormal laboratory tests.

For all of these reasons, expectations are adjusted. Age group criteria have been created regarding when to consider CIRS and how to make the diagnosis. With the former, a child <8 years old with 5 of the 37 diagnostic symptoms would be highly suspect. In another youth, aged between 8 and 11 years, 8 positive symptoms would garner attention about a possible diagnosis. For children ≥11 years, somewhere around 13 symptoms would garner CIRS interest. A 12-year-old could have CIRS with 11 or 12 symptoms, as could an adult, particularly if the illness is nascent, but the likelihood is lower with fewer symptoms, as diagnostic criteria are actually based on symptom clusters and not the raw number of symptoms.

Children who meet the aforementioned symptom raw counts should have screening laboratory tests or a full complement of CIRS proteomic testing to establish diagnosis. Do not forget that children approximating 5–6 years or less may present with a single symptom, such as chronic headaches, recurrent abdominal distress, persistent fatigue or enduring myalgias often misdiagnosed as "growing pains." Here lies a golden opportunity to diagnose CIRS early, when treatment is simple and resolution of symptoms is often complete. Proteomic testing confirms or disproves the diagnosis easily. However, these complaints are often ignored or trivialized by pediatricians who are unaware of mold-based illnesses.

4.3 DIAGNOSTIC CRITERIA

Three peer-reviewed diagnostic methods have been published in the medical literature. Dr. Ritchie Shoemaker,[5] the discoverer of CIRS, developed a three-tiered case definition (CD) in 2006. He created it as a direct parallel from the Centers for Disease Control (CDC)'s CD regarding PEAS (Possible Estuarine-Associated Syndrome), the very first[6] CIRS discerned. In 2008, the U.S. GAO (Government Accountability Office) published their treatise on water damage in interior spaces[7] and contributed a three-tiered algorithm (CD) to determine causation of any mold-based illness. This CD exactly paralleled Shoemaker's diagnostic criteria published 2 years earlier.

For both the Shoemaker and GAO CDs, the first criterion to establish is that there is an indoor mold exposure. This is confirmed by any of the following three: presence of visible mold, presence of musty or mildewy odors, or commercial testing revealing amplified levels of mold inside the structure in question. One of the CDC's guidance documents indicates that if you can see the mold or smell the mold, then remediation is required,[8] and commercial testing is usually not needed. As a side note, an Environmental Protection Agency (EPA) guidance document suggests proper remediation requires donning the equivalent of a Hazmat suit and respiratory tract protection.[9] Do not assume the U.S. government is not aware of the mold problem!

The second criterion for both CDs is demonstrating the patient has (subjective) symptoms and (objective) signs consistent with what the proposed mold-based illness has been documented to show in the peer-reviewed animal or human medical literature. Shoemaker's group has published 31 peer-reviewed articles with many defining the 37 diagnostic symptoms, the 7 common physical exam findings and 10 diagnostic laboratory tests along with >10 other non-diagnostic biomarkers. The signs and symptoms of CIRS are well established in the peer-reviewed literature.

The final CD criterion is to show improvement with appropriate therapy. The first two steps in CIRS treatment are removal from (or remediation of) the offending exposure (typically one or more WDBs) and use of a binder, usually cholestyramine (CSM) or Welchol (colesevelam), though some use potentially weaker agents like clays, Chlorella, charcoal or nostrums sold as "detoxes." Showing significant improvement in symptoms after one or more of these interventions meets this criterion, as does improvement of abnormal laboratory tests. Careful evaluation of potential confounders is indicated. Illnesses that might confound the symptoms are rarely found in the pediatric age group. Further, the presence of abnormal laboratory tests showing disruptions in the innate immune system effectively rules out all potential confounders save those that demonstrate biologically produced toxins and inflammagens.

CDs are excellent at defining an illness; Meeting these criteria ensures one has CIRS to a very high degree of likelihood, approximating 100% (almost nothing in medicine is absolute). However, the CDs suffer from the drawback of the third criterion – establishing improvement with appropriate therapy. The first step toward healing requires moving out of or remediating the offending space. Sometimes, this step is not possible. Further, in day-to-day medical practice, diagnoses are rarely made *after* successful treatment. While evaluating the response to therapy is an important part of the differential diagnosis process, and therapeutic trials may be used for diagnostic purposes, few illnesses actually *require* a therapeutic trial to make the diagnosis. For this reason, an alternate means of making the diagnosis of CIRS was developed.

The third diagnostic approach[10] requires demonstrating ≥6 symptom clusters and ≥4 abnormal results of the 10 diagnostic lab tests in children <11 years. The method uses highly sensitive symptom clusters with highly specific abnormal laboratory tests to create a very effective tool for differentiating CIRS from other illnesses. These two criteria are combined, yielding the diagnosis of CIRS with an alpha error rate of 1.10 in 1,000,000 for small kids. Children ≥11 years, and adults, are diagnosed with at least 8 symptom clusters and at least 5 abnormal diagnostic labs with an alpha error rate of just under 1 in 5000 ($p = 1.94 \times 10^{-4}$).

There are other symptoms, in other body systems, that appear associated with CIRS but are not considered diagnostic. For instance, orthostatic hypotension is commonly found. A history of cold hands and/or feet is often elicited. Sleep issues such as difficulty falling off to slumber, frequent episodes of waking each night and non-restorative sleep are typical. Episodes of tachycardia, palpitations, anxiety and even panic attacks are common. In women, irregular menses, severe cramping pain with menses (so bad the patient does not want to get out of bed) and extremely large flow (menometrorrhagia, >10 pads a day) are often experienced. Other symptoms are noted but are not tracked. Anosmia, loss of taste and tinnitus are such symptoms of the special senses, whose frequency has not been calculated but which appear frequently. These "complete" the abnormalities of all five sensual senses, which include the diagnostic symptoms of skin sensitivity, neuropathic (unusual, burning) pains, metallic taste and photophobia/blurry vision. Diseases such as hypothyroidism and

Hashimoto's thyroiditis appear more frequently than in the general population. Symptoms related to histamine release are also commonly described.

Most diagnostic symptoms are more frequent in older age groups. A reporting bias exists in the very young, as they are unable to articulate some experiences. The frequency of most symptoms should increase due to the progressive nature of the illness. In other words, when one is born, there are likely no symptoms and no systems involved. (One might have symptoms as a newborn, as intrauterine involvement is a possibility, but this has yet to be documented.) Teens with CIRS will typically have problems in at least six body systems with at least eight symptom clusters. Adults have more symptoms and on average, more systems involved. Looking at the age groups of 0–4.9 years, 5–10.9 years, 11–18.9 years and ≥19 years, the average number of symptoms in untreated CIRS patients is 13.9, 17.9, 22.0 and 26.2, respectively.[3] Clearly, there is an increase in abnormalities with time, demonstrating the progressive nature of CIRS. The most probable reason is persisting and recurring exposure chronically affecting the innate immune system.

Diagnostic symptoms by age group are shown in Table 4.1.

4.4 PATHOPHYSIOLOGY

Before continuing the discussion of CIRS differences between adults and kids, it would be useful to survey the most likely pathophysiology. First, note CIRS can be triggered by several different exposures, including WDB,[11] Lyme disease,[12] cyanobacteria,[13] *Pfiesteria*[14] and *Ciguatera*.[15] The common cold is caused by numerous viruses, all acutely activating the immune system with the "side effects" of overproduced cytokines causing the common cold symptoms. Likewise, toxins, inflammagens and microbes from WDB, and the other CIRS-causing microbes listed above, elicit the symptoms of CIRS through chronically overproduced innate immune system cytokines and their actions.

The properly functioning immune system includes adaptive and innate components. The former consist primarily of antibodies with which one is born, like isohemagglutinins, and antibodies that are created after birth. The latter are fashioned after an exposure with complex interactions between T- and B-lymphocytes, antigen presentation cells and more. This system evolves and is called the adaptive, or acquired, immune system. Humans are born with their innate immune system, which includes physical barriers to invasion (skin, mucous membranes and more), cells (neutrophils, macrophages, lymphocytes, mast cells and natural killer cells, for example), chemicals (cytokines, chemokines, defensins and others) and receptors (pattern recognition receptors, or PRRs, of various types). The innate immune system serves to block infection, detect invasion of foreign particles once it occurs, eliminate invading organisms and activate the adaptive immune system. Effector mechanisms like phagocytosis, pinocytosis, antigen presentation, Complement, lysosomes, opsonization and more can be used by the innate and adaptive immune systems.

Should someone, with an active novel COVID-19 infection, cough or sneeze on someone who had never been exposed or immunized, hundreds or even thousands of viral particles could invade the latter's body through the mouth and nose. Defensive units on the mucosa of the entire respiratory tract monitor each landing particle, evaluating markers on each particle's surface indicating whether the particle is "self" or "foreign." Particles identified as self are not harassed. Some foreign particles may have already worked out a peace treaty, or so-called "tolerance," with the innate immune system and are tolerated. *Candida albicans* is an example. Other particles are deemed pathogenic. Markers are then placed on their surfaces indicating the need for destruction.

Since COVID-19 is a novel virus, scientists believe nobody, or very few people, has native antibody protection against it. As such, the innate immune system handles the fight alone using a variety of immunologic techniques. At the same time, the virus is replicating and trying to have its way. A figurative battle ensues, and it may take the human host several days, or several weeks, to get the upper hand. During this time, overproduction of pro-inflammatory cytokines and chemokines leads to various reactions of immune cells, and the results are the side effects of such interactions. Headaches, fevers, myalgias, chills, arthralgias and more are common. Communication between

TABLE 4.1
Average Percentage, by Age Group, of Each Symptom

Symptom	0–4.9 years	5–10.9 years	11–18.9 years	≥19 years
Fatigue	60.7	73.3	87.9	97.0
Weakness	39.3	49.2	76.4	93.5
Aches (Myalgias)	64.3	60.0	65.0	85.9
Cramps	10.7	25.0	56.1	68.4
Unusual pains	10.7	32.5	35.0	63.2
Ice pick pains	7.1	27.5	45.2	54.6
Lightning bolt pains	14.3	20.8	41.4	54.3
Headaches	60.7	71.7	84.1	80.4
Light sensitivity	60.7	63.3	70.7	84.2
Red eyes	42.9	38.3	40.8	54.3
Blurry vision	25.0	51.7	75.2	81.3
Tearing	14.3	41.7	62.4	60.7
Sinus problems	71.4	56.7	66.2	69.0
Cough	60.7	50.0	55.4	62.9
Shortness of breath	28.6	38.3	59.2	76.4
Abdominal pains	67.9	76.7	65.6	68.2
Diarrhea	50.0	33.3	29.9	45.4
Joint pains	35.7	37.5	57.3	81.5
Morning stiffness	17.9	20.8	39.5	67.0
Numbness	7.1	35.8	49.0	71.4
Tingling	7.1	29.2	51.6	71.4
Metallic taste	3.6	27.5	31.2	50.7
Vertigo	7.1	21.7	39.5	58.6
Memory loss	14.3	50.0	73.9	87.8
Focus/concentration issues	50.0	72.5	79.0	83.2
Easily confused	28.6	60.8	75.2	71.7
Difficult assimilation of new knowledge	17.9	52.5	54.8	67.7
Loss of word finding	50.0	62.5	81.5	89.4
Disorientation	3.6	18.3	39.5	48.0
Skin sensitivity	39.3	40.8	46.5	63.4
Excessive drinking	71.4	71.7	74.5	76.0
Excessive urination	75.0	65.0	57.3	84.1
Static shocking	25.0	40.0	41.0	58.3
Excessive sweating	57.1	50.8	54.8	68.3
Mood swings	67.9	85.8	84.1	82.3
Temperature dysregulation	57.1	56.7	70.1	83.7
Appetite swings	78.6	74.2	78.8	63.1
Tremors	0.0	30.0	62.6	62.5

Source: McMahon SW, Experience with the first six years, Oral presentation at: State of the Art CIRS III; October, 2016; Irvine CA.

Note: The average percentage of persons in each CIRS age group experiencing the indicated symptom before treatment.

T-lymphocytes and B-lymphocytes, via antigen presentation, leads to eventual antibody production, but it will be far too late for this fight. As the innate immune system wins the war, and viral particles are cleared, anti-inflammatory substances such as VIP (vasoactive intestinal polypeptide) and MSH (α-melanocyte stimulating hormone) are released to bring the state of the immune system out of "battle mode" and back into more of a "surveillance mode." Even after the infection has been defeated, the development of novel antibody continues for a season, then starts to wane, as all new antibodies do, at around 3 months out.

Should the same person be coughed or sneezed upon again, with the same COVID strain, 4 months later, the same process begins again. Invading viral particles are detected, markers are placed and the innate immune system revs up its war machine. However, circulating monoclonal antibodies specific for this virus's antigen(s), like snipers, take out the threat in a matter of hours instead of days or weeks. Additionally, as antigen is detected by the innate immune system and presented to B-cells, additional specific antibody is produced. If it has been a very long time since the initial infection, there may need to be a short period of ramping up of specific antibody production first, as natural immunity wanes significantly after about 3 months.

Five important concepts arise from this scenario. 1) These systems as described employ numerous cascades. Cascades, by definition, do not respond linearly, but geometrically. 2) The innate immune system is looking at markers with its PRRs, like TLRs (Toll-like receptors) and CLRs (C-type lectin receptors). TLRs sense a number of different microbial types by identifying PAMPs or the host's DAMPs (pattern-associated molecular patterns and danger-associated molecular patterns); CLRs sense sugar moieties commonly found on either bacteria or fungi. PRRs detect molecular patterns;[16] they do not determine whether the possessor of such a pattern is a living microbe bent on propagating or a chemical in the fragment of an old, dead microbe's cell wall. 3) If a PRR detects the molecular pattern (PAMP) of an offending organism, or a DAMP, the PRR activates the innate immune system regardless of whether the offender is an active microbe or the fragment of a microbe. 4) If there is no antigen presentation, if antigen presentation is defective or if the result of antigen presentation creates a subpar antibody (a permissive epitope), then the adaptive immune system's cavalry (antibody snipers) will not ride in and save the day. When this happens, and invasion of fragments or live microbes occurs, the innate immune system must handle the situation by itself. 5) Initial and prolonged activation of the innate immune system releases cytokines and triggers inflammation. If antibodies quell a response in hours, generated inflammation will be significantly less than if the innate immune system stops a perceived threat over days to weeks.

This background serves as a series of building blocks for understanding how CIRS is initiated. The countdown to CIRS begins in most people with a predisposition toward the illness found in the HLA DR region of chromosome 6. Looking specifically at the alleles found in HLA DRB1, HLA DQ and the presence or not of HLA DRB3, B4 or B5, a few haplotypes emerge as being found in >88% of persons[17] diagnosed with CIRS. In fact, these haplotypes are so frequent that they describe a relative risk >2.0 for developing CIRS over persons with "good" haplotypes. Three other allele combinations provide a lower, but still substantial, relative risk, such that only 1.2% of persons developing full-blown CIRS do not have at least one of these highest- or higher-risk haplotypes. Additionally, only around 25% of the normal population carries a high-risk haplotype. Put another way, 75% of the population carry two low-risk haplotypes and only 1.2% of CIRS patients carry two low-risk haplotypes. The undesirable haplotypes lead to faulty antigen presentation (no antibody) or production of permissive epitopes of the key antibody. Faulty antigen presentation, by itself, is not sufficient to develop CIRS.

Without exposure, no one acquires CIRS. Neither the presence nor absence of a predisposing haplotype confers CIRS. There MUST be one or more exposures. With Lyme, cyanobacteria, *Pfiesteria* and *Ciguatera*, the exposure can be one-time, or perhaps some portion of the exposing antigen persists in the host. With WDB, chronic exposure is the rule, with massive one-time exposures the exception. It is not yet clear whether the major offender comes from molds, bacteria,

Actinomycetes or some combination of two or three. Initial transcriptomics data suggests that bacterial endotoxin and *Actinomycetes* are involved in ~80% of CIRS cases and mycotoxins in around 7%. Further study and improved analytics in air and body fluids will eventually narrow down the specific culprits. Regardless of the microbe, the source is the WDB.

Most chronic exposures occur in the home, in the workplace or at school. Imagine spending 6–12 hours in a place, 4–7 days a week, where one has a sensitivity to a particular offending particle in the air. With every breath, this substance, or these substances, is (are) inhaled. The offending particles are much more common in WDB because water, along with the microbial food found in cellulose-containing building materials, allows amplification of numerous microbial strains. Molds, previously sporulated because of minimal access to the resources required to produce energy, now become metabolically active and thus reproduce by a factor of thousands and make secondary metabolic products, a.k.a., toxins. Bacteria and *Actinomycetes* undergo similar processes. As the offending substance is inhaled, antigenic particles will reach respiratory mucous membranes and trigger innate immune recognition. If the host has previously arranged tolerance conditions with this type of particle, all will be well. If the host has developed effective antibody against the invader, all will be well. However, if the host is one of the 25% of the population with a predisposing HLA haplotype, and is relegated to constantly respiring offending toxic and/or antigenic material, the innate immune system will kick in. Since defective antigen presentation insists on little, no or ineffective antibody, the innate immune system will handle the burden … every day of exposure … as long as exposures exist. In addition, some people will have multiple chronic exposures, such as a WDB home and workplace.

It was long thought that the innate immune system lacked a discernible memory. The Medical Arts now know that memory T cells exist, though their contribution, or potential lack thereof, in CIRS is unknown. Regardless, constant repeated exposures of antigenic material found in WDB in HLA-predisposed persons cause continual immune response. Across all age groups, over 68% of untreated CIRS patients have depressed levels of VIP, and ~93% have low MSH levels. These peptides work to suppress an overactive innate immune system, counterbalancing a chronic overproduction of cytokines. It is possible these values are low at birth, but unpublished data suggests they become elevated early in CIRS illness and then fall off later, likely coinciding with an increase in symptom number.

The low VIP and/or MSH levels in almost all CIRS patients also explain why removal from an offending environment does not effectively reverse the syndrome as, say, removal from exposure to cats in a feline allergic person might. VIP and MSH provide major down-regulatory influences on numerous pro-inflammatory cytokines. Lack of sufficient VIP and MSH means the immune system is not only "broken" but unable to adequately regulate itself. As such, proper treatment for CIRS patients requires more than simple removal, because the immune system damage has been done and leads to secondary damage. It is under these conditions, chronic exposure and inadequate circulating VIP and/or MSH, that CIRS cytokine storms prevail. More on these to follow.

In sum, a genetic predisposition sidelines adaptive immune response to chronic inhaled exposure to one or more amplified amounts of toxins, inflammagens and microbes found in WDB. Since exposure is daily, or nearly daily, and often occurs for many hours on each exposed day, the onslaught of antigen leads to near-constant activation of innate immune effector systems and chronic overproduction of cytokines, creating chronic low-level systemic inflammation by definition. Initially, VIP and MSH levels are sufficient to counter this inflammation; however, subsequent loss of circulating levels of these anti-inflammatory neuroimmunoregulatory peptides reduces the host's ability to suppress inflammation. The result is chronic low-level systemic inflammation even when removed from the offending WDB. Rheumatologic illnesses are commonly developed by production of autoantibodies. CRP (C-reactive protein) and ESR (erythrocyte sedimentation rate) are usually reliable markers of these inflammatory diseases. However, in CIRS patients, the inflammation stems from innate immune dysregulation, and elevations in CRP and ESR occur in only about 10% of patients. This is consistent with what is found in many viral infections.

Chronic, low-level inflammation causes symptoms over time and through a few known mechanisms. First, capillary hypoperfusion, due to cytokine effects or vascular congestion from WBC demargination, causes decreased perfusion at the capillary beds, especially in peripheral aspects. As such, cold hands and/or feet are seen frequently, with associated pains and even discoloration/cyanosis in some (which resolves with CIRS treatment). In presented but unpublished data, Shoemaker used magnetic resonance spectroscopy[18] to demonstrate capillary hypoperfusion in the CIRS patients' brains via increased lactic acid levels and altered glutamine/glutamate ratios. Reduced perfusion means less oxygen delivery, at any given time, and cells suffer from decreased ATP production via the Krebs cycle and the electron transport chain (ETC). Brain and other cells with insufficient energy are likely to underperform, leading to symptoms of "brain fog," hand pains, cramping, chronic fatigue and more. Capillary hypoperfusion may occur in the lungs too, limiting oxygen–CO_2 exchange, but a more likely explanation for the shortness of breath and dyspnea on exertion, seen even in children, is found with transient exercise-related rises of PASP (pulmonary artery systolic pressure), suggesting pulmonary hypertension, treatable with intranasal VIP.

In addition, transcriptomics studies and a recent metabolism publication[19] show "molecular hypometabolism" (MHM), first discovered by Dr. Jimmy Ryan and taught by Dr. Shoemaker. MHM is found in untreated CIRS patients and refers to a proliferative physiology where even in the presence of oxygen, aerobic glycolysis (the Warburg effect) is primarily used to generate cellular ATP. Per Shoemaker 2020,

> MHM is characterized by the suppression of ribosomal mRNA for both large and small subunits; suppression of mitoribosomal mRNA in both large and small subunits; and suppression of mRNA from nuclear-encoded mitochondrial genes including ATP synthases, electron transport chain genes (ETC), and translocases.

Each of these levels of down-regulation works to shunt cellular energy production to aerobic glycolysis rather than using the much more efficient Krebs cycle and ETC.

The effect is magnified when VDAC (voltage-dependent anion-selective channels) of the mitochondrial outer membrane are closed. Closure does not allow pyruvate to enter the mitochondria for use in the Krebs cycle and ETC. Some azoles, such as itraconazole, are known to close VDAC. Indiscriminate treatment with systemic antifungals, treating fungal *colonization*, worsens (or causes) proliferative physiology through this mechanism. Fungal nasal colonization has been demonstrated in nearly 98% of the general population. As such, systemic azoles should only be used in CIRS patients with documented infection and not merely with colonization.

Ryan hypothesized the reason for the shunt to MHM in untreated CIRS patients is likely due to the innate immune system sensing foreign antigenic particles and presuming an infecting invasion is occurring. Viral infections, in particular, take over cellular mechanisms and highjack them to produce viral products, allowing mass viral reproduction, lysis of the human cell and subsequent invasion of many other human cells with the new virions. The host's advantage when creating a metabolic slowdown is that minimizing available energy might eventually sacrifice the already doomed cell but would limit the virus's reproductive efforts, theoretically slowing the spread of new virions to many other cells. This delay tactic could allow the innate immune system adequate time to get the upper hand in the war by allowing the orchestrated process of apoptosis instead of unplanned cellular lysis and the release of newly produced virions. However, in CIRS, there is not an infection but rather, the presumption of attack (detection of toxic and/or antigenic material from microbial fragments) due to the presence of inhaled antigen. The immune system does not know the difference. If inhalation of antigen is chronic, this could be interpreted as an ongoing war (infection), and ongoing energy reduction could be a valuable strategy. If energy production reduction occurred in a large number of cells, this surely would have consequences for the host.

Another mechanism of host injury may come directly from toxic effects of mycotoxins. Some mycotoxins, such as T-2 toxin, macrocyclic trichothecenes, fumonisin B_1 and ochratoxin A, are known to be neuropathic[20] in rodents. Direct exposure to peripheral nerve cells could cause the host to suffer neuropathic pains and altered peripheral nervous symptoms such as numbness, tingling, abnormal skin sensations and other neurologic conditions. Neural autoantibodies and neurophysiologic abnormalities[21] have also been documented in persons exposed to WDB. Mycotoxins, bacterial endotoxins and other secondary metabolic products of amplified microbes found in WDB may have additional detrimental effects.

Blood–brain barrier (BBB) integrity is affected by numerous cytokines and inflammatory conditions.[22] These can cause disruptive BBB changes, where permeability is directly affected by creating BBB breaches, and non-disruptive changes, where the structural integrity of the BBB remains intact but permeabilities to some substances are altered, allowing access to the brain parenchyma for cytokines, toxins, cells and more.[20] Systemic inflammation, caused by overproduction of cytokines, can then spread to the parenchyma, conceivably triggering cognitive deficits and central nervous system symptoms such as vertigo and metallic taste. In addition, some areas of the brain are not covered by the BBB. These include the median eminence of the hypothalamus, the pineal gland, the area postrema and the posterior portion of the pituitary.[23] Systemic cytokine overproduction could affect these areas directly and without BBB deficiencies. Published NeuroQuant® (NQ) volumetric brain magnetic resonance imaging (MRI) data[24] show a pattern of structural brain damage that occurs in untreated CIRS patients. Forebrain parenchyma and cortical gray volumes are typically enlarged (probable microinterstitial edema), and caudate nucleus volumes are decreased (probable atrophy due to neuronal death or dendritic pruning). Treatment with the Shoemaker Protocol, not including intranasal VIP, has demonstrated a return to control values for the enlarged volumes.[25] Use of VIP, the final protocol step, has demonstrated improvement not only of depleted caudate volumes but of other gray matter nuclei[26] that were also atrophic on previous NQ.

Preliminary evaluation of teenaged NQ results shows enlarged caudates, even before other structures are affected, in unpublished and non-presented data. One possibility is that early inflammation, and microinterstitial edema, is more caudate specific. Subsequent damage leads to the same changes in the forebrain parenchyma and cortical gray. By this time, the caudate may be experiencing cell death or pruning from continued stresses of chronic inflammation, yielding the common pattern seen in untreated CIRS patients. As more time passes, caudate loss becomes greater, and cortical gray matter can atrophy. This hypothesis needs research support, preferably from biopsy samples and serial NQ studies. As a side note, the caudate nucleus is involved in mood, language acquisition, attention, motor planning and execution, romance, emotion, motivation and reward operations. Each of these functions can be impaired in CIRS.

Late-onset cortical gray atrophy is commonly noted in conjunction with enlargement of the superior lateral ventricles. Shoemaker has proposed "the vascular hypothesis of CIRS" based on the eminent work of Sidney Strickland. Abnormalities of von Willebrand's factor (vWF) profile and transcriptomic coagulation values are frequently seen in CIRS. In fact, CIRS patients are 300 times more likely to develop acquired vWF disease, or low levels of these factors, than the normal population. This author has seen three ~14-year-old girls with CIRS have menses lasting 30 days or longer. The first two did not come to medical attention until after 30 days of bleeding, and both required a blood transfusion. Menstruation in the third was stopped with progesterone. Abnormalities in vWF go in both directions, however, also setting the stage for clotting abnormalities. The vascular hypothesis of CIRS suggests that microemboli form as a result of clotting irregularities, and these occlude capillaries feeding small areas of brain parenchyma. Over time, these occlusions accumulate and lead to the atrophy seen in cortical gray, caudate and other gray matter nuclei. More supporting data are needed.

Tight junctions in the gut are MSH dependent, and most CIRS sufferers have depleted MSH levels. Elevated amounts of the cytokines transforming growth factor (TGF)-β1, matrix metalloproteinase (MMP)-9 and C4a, in concert with low levels of MSH, likely allow damage to these tight junctions. Multiple food sensitivities and allergies, bloating, pains and frequent diarrhea are often seen.

Finally, multiple hypothalamic-pituitary-end organ axis dysregulations are seen in CIRS. The brain takes inputs from around the body, and the hypothalamus takes inputs from around the brain. It also samples the blood to determine levels of cortisol, osmolality and other hormone measures. The hypothalamus integrates all this information and determines what the body needs in response. It is the primary organ of regulation. It monitors and modifies global settings like hunger/appetite, sleep cycles, body temperature and temperature perception. The hypothalamus sets the tone between the sympathetic and parasympathetic nervous systems affecting heart rate, stroke volume, blood pressure, vasoconstriction or dilation, respiratory rate, depth of respiration, pupillary diameter and every autonomic function in the body.

The hypothalamus also gives marching orders to the pituitary, which in turn, dictates the function of much of the endocrine system. Abnormalities of ADH (antidiuretic hormone) and osmolality are seen in >85% of untreated CIRS sufferers, leading to polyuria causing polydipsia, fluid imbalance, excessive thirst, static shocking, orthostatic hypotension and likely POTS (postural orthostatic tachycardia syndrome) in conjunction with dysautonomia. Just over half of untreated CIRS patients have abnormal ACTH/cortisol (adrenocorticotropic hormone) regulation leading to fatigue. Nearly 60% of adult women, and 80% of teens having passed menarche >18 months prior, have at least one of irregular menses, severe cramping with menses or menometrorrhagia, suggesting possible luteinizing hormone/follicle stimulating hormone (LH/FSH) dysfunction. MSH is low in 93.2% of adult patients (92.8% across all age groups) and is involved in multiple regulatory efforts including sleep, appetite and pituitary function. In unpublished data, hypothyroidism and Hashimoto's thyroiditis are significantly more common in CIRS patients than those without CIRS. No data have been gathered or presented regarding prolactin, growth hormone or oxytocin. The hypothalamus and/or pituitary appear to be under attack, most likely from neuroinflammation damaging hypothalamic structures or the portal system, which connects the hypothalamus to the pituitary. The median eminence (not protected by the BBB) is the central depot from which portal system trains depart. The posterior pituitary is also unprotected by the BBB. Brain biopsy information or other supporting data is needed to confirm this theory.

Every CIRS patient will have immune system dysfunction, evidenced by multiple immune system abnormal laboratory tests. Over 90% of CIRS patients will demonstrate endocrine system dysfunction, also documented by discrepant laboratory testing. Neurological damage, demonstrated by toxic encephalopathy, cognitive decline, cognitive changes and/or reproducible NQ abnormalities, also occurs in >90% of CIRS sufferers. These mechanisms of injury, taken as a whole, account for all of the CIRS diagnostic symptoms and many other non-diagnostic ones. These processes also explain the multisystem aspect and seemingly global effect of CIRS. However, cytokine storms also need to be discussed.

4.5 CYTOKINE STORMS AND CIRS OVERLAPS

The prototypical cytokine storm comes from sepsis. An overwhelming bacterial infection causes the innate immune system to throw everything it has at the source in an attempt to save the host. Acute and massive cytokine overproduction with concomitant side effects accompanies sepsis. Tremendous increases in vascular permeability, decreased perfusion, blood shunting, end organ failures, third spacing and paradoxical reactions like disseminated intravascular coagulation are frequent in septic shock. More people die from sepsis each year than from prostate cancer, breast cancer and HIV/AIDS combined.[27] One in three hospital deaths is caused by sepsis each year.[28] In the analogy to be presented, the cytokine storm of sepsis is like a Category 5 hurricane.

COVID-19 is the new player. In severe COVID disease, there is also an acute cytokine storm where floods of cytokines are released to overcome the infection. Side effects from the release are also apparent. Acute, but less potent, the cytokine storm of COVID-19 would be akin to an F5 tornado.

SIRS (systemic inflammatory response syndrome) is typically a non-infectious illness but otherwise phenotypically identical to sepsis. SIRS also causes a cytokine storm. Sepsis always is instigated by infection, which is most commonly bacterial but can be of fungal, viral or amoebic origin;

for example, SIRS can be set in motion by trauma, burns, pancreatitis and other etiologies.[29] The fact that sepsis and SIRS look the same suggests that the same, or similar, pathways are triggered.[25]

CIRS has long been compared to SIRS and is considered a chronic, rather than acute, form of SIRS. CIRS is a more plodding, non-infectious, dysregulation of the immune system that leads to chronic overproduction and release of cytokines. By definition, CIRS is a more chronic and less severe cytokine storm than SIRS. CIRS is like constant 60 MPH winds, 24 hours a day, 7 days a week.

A Category 5 hurricane is devastating with extremely high-velocity winds. An F5 tornado also destroys most everything in its path, though its wind speed may be considerably lower than that of the hurricane. CIRS, with its continuous gale force winds, does not cause immediate damage. However, the constant pelting of and stresses upon a structure will eventually cause some wear and tear, like a few roof shingles being torn off here and there. If the roof is not repaired (or the inflammation is not quelled), from that relatively minor injury comes secondary impairment, and given enough time, the structure will no longer be usable. This is an important concept to understand.

A recent understanding is that severe sepsis survivors also have sequelae. PSS,[30] or post-sepsis syndrome, affects up to half of survivors with sleep problems, cognitive difficulties, anxiety and panic issues, debilitating muscle and joint pains, concentration problems, depression and post-traumatic stress disorder. Many mechanisms are proposed, including increases in MMPs (like MMP-9) and BBB disruption.

Novel COVID-19 has been around for a couple of years, and reports about post-COVID syndrome (PCS) are flourishing. Symptoms include fatigue, dyspnea, chest pain, cough, arthralgias, myalgias, headache, chest pains and palpitations.[31] Considered more serious are also cognitive issues, rashes, olfactory and gustatory dysfunction, depression, anxiety and sleep impairments. Chronic renal, pulmonary and cardiac damage has also been noted.

The overlaps between symptoms of PSS and CIRS, and between PCS and CIRS, are astounding and should catch the readers' attention. Could these all be phenotypic variants of the same pathways triggered, albeit hyperacutely in severe sepsis, acutely in COVID and chronically in CIRS? No one will know for sure until this is studied, but … one pediatric survivor, known to this author, of H1N1 influenza severe sepsis has suffered fatigue, cognitive deficits, behavioral issues, lack of motivation, myalgias and stomach problems for years after illness. Another teen survivor of HSV severe sepsis had similar symptoms. Both were tested for CIRS biomarkers roughly 2 years after their recoveries and had sufficient abnormal tests to be diagnosed with CIRS. Intriguing. When comparing post-COVID survivors who developed PCS with those who did not develop PCS, the long-haulers were shown by transcriptomics to have molecular hypometabolism and exposure to *Actinomycetes*[32] (as seen in untreated CIRS patients), while the non-PCS group had neither. Post-viral illness typically involves proliferative physiology too.

Pediatric CIRS also overlaps with other illnesses. In 2009, Shoemaker et al. published a retrospective case control[33] looking at 163 children who met the diagnostic criteria of chronic fatigue syndrome (CFS/ME, now called SEID or systemic exertion intolerance disease) and 55 controls. The CFS diagnosis had no biomarker that could distinguish this diagnosis from controls, though symptoms clearly separated cases from controls. Shoemaker performed a CIRS symptom and biomarker analysis on each case and control and found that the 163 cases had CIRS laboratory test positive results and the 55 controls did not. The children who met the CFS diagnostic criteria also met the CIRS diagnostic criteria. The caveat was that the CIRS diagnosis has biomarkers and the CFS diagnosis did not. Hence, these children should have originally been diagnosed with CIRS.

In a study by McMahon et al., pending publication, 33 children meeting the strict diagnostic criteria of PANS (pediatric acute-onset neuropsychiatric syndrome) or the closely related PANDAS (pediatric autoimmune neuropsychiatric disorder associated with *Streptococcal* infections) were retrospectively evaluated by symptoms and CIRS laboratory biomarkers. All 33 children met the symptom and laboratory test diagnostic criteria of CIRS. Twelve had NQ brain MRIs showing the classic changes of CIRS and enlarged hippocampi typically found in PANS/PANDAS patients.[34] CIRS treatment was offered, demonstrating improvement in 94% of CIRS symptoms, 94% of overall

PANS/PANDAS symptoms and 75% of PANS/PANDAS neuropsychiatric symptoms. Again, the overlap is stunning and suggests that common pathways are involved. Other illnesses, and patients with most medically unexplained symptoms, also demonstrate CIRS abnormal biomarkers or outright qualify for a CIRS diagnosis.

4.6 DIFFERENCES BETWEEN CIRS IN ADULTS AND CHILDREN

Now that the foundation of pathophysiology has been laid, offering the reader a framework to digest, it is time to discuss differences between pediatric CIRS and adult CIRS cases. Symptoms were discussed earlier and tend to be fewer and less severe in younger patients. Seven physical exam findings are often seen in CIRS patients.[35] These include tremors, facial pallor, red sclerae, erythematous cheeks (similar to rosacea), weakness in the antigravity shoulder muscles in the dominant arm, cold hands and/or feet, and flexibility bordering on hyperflexibility. The exam can be difficult with young children as cooperation is often lacking. It may be impossible to perceive tremors, test for shoulder weakness and measure flexibility. In young and cooperative children, flexibility may be exaggerated, because of age, compared with adults.

Table 4.2 describes diagnostic laboratory testing variances by age group. Adults with CIRS average more abnormal laboratory tests than youngsters. VCS (visual contrast sensitivity) testing can be performed on children as young as 7 years, but significant cooperation is required. Nearly all 9-year-olds are up to the task. A prospective study measured pediatric norms in healthy children using the APT VCS tester.[36] These norms were found to be the same for children aged 7–18 years as for adults (the latter determined by the manufacturer).

Table 4.3 demonstrates treatment improvements by symptom in three different cohorts. VIP and MSH levels can still be low in children but are also frequently elevated, a finding rarely seen in adults and teens.

TABLE 4.2
Average Percentage Abnormal, by Age Group of CIRS Patients, of Each Test

Laboratory test[b]	0–4.9 years	5–10.9 years	11–18.9 years	≥19 years
HLA abnormals[c]	96.2	76.3	86.7	92.2
VIP	66.7	60.6	66.7	71.5
MSH	87.0	92.4	93.2	93.2
TGF-β1	65.2	69.0	73.2	79.8
MMP-9	31.8	26.3	38.0	68.1
C4a	50.0	57.6	63.9	73.5
ADH/osmolality[d]	57.1	54.4	80.1	87.9
ACTH/cortisol[e]	48.2	47.8	62.5	46.4
MARCoNS	66.7	68.8	67.7	73.1

[b] Average percentage of each listed abnormal diagnostic lab in untreated patients by age group and test.

[c] "Dreaded" (multisusceptible) or "Mold."

[d] Absolute high or low ADH or osmolality and dysregulated ADH with respect to simultaneously drawn osmolality.

[e] Absolute high or low ACTH or cortisol and dysregulated ACTH with respect to simultaneously drawn cortisol.

Source: McMahon SW, Experience with the first six years, Oral presentation at: State of the Art CIRS III; October, 2016; Irvine CA.

TABLE 4.3

Average Percentage Symptom Improvement, Three Cohorts, by Symptom

Symptom Improvement[a]	Shoemaker	McMahon[3] 2016	McMahon[4] 2020
Fatigue	50	80.6	68.0
Weakness	86	89.7	76.8
Aches	87	89.5	78.4
Cramps	91	90.2	84.5
Unusual pains	100	89.9	86.6
Ice pick pains	94	73.5	84.5
Lightning bolt pains	100	87.0	73.2
Headaches	56	81.6	77.3
Light sensitivity	90	85.3	88.7
Red eyes	100	87.6	76.3
Blurry vision	93	88.5	75.3
Tearing	100	87.5	76.3
Sinus problems	86	77.9	82.5
Cough	88	88.2	83.5
Shortness of breath		81	80.6
Abdominal pain	100	88.3	80.4
Diarrhea	87	87.5	84.5
Joint pains	75	87.8	81.4
Morning stiffness	100	88.9	70.1
Numbness	85	86.0	76.3
Tingling	86	83.2	76.3
Metallic taste	-	65.5	74.2
Vertigo	67	86.0	70.1
Memory loss	64	80.7	81.4
Focus/concentration issues	91	82.0	85.6
Easily confused	94	83.7	87.6
Difficult assimilation of new knowledge	94	80.0	87.6
Loss of word finding	94	85.2	77.3
Disorientation	100	82.1	59.8
Skin sensitivity	100	90.6	74.2
Excessive thirst	88	80.3	78.4
Excessive urination	100	62.3	81.4
Static shocking	100	86.5	90.7
Excessive sweating	–	53.4	79.4
Mood swings	79	81.6	96.9
Temperature dysregulation	72	83.0	89.6
Appetite swings	83	82.6	69.0

[a] Average percentage of symptom improvement after the first two steps of the Shoemaker Protocol in three data sets, listed by symptoms. One data set is from Dr. Shoemaker and the other two from different cohorts by Dr. McMahon.

Source: McMahon SW, Experience with the first six years, Oral presentation at: State of the Art CIRS III; October, 2016; Irvine CA.

As stated earlier, younger patients tend to have fewer symptoms and better, faster recovery. Management of the protocol can differ with children also. For instance, very young patients cannot tolerate the large blood draws needed for diagnostic tests all at one sitting. For children 2 years and younger, the blood testing may need to be broken into two separate draws at least a week apart. A phlebotomist with great skill is required to obtain pediatric samples. Also, since adults are more likely to develop "adult diseases," which could potentially confound, a much larger array of tests is usually performed on older patients. Children often have just the basic diagnostic labs drawn.

MARCoNS (multiply antibiotic resistant coagulase negative *Staphylococci*) are common in CIRS adults (>80% in some studies)[17] but far less common in children. MARCoNS testing is obtained by a deep nasal swab, much deeper than that performed for COVID testing, and is really quite obnoxious for patients even in skilled hands. This diagnostic test is not usually obtained at the initial visit in children aged <15 years but will be obtained later if the youth is not responding adequately to treatment.

Very young children may only possess symptoms in a single system, such as only headaches, only myalgias, only chronic fatigue or only recurring abdominal pains. If the standard pediatric evaluation and workup for these symptoms is negative, screening for CIRS should be the next step. This is accomplished with an HLA test, VIP and MSH levels, ADH/osmolality and ACTH/cortisol. If all tests are negative, CIRS is an unlikely diagnosis. If two or three tests are abnormal, CIRS is usually the correct diagnostic choice, and the rest of testing should be completed (TGF-β1, MMP-9, C3a and C4a, and anti-cardiolipin [ACLA]/anti-gliadin [AGA] antibodies). VEGF (vascular endothelial growth factor) levels are likely more useful in diagnosis than ACLA/AGA, as abnormalities occur much more often with VEGF, but VEGF as a diagnostic test has not been evaluated in the literature yet.

While the treatment protocols for both adult and pediatric CIRS center on the Shoemaker protocol,[37] implementation may vary because of age. The protocol hinges on removal from or proper correction of the offending WDB and use of a binder medication, such as CSM or colesevelam, for one to several months. The protocol then pivots based on presence or absence of MARCoNS and which biomarkers are still abnormal. A specific step in a specific order[38] is indicated for each persistently abnormal laboratory test. The final step, offered to some based on clinical indicators, is VIP intranasal spray. Some of the intermediate therapies include allopathic medicines typically used in adult populations, such as losartan. These medicines may have untoward side effects in small children. Monitoring of abnormal labs may be instituted, in lieu of medication, unless the particular laboratory abnormality is so excessive it demands a response. Careful dosing is used in these circumstances, with risks versus benefits detailed to parents. Written informed consent and assent documents are used if VIP dosing in children is considered.

4.7 PREVALENCE

CIRS prevalence has been determined in two pediatric studies but not yet in adults. One study[9] looked at all previously identified CIRS patients in a pediatric practice and divided by the total number of peds patients in the practice. The result was a prevalence of 7.01%. This is likely low, as the numerator included only patients already identified with CIRS. A second study[36] looked at 157 consecutive children presenting for well checks or sports physicals. A screen was given looking for multisystem illness. Five of the 157 had already been diagnosed with CIRS. Another 15 failed the multisystem illness screen, indicating symptoms in at least 3 systems. At the time of publication, 7 of the 15 had been worked up for CIRS, and all 7 had positive histories and sufficient abnormal diagnostic lab tests to achieve CIRS diagnosis. If the other eight were all negative for CIRS, the prevalence would have been 7.6%. If all of the other eight were diagnosed with CIRS, the prevalence of pediatric CIRS would have been 12.7%. A prevalence of at least 7.6% was reported. It is presumed that the true pediatric prevalence is higher, based on the methods by which these prevalences were determined. It is also likely that the adult prevalence is even higher, based on the progressive nature of CIRS. The ceiling for prevalence would lie around 25% – the frequency of abnormal haplotypes in the general population.

4.8 DOUBLES

Over 88% of CIRS patients have one or two predisposing haplotypes and all have exposure. Patients with "bad" haplotypes from both parents are referred to as "doubles." Doubles do not necessarily have worse disease, but they do tend to present at an earlier age. Unpublished data show 37.8% of CIRS adults are doubles, while 50.0% of CIRS children aged <5 years have two predisposing haplotypes.

4.9 CIRS IN UTERO

Taking this concept to the earliest of days, some consideration should be given to what happens in utero. Assume a stay-at-home mother is a double with a gestating baby, also a double, living in a WDB – what protections are available to the child? The placenta likely filters most mycotoxins, microbial fragments, cytokines and inflammatory cells. However, aflatoxins, fumonisin and deoxynivalenol are mycotoxins all known to cross[39] the placenta. Ochratoxin A also crosses[40] the human placenta. Fumonisin B1 and Ochratoxin A are known to be neurotoxic in rodents. Are standard half-lives of mycotoxin activity and LD_{50} doses the same in a developing fetus as in older humans? Would infiltration of these toxins cause an immune response in the fetus? Could prenatal exposure to neuropathic mycotoxins cause developmental problems or predispose to autism spectrum disorders? The answer to these questions are as yet unknown.

Interleukin-6 (IL-6) crosses the placenta,[41] whereas IL-1α and tumor necrosis factor-alpha (TNF-α) do not. TGFβ-1, MMP-9 and C4a all have roles in maintaining pregnancy, but it is not clear what happens with excess levels of these cytokines or if they cross the placenta. Elevated TGFβ-1 levels, especially in association with increased IL-6, cause naïve CD4[+] cells to differentiate into Th17 (autoimmune promoter) cells instead of T_{regs} (autoimmune suppressors) in adults. Could the same process be occurring in the fetus? If so, would this interfere with normal fetal development? Intelligence? Behavior? Miscarriage, premature birth or pre-eclampsia? Inflammatory cells,[42] such as neutrophils, T- and B-lymphocytes, macrophages, mast cells and to some degree, natural killer cells, aggregate in the placenta, guarding the interface between the chorion and the decidua basalis, but it is not clear that these cells infiltrate into the fetus. When one factors in consideration of differential gene activation of the fetus induced by cytokine exposure, the likelihood of inflammatory illness occurring before birth is even more likely. These answers are also not known, and more research is needed.

Levels of T_{reg} cells, also known as CD4[+]CD25[+] lymphocytes, are elevated in early (and throughout) pregnancy,[43] are low in women with recurrent miscarriages[44] and decrease around the time of delivery.[45] It is thought T_{reg} cells promote tolerance of the developing fetus. A decrease in T_{regs} may be a stimulus to facilitate labor. Untreated CIRS patients are known to have low levels of T_{reg} cells. This appears to be a mechanism whereby maternal CIRS may lead to miscarriage, premature birth, pre-eclampsia[46] and/or placental insufficiency. ACLA IgM antibodies also are more common in CIRS women with miscarriages (unpublished). More study is needed.

4.10 AUTISM AND SEVERE COGNITIVE DEFICITS

Severe cognitive delays can be seen in children with CIRS. In one case, a 4-year-old with average intelligence and behavior endured water damage and mold growth in her apartment in post-hurricane flooding. Within 6 months, she had significantly regressed in behavior and speech. She was diagnosed by a neuropsychologist as autistic and started in special education classes at her school. The child's mother reached out to this author, who after CIRS evaluation, started the child on CSM. Within 2 months, the young girl showed a marked change and near full return to her previous cognitive and behavioral state. She was re-examined by a neuropsychologist and declared autism free with only a mild speech delay. She was placed in mainstream classes and has continued there for the last 8 years.

Another case, contributed by Dr. Jodie Dashore (personal communication, November 5, 2020), creator of the BioNexus Approach, highlights cognitive and other improvements in a 4-year-old girl diagnosed with CIRS, autism, global developmental delays and other ailments. This clinical vignette demonstrates how complicated a pediatric presentation might be, and yet significant improvement is still possible.

Four year old patient diagnosed with Autism Spectrum Disorder (ASD), Task Specific Seizure Disorder, Primary Ciliary Dyskinesia, Microduplication of Chromosome 15 and Chronic Inflammatory Response Syndrome (CIRS) demonstrated significant cognitive, behavioral, gastro-intestinal, fine motor, gross motor, receptive and expressive language and academic progress using compounded herbal formulations, camel milk therapy, detoxification therapy, and other dietary supplements.

Betsy was born full term via C section to 37-year-old Erica (names changed for confidentiality) with a history of two miscarriages. According to her parents, around 2 years of age, Betsy had one episode of myoclonic seizure related to a fever spike after vaccination and soon after started exhibiting behavioral challenges like head banging and aggression, moderate delay in developmental milestones, severe eczema, numerousfood sensitivities, moderate constipation, gastro-intestinal distress, poor socialization, poor expressive and receptive language, and regression in her gross and fine motor skills. Betsy was diagnosed with ASD at 2.4 years of age. Betsy's parents obtained a religious exemption and she has not been vaccinated since then. Additionally, for a year they diligently adhered to the treatment regimen suggested by the neurodevelopmental physician which consisted of speech and language therapy along with sensory integration therapy and ABA sessions 3 to 4 times a week. Betsy's progress was minimal.

Erica also mentioned Betsy having had chronic sinus distress and "this constant little sniffle and cough that never seems to go away. It's like she's had a cold since she was 3 months old". At age 3 Betsy started mouth breathing that affected her sleep patterns with waking up every 3-4 hours. She was referred to a pulmonologist at Stanford Children's hospital and diagnosed with Primary Ciliary Dyskinesia. She was prescribed airway clearance therapy and nebulizer treatments with Acetylcysteine (1ml,10% solution) and levalbuterol (3ml) twice a day for 30 minutes each. Betsy also underwent a tonsillectomy along with adenoidectomy which was a traumatic experience for the whole family. They found a local naturopathic MAPS (Medical Academy of Pediatric Special Needs) practitioner and started with a gluten free, casein free diet. The practitioner also recommended a DAN protocol which consisted of Fish oil, GAPS diet, and vitamins. The parents saw some gastro-intestinal benefit but no other progress.

At age 3.5 years, still minimally verbal, Betsy had two episodes of petit mal seizures during sleep and was diagnosed with Task Specific Epilepsy. Her pediatrician ordered chromosome microarray test and Betsy was found to have microduplication of 15th chromosome which is related to autism. At that time Betsy had started displaying severe anxiety with previously well tolerated activities and on a daily basis for presumably no reason along with frequency of urination. The pediatrician suggested psychotropic medication and the family refused. Erica recalled that Betsy's anxiety had started a few weeks after a bathtub leak and having had mold issues with their basement in the past they proceeded with in-depth online research. They came across Dr Ritchie Shoemaker's body of work and Dr Jodie A. Dashore's various conference lectures about the CIRS and autism connection. Finally convinced they may have found the missing link, they decided to invest their time, effort and resources into a natural approach and contacted BioNexus Health and Dr. Jodie A. Dashore soon after. The family is Asian-American and Erica has a strong background in traditional Chinese medicine. Additionally, the parents felt a plant-based natural approach would be a gentler and better fit due to Betsy's persistent leaky gut, and other gastro-intestinal complaints. Betsy's pediatrician was brought into the loop and an initial consult with Dr Dashore was scheduled.

In January 2019, the initial appointment was a virtual consult via Zoom video conferencing. The appointment lasted approximately for 2.5 hours wherein a detailed medical, social, academic and environmental history was obtained. In collaboration with the pediatrician, additional testing was done that included urine, stool, and blood tests. Urine tests revealed high levels of Glyphosate (75th percentile), moderately high levels of industrial toxins like phthalates and organophosphates, (50th- to 60th percentile). The stool test revealed imbalanced flora Gamma streptococcus, Klebsiella pneumoniae and Citrobacter fruendii along with high levels of Lysozyme and secretory IgA. A hair minerals and toxic metals analysis revealed mercury at 65th percentile, arsenic at 45th percentile and low levels of magnesium.

The parents requested all four family members be tested for MARCoNS with microbiology labs deep nasal swab test. They all tested positive. Betsy tested positive for MARCoNS, large amount, resistant to four antibiotics.

All family members failed the VCS on the website www.survivingmold.com. Betsy was unable to perform the test.

Blood tests including the Shoemaker panel were attempted but due to Betsy's severe sensory challenges only a limited amount of blood was obtained for a few prioritized tests. Betsy's HLA-DR haplotype is 7-3-53 (Mold susceptible), VEGF 12 (low), TGF-beta-1 was 1059, ADH 1.2, osmolality 289, MSH 12 (low), MMP-9 was 774 (high), IgG subclasses 1-4 were all lower end of the reference ranges, Mycoplasma pneumoniae IgM 1178 (high), MTHFR – compound heterozygous for C677 and A1298 variants. Additionally, the Cunningham panel test for anti-neuronal antibodies for the diagnosis of PANS (pediatric autoimmune neuropsychiatric syndrome) revealed high levels of CaM kinase II, Anti-dopamine D2 antibodies and anti-lysoganglioside antibodies.

HERTSMI analyses [mold DNA PCR testing] scores for the two levels of the house were 10 [upper limit of normal] for the upper level and 18 [elevated] for the basement. The finished basement had a history of water damage and frank mold growth on a section of the wall from a refrigerator leak which was apparently "remediated" 7 years ago. The Berber carpet was not replaced and the basement has served as a play area for Betsy and her younger sister. The HVAC is located in the basement and the heating and cooling is one zone, central with gas heated forced hot air and regular central air conditioning. The laundry was also in the basement with a front-loading washer. Additionally, the girls' bedroom was a dormer extension. The double windows were located directly below the roofline without an overhang and no gutter had been installed. The window capping was rotted outside and the windowsill discolored on the inside.

A CIRS diagnosis was secured through history and several abnormal laboratory tests including a predisposing HLA. Treatment ensued, and the results, as follows, were nothing short of inspiring. Dr. Dashore continued:

Progress at 4 months follow up: Betsy's parents report all head banging, anger, and GI distress has been eliminated with regular well-formed bowel movements 1-2 times a day. Betsy's food sensitivities have greatly reduced and she sleeps well for 8 hours at a stretch. Her teachers report zero meltdowns, improved participation in group activities, improved receptive language and following directions, reduced tactile and auditory sensory challenges and much improved gross motor skills. Upon retesting, her MARCoNS have cleared as have her sister's and her parents' as well. They all passed the VCS test upon retesting.

Progress at 8 months follow up: Betsy's is talking in small sentences, she imitates television characters but uses the phrases appropriately, her anxiety and aggression have greatly reduced, she is affectionate towards her family members, plays with her sister, is able to complete her homework unassisted. Her school is considering mainstream classes for Betsy for gym, music and math. Her appetite is improved and she has gained 4 lbs in weight and half an inch in height. She is no longer a mouth breather and her frequency of urination is greatly reduced.

It is necessary to point out that "Betsy's" improvement in cognition, behavior, bowel function, development, anxiety and sensory challenges did not occur as a function of the child growing older. It was her treatment for CIRS, coordinated by Dr. Dashore, lifting the fog off Betsy's brain, that made all the difference. These two cases, many more of which could have been presented, highlight the extent to which CIRS can affect cognition in children already born. What can it do to a developing fetus's brain?

4.11 HEADACHES

The prevalence of chronic headaches in U.S. children from 4 to 18 years old is reported[47] at an astounding 17%. Assuming roughly 4 million American children are born per year leads to a staggering 10 million children with chronic headaches of all types. This includes migraines, tension headaches, cluster headaches (older children) and chronic daily headaches. While numerous pharmacologic agents are prescribed to treat, little is known about the cause of these headaches. Stress is often offered as an etiology. Unpublished data looking at 400 children with CIRS revealed that around 90% of pediatric patients with chronic headaches had sufficient symptoms and abnormal biomarkers to be diagnosed with CIRS. Prevalence in CIRS patients varied by age group, with 56.0% of children aged <5 years, 75.7% of kids aged 5–10.9 years and 80.8% of youth aged 11–18.9 years having chronic headaches. Appropriate CIRS therapy led to the eradication or significant diminution of severity and/or frequency of headaches in 92.1% of all CIRS children and 100% of children <11 years old. While more study and prospective trials are needed, this represents a potential breakthrough in the understanding of pediatric chronic headaches literally affecting millions.

4.12 FUNCTIONAL ABDOMINAL PAINS

One of the most common reasons for pediatric (and adult) visits to the primary care practitioner is recurrent abdominal discomfort. This presents with numerous faces, including frank pains, frequent nausea, recurring bloating, gas and distention, and the ever so common "I'm not hungry, Mom, my stomach hurts." After a month or so of these symptoms, an extensive workup at the pediatric office awaits. A thorough history excludes constipation, chronic diarrhea, travel, overeating, reflux, food allergies and more. A complete blood count (CBC) is performed to rule out anemia, leukemia and possible infection. ESR, CRP and even ANA (antinuclear antibody) are tested to eliminate potential inflammatory and rheumatologic causes. CMP (complete metabolic profile) screens the abdominal viscera. AGA tests for possible celiac disease. A normal *Helicobacter pylori* assay jettisons the diagnosis of peptic ulcer disease, and occasionally, upper gastrointestinal tract imaging will be performed. A negative UA (urinalysis) and culture reject possible urinary tract abnormalities.

When right upper quadrant pain made worse with eating fatty foods occurs, an abdominal ultrasound can remove gall bladder disease from the differential. Persistent left upper quadrant pain, pain that radiates to the back or splenomegaly may warrant amylase, lipase and Monospot assays. Food diaries and removal of dairy for a few days occasionally yield results. When all these tests are exhausted, all that is left is a visit to the pediatric gastroenterologist for endoscopy. This typically results in normal studies or the irritating "non-specific gastritis" or "non-specific colitis." Gut inflammation of unknown etiology!

These children (and adults) are commonly told their distress is functional – a nice word for "it's all in your head." Pediatric residents are taught this pain usually emanates from a primary gain or secondary gain the child desires. As such, there is no abdominal pathology (as indicated by all the normal tests), and while the children actually feel the pain, it is no more than a projection of the mind. This is the case for roughly 90% of children complaining of chronic abdominal pains. Indeed, 13.5%, or ~10 million U.S. children[48] 0–18 years old, suffer from chronic abdominal issues.

Enter the CIRS knowledgeable physician. Clearly, 90% of these 90% of children with so-called functional abdominal pain will have several abnormal CIRS biomarkers and qualify for the diagnosis. The prevalence of chronic abdominal issues in CIRS children is 63.2%. Treatment with 1–2 months of CSM (or even 2 weeks if <5 years old) will eradicate or significantly decrease abdominal discomforts that have lasted for months to years in 85.1% of these CIRS sufferers. Similar data exist for adults (90.3%). It is time for allopathic medicine to take another look at "functional" complaints and consider innate immune system dysregulation in the differential. Most medically unexplained symptoms (MUS)[49] are explained by CIRS, but that is of no value to a clinician or patient if the physician is not looking for CIRS. Indeed, it was predicted in 1999 that most, if not all, MUS were caused by a single illness.[50] This author believes CIRS is that illness.

4.13 CONCLUSIONS: THE FUTURE

CIRS is an incredibly common, frequently missed illness, which most physicians see every day in their office. It is easy to pick up in the pediatric setting and very easy to treat at younger ages. One must be looking for it, however. Additional studies to verify and extend understanding of pathology are needed. More studies should look at MUS, evaluating persons for CIRS as a possible cause. Medical education needs to be updated. Every physician needs to be aware of CIRS.

CIRS is also completely, totally, 100% preventable. Newborn screening programs are already in effect in every state looking for rare inborn errors of metabolism. Why not screen newborns for a much more frequently found illness – CIRS? Only an HLA-DR-DQ haplotype is needed. Why not incorporate screening MSH levels in kindergarten or non-invasive and inexpensive VCS testing in school on third- or fourth-graders? Then, providers, parents, schools and eventually, patients would be aware of the need to avoid WDB. Building science would change, maintenance practices could be encouraged, and a tremendous amount of human suffering would be eliminated, worldwide.

REFERENCES

1. McMahon SW. CIRS: Adults vs. Peds. Oral presentation at: Symposium on CIRS; October, 2014; Salisbury, MD.
2. McMahon SW. CIRS: Headaches and abdominal pains in children and adults. Oral presentation at: State of the Art CIRS II; November, 2015; Phoenix, AZ.
3. McMahon SW. Experience with the first six years. Oral presentation at: State of the Art CIRS III; October, 2016; Irvine CA.
4. McMahon SW. Research update: 10 years' data & more. Oral presentation at: When Data Matters; May, 2020; Virtual Mold Congress Conference.
5. Shoemaker R, Rash J, Simon E. Sick Building syndrome in water damaged buildings: Generalization of the chronic biotoxin associated illness paradigm to indoor toxigenic fungi. Bioaerosols, fungi, bacteria, mycotoxins and human health. Dr med Eckhardt Johanning MD editor, 2006.
6. Surveillance for possible estuary-associated syndrome – Six states, 199801999. *MMWR Weekly.* 2000;49(17):372–373.
7. GAO Report to the Chairman, Committee on Health, Education, Labor and Pensions, U.S. Senate, Indoor Mold. In: 2008.
8. Centers for Disease Control and Prevention. Basic facts about mold and dampness. MOLD. https://www.cdc.gov/mold/faqs.htm#:~:text=Mold%20growth%20can%20be%20removed,ammonia%20or%20other%20household%20cleaners. Accessed 11/10/2020.
9. United States Environmental Protection Agency. Mold course chapter 6: Containment and personal protective equipment (PPE). MOLD. https://www.epa.gov/mold/mold-course-chapter-6#:~:text=Use%20minimum%20PPE%20when%20cleaning,available%20in%20most%20hardware%20stores. Accessed 11/10/2020.
10. McMahon SW. An evaluation of alternate means to diagnose chronic inflammatory response syndrome and determine prevalence. *Medical Research Archives.* 2017;5(3):1–18.
11. Shoemaker R, House D, Ryan J. Vasoactive intestinal polypeptide (VIP) corrects chronic inflammatory response syndrome (CIRS) acquired following exposure to water-damaged buildings. *Health.* 2013;5(3):396–401.
12. Shoemaker R, Giclas P, Crowder C, House D. Complement split products C3a and C4a are early markers of acute Lyme disease in tick bite patients in the United States. *International Archives of Allergy Immunology.* 2008;146:255–261.
13. Shoemaker R, House D. Characterization of chronic human illness associated with exposure to cyanobacterial harmful algal blooms predominated by Microcystis. 2009 Cyanobacterial harmful algal blooms, p. 653.
14. Shoemaker R. Treatment of persistent Pfiesteria-human illness syndrome. *Maryland Medical Journal.* 1998;47:64–66.
15. Shoemaker R, House D, Ryan J. Defining the neurotoxin derived illness chronic ciguatera using markers of chronic systemic inflammatory disturbances: A case/control study. *Neurotoxicology Teratology.* 2010;32(6):633–639.
16. Chu H, Mazmanian SK. Innate immune recognition of the microbiota promotes host-microbial symbiosis. *Nature Immunology.* 2013;14(7):668–675.
17. Shoemaker, R. Differential association of HLA DR genotypes with chronic, neurotoxin mediated illness: Possible genetic basis for susceptibility. *American Journal of Tropical Medicine and Hygiene.* 2002;67(2):160.

18. Shoemaker R, Maizel M. Innate immunity, MR spectroscopy, HLA DR, TGF beta-1, VIP and capillary hypoperfusion define acute and chronic human illness acquired following exposure to water-damaged buildings. Oral presentation at: International Society of Indoor Air Quality and Climate Health Buildings Conference; September, 2009; Syracuse, New York.

19. Shoemaker RC. Metabolism, molecular hypometabolism and inflammation: Complications of proliferative physiology include metabolic acidosis, pulmonary hypertension, Treg cell deficiency, insulin resistance and neuronal injury. *Trends in Diabetes and Metabolism*. 2020;3:1–15.

20. Doi K, Uetsuka K. Mechanisms of mycotoxin-induced neurotoxicity through oxidative stress-associated pathways. *International Journal of Molecular Sciences*. 2011;12(8):5213–5237.

21. Campbell AW, Thrasher JD, Madison RA, Vojdani A, Gray MR, Johnson A. Neural autoantibodies and neurophysiologic abnormalities in patients exposed to molds in water-damaged buildings. *Archives of Environmental Health*. 2003;58(8):564–574.

22. Varatharaj A, Galea I. The blood-brain barrier in systemic inflammation. *Brain, Behavior and Immunity*. 2017;60:1–12.

23. Dash Pramod. Chapter 11: Blood brain barrier and cerebral metabolism. Department of Neurobiology and Anatomy, McGovern Medical School. https://nba.uth.tmc.edu/neuroscience/m/s4/chapter11.html. Updated 10/20/2020. Accessed 11/22/2020.

24. Shoemaker R, House D, Ryan J. Structural brain abnormalities in patients with inflammatory illness acquired following exposure to water damaged buildings: A volumetric MRI study using Neuroquant®. *Neurotoxicology Teratology*. 2014;45:18–26.

25. McMahon SW, Shoemaker RC, Ryan J. Reduction in forebrain parenchymal and cortical grey matter swelling across treatment groups in patients with inflammatory illness acquired following exposure to water-damaged buildings. *Journal of Neuroscience Clinical Research*. 2016;1:1.

26. Shoemaker RC, Katz D, Ackerley M, Rapaport S, McMahon SW, Berndston K, Ryan JC. Intranasal VIP safely restores volume to multiple grey matter nuclei in patients with CIRS. *Internal Medicine* Review. 2017;3(4):1–14.

27. The World Sepsis Day fact sheet. https://www.uclahealth.org/sepsis/workfiles/Materials-and-Resources/2017_WSD_FactSheet.pdf. Accessed 11/17/2020.

28. Rhee C, Jones TM, Hamad Y. Prevalence, underlying causes, and preventability of sepsis-associated mortality in US acute care hospitals. *JAMA Network Open*. 2019;2(2):e187571.

29. Boka K. What is the etiology of systemic inflammatory response syndrome (SIRS)? Medscape. https://www.medscape.com/answers/168943-41390/what-is-the-etiology-of-systemic-inflammatory-response-syndrome-sirs#:~:text=The%20etiology%20of%20systemic%20inflammatory%20response%20syndrome%20(SIRS)%20is%20broad,trauma%2C%20medications%2C%20and%20therapies. Updated 11/12/2020. Accessed 11/17/2020.

30. Post-sepsis syndrome. Sepsis alliance. https://www.sepsis.org/sepsis-basics/post-sepsis-syndrome/. Updated 6/16/2020. Accessed 11/17/2020.

31. Post-sepsis syndrome. The UK Sepsis Trust. https://sepsistrust.org/get-support/support-for-survivors/post-sepsis-syndrome/. Accessed 11/17/2020.

32. Shoemaker R, McMahon S, Heyman A, Lark D, van der Westhuizen M. Treatable metabolic and inflammatory abnormalities in post COVID syndrome (PCS) define the transcriptomic basis for persistent symptoms: Lessons from CIRS. *Medical Research Archives*. 2021;9(7):1–18.

33. Shoemaker R, Maizel M. Exposure to interior environments of water-damaged buildings causes a CFS-like illness in pediatric patients: A case/control study. *Bulletin of the IACFS*, January 2009.

34. Giedd J, Rapoport J, Garvey M, Perlmutter S, Swedo S. MRI assessment of children with obsessive-compulsive disorder or tics associated with streptococcal infection. *American Journal of Psychiatry*. 2000;157(2):281–283.

35. Shoemaker RC, Johnson K, Jim L, Berry Y, Dooley M, Ryan J, McMahon SW. Diagnostic process for chronic inflammatory response syndrome (CIRS): A consensus statement report of the consensus committee of surviving mold. *Internal Medicine* Review. 2018;5(4):1–47.

36. McMahon SW, Kundomal KA, Yangalasetty S. Pediatric norms for visual contrast sensitivity using an APT VCS tester. *Medical Research Archives*. 2017;5(5):1–9.

37. Shoemaker RC. What do I do? https://www.survivingmold.com/treatment. Accessed 11/14/2020.

38. Vosloo W. Steps of the Shoemaker Protocol for treating chronic inflammatory response syndrome acquired following exposure to water damaged buildings [CIRS-WDB]. https://www.survivingmold.com/docs/12_STEP_SHOEMAKER_PROTOCOL_FOR_CIRS.PDF. Accessed 11/14/2020.

39. Stoltzfus R. Mycotoxin exposure in pregnancy and birth outcomes in Zimbabwe. Exploratory/ Developmental Grants (R21) from NIEHS. Project #1R21ES023980-01A1. 2015. https://grantome.com /grant/NIH/R21-ES023980-01A1. Accessed 11/17/2020.

40. Malir F, Ostry V, Pfohl-Leszkowicz A, Novotna E. Ochratoxin A. Developmental and reproductive toxicity – An overview. *Birth Defects Research Part B Developmental and Reproductive Toxicology.* 2013;98(6):493–502.

41. Zaretsky MV, Alexander JM, Byrd W, Bawdon RE. Transfer of inflammatory cytokines across the placenta. *Obstetrics & Gynecology.* 2004;103(3):546–550.

42. Gomez-Lopez N, Guilbert LJ, Olson DM. Invasion of leukocytes into the fetal-maternal interface during pregnancy. *Journal of Leukocyte Biology.* 2010;88(4):625–633.

43. Sharma S. Natural killer cells and regulatory T cells in early pregnancy loss. *International Journal of Development Biology.* 2014;58:219–229.

44. Keller CC, Eikmans M, van der Hoorn, MP, Lashley L. Recurrent miscarriages and the association with regulatory T cells: A systematic review. *Journal of Reproductive Immunology.* 2020;139:103105.

45. Shima T, Sasaki Y, Itoh M, Nakashima A, Ishii N, Sugamura K, Saito S. Regulatory T cells are necessary for implantation of early pregnancy but not late pregnancy in allogenic mice. *Journal of Reproduction and Immunology.* 2010;85(2):121–129.

46. Tsuda S, Nakashima A, Shima T, Saito S. New paradigm in the role of regulatory T cells during pregnancy. *Frontiers in Immunology.* 2019;10:573.

47. Lateef TM, Merikangas KR, He J, Kalaydjian A, Khoromi S, Knight E, et al. Headache in a national sample of American children: Prevalence and comorbidity. *Journal of Child Neurology.* 2009;24(5):536–543.

48. Korterink JJ, Dierderen K, Benninga MA, Tabbers MM. Epidemiology of functional abdominal pain disorders: A meta-analysis. *PLoS One.* 2015;10(5):e0126982.

49. Edwards TM, Stern A, Clarke DD, Ivbijaro G, Kasney LM. The treatment of patients with medically unexplained symptoms in primary care: A review of the literature. *Mental Health Family Medicine.* 2010;7(4):209–221.

50. Wessely S, Nimnuan C, Sharpe M. Functional somatic syndromes: One or many. *Lancet.* 1999;354:936–939.

5 Mechanisms of Potential Central Nervous System Injury in Chronic Inflammatory Response Syndrome

April Vukelic

CONTENTS

DOI: 10.1201/b23304-6

5.1   INTRODUCTION

Chronic inflammatory response syndrome (CIRS) impacts multiple systems, causing multiple symptoms, and the central nervous system (CNS) demonstrates this dramatically. There are a host of diverse symptoms, which can imitate or contribute to several neurologic diseases. Because CIRS is both exceedingly common and vastly underdiagnosed, it is essential to describe and define its impact on the nervous system.

If 8 or more clusters out of 13 are present, there is a 95% certainty of CIRS. The accuracy jumps to 98.5% if the Visual Contrast Sensitivity test (VCS) screen is also positive.[1] The cluster categories are: General, musculoskeletal, eye, respiratory, gastrointestinal, cognitive, hypothalamic and neurologic. Many symptoms originate in the CNS.[1] It is imperative to be aware of neurologic manifestations in order to adequately screen and treat CIRS patients.

5.1.1   IMMUNE PRIVILEGE OF THE BRAIN

Historically, scientists thought the brain was "immune privileged" and not subject to inflammation in the way the rest of the body is. Recent advancements in the understanding and mechanisms of neuroinflammation have changed this paradigm. We now know the brain responds to inflammation and can promote inflammation. The brain shows inflammation by releasing proinflammatory cytokines, complement and prostaglandins, amyloid β(Aβ) formation, glial activation, edema and increased expression of adhesion molecules.

These issues are amplified with an insult to the blood–brain barrier (BBB).Interleukin (IL)-1 is released from activated glia and shows a decrease in glutamate release, upregulation of inducible nitric synthase (iNOS), modulated neuron response to glycine and mitochondrial DNA (MDNA), and enhanced gamma-aminobutyric acid (GABA) effects. There are notable effects on neuroendocrine, cardiovascular and sympathetic nervous systems.[2]

5.2   PHYSICAL FINDINGS

5.2.1   CIRS AND THE CRANIAL NERVES

Cranial nerves are technically part of the peripheral nervous system, but it is essential to discuss them to be complete. All cranial nerves, 1–12, can be affected by CIRS. CN9 and 11 have the weakest associations, primarily from case reports. There has been conjecture from research at Michigan State whether biotoxin exposure damages the olfactory nerve itself. Certainly, inhalation of biotoxins is a rapid and direct route to the olfactory nerve. It is unknown precisely how multiple chemical sensitivity relates to the olfactory nerve.[3] Olfactory dysfunction is also very common in patients with cognitive decline and dementia.[4] CN2 is directly affected, as evidenced by impaired VCS and blurred vision. Blurred vision is a common symptom on the CIRS roster. Common complaints are floaters, tearing issues, visual disturbances and dry eye symptoms. Lacrimal duct problems, which cause underproduction or overproduction of tears, can involve CN7.[5, 6] CN3, 4 and 6 can be associated with double vision, since they control extraocular movement.[7]

CN5 can be affected by multiple antibiotic-resistant coagulase-negative staphylococci (MARCoNS) and may lead to facial pain. Trigeminal neuralgia is rare in CIRS. Yearly tests for MARCoNS and looking for cavitations in root canals are necessary for CIRS patients. Ozone treatment and surgery can be beneficial for those with dental MARCoNS.[3] MARCoNS can also release polycyclic ethers through CN1 and further sicken the patient.[5] CN7 palsies are well known with Lyme but can occur in many CIRS patients. The author noticed facial nerve abnormalities in patients with mold exposure, which can wax and wane. One was so dramatic that the patient went to the emergency room, and a negative computed tomography (CT) ruled out a cerebrovascular accident (CVA).[1, 7]

A metallic taste is present in some patients with CIRS.[3] It can occur in all types of CIRS patients and has a basis in multiple cranial nerves. The metallic taste may be absent in cold drinks but become present as the beverage approaches room temperature.[5] Abnormalities in CN8 can produce acute vestibular neuronitis and unilateral sensorineural hearing loss.[5]

5.2.2 Seizures, Tics, Tremors and Fasciculations

Movement disorders can be harbingers of dreaded neurodegenerative illnesses and may be alarming. Tremors and fasciculations will frequently lead to extensive testing and neurology consults. However, it is unlikely the neurologist will look to increased transforming growth factor β-1 (TGFβ-1) as a factor in the presentation, even after ruling out more sinister causes. Seizures and unusual seizure-like presentations can occur with high TGFβ-1 and low vascular endothelial growth factor (VEGF), biomarkers associated with a leaky BBB. These seizures are less likely to be classic tonic-clonic seizures.[3, 8]

Tics, commonly seen in the face, are more common in CIRS patients than in controls.[3, 8, 9] Caudate abnormalities may correlate with tics.[3] Twitching can take the form of fine fibrillations or coarse fasciculations.[9, 10, 11] Resting tremors can also occur, but take care to distinguish a pill-rolling tremor, which should point the clinician to Parkinson's disease.[5]

5.2.3 Unique Neurological Manifestations of Ciguatera

Interestingly, the symptoms for all causes of CIRS are just about the same, no matter the cause of CIRS or geographic location. Notably, Ciguatera has some unique neurological characteristics in presentation, as it reverses the perception of hot and cold and causes paresthesias. Circumoral paresthesia is one such presentation.[1] The discomfort from the altered perception of hot and cold was also termed "cold allodynia."[12] Ciguatera, a low-molecular-weight ionophore, is typically bound to sodium channels on neural axons instead of circulating in the blood. Sodium floods the neuron, and potassium exits. Ciguatera has a low dissociation constant, which will lead to a more protracted course of excretion using cholestyramine (CSM) binding.[13]

5.2.4 NeuroQuant® Findings in CIRS

Dr. Scott McMahon's work with teenage patients with WDB-CIRS (CIRS from water-damaged buildings) typically demonstrates caudate enlargement early on, followed by atrophy. He believes the caudate nucleus is the first structure damaged by CIRS.[14] Enlargement in microscopic interstitial edema in the forebrain parenchyma and cortical grey areas occurs in CIRS patients with age-matched parameters. Post-Lyme syndrome shows putamen atrophy. Antifungals pose a threat in the form of grey matter atrophy seen on NeuroQuant® via disruption of microtubules.[5] Tubulin elevation on GENIE (Gene Expression: Inflammation Explained) can correlate with the dangers of azoles. Changes in platelet conformation further compromise blood flow to the brain.[15] Concomitant use of GENIE demonstrated that actinomycetes and endotoxins had a tremendous impact on transcriptomics and brain injury via metabolic and inflammatory bases. Coagulation markers on GENIE can show an increased risk of vascular dementia and microclots. Oxidation stress, tau phosphorylation and formation of amyloid β can occur and compound neuronal damage.[15] Once again, this points to evidence of proliferative physiology in the brain and the damage from this intersection of physiology.[5, 8, 11] Transcriptomics has been pivotal in identifying the source of illness, personalizing treatment and demonstrating recovery. VIP (vasoactive intestinal polypeptide) has been the only medication shown to reduce multinuclear atrophy of grey matter.

In the case of enlarged superior lateral ventricles, one must consider normal pressure hydrocephalus (NPH) and look at Evan's Index. A ratio of greater than 0.31 maximum width of both horns of the lateral ventricle to the inner table of the cranium indicates possible NPH.[16] Dr. Shoemaker has found post-traumatic stress disorder (PTSD) on NeuroQuant to be associated with a small amygdala. PTSD is an inflammatory condition that responds poorly to treatment with standard psychiatric interventions. On the other hand, PTSD can improve dramatically with VIP.[1, 17]

5.3 HYPOTHALAMIC ISSUES

5.3.1 Headaches

Headaches are a frequent complaint in both CIRS patients and the general population. Some patients no longer require daily medications from the neurologist when they implement the Shoemaker Protocol. All factors that produce musculoskeletal aches and pain in CIRS patients may also be present with headaches. These factors include capillary hypoperfusion and muscle cramping, which contribute to tension headaches. Patients may also describe "migraines" that last for days and result from dehydration and hypovolemia from antidiuretic hormone (ADH) dysregulation.[1] Falling melanocyte stimulating hormone (MSH) may also contribute to headaches.[1, 6] Additionally, CIRS patients may have increased sensitivity to bright lights and loud noises, which mimics migraines.[11, 18] Sinus problems may be a contributor as well, but a good history is essential, because "sinus" issues often tend to be overstated. Remarkably, Dr. Scott McMahon has found CIRS to be the most common cause of pediatric headaches.[5] Lyme meningitis could be an unusual cause of headaches. Facial palsy may also accompany these headaches.[1]

5.3.2 ADH Dysregulation

ADH is a hormone secreted from the hypothalamus. Falling ADH is frequently seen in CIRS patients and causes increased thirst, increased urination, increased sweating (especially in night sweats), neurally mediated hypotension, hypovolemia and increased static shocks. ADH and osmolality must be measured simultaneously to evaluate their relationship. ADH dysfunction occurs in over 60% of CIRS patients.[1] In addition, MSH, another hormone made in the hypothalamus, impacts ADH regulation.[6, 10]

5.3.3 POTS, Pre-Syncope and the Dangers of Steroid Use in CIRS Patients as It Relates to the HPA Axis

Anyone who has spent time in an emergency room can say the complaints of pre-syncope, syncope and dizziness are incredibly common, and the etiology is frequently unknown. Keeping CIRS in the differential diagnosis is essential. Dehydration and ADH dysregulation occur in patients with misdiagnosed postural orthostatic tachycardia syndrome (POTS). Damage to the hypothalamus can cause neurally mediated hypotension (NMH), a form of dysautonomia, which can produce lightheadedness and fatigue.[11] These patients become lightheaded when they stand up due to dehydration and increased pulmonary artery systolic pressure (PASP). Requesting a PASP on every stress echocardiogram is critical in diagnosing pulmonary hypertension. A rise of PASP following exercise by 8 mmHg or more is diagnostic for pulmonary hypertension, which may normalize with VIP. CIRS patients may experience dizziness or vertigo. The source of this dysregulation can be central, and certainly, hypovolemia can induce tachycardia and decreased blood pressure. Calling this phenomenon "POTS" fails to acknowledge the mechanism of reduced volume from ADH dysfunction, hypothalamic damage or the accompanying PASP. Patients may describe having "low blood sugar," which is actually low blood pressure. In these cases, patients should measure orthostatic blood pressures with an automated cuff and blood glucose levels when symptomatic. It is essential to look for hypermobility and increased TGFβ-1 because these patients frequently have the 11-3-52B HLA.[3, 5]

CIRS can cause lightheadedness, syncope and even head injuries from falls. When patients describe daily headaches or long-standing headaches and lightheadedness, it is crucial to take a good history of falls, syncope and concussions. Syncope is a diagnosis that prompts neurology and cardiology consults, and the patient may have a positive tilt-table test and receive a prescription for fludrocortisone.[5]

Fifty percent of CIRS patients with low MSH have adrenocorticotropic hormone (ACTH) and cortisol dysregulation. Hypothalamic-pituitary-adrenal (HPA) axis dysfunction from CIRS affects cortisol, ACTH and also androgens.[19] ACTH is released from the anterior pituitary and stimulates the production of cortisol from the adrenal cortex. ACTH is a melanocortin like MSH, and they both come from proopiomelanocortin.[3] ACTH can rise early in CIRS and then fall.[20] If there is an actual reduction of inflammation, cortisol should drop, and ACTH should be stable. A falling ACTH with unchanged cortisol levels signifies the need to taper the steroid because the steroid is causing further hormonal dysregulation. Consequently, failure to diagnose CIRS will result in a lack of improvement and failure to self-heal, and a potential worsening of the condition. Low cortisol and simultaneously suppressed ACTH are strong predictors of poor outcomes.[20] Consequently, one must first test for MSH and closely monitor cortisol and ACTH levels while the patient is on steroids.

5.3.4 Vertigo

Vertigo is a common complaint for both a primary care provider and a neurologist. One must be specific in defining the term, as many lightheaded people will report feeling "dizzy." Vertigo is either objective or subjective, with the room spinning or the patient spinning. CIRS patients can have unilateral neuronitis or vestibular neuronitis. Cranial nerves should also receive a good examination.[5] Checking ADH with osmolality and orthostatic blood pressures is in order.

5.3.5 Leptin Dysregulation and Weight Gain

Leptin is produced in the adipocytes and acts as a hormone and cytokine. As MSH falls, damage to leptin receptors causes leptin resistance and disruption at the gp-130 cytokine receptor. IL-6, IL-11 and IL-12 are some cytokines that compete for the leptin receptor due to similar conformation.[19] Leptin acts to create tumor necrosis factor-α (TNF-α), IL-1 and IL-6. Leptin receptors are in the arcuate nucleus of the hypothalamus. Leptin binding to healthy receptors causes the prohormone proopiomelanocortin (POMC) to stimulate the formation of endorphins, MSH and ACTH. Consequently, these crucial hormones are not released at normal levels when leptin resistance occurs, and leptin levels rise. Cytokines can obstruct leptin receptors, and the result is weight gain that is resistant to traditional methods of weight loss. The patient experiences fatigue, and the mitochondria starve for oxygen. Sugar is metabolized in the cytoplasm, producing 2 ATP and lactate and pyruvate, which are shunted to the mitochondria. Due to capillary hypoperfusion in the absence of oxygen, the cells cannot create the theoretical 36 ATP that should be present. Instead, the body burns glucose and glycogen stores, and it takes 2 days to replenish glycogen reserves. CIRS patients also frequently have appetite swings with low MSH, as outlined on the symptom roster. Measure baseline leptin levels at intake. One important reason to measure leptin is that rapid leptin reduction (by pioglitazone, for example) can reduce MSH dramatically. MSH must be monitored on pioglitazone.[3]

If the patient surpasses the anaerobic threshold and has leptin resistance from cytokine response, protein stores will be tapped in the form of alanine and glutamine instead of burning fatty stores. So, the patient can rapidly gain weight and burn through protein stores, which drive basal metabolism down. Lack of adiponectin contributes to this vicious cycle.[21] As a result of these changes in the CNS, the patient may have significant, otherwise unexplained weight gain with far-reaching implications for health.[1] In this way, the direct CNS assault can affect the rest of the body and feedback to further CNS damage.[6] Daily, timed, graded exercises help to increase adiponectin and increase oxygen delivery to patients with capillary hypoperfusion.[22]

Weight loss and muscle wasting is also a frequent occurrence. Male patients may report an inability to build muscle or suffer a weight loss that coincides with muscle atrophy. Physicians should rule out malignancies with unexplained or unintentional weight loss and address depression, too.

Interestingly, C-reactive protein, monocyte chemoattractant protein-1 (MCP-1), TNF-α and IL-1β were all elevated in obese Type 2 diabetics. Vascular injury, platelet dysfunction and a greater predisposition for clotting exist in this hyperglycemic state.[19] Obesity may increase the risk factor for clotting and contribute to cognitive decline. This is another example of how CIRS can damage the CNS in profound and complex ways. Recent insights from Dr. Shoemaker and Dr. Ryan have provided even more understanding of these coagulation and metabolic processes.

5.3.6 ANDROGEN DYSREGULATION

MSH regulates androgens, and its decline directly affects androgen levels.[10] Physicians see androgen dysregulation in 40% of patients with low MSH, and erectile dysfunction may occur. In yet another assault on normal physiology, low MSH causes aromatase upregulation, which may result in abnormal total testosterone, dehydroepiandrosterone sulfate and estradiol levels. One of the implications of altered androgens is the risk of atrophic or Type 2 Alzheimer's disease. A deficit in androgens is a risk factor for cognitive decline, as defined by Dr. Bredesen.

5.3.7 THE IMPORTANCE OF VIP AND THE ROLE OF VIP INTRANASAL SPRAY

VIP is another hormone produced in the hypothalamus that is frequently very low because it is severely affected by CIRS. Replacement VIP via nasal spray crosses the BBB. VIP is safe and effective in treating CIRS patients and has been vitally helpful for their recovery. VIP has neuromodulatory and immunomodulatory effects; it works by increasing cyclic AMP and endorphins. VIP decreases cytokines, C4a, matrix metallopeptidase 9 (MMP-9), TGFβ-1, mannan-associated serine protease (MASP2), aromatase (which in turn normalizes androgens) and PASP.[23] VIP also normalizes VEGF and vitamin D levels.

Intranasal VIP has been incredibly important for patients with pulmonary hypertension. Low VIP causes shortness of breath and pulmonary hypertension, contributing to decreased quality of life and deconditioning. Low VEGF can also contribute to shortness of breath and fatigue. VIP can improve low VEGF.[5]

VIP normalizes disturbances in clotting and bleeding, as in the correction of acquired von Willebrand's disease. VIP can normalize ADH and osmolality as well as ACTH and cortisol. VIP has also corrected eIF2. eIF2 abnormalities occur in patients with rheumatoid arthritis, systemic lupus erythematosus (SLE) and colonization of MARCoNS. The benefits of VIP are numerous and impressive. However, the need for the patient to avoid water-damaged buildings continues for life.[23]

Intranasal VIP is the only means to date to demonstrate an improvement of multinuclear atrophy. The Shoemaker Protocol prior to VIP demonstrated normalization in the forebrain parenchyma and cortical grey areas. The addition of VIP and reversal of multinuclear atrophy is a medical milestone. Significant improvements occur in the hippocampus, caudate, putamen, pallidum, thalamus and cerebellum. High-dose VIP increased hippocampal size by a remarkable 61.5%.[24] The implications for Alzheimer's disease are particularly promising.[24] Low-dose VIP improved amygdala volume especially well.[24]

VIP also appears to help normalize MASP2 inflammation through an unknown mechanism.[25] In some patients, ficolin-binding protein MASP2 creates a greater response to less and less exposure, a phenomenon Dr. Shoemaker calls "sicker, quicker." C4a will rise quickly and stay elevated until treatment.[9] VIP blunts C4a elevations and reduces symptoms from baseline.

VIP may even prevent joint damage and reduce pain. TGFβ-1 appears to have an important role in osteoarthritis, and VIP may have a direct benefit in this common and debilitating condition. Also, the normalization of TGFβ-1, VEGF and MMP-9 contributes to improved tendon healing.[12]

5.4 IMPLICATIONS FOR PAIN

MSH dysregulation happens in about 95% of patients with CIRS. MSH contributes to thermal dysregulation, sweats, muscle aches and difficulty with concentration.[1, 5, 19] MSH regulation also impacts the tight junctions of the gut and can result in food intolerances. MSH is an important hormone that promotes cAMP (cyclic adenosine monophosphate) and blocks nuclear factor κ β. MSH inhibits a number of cytokines: TNF-α, IL-1β, IL-6 and interferon (IFN)-γ. Injured intervertebral discs will release some of the same compounds observed in CIRS, namely IL-1β, IL-6 and TNF, which are all proinflammatory.[12] TNF-α may further interfere with perfusion via vasoconstriction or cytokine effect on blood vessels.[5] Falling MSH levels contribute to unusual pain in the CIRS patient, as endorphins also fall.[6] Some of these pains may be described as "icepick" or unusual skin sensitivity. TNF-α may contribute to capillary hypoperfusion via the recruitment of leukocytes.[10] With low MSH, MARCoNS colonization can be acquired, which may cause facial pain, as outlined by Drs. Roberts and Butts.[3] MARCoNS further degrade MSH by the production of exotoxins A and B. MARCoNS secrete hemolysins, produce biofilms and alter transcriptomics, and one must monitor for re-acquisition of MARCoNS.[5, 6]

MMP-9 is generated from macrophages and endothelial cells, contributing to a leaky BBB, inflammation and pain. The inflammation can occur in the brain, lungs, muscles, nerves and joints.[1, 6, 19, 26] No single marker causes any single symptom, but MMP-9 contributes to chronic pain and fatigue as muscles, joints and nerves are affected. We know MMP-9 rises after exposures, as VCS scores fall in rows D and E. Low VEGF can contribute to muscle cramps and cytokine release. MMP-9 may correlate with T1 imbalances.[27] High C4a levels also contribute to musculoskeletal issues, fatigue, capillary hypoperfusion and muscle cramps.

Peripheral neuropathy is a common symptom of CIRS, and patients frequently report numbness and tingling in the extremities, particularly fingers and toes, as listed in the symptom roster for CIRS. GENIE may demonstrate upregulation of the vanilloid series in patients with peripheral neuropathy and chronic pain.[5, 12] There is also evidence that thrombin is instrumental in the occurrence of diabetic neuropathy of the peripheral nervous system. Rat studies performed by Joab Chapman showed increased thrombin activity in the sciatic nerve of diabetic rats compared with controls.[28] This may indicate an interplay between coagulation, metabolism, inflammation and pain.[29]

Once again, patients with chronic pain may be put on steroids for back pain and headaches by those unfamiliar with CIRS without regard for the resulting dysregulation of cortisol production. Misdiagnosed CIRS patients with chronic pain may even receive unnecessary prescription pain medication.

5.5 PEDIATRIC ISSUES

5.5.1 LEARNING DISABILITY AND ADHD

Anecdotal cases of improvement in learning disability have resolved with an improvement of CIRS, but no statistically significant data exists. One such example is the Aiello legal case from

Michigan, which demonstrated in utero exposure, evidence of altered biomarkers and resolution of illness by treatment with CSM alone. It stands to reason that optimizing health and reducing dysfunctional inflammation is a good goal for these patients and anyone wishing to focus on brain health.[3] A small study in Poland correlated 6-year-old children living in homes with visible mold and a loss of 10 IQ points.[30]

Attention deficit hyperactivity disorder (ADHD) is a clinical diagnosis, and Dr. McMahon has noted that many children with ADHD will have their symptoms resolve as the inflammation of CIRS normalizes.[14] Once again, this organic dysregulation should be evaluated and treated before a psychiatric diagnosis.[3] Patients with ADHD and manic patients can demonstrate high glutamate to glutamine ratios on magnetic resonance (MR) spectroscopy.[31]

Before prescribing a controlled medication, screening children with learning difficulties with VCS, inflammatory biomarkers and environmental studies makes sense. It can be detrimental to send children to playrooms in "finished basements" or a basement nursery at church. How many children with treatable psychological conditions are adversely impacted by water-damaged buildings?

5.5.2 PANS/PANDAS AND OCD

Dr. Scott McMahon recounts an exceptional case where a child with seizures was diagnosed with pediatric acute-onset neuropsychiatric syndrome (PANS) and CIRS in *The Art and Science of CIRS*. PANS can manifest as serious behavioral changes which exhibit sudden and acute symptoms of the following: Obsessive-compulsive disorder (OCD), rage, psychotic reactions, mood and behavior changes, eating avoidance, facial tics and others. The symptoms may recur irregularly. These behaviors may lessen in intensity but do not disappear permanently and may exacerbate within only 2–3 days after the onset of another acute illness.[5]

PANS can occur after any illness, and pediatric autoimmune neuropsychiatric disorder associated with streptococcal infections (PANDAS) describes only Group A beta-hemolytic streptococcal infections. Dr. McMahon certainly sheds a different light on the ubiquitous pediatric illnesses like colds and strep throat, because some of these changes can be permanent and life-altering. Dr. McMahon references his exciting work in The Art and Science of CIRS Medicine, which describes 33 out of 33 children with PANS/PANDAS who each met the criteria for CIRS. CSM alone reduced 75% of neuropsychiatric symptoms and 94% of CIRS symptoms. The connection between CIRS and PANS/PANDAS and the resolution of symptoms is nothing less than revolutionary.[5]

In addition, Dr. McMahon has found that abdominal pain, headaches and growing pains are frequently caused by CIRS. He suggests screening for CIRS if a child has chronic fatigue, inattention after 6 years of age, or failure to "potty train" by 6 years.[14] The scope of CIRS continues to grow, and one can look forward to the day when every physician will readily recognize it, because these are treatable common complaints.[5]

5.6 MENTAL HEALTH CONSIDERATIONS

5.6.1 AUTOIMMUNE DISEASE AND MENTAL HEALTH

A study conducted in Denmark showed a 45% increase in mood disorders after an autoimmune diagnosis. Recent hospitalization for an infectious disease also conveyed a 62% increase in mood disorders. An autoimmune diagnosis and a recent hospitalization more than doubled the mood disorder risk.[32] This study is thought-provoking. Infections were associated with both unipolar depression and bipolar disorder.[33] We know severe illnesses like sepsis can produce lingering dysregulation in the innate immune system, coagulation and T-regulatory dysfunction (with Th1, Th2 and Th17) in the form of systemic inflammatory response syndrome (SIRS). As TGFβ-1 increases, CD4+CD25+ falls. IL-6 augments the decrease. As this occurs, naive T4 cells favor producing Th17 instead of T-regulatory cells.[14] Autoimmune disease, namely SLE, Type I diabetes and celiac disease, is more strongly associated with unipolar depression. Although not necessarily causal, the correlation between autoimmune disease and mood disorder raises questions regarding the connection between illness and mental health, particularly the T-regulatory dysfunction in CIRS that patients can correlate with autoimmunity. Interestingly, patients with schizophrenia have shown increased C4a.[34] It is standard of care to always look for organic illness before making a psychiatric diagnosis. Screening all patients with new-onset psychiatric disorders for CIRS would be a fascinating way to see what physiology we are missing.[18]

5.6.2 SLEEP DISTURBANCES

Sleep difficulties are a frequent complaint among CIRS patients, and the sleep they do get is typically non-restorative. In CIRS, MSH and melatonin levels fall, and the circadian rhythm is disrupted, which may lead to poor sleep quality.[5, 6, 10] Patients may complain of waking with "clawing" of the feet, "charley horses," night sweats, roving aches, and increased thirst and nocturia from ADH dysregulation.[1, 10] VIP dysregulation leads to a disturbance in the circadian rhythm. Additionally, as previously stated, cortisol is frequently dysregulated, and sleep quality deteriorates further: The combination of symptoms plus the stresses that accompany CIRS add up to poor sleep quality. Anecdotally, the author has noted that CIRS patients may not recall their dreams well and report violent or oppressive nightmares.

5.6.3 MOOD

Mood swings are also common and listed on the symptom roster. The combination of cognitive symptoms and fatigue with emotional dysregulation creates a very challenging situation for CIRS patients. They may have to change homes and jobs, alter their social lives drastically and part with many of their belongings. Dealing with CIRS calls for a high degree of order, organization and learning a great deal of challenging and expansive new information when the patient may feel least capable of it.[10] MSH has implications for mood disorders and mood swings. MMP-9 and TGFβ-1 can also contribute to increased BBB permeability and depression.[18] TGFβ-1 and C4a levels can rise minutes after exposure.[35] VEGF dysregulation may occur during periods of stress and depression.[36]

5.6.4 ANXIETY

Anxiety is an incredibly common, although non-specific, symptom that many face, and it is not part of the symptom roster. Many CIRS patients report anxiety and depression, which can be quite severe. Data from Dr. McMahon's 2016 CIRS lecture in Irvine cited that 32.9% of adults with CIRS had issues with anxiety.[14] There has been conjecture on whether or not caudate size is causative or at least, a factor in anxiety.[37] Part of increased anxiety may correlate with the excitotoxicity effects of inflammation.[18] Decreased VIP may contribute to anxiety and depression.[18]

5.6.5 SUICIDE

Suicide is the 14th largest cause of years of life lost according to the World Health Organization, 2014.[38] Suicide attempts outnumber completed suicide cases 10- to 20-fold. Suicidality is a major problem in patients with CIRS. Dr. Shoemaker cited an unpublished chart review that states 95% of CIRS patients had contemplated suicide.[37] Many CIRS patients are sick for years prior to diagnosis and are unaware of how that exposure worsens their illness and mental health. For example, a CIRS patient who is told they have fibromyalgia, and continues to live in a moldy home, is unlikely to recover. Patients can spend years and significant sums of money on treatments that do not work while suffering out-of-control inflammation and remaining undiagnosed. Recovery is no accident and requires a proper diagnosis and, step-wise, methodical interventions. Almost half of suicidal patients seek care from a mental health or primary care provider in the month preceding suicide.[38] Most psychiatrists, emergency room doctors and primary care physicians will overlook CIRS as a risk factor for suicide. The patients are reaching out but still dying.[38] A European study linked moldy homes with depression.[39] We should also be screening known CIRS patients carefully as a secondary prevention measure. Psychiatric treatment could accomplish much more through environmental exposure management, and the underlying inflammation decreases.[37]

Inflammation causes activation of the kynurenine pathway of tryptophan, which degrades tryptophan and creates quinolinic acid.[5] Quinolinic acid is an N-methyl-d-aspartate (NMDA) agonist, which increases excitatory glutamate uptake. Kynurenic acid is made in the astrocytes and is an antagonist at the NMDA receptors. Activated microglia produce quinolinic acid. This is an excitotoxin with neurotoxic and gliotoxic effects, has inflammatory properties and is associated with neuronal loss. Quinolinic acid may contribute to hippocampal loss seen in depression.[40] The cerebrospinal fluid (CSF) of patients who attempted suicide had quinolinic acid levels 300% higher than controls. High levels of quinolinic acid also correlate with the cytokine IL-6 and increased Suicide Intent Scale. Postmortem analysis demonstrates microglia activation and increases in IL-6.[40] Quinolinic acid levels in CSF in patients with prior suicide attempts fell in the 6 months following the attempt but were still increased by 150% in patients for 2 years following a suicide attempt. Quinolinic acid was also higher in violent suicide attempts.

Immunotherapy with cytokines can induce depression.[38] This is accepted widely, and psychological clearance for patients receiving interferon can be a prerequisite for treatment. Patients receiving interferon treatment who were previously healthy individuals and without a history of depression have had new-onset suicidal ideation within 1 month of interferon treatment. If it is established within the scientific community that a flood of cytokines can cause precipitous and severe depression, why are physicians overlooking the inflammatory response from CIRS patients with depression?[41]

In completed suicide cases, elevated quinolinic acid occurs in the cortical and subcortical regions of the brain, specifically in the subgenual anterior cingulate cortex and anterior midcingulate cortex. Increases in quinolinic acid also occur in Alzheimer's disease (AD), Parkinson's disease (PD) and Huntington's disease (HD).[18] A challenge of studying quinolinic acid lies in its 20-minute half-life in blood; hence the need to obtain levels via CSF.[38]

Small studies have shown decreased suicidality in patients with administration of the NMDA antagonist ketamine and may further our understanding of quinolinic acid's role in depression. Interestingly, ketamine has decreased suicidality within 40 minutes, and this may last 10 days.[38] This helps elucidate the role of the NMDA receptor in suicide. The NMDA antagonist kynurenic acid is neuroprotective and has anticonvulsant attributes.[42] However, too much kynurenic acid may cause cognitive issues and psychosis, as in the case of people with schizophrenia, who have 50–70% more kynurenic acid than controls. Low levels of CSF kynurenic acid correlated with more severe depressive symptoms and were reduced by 35% 2 years later in patients following a suicide attempt.[38, 42]

In a cohort of 51 individuals who attempted suicide, plasma VEGF levels were significantly lower than in controls. This study looked at IL1-α, IL 1-β, IL-2, IL-4, IL-6, IL-8, IL-10, IFN-γ, TNF-α, MCP-1, epidermal growth factor (EGF) and VEGF. Despite the psychiatric intervention, 14 of the 51 patients eventually committed suicide. The study lasted 13 years. VEGF levels were significantly lower in cases of completed suicide versus cases of attempted suicide. VEGF levels for completed suicides were 14.58 ± 6.03 pg/mL. Patients with the lowest VEGF made more suicide attempts. VEGF is frequently low in CIRS patients. Dr. Shoemaker cites VEGF levels of 31–86 pg/mL as normal. VEGF has a neurotrophic factor with roles in neuroprotection and neurogenesis that may protect the hippocampus in electroconvulsive treatment. Higher IL-6 correlates with low VEGF. Those with suicide attempts had a trend toward decreased IL-2 levels, but it did not correlate with suicide planning and intent. High IFN-γ also correlated with higher suicidal intent. Some studies suggest corticosteroids may also reduce VEGF, and that may be another reason for a CIRS patient to avoid oral steroid use.[28, 36]

The issue of having a serious illness that affects neurologic function is compounded by several factors, including not getting a timely diagnosis, not being treated appropriately and not recovering in a timely manner, financial difficulties due to treatment and lost productivity, lost homes and jobs, executive function difficulties, and the stress of not being understood by friends and family. The overall effect is that patients are frequently isolated, unwell and overwhelmed and have little social support. Universal screening for CIRS in the general population and all patients presenting with depression, anxiety and suicidal ideation would save lives. One can imagine a future where depressed patients at the primary care provider's office receive a VCS and symptom screening and instructions to obtain a Health Effects Roster of Type-Specific Formers of Mycotoxins and Inflammagens (HERTSMI) of their home and work.

5.7 NEURODEGENERATIVE ILLNESSES

5.7.1 Cyanobacteria and BMAA

Dr. Paul Cox has theorized that β-N-methylamino-L-alanine (BMAA) links to amyotrophic lateral sclerosis (ALS). An earlier hypothesis that fell out of favor was focused on cycad flour in the diet of the Chamorro people of Guam, causing neurodegeneration in the form of ALS/PDC (Parkinson's dementia complex).[43] The BMAA concentrates in seeds used to create flour.[1] This theory was amended to account for the much more concentrated Nostoc from the native diet of flying fox meat. The theorized mechanism revolved around the idea that BMAA could damage NADPH motor neurons by activating glutamate receptors α-amino-3-hydroxyl-5-methyl-4-isoxazole-propionate (AMPA) and NMDA. Dr. Cox further proposed that BMAA was mistaken for L-serine and incorporated into proteins, which caused the formation of hyperphosphorylated tau. Dr. Cox has promoted L-serine ingestion to counter the BMAA inclusion in proteins. Perhaps more compelling is that two replicated experiments with BMAA in vervet monkey feed for 140 days produced hyperphosphorylated tau and some (Aβ) deposits that were not present in controls.[43] Feeding the monkeys L-serine reduced reactive astroglia in the anterior horn of the lumbar spinal cord and neurofibrillary tangles in the upper motor neurons of the primary motor cortex.[44]

5.7.2 ALS and MMP-9

Dr. Christopher Henderson, professor of pathology at Columbia, said of MMP-9 and ALS at the moment of discovery that he was sure that MMP-9 was, at the minimum, the first marker they had for the vulnerable motor neurons in the current model of ALS. In a mouse model of ALS, MMP-9 in nerves leads to neurodegeneration. In genetically predisposed mice, genetic reduction of MMP-9 in MMP-9 knockout mice resulted in a 25% longer life and a delay in neuron loss. MMP-9 elevation occurs in AD, HD and PD.[45] This is not to say CIRS causes these illnesses, and an elevated MMP-9 alone is never diagnostic of CIRS, but one could make a case for targeted screening in those with neurological issues. If a patient has both CIRS and serious neurodegenerative illness, correcting the biomarkers and cellular dysfunction associated with CIRS will likely benefit the quality of life.

5.7.3 Parkinson's Disease and the Role of Thrombin

Thrombin acts on protease-activated receptors (PARs) and increases neuroinflammation. Increases in PAR1 have been seen in astrocytes in substantia nigra in Parkinson's patients. PAR1 occurs in neurons and astrocytes in the human hippocampus, cerebral cortex and striatum. PAR1 deficient animal studies demonstrate memory and learning issues associated with the hippocampus. Thrombin and activated PAR1 may induce seizures in rats.[46] Lower levels of thrombin appear to be protective in cases of PD.[47]

5.7.4 Gadolinium and Parkinson's Disease

Dr. Shoemaker presented a case study where a patient had magnetic resonance imaging (MRI) with gadolinium, resulting in skin thickening and symptoms of PD. The patient also had scleroderma-like esophageal dysmotility and abnormal lung diffusion capacity but no markers for scleroderma. The patient had increased TGFβ-1, which causes epithelial to mesenchymal transformation (EMT). Losartan successfully corrected TGFβ-1. The patient's symptoms of PD resolved.[48] Of note, anti-cardiolipin antibodies (ACLA) can be elevated in lupus and scleroderma and also in CIRS patients.[5]

5.7.5 Multiple Sclerosis, Thrombin and Hypercoagulability

The innate immune system and the presence of thrombin may impact multiple sclerosis (MS). MS patients have a higher risk of venous thromboembolism in the form of pulmonary embolism, deep vein thrombosis and stroke. Genomic studies found a higher vascular cell adhesion molecule (VCAM1) level, which thrombin may mediate. Hypoperfusion, disturbances in the BBB and increases in hypoxia-inducible factor (HIF) occur in MS.[49] Single-photon emission computerized tomography (SPECT), positron emission tomography (PET) and dynamic susceptibility contrast-enhanced MRI also demonstrate cerebral hypoperfusion. Dr. Tatiana Koudriavtseva posits that cerebral hypoperfusion, slowed blood flow and changes in hypoxia-inducible factors may contribute to hypercoagulability. Innate immune system activation and the coagulation system play a role in allergic encephalomyelitis (EAE). EAE shows increased brain protease nexin-1 and thrombin-antithrombin complexes. Damage to the BBB, fibrin and activated microglia have a role in the demyelination of rats with EAE. MS correlates with higher antiphospholipid antibodies, and the mechanism of injury may involve thrombotic processes. Neuromyelitis optica (NMO) coincides with greater anti-thrombin III activity and D-dimer levels, which confer thrombotic risk.[29, 50, 51] It could be fruitful to look at transcriptomics in patients with neurodegenerative illness and coagulation abnormalities.[29, 50, 51]

Increases in TGFβ-1 can be associated with gliosis.[9] Gliosis is a form of scarring indicative of inflammation; it is a non-specific finding seen more commonly in CIRS patients. Gliosis occurs in 45% of cases of CIRS and only 5% of controls. Gliosis also occurs in MS, and although we cannot point to CIRS as a cause of MS, the commonality of gliosis is interesting to note. Myoinositol is seen in MS yet not associated with CIRS cases on MR spectroscopy. A notable finding for CIRS patients on MR spectroscopy is a rise in lactate.[52, 53]

Dr. Strickland says gliosis, or white matter hyperintensities, demonstrates small vessel cerebrovascular disease, which includes microbleeds and microinfarcts, lack of BBB integrity, and hypoperfusion, and can result in hippocampal atrophy.[54]

5.7.6 Case Study of MS and CIRS from Dr. Shoemaker

Another fascinating case that Dr. Shoemaker presented is that of a teenage girl with a definitive MS diagnosis. The patient had oligoclonal bands in CSF and plaques on MRI. The patient started to go blind and received steroids. Her TGFβ-1 was over 40,000. The home underwent successful remediation. The patient improved dramatically on CSM alone, and TGFβ-1 dropped to under 3000. The lesions resolved on imaging. The family declined a confirmatory CSF sample.[52] High TGFβ-1 can contribute to MS-like symptoms.[9]

5.8 COGNITION AND ALZHEIMER'S DISEASE

5.8.1 Executive Function Difficulties in CIRS Patients

One of the most striking and troublesome ways CIRS expresses itself is through cognitive difficulties, especially in executive function. Difficulties with focus and short-term memory, dyscalculia, confusion, disorientation and problems with assimilation of new information are all hallmarks.

These cognitive issues occur in an astounding 90–95% of CIRS patients.[55] For example, patients who are normally high-functioning can experience alarming disorientation and difficulty navigating familiar routes; it is common for a patient history to include getting lost on the way to a doctor's appointment even after visiting the location for years. One common cognitive problem in CIRS patients is difficulty with word-finding, including very basic terms for household items and familiar terminology in their profession.[10] Patients also experience intrusive thoughts and may impulsively interrupt conversations as executive function wanes.[8] This constellation of executive function issues may at times bias a physician unfamiliar with the challenges of CIRS to dismiss the concerns of a CIRS patient.

5.8.2 Cognition, Hypoperfusion and the Blood–Brain Barrier

Frequently, "brain fog" describes the cognitive difficulties accompanying CIRS. The colloquial term "brain fog" is too general, innocuous-sounding and vague to convey the condition's profound, progressive and disabling potential. "Brain fog" does not even hint at the association with AD, as outlined by Dale Bredesen, MD. On the contrary, we find that "brain fog" is associated with nuclear atrophy, mitochondrial underperformance (due to anaerobic respiration) and cytokine release causing capillary hypoperfusion and reduced oxygen delivery.[12, 31] CIRS causes defects in gene regulation in glycolysis, as well as abnormalities in ribosomal and mitochondrial activity.[24] Glutamate (excitatory) to glutamine (inhibitory) ratios, as seen in MR spectroscopy, are typically depressed in patients with CIRS who exhibit cognitive challenges.[31] Lactate elevations and glutamate to glutamine ratio abnormalities can even correlate with Environmental Relative Moldiness Index (ERMI) scores and C4a levels in patients with low MSH.[31] Dr. Shoemaker states that elevated lactate and change of glutamate to glutamine ratios are more evidence of proliferative physiology and metabolic disturbance at work.[5] Dr. James Ryan has discovered molecular hypometabolism (MHM) in 80% of CIRS cases.

A dysfunctional BBB with high TGFβ-1, low VEGF and high MMP-9 leads to capillary hypoperfusion, disturbances in glycolysis, reactive microglia, reactive astrogliosis and worsening cognition.[8, 10, 11] Additionally, failure to eradicate MARCoNS will further reduce MSH and increase risk of brain atrophy.[6] MMP-9 and plasminogen activator inhibitor-1 (PAI-1) increase clot formation and arterial blockage, leading to atherosclerotic plaques and potential for rupture.[3]

TGFβ-1 may also cause pathologic hardening of arterial vessels, resulting in blockage.[56] Some of the inflammatory cytokines implicated in BBB permeability are IL-1, IL-6 and TNF.[18] Higher levels of TGFβ-1 occur in the CSF of Alzheimer's patients compared with controls. In a meta-analysis of 40 studies, higher levels of IL-6, TNF-α, IL-1β, IL-12, IL-18 and TGF-β may occur in the peripheral blood of patients with AD.[57]

High C4a and low VEGF are also associated with cognitive dysfunction and reduced oxygen delivery to the capillary beds, as verified on MR spectroscopy.[9, 58, 59] VEGF is frequently dysregulated in CIRS.[59] As HIF increases, VEGF and TGFβ-1 are released. VEGF promotes new vessel growth and vasodilation to increase perfusion. The resulting oxygen increase attempts to compensate for capillary hypoperfusion from cytokine release. The increase in VEGF is short-lived; it rises on day one and then falls by day three following a rise in TGFβ-1. Loss of VEGF may weaken the BBB and worsen cognition, because VEGF has neuroprotective properties.[1, 60, 61]

In Dr. Shoemaker's landmark paper in *Trends in Diabetes and Metabolism*, he ties together the genomic effects of CIRS, proliferative physiology (aerobic glycolysis) and disturbances in coagulation by noting that there is a commonality of complexity and an almost universal response of inflammation and coagulation genes, including the relationship of suppression of ribosomal mRNA production and nuclear-encoded mitochondrial genes to multiple characteristics of glucose metabolism (especially aerobic glycolysis).[56] Increased PASP happens in over 80% of patients with molecular hypometabolism and IRS (insulin receptor substrate) elevations. Closed voltage-dependent anion channels (VDAC) lead to increased lactic acid and metabolic acidosis. There is T-regulatory cell suppression. Common changes in the brain on NeuroQuant® include increased superior lateral ventricle size, grey matter nuclear atrophy and suppression of cortical grey, which result in cognitive impairment.[15]

This constellation of abnormalities caused by CIRS resembles those found following an acute, severe illness in the form of SIRS. Both SIRS and CIRS cause widespread damage in the forms of the immune response, coagulation and inflammation. The disruption of cellular function is more far-reaching and complexly intertwined than most could have imagined. Dr. Shoemaker and Dr. Ryan's visionary work made these unifying connections.

5.8.3 Dr. Heyman's Neurodegenerative Model of Hypercortisolism

Dr. Andy Heyman states that the hippocampus has the greatest density of cortisol receptors in the brain. He observes that at first, there is swelling of the hippocampus due to increased (and chronic) cortisol activity, a condition common in the early stages of CIRS. The hippocampus and hypothalamus are adjacent and functionally connected, and we recognize frequent hypothalamic dysregulation in CIRS. Catabolic activity from increased cortisol inside the hippocampus eventually causes atrophy. Impaired HPA axis feedback results in further dysregulation of inflammation.[27] Cortisol levels may subsequently plummet, which is common as CIRS progresses.[27]

5.8.4 Bredesen Classification

AD affects more than 5 million Americans right now. Forty-five million Americans currently alive, or 15% of the population, will develop AD during their lives, and the frequency is increasing. AD costs the US economy $300 billion per year and causes untold human suffering. AD is cruel and relentless. The work of Dr. Bredesen and Dr. Shoemaker has been instrumental in providing a framework of hope for this population.[62] Dr. Bredesen states that amyloid β (Aβ) is part of the innate immune system, and the role of the innate immune system is crucial in the treatment of AD.

Dr. Bredesen cites AD as the third largest cause of death in America, and Type 3 Toxic (mold is the most common cause) accounts for 20% of Alzheimer's cases as the primary subtype. Even more startlingly, Dr. Bredesen has found Toxic contributors such as mold to be a factor in 60% of AD cases.[62] Subjective cognitive decline can occur a decade or more before AD is diagnosed. It is alarming that susceptible individuals exposed to water-damaged buildings for years or decades may be dismissing this preventable progressive decline as "brain fog." Implementing Dr. Shoemaker's work in every doctor's office and hospital in America may prevent illness progression.

Dr. Bredesen finds his average Type 3 Toxic subtype patients are typically younger than 65. On average, these patients are about 52\years old (it can occur in people as young as in their 40s), are more likely to be ApoE4 negative and typically have a negative family history of AD. He has found this subtype to be more difficult to treat than other Alzheimer's subtypes. Dr. Bredesen supports Dr. Shoemaker's idea that executive function is severely affected by CIRS. Dyscalculia, word-finding issues, tangential speech and poor fluency, co-morbid depression, low triglycerides and low zinc are typically present, according to Dr. Bredesen. He says the poor organization is a hallmark, as opposed to amnesia. Dr. Bredesen says he can often predict which patients are Type 3 from the quality of the phone conversations. For example, the physician might notice frequent interruptions, word-recollection issues and loss of focus in Type 3 patients with CIRS. When a family member with shared genetics and/or environment calls on behalf of a loved one, the conversation often leads to a screening and eventual discovery of CIRS in the "healthy" relative. Dr. Bredesen also remarks that Type 3 patients cope poorly with stress and travel, and have a non-restorative sleep, common in CIRS patients. These frontal lobe abnormalities resemble Lewy body disease more closely than other forms of dementia.[62]

Interestingly, CIRS itself can contribute to every type of AD outlined by Dr. Bredesen. AD correlates with atherosclerosis, hypertension, dyslipidemia, diabetes mellitus, CVAs, atrial fibrillation, factor V Leiden mutation, elevated D-dimer and increased homocysteine.[48, 63] Type 1 is Inflammatory, and there can be increases in IL-6, IL-8 and TNF-α. Type 1.5 is Glycotoxic, and CIRS may exacerbate leptin resistance, low adiponectin levels and protein wasting (which affects basal metabolic rate). The result is aberrations in weight and metabolism.[22, 64] Falling cortisol, androgens and hormonal dysregulation could correlate with Type 2 or Atrophic AD. Type 3, or Toxic Alzheimer's, is the subtype most associated with CIRS, and rigorous application of the Shoemaker Protocol is essential for recovery. Type 4 is Vascular and dovetails nicely with Dr. Strickland's work on the vascular theory of dementia. There is even a link to Type 5 or Traumatic cases through ADH dysregulation and low blood pressure, which may lead to falls and subsequent head trauma. Concussions are a hidden danger in CIRS that may contribute to future cognitive issues, as described by Dr. Bredesen as a Type 5 subtype of AD. They do not all apply to every patient, but the diagnosis and scope of CIRS, as it relates to the Bredesen Protocol, should be considered in each patient treated for cognitive decline.

5.8.5 Dr. Strickland's Vascular Theory of Dementia

The potential role of CIRS in AD is a fascinating one. Treatment of CIRS may unlock part of this complex and dreaded disease. Pathological changes in AD include amyloid β(Aβ) peptide plaques, tau tangles, neuroinflammation, cerebral amyloid angiopathy (A β deposition on vessel wall), vessel lumen narrowing, damage to the microvasculature, white matter lesions, ischemia, subcortical infarcts and neural loss resulting in gross atrophy.[17, 65, 66] Early on, microglial activation, which may help clear plaques, eventually becomes counter-productive with increased inflammation.[65] PAI-1 may increase in AD patients.[65] Coagulation factor XIIIa cross-linking may cause Aβ peptide deposits in the vascular lumen and contribute to clotting and cerebral amyloid angiopathy (CAA) (Figure 5.1).[67]

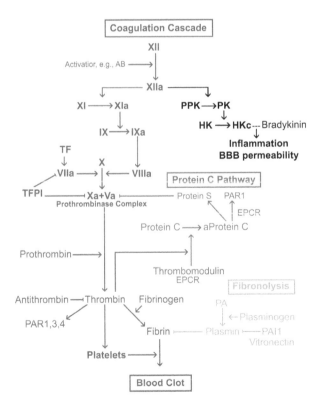

FIGURE 5.1 Coagulation cascade.

A mechanism that may be causing dementia is hypoxia in the form of increased tau hyper-phosphorylation. Postmortem brains of AD patients with subcortical ischemic disease demonstrate reduced hippocampal volumes and cortical shrinking. These findings parallel neuronal death in rats with salt-induced hypertension. The rats demonstrate disruption of BBB, narrowed lumen walls, microglial activation, CAA, white matter damage and hippocampal atrophy.[68] Alteration of micro-tubules is a proposed mechanism of injury in the tau hyperphosphorylation model. These changes should warrant caution against indiscriminate azole use.

Over 2000 postmortem cases of AD strongly correlate with vascular abnormalities.[69] CAA is found in between 80% and 95% of patients with AD and can cause vessel occlusion, ischemia, microbleeds and inflammation.[54] Postmortem human brains from patients with AD also had more fibrinogen in the parenchymal vessels than controls.[47]

A proposed mechanism of cognitive decline in Alzheimer's patients is from the interaction of Aβ and fibrinogen and factor XII. Fibrinogen could mechanistically connect both the vascular hypoth-esis and amyloid hypotheses of AD. Aβ forms when amyloid-β precursor protein (APP) is cleaved by β and γ secretases. Aβ accumulates in the plasma and CSF. Fibrinogen is cleaved by thrombin to form fibrin. Fibrinogen activates platelets to form microinfarcts that obstruct capillaries and reduce blood flow. Fibrinogen forms with higher levels of IL-2.[46] A proposed mechanism of injury is the presence of amyloid angiopathy damaging the vessels and increasing vascular dysfunction by cere-bral microbleeds and infarction. Dr. Strickland theorizes that fibrin's role in neuronal degeneration may be due to a mechanical occlusion and chronic inflammation.[54] This may beget more hypoperfu-sion, clotting, inflammation and BBB degradation, and the cycle of neuronal damage continues.[70, 71]

Aβ-fibrinogen clots are denser and resist degeneration. Aβ decreases fibrinolysis through three proposed mechanisms:[71, 72]

1. Aβ-fibrinogen creates thinner and tighter fibrin fibers, resulting in a dense structure.
2. Aβ-fibrinogen mechanically reduces plasminogen interaction in the form of steric interference.
3. Aβ-fibrinogen blocks plasmin from cleaving fibrin.

Aβ-fibrinogen clots also deposit in the brain parenchyma itself. This process could precipitate microinfarcts, leading to hemorrhage, inflammation and BBB disruption, all of which regularly occur in AD.[71] Dr. Shoemaker recommends using a 9 Tesla Coil MRI to diagnose transient ischemic attacks (TIAs) or microclots. Microclots can then transform into microbleeds. Microbleeds can, in turn, create hypoxia and tau protein.[15]

Aβ42 (the 42-residue isoform) in plasma increases thrombin generation. Aβ42 not only induces clot formation but can also form over preformed clots. The more Aβ42, the more thrombin it gener-ates. Aβ42 works via the factor XII(FXII) intrinsic pathway and will not initiate thrombin genera-tion in FXII-deficient plasma. Longitudinal studies show that higher levels of Aβ42 are found in early AD cases and even before symptoms occur.[73, 74, 75] The Aβ42 decreases as Alzheimer's pro-gresses. Aβ42 may be the first marker, up to 15 years before the onset of first symptoms.[76]

Aβ-fibrinogen clots are resistant to tissue plasminogen activator (tPA) degradation. Also, PAI-1 blocks tPA and urokinase-type plasminogen activator (uPA) from breaking down clots via plasmin-ogen and plasmin.[6] AD patients also have decreased plasmin and increased levels of plasminogen activation inhibitors. Activation of complement proteins also decreases the ability to clot. Aβ also promotes coagulation through interaction with factor XII and increased inflammation in the form of bradykinin release. Increased high-molecular-weight kininogen cleavage, kallikrein and activated factor XIIa may occur.

Rat studies demonstrated that fibrinogen injections in the hippocampus caused neuronal death, increased BBB permeability and microgliosis.[63] To establish a possible mechanism, mice were treated with an antisense oligonucleotide to reduce high-molecular-weight kininogen. Removing the fibrinogen in mice reduced cerebral amyloid angiopathy, BBB permeability, amyloid deposition and microglial activation. The mice displayed improved cognitive function as the inflammation and fibrin decreased. Mice with AD had a higher risk of thrombosis.[63, 77] Lipopolysaccharides (LPS) also induced fibrin. Coagulation induces the amyloid formation and further defines the connection between coagulation, inflammation and AD.[78]

Vascular disease correlates strongly with the cognitive decline seen on Mini-Mental State Exam (MMSE). Patients with AD form more than twice the number of spontaneous clots by transcranial Doppler versus age-matched controls. Patients with AD who are clot formers are more likely to have rapid cognitive decline 6 months after the study. Interestingly, 20–30% of AD patients suffer from cerebral microbleeds. CIRS patients also experience a predisposition both to clot and to bleed in numbers greater than control. Universal screening for CIRS and performing GENIE in a large cohort of AD patients would be fascinating.[65]

A study in China examined patients with and without cerebral microbleeds in the form of lacunar infarcts and found greater cognitive impairment in patients with the microbleeds. These patients had greater cognitive impairment in executive function, memory, and spatial and abstract thinking. All patients had MRIs and Montreal Cognitive Assessment (MOCA) testing, and there was a positive correlation between the severity of cerebral microbleeds and decreasing MOCA scores. It is worth noting that patients with cerebral microbleeds had more endothelial dysfunction and BBB damage.[79]

Anticoagulants may have a role in the treatment of AD. AD mice were treated with enoxaparin and showed improved spatial memory. Human studies show that AD patients do better on warfarin than controls. Patients with atrial fibrillation on warfarin have a lower risk of AD. Studies suggested that Dabigatran may be a possible therapeutic medication for AD. It conveys a lower risk of cranial bleeding and has fewer drug interactions than warfarin. Dabigatran was able to aid memory, reduce Aβ burden, reduce fibrin deposition and increase cerebral perfusion in AD mice (TgCRND8). Of course, these medications come with serious risks, and they could exacerbate those more prone to bleeding, especially given the tendency for microbleeds in AD patients.[63] This benefit of anticoagulants is, of course, tempered by the threat of bleeding.[63] Could transcriptomics identify patients who are prone to microbleeds? Could decreasing innate immune system dysfunction be the better and more proximal route for some of these patients who tend to bleed or clot?

Thrombin works via protease-activated receptors or PARs. Thrombin may also lead to increased platelet secretion.[46] With a high dose of thrombin, the astrocytes and microglia become reactive. The glutamate function is lost, and there is an increase in reactive oxygen species or ROS. Inducible nitric oxide (iNOS), inflammatory cytokines IL-1β and TNF-α increase. There is increased neuritis reaction, increased Ca++ and cell death. The BBB is compromised, and MMP-9 damages the extracellular matrix. Increased thrombin contributes to the pathways of dysfunction that lead to neuronal death. Thrombin plays a role in ALS in activation of PAR1, which leads to increased glutamate metabolism and motor neuron damage by an unknown mechanism. Aβ increases MMP-9, which may have a role in spontaneous intracerebral hemorrhage or cerebral amyloid antipathy. Factor XIIIa and thrombin occur in Aβ deposits in CAA.[46]

Plasma protein factor XII leads to kallikrein-mediated cleaving of high-molecular-weight kininogen and releases bradykinin. Aβ plaques may contain factor XII, and more kallikrein activity occurs in the parenchyma of AD brains.[76] Plasma kallikrein cleaves intact high-molecular-weight kininogen (HKi) into *cleaved* high-molecular-weight kininogen (HKc) and bradykinin. Increased HKc in AD plasma correlates with cognitive dysfunction and plaques on autopsy. HKc plasma levels correlate with Aβ42 and may be a helpful biomarker for early detection of AD.[80] Bradykinin is associated with increased inflammation, BBB permeability, edema and cytokines. In mice models, decreases in bradykinin reduce AD and neuroinflammation.[76]

Dr. Shoemaker has postulated that VIP can benefit cognitive decline by normalizing the coagulation genes responsible for neuronal loss. Dr. Shoemaker's and Dr. Ryan's work fits beautifully with the work of Dr. Strickland and his vascular theory of dementia. Dr. Shoemaker has found that 66% of CIRS patients have clotting abnormalities, with 60% of those patients being at risk for excessive clotting and 40% at risk for excessive bleeding. In contrast, only 5% of controls have clotting/bleeding abnormalities. There is a predisposition for CIRS patients to have abnormalities with D-dimer, PAI-1 and von Willebrand's, factor VIII, and a clinical predisposition to clotting and bleeding abnormalities.[1, 81]

Dr. Strickland notes both increased clotting and bleeding in AD patients as well. Microbleeds and microclots may have a role not only in worsening dementia but also in the promotion of dysregulation of coagulation and the promotion of ever-increasing inflammation and injury.[77, 81] Dr. Strickland theorizes that patients with mild cognitive impairment and BBB damage could allow fibrinogen to enter brain parenchyma and perpetuate neuronal injury. He also states that hypoxia-inducible factor HIF-1α may be increasing Aβ. The overlap with CIRS is striking.

5.9   SUMMARY

The recent work by Dr. Shoemaker and Dr. Ryan has profound implications for entire fields in medicine. Some of the effects of CIRS on the CNS come from issues with BBB, hypothalamic dysfunction and hormonal dysfunction. There are far-reaching consequences of CIRS on the CNS that have implications for illnesses with social implications such as chronic pain, dementia, obesity and mental health. The intersection of inflammation, coagulation and metabolism is on the cutting edge of understanding many of these issues. Certainly, CIRS can worsen many seemingly unrelated issues and be essential in improving others.

REFERENCES

1. Shoemaker, Ritchie, K. Johnson, L. Jim, Y. Berry, M. Dooley, J. Ryan, and S. McMahon. "Diagnostic Process for Chronic Inflammatory Response Syndrome (CIRS): A Consensus Statement Report of the Consensus Committee of Surviving Mold Authors." *Internal Medicine Review*, May 2018.
2. Lucas, Sian-Marie. "The Role of Inflammation in CNS Injury and Disease." *British Journal Pharmacology*, January 9, 2006, pp. 232–240. www.ncbi.nlm.nih.gov/pmc/articles/PMC1760754/.
3. Shoemaker, Ritchie. "State of the Art Answers to 500 Mold Questions." *BookBaby*, 2014.
4. Alves, Jorge. "Olfactory Dysfunction in Dementia." *World Journal of Clinical Cases* 2, no. 11 (2014): 661. http://doi.org/10.12998/wjcc.v2.i11.661.
5. Shoemaker, Ritchie W., Scott W. McMahon, and Andrew W. Heyman. *The Art and Science of CIRS Medicine*, 2020.
6. Berry, Yvonne. *A Physician's Guide to Understanding & Treating BiotoxinIllness Based on the Work of Ritchie Shoemaker*, 2014.
7. "Cranial Nerves and CIRS From Dr. Shoemaker." *E-mail*, October 14, 2020.
8. Welcome to NeuroQuant. https://www.youtube.com/watch?v=q5mirRc8Ppo&t=6s. March 3, 2014. https://www.youtube.com/watch?v=q5mirRc8Ppo&t=6s.7,=.
9. Laboratory Test Instructions Part 2. May 8, 2014. https://www.youtube.com/watch?v=5TQ92uEHxVI.
10. McMahon, S. W., R. C. Shoemaker, and J. C. Ryan. "Reduction in Forebrain Parenchymal and Cortical Grey Matter Swelling Across Treatment Groups in Patients With Inflammatory Illness Acquired Following Exposure to Water-Damaged Buildings." *Journal of Neuroscience and Clinical Research* 1, no. 1 (2016): 2. http://doi.org/10.4172/jnscr.1000102.
11. Shoemaker, Ritchie C. *Surviving Mold: Life in the Era of Dangerous Buildings*. Baltimore, MD: Otter Bay Books, LLC, 2010.
12. Shoemaker, Ritchie C., and James C. Ryan. "Inflammatory Responses Acquired Following Environmental Exposures Are Involved in Pathogenesis of Musculoskeletal Pain." In *Metabolic Therapies in Orthopedics*, 2nd ed., 159–84. Boca Raton: CRC Press, 2018. http://doi.org/10.1201/9781315176079-8.
13. "Molecule Shape and Size Makes a Difference in Biotoxin Diagnosis." March 4, 2014. https://www.youtube.com/watch?v=Kdsq3CgaLxU.
14. McMahon, Scott. *E-Mail Message to Author*, December 26, 2020.
15. CIRS Webinar 2/17/21. "Performed by Andy Heyman/Ritchie Shoemaker." *YouTube*, February 17, 2021. Accessed February 20, 2021. https://www.youtube.com/watch?v=1AHiLqG7u04.
16. Shoemaker, Ritchie. "NeuroQuant and CIRS." Lecture, Mold Congress, Fort Lauderdale, January 2019.

17. When Inflammation Becomes Chronic. September 18, 2015. https://www.youtube.com/watch?v=Nlsecg_kNtY&t=3521s.

18. Ackerley, Mary. "Brain on Fire: The Role of Toxic Mold in Triggering ..." Accessed October 28, 2019. https://paradigmchange.me/wp/wp-content/uploads/2014/11/Mary-Ackerley-Brain-On-Fire-Talk-References.pdf.

19. Randeria, Shehan N., Greig J. A. Thomson, Theo A. Nell, Timothy Roberts, and Etheresia Pretorius. "Inflammatory Cytokines in Type 2 Diabetes Mellitus as Facilitators of Hypercoagulation and Abnormal Clot Formation." *Cardiovascular Diabetology* 18, no. 1 (2019): 1–15. http://doi.org/10.1186/s12933-019-0870-9.

20. Laboratory Test Instructions Part 3. April 9, 2014. https://www.youtube.com/watch?v=oFOfMe1bcVU.

21. Exercises and Capillary Hypoperfusion. March 3, 2014. https://www.youtube.com/watch?v=SQYYcyLCFYU.

22. Anaerobic Threshold Exercise Program. March 3, 2014. https://www.youtube.com/watch?v=jjEDcBbpS_0.

23. VIP My New Friend. February 4, 2014. https://www.youtube.com/watch?v=PiBtYMeH95c&t=1s.

24. Shoemaker, Ritchie. "Intranasal VIP Safely Restores Volume to Multiple Grey Matter Nuclei in Patients With CIRS." *Internal Medicine Review* 3, no. 4 (2017). http://doi.org/10.18103/imr.v3i4.412.

25. MASP2 and Biotoxin Illness. April 23, 2014. https://www.youtube.com/watch?v=7nMQCT3AOvs&t=206s.

26. MMP9 and Biotoxin Illness. March 3, 2014. https://www.youtube.com/watch?v=Xnzg8DRdNG0&t=1s.

27. CIRS (Part 1). "Overview Of Chronic Inflammatory Response Syndrome." *Wholistic Matters*, August 30, 2018. https://www.youtube.com/watch?v=31Ftaa_PBRk&t=73s.

28. Koudriavtseva, Tatiana. "Thrombotic Processes in Multiple Sclerosis as Manifestation of Innate Immune Activation." *Frontiers in Neurology*, May 5, 2014. http://doi.org/10.3389/fneur.2014.00119.

29. Shavit-Stein, Efrat. "The Role of Thrombin in the Pathogenesis of Diabetic Neuropathy." *PLoS*, July 5, 2019. https://doi.org/10.1371/journal.pone.0219453.

30. Jedrychowski, Wieslaw, Umberto Maugeri, Frederica Perera, Laura Stigter, Jeffrey Jankowski, Maria Butscher, Elzbieta Mroz, Elzbieta Flak, Anita Skarupa, and Agata Sowa. "Cognitive Function of 6-Year Old Children Exposed to Mold-Contaminated Homes in Early Postnatal Period. Prospective Birth Cohort Study in Poland." *Physiology & Behavior* 104, no. 5 (2011): 989–95. http://doi.org/10.1016/j.physbeh.2011.06.019.

31. MR Spectroscopy in Biotoxin Illness. April 24, 2014. https://www.youtube.com/watch?v=tLUnRQwFzS4.

32. Benros, Michael E., Berit L. Waltoft, Merete Nordentoft, Søren D. Østergaard, William W. Eaton, Jesper Krogh, and Preben B. Mortensen. "Autoimmune Diseases and Severe Infections as Risk Factors for Mood Disorders." *JAMA Psychiatry* 70, no. 8 (2013): 812. http://doi.org/10.1001/jamapsychiatry.2013.1111.

33. Benros, Michael E., Berit L. Waltoft, Merete Nordentoft, Søren D. Østergaard, William W. Eaton, Jesper Krogh, and Preben B. Mortensen. "Autoimmune Diseases and Severe Infections as Risk Factors for Mood Disorders." *JAMA Psychiatry* 70, no. 8 (2013): 812. http://doi.org/10.1001/jamapsychiatry.2013.1111.

34. Yilmaz, Melis, Esra Yalcin, Jessy Presumey, Ernest Aw, Minghe Ma, Christopher W. Whelan, Beth Stevens, Steven A. Mccarroll, and Michael C. Carroll. "Overexpression of Schizophrenia Susceptibility Factor Human Complement C4A Promotes Excessive Synaptic Loss and Behavioral Changes in Mice." *Nature Neuroscience*, 2020. http://doi.org/10.1038/s41593-020-00763-8.

35. Laboratory Test Instructions Part 1. May 19, 2014. https://www.youtube.com/watch?v=HDuUCGZXi2I.

36. "Low Plasma Vascular Endothelial Growth Factor (VEGF) Associated With Completed Suicide." *The World Journal of Biological Psychiatry*, November 2011: 468–73.

37. Shoemaker, Ritchie. "Cause of Death in CIRS." October 30, 2019. https://www.survivingmold.com/physicians/dashboard/faq/daily-member-questions/10-30-2019-cause-of-death-in-cirs.

38. Bryleva, Elana. "Kynurenine Pathway Metabolite and Suicidality." *Neuropharmacology* 112, no. Part B (January 2017): 324–30. http://doi.org/10.3109/15622975.2011.624549.

39. Shenassa, Edmond D., Constantine Daskalakis, Allison Liebhaber, Matthias Braubach, and Maryjean Brown. "Dampness and Mold in the Home and Depression: An Examination of Mold-Related Illness and Perceived Control of One's Home as Possible Depression Pathways." *American Journal of Public Health* 97, no. 10 (2007): 1893–899. http://doi.org/10.2105/ajph.2006.093773.

40. Erhardt, Sophie, Chai K. Lim, Klas R. Linderholm, Shorena Janelidze, Daniel Lindqvist, Martin Samuelsson, Kristina Lundberg, Teodor T. Postolache, Lil Träskman-Bendz, Gilles J. Guillemin, and Lena Brundin. "Connecting Inflammation With Glutamate Agonism in Suicidality." *Neuropsychopharmacology* 38, no. 5 (2012): 743–52. http://doi.org/10.1038/npp.2012.248.

41. Lotrich, Francis. "Management of Psychiatric Disease in Hepatitis C Treatment Candidates." *Current Hepatitis Reports* 9, no. 2 (2010): 113–18. http://doi.org/10.1007/s11901-010-0035-5.

42. Erhardt, Sophie, Chai K. Lim, Klas R. Linderholm, Shorena Janelidze, Daniel Lindqvist, Martin Samuelsson, Kristina Lundberg, Teodor T. Postolache, Lil Träskman-Bendz, Gilles J. Guillemin, and Lena Brundin. "Connecting Inflammation With Glutamate Agonism in Suicidality." *Neuropsychopharmacology* 38, no. 5 (2012): 743–52. http://doi.org/10.1038/npp.2012.248.

43. "Why Reducing MMP-9 Could Be a "Good Thing" for ALS." *Neurology Today Online*, March 6, 2014. https://journals.lww.com/neurotodayonline/Fulltext/2014/03060/Why_Reducing_MMP_9_Could_Be _a__Good_Thing__for_ALS.7.aspx.

44. Davis, David A., Paul Alan Cox, Sandra Anne Banack, Patricia D. Lecusay, Susanna P. Garamszegi, Matthew J. Hagan, James T. Powell, James S. Metcalf, Roberta M. Palmour, Amy Beierschmitt, Walter G. Bradley, and Deborah C. Mash. "L-Serine Reduces Spinal Cord Pathology in a Vervet Model of Preclinical ALS/MND." *Journal of Neuropathology & Experimental Neurology* 79, no. 4 (2020): 393–406. http://doi.org/10.1093/jnen/nlaa002.

45. Cox, Paul Alan. "BMAA and Neurodegenerative Illness." *Neurotoxicity Research*, January 2018: 178–83. http://doi.org/10.1007/s12640-017-9753-6.

46. Shimon, Marina Ben, Maximilian Lenz, Benno Ikenberg, Denise Becker, Efrat Shavit Stein, Joab Chapman, David Tanne, Chaim G. Pick, Ilan Blatt, Miri Neufeld, Andreas Vlachos, and Nicola Maggio. "Thrombin Regulation of Synaptic Transmission and Plasticity: Implications for Health and Disease." *Frontiers in Cellular Neuroscience* 9 (2015): 151. http://doi.org/10.3389/fncel.2015.00151.

47. Cortes-Canteli, Paul, and Sidney Strickland. "Fibrinogen and Beta-Amyloid Association Alters Thrombosis and Fibrinolysis: A Possible Contributing Factor to Alzheimer's Disease." *Neuron* 66, no. 5 (May 14, 2010): 695–709.

48. Biotoxin Illness Case Studies 3 & 4. July 9, 2014. https://www.youtube.com/watch?v=M5FBAHcTKKw &t=298s.

49. Juurlink, Bernhard. "The Evidence for Hypoperfusion as a Factor in Multiple Sclerosis Lesion Development." *Multiple Sclerosis International*. Article ID 598093 2013: 1–6. https://doi.org/10.1155 /2013/598093.

50. Koudriavtseva, Tatiana, Rosaria Renna, Domenico Plantone, and Caterina Mainero. "Demyelinating and Thrombotic Diseases of the Central Nervous System: Common Pathogenic and Triggering Factors." *Frontiers in Neurology* 6 (2015): 63. http://doi.org/10.3389/fneur.2015.00063.

51. Plantone, Domenico, and Tatiana Koudriavtseva. "A Perspective of Coagulation Dysfunction in Multiple Sclerosis and in Experimental Allergic Encephalomyelitis." *Frontiers in Neurolog* 9 (January 14, 2018). http://doi.org/10.3389/fneur.2018.01175.

52. Identifying Mold Illness. January 30, 2014. https://www.youtube.com/watch?v=yV4AkIB0z30&t=1s.

53. Identifying Mold Illness 2. February 24, 2014. https://www.youtube.com/watch?v=qm-qNmjImOQ.

54. Strickland, Sidney. "Blood Will Out: Vascular Contributions to Alzheimer's Disease." *Journal of Clinical Investigation* 128, no. 2 (2018): 556–63. http://doi.org/10.1172/jci97509.

55. Strickland, Sidney. "Blood Will Out: Vascular Contributions to Alzheimer's Disease." *Journal of Clinical Investigation* 128, no. 2 (2018): 556–63. http://doi.org/10.1172/jci97509.

56. Shoemaker, Ritchie C. "Metabolism, Molecular Hypometabolism and Inflammation: Complications of Proliferative Physiology Include Metabolic Acidosis, Pulmonary Hypertension, T Reg Cell Deficiency, Insulin Resistance and Neuronal Injury." *Trends in Diabetes and Metabolism* 3 (2020): 4–15. http://doi .org/10.15761/TDM.1000118.

57. Swardfager, W., K. Lanctôt, L. Rothenburg, A. Wong, J. Cappell, and N. Herrmann. "A Meta-Analysis of Cytokines in Alzheimer's Disease." *Biological Psychiatry*. Accessed October 28, 2020. https:// pubmed.ncbi.nlm.nih.gov/20692646/.

58. C4a and Biotoxin Illness. March 2, 2014. https://www.youtube.com/watch?v=1VGm3mRzsbI.

59. VEGF and Biotoxin Illness. March 5, 2014. https://www.youtube.com/watch?v=qB0T5wROv6U.

60. Brain on Fire Webinar - Brain Changes in Mold Illness With Dr. Mary Ackerley. January 19, 2017. https://www.youtube.com/watch?v=cB7X-bCkd7c&t=1122s.

61. Measuring VEGF in Biotoxin Illness. March 24, 2014. https://www.youtube.com/watch?v=G -K4B7SYu4c.

62. Bredesen Training 2.0 by Dale Bredesen. Apollo Health, 2020.

63. Cortes-Canteli, Marta, Anna Kruyer, Irene Fernandez-Nueda, Ana Marcos-Diaz, Carlos Ceron, Allison T. Richards, Odella C. Jno-Charles, Ignacio Rodriguez, Sergio Callejas, Erin H. Norris, Javier Sanchez-Gonzalez, Jesus Ruiz-Cabello, Borja Ibanez, Sidney Strickland, and Valentin Fuster. "Long-Term

Dabigatran Treatment Delays Alzheimer's Disease Pathogenesis in the TgCRND8 Mouse Model." *Journal of the American College of Cardiology* 74, no. 15 (2019): 1910–923. http://doi.org/10.1016/j.jacc .2019.07.081.

64. Bredesen, Dale E. *The End of Alzheimers: The First Program to Prevent and Reverse Cognitive Decline.* New York: Avery, an Imprint of Penguin Random House, 2020.

65. Suidan, Georgette L., and Sidney L. Strickland. "Abnormal Clotting of the Intrinsic/Contact Pathway in Alzheimer Disease Patients is Related to Cognitive Ability." *Blood Advances*, April 26, 2018: 954–63. https://doi.org/10.1182/bloodadvances.2018017798.

66. Luca, Ciro De, Assunta Virtuoso, Nicola Maggio, and Michele Papa. "Neuro-Coagulopathy: Blood Coagulation Factors in Central Nervous System Diseases." *International Journal of Molecular Sciences* 18, no. 10 (2017): 2128. http://doi.org/10.3390/ijms18102128.

67. Sur, Woosuk. "Coagulation Factor XIIIa Cross-Links Amyloid β into Dimers and Oligomers and to Blood Proteins." *Journal of Biological Chemistry*, November 8, 2018: 390–96. http://doi.org/https://doi .org/10.1074/jbc.RA118.005352.

68. Limor, Raza. "Hypoxia Promotes Tau Hyperphosphorylation With Associated Neuropathology in Vascular Dysfunction." *Neurobiology of Disease*: 124–36. Accessed June 2019. https://doi.org/10.1016/j .nbd.2018.07.009.

69. Hyung, Jin Ahn, and Sidney Strickland. "Interactions of β-Amyloid Peptide With Fibrinogen and Coagulation Factor XII May Contribute to Alzheimer's Disease." *Current Opinion in Hematology* 24, no. 5 (September 2017): 427–31. http://doi.org/10.1097/MOH.0000000000000368.

70. Cortes-Canteli, Marta, Daria Zamolodchikov, Hyung Jin Ahn, Sidney Strickland, and Erin H. Norris. "Fibrinogen and Altered Hemostasis in Alzheimer's Disease." *Journal of Alzheimer's Disease* 32, no. 3 (June 17, 2017): 599–608. http://doi.org/10.3233/JAD-2012-120820.

71. Wolberg, Alisa S. "Aβ and C(lot), But Not D(egradation)." *Blood* 119, no. 14 (2012): 3196–197. http://doi .org/10.1182/blood-2012-02-406660.

72. Zamolodchikov, Daria, and Sidney Strickland. "Aβ Delays Fibrin Clot Lysis by Altering Fibrin Structure and Attenuating Plasminogen Binding to Fibrin." *Blood* 119, no. 14 (2012): 3342–351. http://doi.org/10 .1182/blood-2011-11-389668.

73. Zamolodchikov, Daria, Hanna E. Berk-Rauch, Deena A. Oren, Daniel S. Stor, Pradeep K. Singh, Masanori Kawasaki, Kazuyoshi Aso, Sidney Strickland, and Hyung Jin Ahn. "Biochemical and Structural Analysis of the Interaction Between β-Amyloid and Fibrinogen." *Blood* 128, no. 8 (August 25, 2016): 1144–151.

74. Zamolodchikov, Renne, and Sidney Strickland. "The Alzheimer's Disease Peptide β -Amyloid Promotes Thrombin Generation Through Activation of Coagulation Factor XII." *Journal of Thrombosis and Haemostasis* 14 (November 28, 2015): 995–1007. https://doi.org/10.1111/jth.13209.

75. Zamolodchikov, Daria, and Sidney Strickland. "A Possible New Role for Aβ in Vascular and Inflammatory Dysfunction in Alzheimer's Disease." *Thrombosis Research* 141, no. suppl. 2 (May 2016): S59–61. https://doi.org/10.1016/S0049-3848(16)30367-X.

76. Zamolodchikov, Daria, and Sidney Strickland. "Factor XII Activation in Alzheimer Disease Plasma." *Proceedings of the National Academy of Sciences* 112, no. 13 (March 2015): 4068–73. http://doi.org/10 .1073/pnas.1423764112.

77. Cortes-Canteli, Marta. "Fibrin Deposited in the Alzheimer's Disease Brain Promotes Neuronal Degeneration." *Neurobiology of Aging* 36, no. 2 (October 31, 2014): 608–17. http://doi.org/10.1016/j.neu-robiolaging.2014.10.030.

78. Page, Martin J., Greig J. A. Thomson, J. Massimo Nunes, Anna-Mart Engelbrecht, Theo A. Nell, Willem J. S. De Villiers, Maria C. De Beer, Lize Engelbrecht, Douglas B. Kell, and Etheresia Pretorius. "Serum Amyloid A Binds to Fibrin(ogen), Promoting Fibrin Amyloid Formation." *Scientific Reports* 9, no. 1 (2019): 1–14. http://doi.org/10.1038/s41598-019-39056-x.

79. Jianjun, Yang. "Relationship Between Cerebral Microbleeds Location and Cognitive Impairment in Patients With Ischemic Cerebrovascular Disease." *Clinical Neuroscience* 29, no. 14 (September 26, 2018): 1209–213. http://doi.org/10.1097/WNR.0000000000001098.

80. Yamamoto-Imoto, Hitomi, and Sindey Strickland. "A Novel Detection Method of Cleaved Plasma High-Molecular-Weight Kininogen Reveals Its Correlation With Alzheimer's Pathology and Cognitive Impairment." *Alzheimer's & Dementia: Diagnosis, Assessment & Disease Monitoring* 10 (2018): 480–89. https://doi.org/10.1016/j.dadm.2018.06.008.

81. Shoemaker, Ritchie. "Additonal Uses of VIP." November 22, 2019. https://www.survivingmold.com/ save-vip/additional-uses-of-vip.

6 Chronic Inflammatory Response Syndrome (CIRS) and Metabolism

Proliferative Physiology and Insulin Resistance

Ritchie Shoemaker and April Vukelic

CONTENTS

DOI: 10.1201/b23304-7

6.1 REVIEW

Metabolism is the group of biochemical processes needed to maintain cellular life.[1] This broad term classifies all metabolic processes into a single over-arching, process-interacting system. Such an all-encompassing term does not define the distinct bases of metabolism or their interplay with other systems, including inflammation. Specific elements of the definition of metabolism support an enhanced understanding of unique metabolic functions, but lost is the cohesive consideration of all metabolic processes acting in concert to maintain life and health.[1] New data on the interaction of metabolism with inflammation, combined with transcriptomic findings in syndromes characterized by chronic inflammation, are uncommon.

An indirect understanding of research foci in metabolism comes from the prevalence of search words on PubMed. Citations assessed on February 15, 2020 included 7,914,000 that were devoted just to [metabolism], with over half of those citations (4,819,000) indexed to [metabolism, protein]. [Disorders of protein metabolism] brought up nearly 1,000,000 hits. [Metabolism, glucose] brought 435,000 matches, but [disorders of glucose metabolism] had only 177,000 matches. So, here is a massive scientific database on metabolism and disorders of metabolism of proteins and sugars, but there is a discrepancy between general and specific topics in metabolism.

Against this dense background of the discussion of the essential elements of metabolism, we have the new transcriptomic findings of "molecular hypometabolism" (MHM), coined by Dr. James Ryan in 2016. The findings describe the simultaneous reduction in the number of copies of ribosomal mRNA and mitoribosomal mRNA made by individuals with a chronic, multisystem, multisymptom illness. Chronic fatigue[2–4] of a particular type called chronic inflammatory response syndrome (CIRS) is a hallmark of MHM. Of note is the increased production of inflammatory compounds that accompanies the suppression of the production of ribosomal mRNA.[4]

Nearly all CIRS cases also meet the case definition for Chronic Fatigue Syndrome (CFS)[5] and Severe Exercise Intolerance Disease (SEID), though CFS and SEID have no specific biomarkers.[6] CIRS has at least 15 biomarkers.[7] For these individuals, compromise of metabolism may be adaptive, providing the potential for cell survival in an inflammatory or ribotoxin-mediated attack on protein synthesis at the sarcin-ricin loop (SRL),[8] an evolutionarily conserved structure located between the large and small subunits of ribosomes. As it is found in all living organisms and directly involved with initiation, elongation and termination of amino acid chains, one may speculate as to the source of the paucity of papers on the incredibly important role in the metabolism of ribosomal protein production played by the SRL (number of papers on [metabolism, SRL] = 177) compared with [metabolism, ribosomes] (= 44,400).

The severe cellular impairment created by the simultaneous suppression of nuclear-encoded mitochondrial genes adds to decreased protein production and innate immune inflammation in MHM. While putative mitochondrial dysfunction in CFS and CIRS has many proponents, we must account for differential gene activity for mitochondrial genes that have migrated to the nucleus over several billion years. Nuclear-encoded mitochondrial genes number in the hundreds, but only 37 genes remain in the mitochondrial genome.[9]

Specifically, genes for electron transport chain (ETC) and ATP synthases were noted by Dr. Ryan to be suppressed, as were translocases. Translocases move nuclear gene–encoded products out of the cytosol, across the outer mitochondrial membrane, in conjunction with porins, small electrically charged channels (voltage-dependent anion channels, VDAC) that permit entry of ions, solutes, ADP and pyruvate against a gradient into the intermembranous space.[10–12] Specific carriers will complete delivery across the inner mitochondrial membrane to the matrix.

Failure to enter pyruvate into the mitochondrial matrix compartment from the cytosol has very important consequences for metabolism. However, survival adaptations using MHM are maintained at a cost, as organisms with MHM are alive but might not be vigorous in two main cellular energy processes:

1. Proliferation.
2. Conservation.

The literature is relatively silent on survival with MHM. Indeed, with mitochondrial gene suppression, as shown by measurable abnormalities in the amount of mRNA produced by nuclear-encoded mitochondrial genes, little is published on energy production in patients with CIRS or SEID. They have a deficiency of translocases. For perspective, while [metabolism, mitochondria] yields 167,000 papers, nuclear-encoded mitochondrial genes are only referenced by 1471 papers under [metabolism, nuclear-encoded mitochondrial genes] and only 4 for [metabolism, fatigue, and voltage-dependent anion channels (VDAC)]. Given that the estimates of the prevalence of chronic fatiguing illnesses in the United States alone exceed 50,000,000 cases, with that number increasing yearly, it was disturbing to find the dearth of papers on [metabolism, CIRS] (=1334) and [metabolism, ribotoxins], the source of SRL injury (= 72). Fortunately, a diagnostic and treatment protocol that identifies and corrects the transcriptomic abnormalities of MHM has been in wide use[2, 4] since 2010, with correction of MHM noted in over 90% of cases.

This chapter will review the impact of MHM on metabolism as those pathways interact with inflammation seen in CIRS, with particular attention to aerobic glycolysis and VDAC effects on metabolic acidosis, grey matter nuclear atrophy and pulmonary hypertension in CIRS. We follow that thread with study data on 112 patients with CIRS.

6.2 SEVERE EXERCISE INTOLERANCE DISEASE (SEID), CHRONIC INFLAMMATORY RESPONSE SYNDROME (CIRS) AND METABOLISM

The recent addition of transcriptomic testing as an approach to patients with chronic fatiguing illnesses, defined as multisystem, multi-symptom illnesses, including SEID, fibromyalgia, post-Lyme disease, and CIRS, is demonstrated by the following:

1. A commonality of the complexity and near universality of responses of genes of inflammation and coagulation.
2. The relationship of suppression of production of ribosomal mRNA and nuclear-encoded mitochondrial genes to multiple facets of glucose metabolism, especially aerobic glycolysis,[13, 14] resulting in neuronal injury, including cognitive impairment,[15-19] and pulmonary hypertension.

These findings in chronic illnesses parallel the findings of acute sepsis (systemic inflammatory response syndrome, SIRS), with excessive inflammation, coagulation and immunosuppression persisting beyond the treatment of infection.[20]

Each of these elements is consistent with the classic observations of Lewis Thomas that the host immune response, once initiated, can become the disease. When combined with disturbances in glycolysis and pyruvate uptake into mitochondria through VDAC, it is clear that ongoing maladaptive responses to immune and metabolic initiators underlie multiple sources of SEID (excluding CIRS). The absence of objective diagnostic parameters, without which there are no guides to physiology-based therapies, typifies SEID. Transcriptomics helps with a better understanding of the role of VDAC.

A chronic illness called persistent inflammation and catabolism syndrome (PICS)[20] often develops in patients who survive sepsis. While we have chosen the term CIRS to describe "chronic PICS" and other associated illnesses related to chronic inflammation, the illness concepts are the same. The difference is that CIRS literature has data on many recognized biomarkers and a published treatment protocol,[7] but PICS does not.

These biomarkers include symptom clusters for CIRS acquired following environmental exposures to biotoxins and inflammagens in water-damaged buildings (WDB), finding at least 8 of 13 clusters present. Proteomic biomarkers compared with controls[4] include:

1. The increased relative risk for specific HLA haplotypes.
2. Presence of a distinctive deficit seen in visual contrast sensitivity (VCS).

3. Reduction of mean levels of melanocyte-stimulating hormone (MSH).
4. Dysregulation of ACTH to cortisol.
5. Dysregulation of ADH to osmolality.
6. Elevated C4a.
7. Transforming growth factor β-1 (TGFβ-1).
8. Matrix metallopeptidase 9 (MMP-9).
9. Suppression of vascular endothelial growth factor (VEGF).
10. Increased incidence of antigliadin antibodies.
11. Increased incidence of anticardiolipin antibodies.[7]

Functional CIRS-WDB biomarkers include:

1. A distinctive "fingerprint" of volumetric abnormalities[21–23] seen on NeuroQuant®.
2. Reduction of VO_2 max shown by pulmonary stress testing.
3. Reduction of anaerobic threshold shown by pulmonary stress testing.
4. Elevated pulmonary artery pressures at rest on echocardiogram.
5. Elevated pulmonary artery pressures after exercise on echocardiogram.
6. Transcriptomics.

6.3 MOLECULAR HYPOMETABOLISM

The advances in understanding the physiology associated with MHM are brought to light by transcriptomics. These advances highlight the application of differential gene activation, stratified by age, comparing cases with controls for ribosomal mRNA genes for the small ribosomal subunit and differentiating those mRNA findings from the large ribosomal subunit. Further, transcriptomics allows us to understand mRNA findings on large and small subunits of mitoribosomes. These findings are important when evaluating NeuroQuant®, looking at the role of commensal multiple antibiotic resistant coagulase negative staphylococci (MARCoNS), now found to make unidentified polycyclic ether toxins (unpublished). The role of mitochondrial gene suppression in association with MARCoNS is fertile ground for continued research.

When taken as a whole, with a correction for the high and the low number of mRNA copies, combined with an adjustment for age, we have seen that transcriptomics will accurately identify molecular hypometabolism in patients with CIRS and SEID. For example, we also see these fundamental abnormalities in less commonly represented illnesses in our data set, including multiple sclerosis and cancer. Disorders of inflammation, metabolism and loss of regulation of differential gene activation, commonly seen in CIRS, SEID and other chronic fatiguing illnesses, hold importance by defining pathological abnormalities in metabolism that may apply to other chronic illnesses.

Changes in MHM with therapy also provide a window on the treatment of CIRS, as the use of a peer-reviewed protocol[4] shows the correction of suppression of ribosomal and nuclear-encoded mitochondrial genes, especially translocases. The completion of initial treatment is marked by an overshoot of the number of copies of targeted genes compared with controls, with a return to control levels using intranasal vasoactive intestinal polypeptide (VIP). The changes in individual mRNA counts seen in each MHM entity are parallel in shape when graphed, describing the "CIRS curve."[24]

6.4 METABOLIC ACIDOSIS

6.4.1 Specifics of Glycolysis and Pyruvate

Once glucose enters the cell, often by the facilitated transport from a family of solute carriers called GLUT-1 (SLC2A1) and GLUT-4 (SLC2A4), it enters into a cytosolic pathway called glycolysis (also called the Embden–Meyerhof pathway). This series of enzymatic steps can generate needed precursors used for other metabolic pathways, small amounts of ATP and pyruvate. Glycolysis is an evolutionarily conserved process used by all living organisms. As seen with the SRL, evolutionary conservation means that all the possible mutations and nucleotide polymorphisms that occurred over three billion years yielded no replacement of the glycolysis genes or pathway.

Glycolysis is a ten-step pathway of intracytoplasmic conversion of a six-carbon ring, glucose, to create two copies of a three-carbon fragment, pyruvate. There are two phases in glycolysis. The first is called the "preparatory phase," and the second is the "payoff phase." The preparatory phase consumes two ATP to place phosphate moieties strategically on metabolites, with the return of a total of four ATP in the payoff phase. Diversion of metabolic precursors to other pathways subtracts from the net four generated ATP.[25, 26]

The conversion of glucose to the first metabolite, glucose 6-phosphate, is accomplished at the cost of one ATP to fuel an important enzyme, hexokinase. As an aside, hexokinase has recently become the focus of much attention in degenerative central nervous system diseases, especially Alzheimer's, as ApoE2 patients will rarely have Alzheimer's and have a rich endowment of hexokinase, but ApoE4 is associated with central nervous system (CNS) deterioration, with reduced hexokinase.[27–29]

Once hexokinase's first change of glucose occurs, the first diversion of glucose from its ultimate goal of producing pyruvate can occur. Here, glucose 6-phosphate can shunt to participate in synthesizing a storage compound, glycogen, a complex carbohydrate. A second diversion occurs when glucose-6-phosphate dehydrogenase (G6PD) is activated to convert G-6-P to ribose-5-P, the first step of the pentose phosphate shunt, a significant source of metabolites, especially nucleotides, needed for added cell division. This shunt is a crucial diversion used in proliferative physiology.

If glycolysis continues, the next step is to make fructose 6-phosphate by the enzyme phospho-hexose isomerase. The new stereochemistry primes fructose 6-phosphate, and at the cost of one additional ATP, the enzyme phospho-fructokinase-1 will add a phosphate group, making fructose 1,6-bisphosphate. The six-carbon ring can now be cleaved into two pieces. Note that fructose-6-phosphate can lead to the hexosamine biosynthetic shunt, part of the cell's metabolic response to stressors such as infection, ischemia or trauma.

This cleavage is accomplished by the enzyme aldolase, known for its role in muscular diseases, to make glyceraldehyde 3-phosphate and dihydroxyacetone phosphate. The latter is then converted by triose phosphate isomerase, thus making two molecules of glyceraldehyde 3-phosphate. If the word glycerol seems similar to glyceraldehyde, it is because there can be a diversion of glyceraldehyde to make glycerol. Alternatively, dihydroxyacetone phosphate can participate in synthesizing lipids.

This step marks the crossover from the preparatory phase to the payoff phase. The two molecules of glyceraldehyde 3-phosphate can be converted by oxidation and phosphorylation using the enzyme glyceraldehyde 3-phosphate dehydrogenase (GAPDH) to make two molecules of 1,3 biphosphoglycerate. GAPDH is a vitally important enzyme that serves as a rate-controlling regulator of pyruvate production, which in turn, serves as a vital component of gamma interferon activated inhibitor of translation (GAIT), as will be discussed. GAIT provides a mechanism for cellular feedback control to downregulate inflammatory cytokine responses and maintain metabolism. GAPDH has other important roles as well.

GAPDH will also generate reduced NADH in this pathway in the next step, facilitating the production of two additional ATP. Step 7 uses phosphoglycerate kinase to make two copies of a single phosphate molecule, 3-phosphoglycerate. Cleaving a phosphate group from each permits conversion of ADP to make a total of two ATP for each pyruvate. Remember, the preparatory phase saw the consumption of two ATP; now, two sets of two ATP are returned, making a net yield of positive two molecules of ATP. Conversion of 3-phosphoglycerate into the amino acid serine fuels the production of other amino acids needed for protein synthesis.

Next, moving one phosphate is a necessary step to manufacture two copies of 2-phosphoglycerate by phosphoglycerate mutase. Enolase converts each 2-phosphoglycerate into phosphoenolpyruvate. Pyruvate kinase further converts this compound to make pyruvate.

If pyruvate can traverse the outer mitochondrial membrane and reach the mitochondrial matrix, it feeds into the Krebs cycle (tricarboxylic acid pathway, TCA), where it can be converted to acetyl-CoA by pyruvate dehydrogenase (PDH), leading to lipid synthesis. Pyruvate kinase (PDK1) can block PDH. Hypoxia-inducible factor 1 alpha (HIF-1α) induces PDK1, a compound that also activates the conversion of pyruvate to lactate. Further, HIF-1α can increase glucose uptake through GLUT-1 and 4 and activate hexokinase, setting off glycolysis. HIF-1α is important in aerobic glycolysis (see the section on PAH later). There is interest in using PDK1 as a possible chemotherapy agent, as the use of aerobic glycolysis typifies many cancers. HIF-1α also has a significant role in suppressing the production of T-regulatory (reg) cells by activating the production of T-effector cells.

As complex as the glycolysis pathway is with its multiple diversions, a basic tenet of metabolism is that the activation of one pathway will change the activity of competing pathways.[30] Metabolism adapts to environmental change, which creates a stimulus for differential gene activation, controlling discrete elements of metabolic pathways and inflammation. These changes create a cellular environment where two consecutive measurements of gene activity and metabolism are rarely similar unless the initiating stressor (exposure to ribotoxins, for example) is constant. Here is the generally considered role for inflammation controlling gene activation, with metabolic changes driven by gene activation regulated by inflammation. An exciting finding is that medications associated with salutary health effects[2, 4, 23] that change gene activation and inflammation will restore regulation of abnormalities of metabolism.

A prime example of gene activation, inflammation and metabolic control comes from a review of the effect of the Randle cycle on glycolysis. As each pathway is mutually reciprocal, an increase in the Randle cycle decreases glycolysis in favor of fatty acid oxidation with its enriched source of ATP production. Increasing fatty acid oxidation, as follows a rise in insulin receptor substrate 2 (IRS 2), activating GLUT-1 and GLUT-4, will suppress glucose catabolism, but at the cost of increasing oxygen consumption: Burning fatty acids costs oxygen. Citrate, part of the Krebs cycle, will suppress phosphofructokinase, increasing glucose-6-phosphate, shunting the glycolysis pathway to increase glycogen storage. This part of the Randle cycle creates the "second wind," as well-trained athletes know, as increased energy (9.3 calories/gram) comes from fatty acid oxidation, compared with 3.4 calories/gram from glucose oxidation.

Simply stated, direct fat-burn stores glycogen. Fatty acid oxidation, in turn, generates acetyl-CoA, which blocks pyruvate dehydrogenase, preventing pyruvate from being converted into acetyl-CoA. This step leads to aerobic glycolysis and production of lactate, especially if pyruvate is also blocked from entering mitochondria across the VDAC by inflammation-induced reduction of translocases. The combination of the development of hypoxemia (from fatty acid oxidation [FAO]) and aerobic glycolysis is the development of pulmonary hypertension.[31] Blocking FAO in isolated myocytes of the right ventricle leads to increased pyruvate burn and lower oxygen consumption.[31] Meanwhile, the Krebs cycle is the site of the conversion of glutamine to glutamate, making available a free amino group crucial to glycosylation, discussed later.

Finding these ten metabolic steps conserved by evolution seems surprising at first glance, yet nature works in predictable ways. The amount of enzymatic work to make just two net ATP seems excessive, but the production of so many building blocks has two important additional benefits:

1. The manufacture of a reservoir of compounds needed for cell proliferation.
2. The speed of ATP production.

A theme in metabolism, both in health and in disease, is the dual role of glucose in

1. Energy conservation.
2. Energy expenditure to support cell proliferation.

Glucose remains the coin of the metabolic realm, as it leads to the production of pyruvate, which can be further processed by an enzyme, lactate dehydrogenase (LDH), to generate lactic acid (lactate).

In turn, transport molecules move lactate out of the cell. We may suspect excessive amounts of lactate production by seeing a widened anion gap in peripheral blood. However, even this seemingly simple calculation can be complicated by further metabolism of lactate in capillary beds adjacent to where it was produced, with reconversion to pyruvate, reducing the anion gap.

Pyruvate is the cellular metabolic treasure; it plays a dominant role in cell proliferation versus cellular conservation of energy, primarily based on where pyruvate is further metabolized. Mitochondrial production of ATP depends on the delivery of pyruvate into the mitochondrial matrix. If delivery is compromised, cytosolic metabolism will be the default site for pyruvate metabolism. If there is too much pyruvate in the cytosol, or too little gets consumed, look for suppression of GAPDH gene(s) to reduce pyruvate production, possibly contributing to insulin resistance.

Some rapidly dividing cells will use the conversion of pyruvate to lactate as their primary source of ATP through "aerobic glycolysis," also called the Warburg Effect.[32, 33] At first glance, this low-yield conversion of pyruvate to make ATP, compared with what Krebs cycle and ETC pathways in the mitochondrial matrix would bring, seems dysfunctional. What benefit does a rapidly dividing cell glean from "wasting" the ability to create molecules used for energy? Cancer cells commonly use this so-called "Warburg physiology" to produce lactate and export it from the dividing cell, creating an adverse microclimate that serves as a defense to prevent T-cells from attacking growing cancer cells. Cells at the surface of the developing tumor use the reverse of cellular fermentation by reconverting lactate back to pyruvate as a source of ATP.[33]

In CIRS, we worry about the Warburg Effect, because it underlies the pathologic development of clinically significant metabolic acidosis and pulmonary hypertension;[34] it underlies abnormalities, including metabolism in branched chain glycans, that will lead to insulin resistance. Further, we also see multiple examples of injury to neuronal tissue associated with the Warburg Effect, both peripherally, creating peripheral neuropathy, and centrally, possibly contributing to dementing illnesses.

The marker for the Warburg Effect that can harm CIRS patients, the anion gap, which is readily calculated but not so readily confirmed, is due to the fermentation of pyruvate to make lactate. Excess lactic acid adds to or widens the normal anion gap. To calculate the anion gap, add values of sodium (Na^+) to those of potassium (K^+), and from that sum, subtract the sum of CO_2 and chloride (Cl^-). If the number is 10-12, that is a normal anion gap. However, beyond a gap of 14 or 15, we become concerned regarding the excessive presence of anionic compounds that contribute to the widened anion gap. The body uses lactic acid and bicarbonate to help regulate pH tightly; metabolic acidosis is common in multiple disease states, including PICS and CIRS, diabetes and renal failure.

6.4.2 Voltage-Dependent Anion Channels (VDAC) and Pyruvate

If pyruvate is not converted to lactate, we expect pyruvate to cross into the mitochondrial matrix for fuel purposes. Unfortunately, there is a channel, 2–3 nm in diameter,[35] which creates a pore in the outer membrane of the mitochondria that is dependent upon the normal presence of translocases to function. As the term[36] suggests, translocases have a role in moving protein compounds from one cellular environment to another. In this case, for mitochondrial concerns, the pore will permit the entry of solutes, ions, ADP and pyruvate through the outer membrane to reach the intermembranous space. ATP will exit the pore after the ETC produces it, and possibly reactive oxygen species (ROS), in the matrix of the mitochondria. This pore, however, is closed by

1. The absence of translocases, commonly seen in MHM, as discussed earlier.
2. The activity of products made by Streptomyces and other actinomycetes,[37] especially valinomycin; it is unknown if another actinomycetes product, piericidin A, an irreversible inhibitor of Complex I, also uses the VDAC.

Other factors closing the VDAC are tubulins,[38] hexokinase[39] and itraconazole.[40, 41] Actinomycetes' metabolites can shut down flow in both directions across the pore, discharging the electrical gradient that maintains the opening.[41] Azole antifungal medications, unfortunately, are widely used by some involved in the management of illness acquired following exposure to the interior environment of WDB. This inappropriate use of azoles creates proliferative physiology; we must recognize it for its significant contribution to adverse metabolic outcomes, especially grey matter nuclear atrophy. Elevated amounts of beta-tubulin are also associated with excessive and premature grey matter nuclear atrophy and the loss of cortical grey in CIRS patients.[42]

If pyruvate can cross the outer membrane of the mitochondria, there is a mitochondrial pyruvate transporter that will move it across the inner mitochondrial membrane into the matrix. There, pyruvate has several possible fates. First, pyruvate is converted by pyruvate dehydrogenase (PDH) to make acetyl-CoA. Acetyl-CoA is also produced from stored fatty acids to make oxaloacetic acid (OAA). In the Krebs cycle, OAA will join acetyl-CoA to make citrate. Citrate and OAA are major components of the cycle that operate in the mitochondrial matrix to regulate energy metabolism. Citrate also has a "shuttle" in which it can be shunted back through the VDAC to be hydrolyzed to remake acetyl-CoA in the cytosol compartment, leading to fatty acid production in the cytosol. Conversely, citrate can be further metabolized in the matrix to make alpha-ketoglutarate in combination with glutamine after an amino acid is split off from glutamine by glutaminolysis. Alpha-ketoglutarate can be metabolized to make succinate, regenerating OAA, repeating the cycle.

Alternatively, alpha-ketoglutarate can enter the ETC for further metabolism. Here, the role of NADH and FADH2 is vitally important. As NADH breaks down into NAD, it releases a hydrogen ion, a proton, which helps balance the electrons transported in the chain to make ATP. Ideally, glycolysis will generate two molecules of pyruvate, which are then shunted through the Krebs cycle to the ETC to generate 36 ATPs.

This process is rarely entirely successful, as the free electrons in the ETC can divert into making superoxides (ROS) that can damage mitochondria by a variant of apoptosis called ferroptosis.[43] It makes sense that the mitochondria "want" to avoid programmed death from ROS. One mechanism mitochondria possibly use to stay functional is not to let pyruvate cross the outer membrane initially and to focus energy production by aerobic glycolysis, thereby avoiding ROS formation.

Multiple complexes function to generate ATP, CO_2 and water in the ETC. Two of these complexes have areas for which interaction with actinomycete metabolites can be disruptive. This is particularly true for Complex III, in which oligomycin can irreversibly bind to ATP synthases, stopping ETC production of ATP. If there is suppression of ATP synthases in MHM, oligomycin could be less toxic to Complex III. As mentioned, piericidin A will bind irreversibly to Complex I.

The interaction of cytosol compartments and the mitochondria with each of their two membranes is extraordinarily complex. Glucose metabolism products in the cytosol versus the mitochondrial matrix are simply one example of compartmental complexity. The difficulty in assessing metabolic needs for each of these interactions is measuring mitochondrial activity within a living cell, understanding that there are thousands of mitochondria functioning in each cell at a given time. Some, but not all, may be affected by other metabolic pathways.

Pyruvate is vitally important in cell proliferation in which the Warburg Effect is active, compared with cell conservation of energy where ETC is involved. The distinct differences in the results of pyruvate metabolism from either cytosol or mitochondrial matrix compartments underlie proliferative versus energy conservation physiology.

6.5   FOCUS ON THE WARBURG EFFECT

Otto Warburg gets less recognition than the theme of this chapter suggests he deserves. Perhaps, if we had made broader advances in the treatment of cancers, Warburg would be better known, since his work defining aerobic glycolysis, as used by many malignant cells, was indeed a seminal event.[13]

The concept that pyruvate is converted to lactate in the presence of oxygen, called aerobic glycolysis, *not in the absence of oxygen* (anaerobic glycolysis), was a radical idea 100 years ago. The fact that cancer cells used aerobic glycolysis made Warburg's observations even more dramatic.

Warburg did not know enough about the role of mitochondria and oxidative phosphorylation, as Hans Krebs published his work on the eponymous Krebs cycle in 1937. He also did not explain the increased ammonia observed in his tissue preparations, now recognized as a marker for active amino acid metabolism, including glutaminolysis. Warburg felt that mitochondria in cancer cells were dysfunctional. Perhaps if he had known about VDAC, he would have recognized that the dysfunction was an indicator of the closure of that pore in the outer mitochondrial membrane and that nothing was wrong with the mitochondria.

Not all cancers use aerobic glycolysis, but this does not detract from the importance of Warburg's discovery. While aerobic glycolysis and oxidative phosphorylation can coexist in a given tumor, we speculate that slower-growing tumors use aerobic glycolysis less than faster-growing tumors. To summarize, rapidly dividing tissue needs more cellular building blocks than energy conservation–driven cells in tissues with normal growth rates. These building blocks include nucleotides (influenced by G6PD) and lipids (influenced by TPI, triose phosphate isomerase) made during the first three steps of glycolysis.

Understanding that CIRS cases comprise the majority of those studied with transcriptomics to date, the finding of upregulation of CD14 and TLR4 correlates with exposure to WDB with elevated levels of endotoxins. Tentative markers of exposure to WDBs with increased species abundance of actinomycetes are ribosomal stress responses, including mitogen-activated protein (MAP) kinases (MAPKs),[44, 45] with normal levels of a version of a building health index called Health Effects Roster of Type-Specific Formers of Mycotoxins and Inflammagens, version 2 (HERTSMI-2).[46] Exposure to mycotoxins also can involve upregulation of MAPKs, among other genes, though greater in number than seen with exposure to actinomycetes.

6.6 TRANSCRIPTOMICS AND METABOLISM

The approach to metabolism in CIRS as a unique entity is complex, with multiple interacting systems of feedback regulation. While that source of complexity is daunting, further complications occur in understanding metabolism in CIRS because of the paucity of papers in the metabolism literature on the inflammatory gene database interacting with MHM. Novel discoveries like MHM form the basis for possible advances in science, but the expansion of the application of new ideas can be a slow, step-by-step journey. The metabolism literature has a paucity of proteomic testing results (TGFβ-1, MMP-9, MSH, and VEGF).

A proprietary transcriptomic assay, GENIE, has shown us the in-depth importance of MHM and its multiple implications for cell physiology and metabolism. With MHM, one will first see issues regarding impairment of protein synthesis by disruption of messenger RNA (mRNA) for ribosomal genes that will impact variously on initiation, elongation and termination of the RNA signal at the SRL wedged between the large and small ribosomal subunits. The second issue is compromised energy production by impairing the synthesis of mitochondrial genes found in the nucleus. Such nuclear-encoded mitochondrial RNA is produced following disrupted signals by transcription factors, epigenetic factors, microRNA and regulatory factors such as ribonuclear proteins. The metabolic importance of regulating nuclear-encoded mitochondrial RNA production parallels the importance of protein interactions and modification of proteins seen in metabolic pathways with such modifications following glycosylation.

Similarly, when ATP synthases are also affected, mitochondrial function is impaired. There is little wrong with the mitochondria in these situations. The energy metabolism is subject to such a diverse series of dysregulations found in MHM that attempting to tease out individual aspects is difficult.

6.7 INSULIN RECEPTOR SUBSTRATE 2 (IRS2)

GENIE shows that patients with MHM may have either up- or downregulated responses to IRS2 activation. IRS2 is part of a group of cytoplasmic proteins that are anabolic, preventing the development of Type 2 diabetes, in part by activating glucose transport channels GLUT-1 and GLUT-4, as well as activating pathways that gear towards protein synthesis, cell proliferation and cell survival.[47] If GLUT-1 and 4 are open, but there are reduced translocases, there will be an increased cytosolic glucose load in the face of reduced pyruvate delivery to the mitochondrial matrix. Aerobic glycolysis and proliferative physiology will follow. IRS2 also helps coordinate extracellular signals via transmembrane receptors that regulate downstream pathways, including FAO, P13K/Akt/mTOR and MAPK.[48]

IRS2 is one of the major mediators that respond to insulin and insulin-like growth factor (IGF1). If IRS2 is upregulated with hypometabolism, creating a "mismatch," one of the mechanisms to control cellular survival during MHM is to downregulate the production of pyruvate by suppressing glycolysis. If IRS2 is upregulated in MHM, activation of Akt and MAPK proceed unchecked, wasting energy and cellular building blocks. This mismatch can be disastrous for the MHM cell metabolism, as it becomes a prescription for enhanced Warburg Effect.

Conversely, if MHM is absent and IRS2 is downregulated, normal cell survival and protein synthesis will again be compromised, as the cell will have compromised delivery of glucose to an intact system of

1. Pyruvate production by glycolysis.
2. Pyruvate delivery into the mitochondrial matrix.

When IRS2 is downregulated, GLUT-1 and GLUT-4 transports are impaired.[49] With such impairment, a major source of glucose delivery becomes an endosome, containing an insulin receptor bound to insulin and bound to glucose, and moving from the cell membrane inside the cell.[50] This endosome, functioning like an insulin bubble surrounded by a membrane, is held intact in the cytoplasm until it becomes acidified. If hydrogen ion enters the endosome, there will be a release or recycling of insulin and insulin receptors back to the cell membrane and glucose delivery for glycolysis.[51] In the presence of polycyclic acid ether toxins made by actinomycetes species, primarily Streptomyces, including monensin and nigericin, there will be *impairment* of acidification of the endosome and absent or reduced release of glucose, with little recycling of insulin and insulin receptors.[52] There is no dearth of insulin, no dearth of insulin receptors, but functionally, insulin resistance is created. This mechanism of enhanced storage of insulin, insulin receptors and glucose inside the cell may be a form of "intracellular insulin resistance"[52] as opposed to the "extracellular" insulin resistance created by glycosylation of proteins in adipose tissue.

6.8   METABOLIC COMPLICATIONS: PULMONARY HYPERTENSION (PAH)

Pulmonary hypertension (PAH), an increase of pressure between the right ventricle and the lung in the pulmonary artery, remains underdiagnosed. The methods used to diagnose pulmonary hypertension are either a static measurement at heart catheterization or a potentially dynamic measurement of baseline echocardiogram measurements that indirectly permit pulmonary artery pressure calculation. Performed as an echocardiogram exam, with the potential to do a stress echocardiogram looking at the rise of pulmonary artery pressure in exercise, confirmation of elevated pulmonary artery pressure is common in CIRS.[7] Rarely is heart catheterization performed to diagnose pulmonary hypertension; measurement of elevated systolic pressure in the pulmonary artery (PASP) is regarded as an ancillary exam when concerns about left ventricular function are dominant. The difficulty of obtaining a stress echo to diagnose acquired pulmonary hypertension is amplified because most cardiology stress test protocols focus on left ventricular ischemia. Coronary artery disease and left ventricle function, especially ischemia in coronary disease and ejection fraction in heart failure, are normally of much greater clinical concern to cardiologists than evaluation for PAH.

During a baseline echocardiogram, the flow velocity moving backward across the tricuspid valve, called the tricuspid jet, is used to calculate pulmonary artery pressure (PASP). Taking the square of the tricuspid regurgitant velocity and multiplying that number by 4 gives us a definable idea of PAH.

$$PASP = 4\left(V_{TR}\right)^{2^2} + RAP$$

Adding the baseline pressure in the right atrium completes the calculated PASP. For adults, any calculation of PASP, measured in four different ways during echocardiography, was found in a 2013 study[4] in nearly 50% of adults with CIRS. In the 2013 study, VIP was provided at four sprays a day (50 µg/dose). At the end of 1 month, if PASP had not returned to normal, the dose of VIP was increased to eight sprays a day. After 2 months, the dose was re-titrated to the lowest dose needed for correction.

Since that study was published, there has been a surge of scholarly publications, notably those from Dr. John Ryan at the University of Utah Medical Center. We now know that aerobic glycolysis remains a fundamental cellular mechanism that results in PAH. In PAH, normal PASP is increased by the proliferation of endothelial tissue both lining blood vessels and in the middle of blood vessels, as well as by vascular stiffening, clotting in small arterials and the presence of an inflammatory lymphocytic infiltrate. If the condition continues undetected, possibly in concert with elevated TGFβ-1, there will be endothelial to mesenchymal remodeling that stiffens small arterial vessels and narrows them to the point of blockage. The complications of pulmonary hypertension include right ventricular failure with a 5-year survival rate of less than 50%.[53]

While PAH relates to toxin exposure, the role of exposure to WDB, especially actinomycetes, is evolving. We must rule out thrombotic sources of PAH, typically pulmonary emboli, when considering PAH due to proliferative physiology.

Now that we know proliferative changes resulting from aerobic glycolysis are common in CIRS, there will be demand for data on the etiology of PAH beyond interstitial lung disease, thrombosis and inflammation. Compared with the evaluation of the Warburg Effect in cancer cells, where proliferation follows increased glucose uptake, in PAH, there are more influences, especially hypoxia and inflammation, all leading to metabolic stress. The role of mitochondrial inputs, while possibly reduced due to closure of VDAC, still includes dysregulation of ETC, leading to ferroptosis.

Oxidative stress, inflammation and hypoxia are threefold stimuli that induce abnormalities of gene pathways involving hypoxia-induced factor 1α. However, the metabolic complexity includes the pentose phosphate shunt, glycolytic programming and mitochondrial-induced apoptosis.[54] These pathways include the pentose phosphate pathway, glutaminolysis, iron, hemostasis and fragmentation of mitochondria themselves. Also, abnormalities of fatty acid metabolism, stimulated in part by IRS2, as discussed previously, can be recognized by increased circulation of free fatty acids and accumulating elements that create lipotoxicity. The interaction of FAO and glucose oxidation is inversely proportional, as evidenced by the function of the Randle cycle, in which oxidation of fatty acids impairs glucose oxidation and vice versa.

CIRS produces excessive use of aerobic glycolysis. The first is in pulmonary hypertension, possibly due to toxic exposure; the second is due to deficient production of T-reg cells in a rapidly expanding pool of immune lymphocytes (see later).

In pulmonary hypertension, HIF-1-dependent upregulation of pyruvate dehydrogenase kinase (PDK1 and PDK2) blocks pyruvate dehydrogenase. This blockade prevents the conversion of pyruvate to acetyl-CoA in the mitochondria, which leads to the failure of the mitochondrial ETC production of ATP. The findings in pulmonary hypertension may well involve pathways focusing on glutaminolysis, including the hexokinase and hexosaminidase pathways.[55–57]

Another central question in pulmonary hypertension and to a lesser extent, T-regulatory cell depletion is the role of hypometabolism. In hypometabolism, with IRS2 suppression genes, there will be reduced stimulus for glycolysis, reduced GLUT-1 and GLUT-4 activity, reduced activation of the Akt pathways, reduced FAO and reduced MAP kinase pathways. When these factors combine with the activation of platelet beta-tubulin genes, either TUBB1 or TUBA4A, especially if combined with the upregulation of multiple coagulant genes, we are looking at a microvascular flood of glucose shunted toward proliferative physiology. Proliferative physiology reduces the Krebs cycle, NADH production, oxidative phosphorylation, and hexokinase and hexosaminidase pathways.

Unlike the classic Warburg Effect, which activates glutaminolysis to initiate the Krebs cycle, molecular hypometabolism suppresses ribosomal and mitochondrial functions and includes enhanced and reduced coagulant gene activity. The difference between Warburg Effect findings and current findings in PAH in CIRS patients is that we now know that treatment of the inflammatory response will reactivate the metabolic pathways and return the patient to normal with a reduction of PAH. With the suppression of HIF-1 pathways, combined with the suppression of Akt and MAP kinase pathways, we have a prescription for the three elements needed to stimulate the production of T-regulatory cells.[57] In the face of stimulation of constant bombardment of innate immune receptors with inflammagens in CIRS, an upregulation of metabolic pathways accompanies a widened anion gap, usually due to increased capillary levels of lactic acid that must be corrected in order for PAH itself to be corrected.

A common path of physiologic features includes endothelial dysfunction, excessive proliferation, impaired apoptosis of vascular cells and mitochondrial fragmentation. The proliferation/apoptosis imbalance relates to the activation of transcription factors, hypoxia-inducible factor-1α, nuclear factor of activated T-cells (NFAT) and apoptosis. Pulmonary hypertension also occurs due to the peripheral inflammatory disruption of adventitial connective tissue and a glycolytic metabolic shift in vascular cells and right ventricular myocytes. These are also seen in target tissue in the right ventricle and skeletal muscle, reflecting the systemic nature of not just glycolysis but the entire metabolic shift driven by nuclear transcription factors. PAH is an obstructive pulmonary vasculopathy characterized by excessive proliferation and apoptosis-resistant inflammation.[58]

Fortunately, the treatment protocol discussed earlier with each of the 12 steps effectively corrects hypometabolism, stops the Warburg Effect, permits correction of PAH, permits restoration of T-cell populations, blocks metabolic acidosis and begins the process of neuronal healing. All these benefits happen from using a measurement of molecular hypometabolism in gene activation by applying transcriptomic testing.

6.8.1 Gamma Interferon Activated Inhibitor of Translation Complex (GAIT) Is One of Many Biologic Controls on Inflammation

The gamma interferon activated inhibitor of translation complex (GAIT) consists of four elements: Glutamyl-prolyl-tRNA synthase, NS1-associated protein 1 (NSAP1), ribosomal protein L13a and glyceraldehyde-3-phosphate dehydrogenase (GAPDH).[59] Perhaps no other feedback system exemplifies the tightly regulated interactions between inflammation and metabolism more than GAIT. This grouping can bind to translation regions of given inflammation genes, including VEGF, to inhibit their translation. While there are differences in the inflammatory response between mice and humans, the well-described regulatory GAIT system in mice is similar to the less well-described human GAIT system.[60]

GAIT is an extraordinary complex negative feedback regulation system that helps slow down the over-translation of inflammatory genes. Moreover, it acts as an additional mechanism to slow down glycolysis by removing GAPDH from the pathway of conversion of glucose to pyruvate. By blocking pyruvate production, the cell can avoid producing lactic acid when problems with molecular hypometabolism affect mitochondrial pathways, including the Krebs cycle and ETC. Specifically, in the absence of normal production of mitochondrial membrane translocases, it teleologically serves the cell well to "hibernate," reducing inflammation and reducing the creation of pyruvate until the hypometabolism resolves.

The GAIT proteins are metabolically expensive to produce and operate. Gamma interferon activates kinases in multiple discrete steps by which a phosphate group is placed on specific amino acids (usually serine or threonine) to change protein structure and function. By linking interferon, produced as a result of inflammation, which controls glycolysis, together with a mechanism to control the initiation of protein synthesis, the cell obtains the ability to handle the potential for multiple adverse effects caused by inflammation.[60]

It is instructive to note that levels of plasma VEGF in CIRS cases fall into three groups: Suppressed, over-expressed and no different from controls.[4] Each result is approximately 33% in prevalence for VEGF in CIRS cases. VEGF increases following interferon-gamma treatment within 8 hours but by 24 hours, has returned to basal levels. We see this phenomenon in the repetitive exposure protocol called SAIIE (sequential activation of innate immune elements). On day 1 of re-exposure, VEGF levels rise rapidly, only to fall by day 3 to nadir. The mechanism here is translational silencing by the GAIT system of VEGF.

There are GAIT effects on other genes of uncertain influence on the progression of CIRS, including ZIPK, CDK5 and ceruloplasmin. DIPK and ZIPK are similar to housekeeping genes in that they mediate phosphorylation of the protein L13a, therefore functioning as GAIT internal regulatory elements.[61]

6.8.2 Myeloid Cells

In CIRS, we see the diverse metabolic effects of myeloid cells during innate immune responses.[62] First studied in a Toll 4, CD14 system looking at the programming of myeloid cells following endotoxin exposure, thought to be replicated in other toxin exposures initially, is now showing the remarkable diversity of "rewiring" that takes place after a diversity of exposures.[62] This emerging field, called immunometabolism, is now a problem in innate immune responses, specifically increasing the availability of small molecules that can manipulate a diverse array of metabolic roots.

Cellular metabolic pathways may serve three major functions:

1. Generation of energy.
2. Production of building blocks necessary for cellular maintenance.
3. Proliferation and modulation of cellular signaling.

Immune cells in forced stimulation are not activated to either proliferate or increase uptake of nutrients. Following antigen presentation to myeloid cells, there is a need to rapidly expand the myeloid cell population. Building blocks, including nucleotides and lipids, are generated by repurposing metabolic pathways. As the immune cell population selectively expands, new signaling molecules organize the inflammatory response.[62]

As expected, aerobic glycolysis coincides with the rapid expansion of cell lines. In the presence of pyruvate dehydrogenase kinase, there will be suppression of the Krebs cycle, reducing the production of acetyl-CoA (and therefore, lipids from citrate). Much of the evidence involved with the metabolism of myeloid cell activation comes from stimulation of Toll receptor 4 (TLR4) by bacterial endotoxin, lipopolysaccharide (LPS).

As discussed previously in this chapter on aerobic glycolysis, this is the function of the rapidly expanding cell lines. New data suggests that in addition to increasing the rate of glycolysis, there are additional metabolic signatures in myeloid cells separate from the Warburg Effect. The diversity of metabolic responses in myeloid cells is remarkably conserved. One of the mechanisms for long-term reduction of innate immune memory involves epigenetic changes involving methylation and demethylation, or acetylation of histones or deacetylation of histones. These epigenetic findings can impact Krebs cycle physiology and differential gene activation.[62]

The presence of chronic inflammatory environmental conditions can not only alter the microenvironment but also alter transcriptomic responses. Both elements can contribute to the migration of macrophages into tissue and T-regulatory cells. While perhaps better studied in tumor cells, lactate can initiate pro-inflammatory effects and prompt tumor angiogenesis. Thus, metabolic changes in immune cells accumulate in blood vessel walls, as in margination, or in joint capsules promoting inflammation as the disease progresses, possibly including atherosclerosis.[63]

Of interest are the associated findings with the pentose phosphate shunt in which accumulation of succinate, brought about by the Krebs cycle's disruption, leads to the stabilization of HIF-1α, which as a transcription factor will induce the production of an inflammatory cytokine, interleukin-1β (IL-1β). Suppose the mitochondrial mechanisms, including translocases, are not adversely impacted, as seen in hypometabolism. In that case, LPS stimulation will cause remodeling of the ETC itself, promoting the generation of mitochondrial ROS, which assists in killing microbes.[64]

Similarly, another element of this Krebs cycle, citrate, can be exported from mitochondria to the cytoplasm following LPS stimulation. The expansion of the endoplasmic reticulum and Golgi bodies, in turn, supports cytokine release from dendritic cells.[62] We see metabolic networks to regulate inflammatory processes throughout the cell, including nuclear transcription and mitochondrial function.

As discussed, IRS2 activation will stimulate the activation of the mammalian target of rapamycin (mTOR), which is an important stimulator of the metabolic response of the cell, affecting nutrient availability and energy demands, together with P13K/Akt. This combination drives aerobic glycolysis to meet the demands of actively dividing cells. The regulatory counter-balance is the activation of 5' AMP-activated protein kinase (AMPK), which enhances the regulation of oxidative phosphorylation, promoting both ATP production and inflammatory properties.[65]

6.8.3 Hexosamine Biosynthetic Pathway (HBP)

The layers of regulatory interaction of the transcriptome, inflammation and glucose metabolism are well exemplified by an important metabolic pathway for glucose (but only affecting 3–6% of intracellular glucose), the HBP. This pathway provides another "side street" for glucose entering glycolysis. Remember that when glucose is converted into glucose-6-phosphate, the body uses the compound to

1. Make glycogen.
2. Enter into the pentose phosphate shunt.
3. Be converted into fructose-6-phosphate.

If 3 applies, glycolysis can continue, or fructose-6-phosphate can enter the HBP, especially in GAPDH suppression. This pathway is intimately involved with the response to stressors, particularly inflammation, ischemia, trauma or oxidative stress from ROS. The HBP is called the survival pathway.[66] It maintains serum glucose higher than normal and leads to insulin resistance. In addition to providing extra nucleotides needed for cell proliferation, HBP provides the needed building block, UDP-GlcNAc, required to produce glycans (O-linked-N-acetyl glucosamines, O-GlcNAc), which in turn, regulate countless proteins and transcription factors.[67, 68]

In the necessary presence of glutamine, we see that the regulatory control that impacts HBP begins at the second step in glycolysis, where fructose-6-phosphate is changed by glutamine-fructose-phosphate amidotransferase (GFAT), especially in the concomitant presence of hypoxia, by adding glutamine to make glucosamine-6-phosphate. Adding an acetyl-CoA makes glucosamine-N-acetyl-6-phosphate, followed by rearrangement of the location of the phosphate. Then, the nucleotide uridine phosphate is added from nucleotide pools to make uridine diphosphate N-acetyl-glucosamine (UDP-GlcNAc).

Posttranslational protein modification to membrane-bound or secreted proteins on serine or threonine moieties on hundreds of nuclear and cytoplasmic proteins via a modulatory process called O-glycosylation involving the enzyme O-GlcNAc transferase (OGT) forms UDP-GlcNAc. OGT is evolutionarily conserved and is the only enzyme that does the actual glycosylation. Acute cellular stress increases UDP-GlcNAc; increasing levels increases cell survival,[66] and feedback suppresses GFAT.[67] O-glycosylation is involved in many feedback control systems. The survival pathway also stimulates O-glycosylation to make defensins, non-specific acute phase neutrophilic peptides used in host defense against bacteria and viruses.

Opposing UDP-GlcNAc and OGT is N-acetylglucosaminidase (O-GlcNAcase; OGA), also evolutionarily conserved, the only enzyme that *removes* the glucosamine from previously O-glycosylated proteins, acting primarily in the cytosol. The flux through the HBP that excessively favors OGT over OGA contributes to the development of insulin resistance. Work on adipocytes shows impairment of insulin-stimulated glucose uptake, caused in part by

1. Increasing glucose toxicity.
2. Decreasing GLUT-4.
3. Increasing glycosylation of IRS-1 and AKT.[69]
4. Blockade by inhibition of GFAT.[67]

A known biological antagonist of OGA is O-(2-acetamido-2-deoxy-D-glucopyranosylidene) amino-N-phenyl carbamate (PUGNAc).[66, 68, 69] PUGNAc blocks the removal of glycans placed by OGT by inhibiting OGA. The presence of PUGNAc impairs glucose utilization; phosphorylation of IRS and Akt was impaired, and insulin resistance markedly increased. Theoretically, downregulating gene activation for PUGNAc could have salutary health effects on insulin resistance and inflammation decrease via OGA activation.

Understanding that the sources of insulin resistance are multifactorial, and returning to the role of capillary hypoperfusion in CIRS, we can speculate to what extent prevention of hypoxia activates HBP, which

1. Reduces metabolic acidosis.
2. Prevents proliferative physiology.
3. Enhances VDAC.
4. Thereby enhances energy conservation from mitochondrial matrix function.

HBP provides salutary benefits in protection from decreased glucose uptake and protection from O-glycan-induced insulin resistance.

6.8.3.1   Inside Insulin Resistance

Using a T3-L1 cell line that expresses the GLUT-4 transporter, a well-characterized model of the study of insulin resistance, Vosseller and Wells show the effect of excessive glycosylation by OTG. A reduction of OTA, or blockade of OTA, by PUGNAc reduces the activation of downstream effectors of insulin receptors.[70] By identifying the glycosylation status of individual members of the insulin signaling cascade, including IRS and B-catenin, insulin resistance was recognized. The study shows that metabolism incorporates posttranslational regulatory modification of proteins, accentuated by the glucose flux through the HBP.

The role of glycosylation extends beyond insulin resistance. Glycosylation is catalyzed by only one enzyme, OGT. Removal of O-GlcNAc from proteins is catalyzed by only one enzyme, OGA. The balance of OGT versus OGA alters the activity of PUGNAc, which preferentially blocks OGA.[68] Abnormalities of proteins, including transcription factors, are linked by glycosylation, which can influence

1. Transcription activity.
2. DNA.
3. Localization.
4. Stability in interaction with cofactors.

The role of regulation of glycosylation affecting transcription factors shows excellent potential for new approaches for the treatment of diabetes and obesity.

Despite the promise of new insights, awareness of O-glycosylation is not new. Indeed, in 2003, Kamemura discussed the balance of glycosylation versus phosphorylation of nucleocytoplasmic proteins as having a role in the metabolic control of signaling and transcription.[71] The role of OGT back then was identified as necessary for stem cell viability, making GlcNAc essential for life in multicellular creatures. The gene encoding OGA maps to a locus important to late-onset Alzheimer's disease. This link of the blockade of glycosylation to neuronal injury underscores the importance of the combination of inflammation, increasing coagulation elements bound to beta-amyloid, with metabolism. The interaction of glycosylation and phosphorylation is important for regulatory proteins, variously including estrogen receptors, Sp1, endothelial nitric oxide synthase and B-catenin. This chapter emphasizes the interaction of protein modifications in metabolism, to which we add the additional role of interactions with known confounders and inflammatory responses.

In 2005,[69] Park extended the cell culture basis of insulin resistance to glycosylation and modification of IRS2 and Akt2 by PUGNAc. PUGNAc does not affect GLUT-4; it has an increased effect on glycosylation of insulin signaling intermediates, reducing the insulin-stimulated phosphorylation on IRS2 and Akt, leading to insulin resistance in adipocytes.

By 2010, additional studies of insulin resistance, focusing on the main tissues involved with glucose clearance, i.e., adipose tissue and striated muscle, added to the understanding of the important role of the hexosamine biosynthesis pathway.[67] Once again, we see protein modifications by glycosylation, which modulates insulin sensitivity in fat cells. Here, we see the interaction of adipose tissue for the disposal of glucose, interacting with leptin as a central element in energy homeostasis. The conclusion is that animal studies show adipose tissue factors are key regulators in maintaining glucose homeostasis. Metabolism focusing on glucose extends to fat cell hormones and adipocytokines. The recurrent theme is that the HBP in glycosylation controls the endocrine function of adipocytes, mediating insulin resistance.

A tantalizing approach to the treatment of insulin resistance has to do with the blockade of the crucial enzyme GFAT. The use of azaserine or 6-diazo-5-oxonorleucine prevented glucose-insulin resistance in fat cells. On the other hand, the treatment of cells with glucosamine showed a reduction in insulin-mediated glucose uptake. Azaserine does not block this effect.

Additional work from Wells and Teo, published in 2014, underscores that while glycosylation is involved in the regulation of adipose cytokine secretion upon induction of insulin resistance in human fat cells, the investigators identified secretion of 190 proteins, as well as 20 upregulated proteins and 6 down-regulated in insulin resistance.[72] Glycosylation can be mediated by more than oxygen; nitrogen and sulfur can contribute to the creation of glycans. Here, 91 glycosylation sites were derived by 51 secreted proteins, and 155 and 29 N-O glycans, respectively, were also identified. Quantification of N-O glycan structures shows how genuinely complex insulin resistance is. None of these studies occurred in cell culture or animals controlled for molecular hypometabolism, which further confuses the issue of precisely what contributes to insulin resistance.

The HBP generates aminosugars and provides building blocks for glycosyl side chains, proteins and lipids. All these effects begin with the regulation of GFAT together with OGT, which catalyzes a reversible, posttranslational protein modification in O-linkage to specific serine/threonine residues.[73] In this sense, HBP acts as a cellular nutrient sensor and plays a role in developing insulin resistance, not to mention the vascular complications of diabetes. Crucial in this last function, complications of diabetes are the induction of TGFβ-1 and plasminogen activator inhibitor-1 in vascular smooth muscle cells, renal cells and aortic endothelial cells. In this era of implantable insulin pumps, there is speculation about titrating inhibitors and activators of GFAT. Still, there are no published studies to confirm a "magic bullet" for the treatment of diabetes and obesity.

6.8.4 T-Regulatory Cells and Proliferative Physiology

The fourth element of CIRS, in which proliferative physiology plays a crucial role, is the balance of production of T-regulatory cells versus T-effector cells. Acquired T-regs were CD4+CD25++.

Thymus-derived T-regs were CD4+CD25++CD127–/lo. The CD25 indicates a binding site for IL2; the CD127 is a binding site for IL7. Having these two types of T-reg cells enumerated by flow cytometry provided a rapid determination of whether CIRS patients had deficiencies of T-regulatory cells or not. It also became clear that treatment with VIP corrected the deficiency of T-regs.

T-regs will interact with retinoic acid orphan receptors (ROR) in tissue to suppress tissue-based inflammation and reduce autoimmunity. If ROR are not present in normal amounts, the T-reg cells are plasticized and made into T-effector cells. These cells make more TGFβ-1, setting up a positive feedback loop leading to a deficiency of T-regs.

For years, the feedback loop idea provided a working hypothesis to explain why low levels of T-regs link to putative deficiencies of ROR. Still, there were no assays to demonstrate ROR without obtaining tissue by biopsy. The unconfirmed idea of assigning causation by ROR had little support. Impairment of normal production of T-reg cells in favor of T-effector cells accrues when lymphocytes proliferate in response to a metabolic or inflammatory stressor.

Indeed, this mechanism has been known for years. Unfortunately, the link between metabolism and inflammation and T-reg suppression is attracting reduced attention in current literature. We find in T-regulatory cells that repression of Akt/mTOR, hypoxia-inducible factor-1 alpha and aerobic glycolysis are important for the suppression of efficient generation of T-reg cells. Those same pathways suppress T-reg cell development and mature T-reg cells.[74]

As discussed in metabolic acidosis and pulmonary hypertension, the link between IRS2 and Akt/mTOR, glycogen, HIF-1α and aerobic glycolysis follows the same pathways in lymphocytes. The net result is a varied effect of the same molecular basis in metabolism that affects human health.

Toll-like receptor signaling will promote T-reg cell differentiation. We also see increases in Akt/mTOR, HIF-1α and aerobic glycolysis. If we add in an additional confounder, a transcription factor, FoxP3 blocks this activation of Akt/mTOR, so that the reduction of glycolysis that follows can increase oxidative metabolism and increase T-regs.

6.8.5 Brain Atrophy

Given the commonality of aerobic glycolysis in proliferative physiology seen in the systemic illness of those with chronic fatigue, a search was extended to the literature looking for evidence for proliferative physiology in the brain. The following observations are consistent with what we would expect to see if there were adverse effects of proliferative physiology in the brain:

1. Grey matter nuclear atrophy.
2. Atrophy of cortical grey.
3. Superior lateral ventricle enlargement, as seen on NeuroQuant®.

Finding such evidence would complete the unifying thread that encircles CIRS as a metabolic disorder causing the end-organ injury seen in chronic fatiguing illnesses.

Work from the lab of Yellen, including Diaz-Garcia, has provided evidence of the extrapolation of systemic proliferative physiology to the brain.[75] Neuronal stimulation triggers neuronal glycolysis, which is not surprising, since normal brain function requires 20% of whole-body energy. Neurons will preferentially use aerobic glycolysis during brain stimulation instead of oxidative phosphorylation and ETC activation in mitochondria. It is unclear whether proliferative physiology is confined to neurons or generalized to other brain cells. The authors used hippocampal slices of mice to show that neuronal metabolic response to stimulation does not depend on astrocytic contribution, nor does it require neuronal uptake of lactate.

This paper from Yellen's laboratory looks for aerobic glycolysis in the brain's transient response to activation.[76] It also addresses possible cellular mechanisms for metabolic resupply of energy and neurons. Unfortunately, without consideration of VDAC, we are left with an open question regarding the continuation of proliferative physiology following stimulation.

An additional question regarding neuronal consumption of oxygen and glucose has to do with the plasticity of activity given a different set of activity patterns. The speculation was that different gene expression programs would be involved. The authors note the crucial role of MAPK/ERK but again, do not discuss MAPK activation following IRS2 activation.[77] Based on MAPK activation of other tissues, one would expect to find IRS2 activation as a precursor. Changes in gene activation will be subject to translocase function and VDAC opening.

From Yellen's laboratory,[78] metabolism will increase during stimulation, but not all energy metabolism is equally affected. An increase in local cerebral blood flow with increased glucose uptake, not matched by a similar increase in oxygen consumption, suggests that glycolysis becomes a dominant metabolic pathway producing energy. These changes in the brain correspond to a temporary increase in lactate production not well measured at the bedside except with magnetic resonance spectroscopy. This paper provides evidence that stimulated neurons become exporters of lactate, suggesting proliferative physiology.

As the preceding review suggests, if proliferative physiology is present, can we extrapolate to adverse effects of proliferative physiology with neurodegeneration, particularly Alzheimer's disease? Here, a variety of central nervous system injuries, including the presence of beta-amyloid, and reactive astrogliosis (which can disrupt normal glycolysis), weakens astrocytes' relationship to neurons in the purported astrocyte shuttle of lactate to neurons. This cascade impairs normal brain homeostasis, impairs clearance of beta-amyloid, promotes cytokine release and inexorably leads to neurodegeneration.[79]

Microglial cell metabolic physiology is similarly at risk for proliferative physiology. Microglial cells routinely use glucose, FAO and glutamine, with glucose transporters expressed, to supply sufficient glucose intake.[80] Microglial-fueled metabolism may be associated with glial reactivity, with a fuel switch contributing to an underlying cause of hypothalamic dysregulation associated with obesity. There is no comment on proliferative physiology.[3]

Supportive cells, including astrocytes and microglial cells, aside, neurons also have cellular metabolic demands at nerve terminals. Neurotransmission requires ATP to support energetic demanding steps, including maintaining ionic gradients or sodium/potassium pumps and reversing changes in intracellular calcium that arise from opening voltage-gated calcium channels.[81] Energy demands in the brain are met by glycolysis and oxidative phosphorylation, with glycolysis dominating the early stages of recovery of synaptic function and dysregulation of glycolysis contributing to neurodegeneration.

Finally, glycogen availability comes into play during the intense activity of the nervous system when energy demand exceeds supply. Glycogen in astrocytes converts to lactate, some of which is transported to neurons, thereby protecting hypoglycemia and preserving neuronal function.[82] If there is impairment of conversion of lactate to pyruvate during cerebral metabolic stress, the protective effect of lactate is lost.

Taken together, we have supportive data on the adverse effects of proliferative physiology in the brain involving neurons, astrocytes, glial cells and synapses. Given the role of molecular hypometabolism in proliferative physiology, the next steps support brain research on metabolic abnormalities found in aerobic glycolysis in SEID and CIRS.

6.9 THE STUDY

Using a retrospective waiver for transcriptomic studies from Copernicus Group IRB, Cary, NC, a collation of clinical charts reviewed 112 consecutive de-identified patients who had transcriptomics testing done, including MHM. Most of the patients also had an anion gap, pulmonary artery pressures and NeuroQuant® testing. Not all cases with transcriptomics had an ancillary study. Control groups were from a single medical clinic.

6.9.1 Methods

We have permission to present molecular methods used for transcriptomic testing.

RNA collection, extraction and labeling PAXgene RNA blood collection tubes (www.pre-analytix.com/product-catalog/blood/rna/products/paxgene-blood-rna-tube/) were filled with venous blood, incubated for 4 hours at room temperature and then frozen at −80 °C until RNA extraction. According to the manufacturer's protocol, the total RNA underwent extraction with the Qiagen PAXgene Blood miRNA System kit. The total RNA was analyzed using an Agilent 2100 bioanalyzer (Agilent Technologies, United States) for RNA integrity and quantified using a NanoDrop ND-2000 (Wilmington, DE). Only samples with Agilent RIN scores ≥8 were sequenced.

6.9.2 SEQUENCING

Sequencing libraries were made from 1 µg of total RNA starting material with the Kapa Biosystems stranded mRNA-Seq kit (www.kapabiosystems.com) according to the manufacturer's instructions for the Illumina platform. The amplified library fragments were purified and checked for quality and concentration using an Advanced Analytical Fragment Analyzer™ to check the size and quality of the individual libraries and a Qubit for concentration. Equimolar amounts of individual libraries formed eight groups with a final round of quantification using an Agilent 2100 Bioanalyzer with a High Sensitivity DNA chip (Agilent Technologies, United States). The pooled samples of eight[8] were sequenced on an Illumina NextSeq 500 DNA sequencer using a Version 2, high output, 75-bp single-end sequencing reagent kit (Illumina, United States) with a target depth of 60 million reads per sample. The raw data files were streamed to the BaseSpace data warehouse (basespace.illumina.com) and de-multiplexed by sample into FASTQ files.

6.9.3 SEQUENCING ANALYSIS

FASTQ sequencing data in CLC Biomedical Genomics Workbench (BGW) analysis software version 4.0 mapped to gene regions of the human genome using the USC hgb37 build. Samples were divided into patient and control classes and subjected to Empirical analysis of DGE, as available in the EdgeR Bioconductor package (Robinson et al., 2010). Empirical analysis of DGE was run using all raw data, as suggested in the user guide, but also after using different quality filters on the data. Data filtering consisted of removing hemoglobin alpha and beta reads and scaling remaining entities into reads per million. Scaled data were then quantile normalized and filtered at four different, increasing expression levels, using genes present in either class at >0.3, 0.5, 0.75 and 1 reads/million. The study selected for significantly expressed genes for gene ontology (GO) and molecular pathway analysis for possible enrichment of genes compared with specific biological themes using Elsevier's Pathway Studio and the Database for Annotation, Visualization, and Integrated Discovery, v6.8 (DAVID).

6.9.4 NANOSTRING

Twenty-four total RNA samples (12 controls and 12 patients) were analyzed using the NanoString platform for direct, multiplexed analysis of mRNA to validate RNA Seq data (www.nanostring.com). This platform captures and detects probes on purified RNA with no enzymatic sample manipulation. The comparison used 100ng of total RNA against a panel of 185 genes. According to the manufacturer's recommendation, NanoString proof of principle laboratory in Seattle, WA, ran the samples.

6.9.5 RESULTS

We identified 4 groups in our total cohort of 112 Stage 1 patients. In Group 1, molecular hypometabolism was present with IRS2 upregulation in this cohort of 62 patients. The combination of metabolic hypometabolism and IRS2 upregulation suggests a mechanism for enhanced grey matter nuclear atrophy in our cases (see Table 6.1). The mean number of atrophic nuclei seen on NeuroQuant® (NQ) was 4.1. The mean IRS2 was 1.78, with 16.1% of patients exhibiting an increased size of a superior lateral ventricle, an untoward finding consistent with one of the following:

1. Obstruction of the flow of cerebral spinal fluid contributing to hydrocephalus (NPH).
2. Loss of substance of cortical grey.

No patients showed an increased Evan's Index, ruling out NPH. Eighty percent of cases had pulmonary hypertension (>30 mm Hg), with widened anion gap seen in 85% of cases.

In group 2, 26 patients had MHM present but IRS2 was negative. Mean atrophic grey matter nuclei were 3.0, suggesting that the enhanced glucose delivery for glycolysis seen in IRS2 positive has an increased incidence of atrophy of grey matter nuclei compared with those with MHM but with IRS2 negative. Mean IRS2 in cohort 2 was −0.97. Superior lateral ventricle enlargement was less common; 7.6% of patients had this abnormality. PAH occurred in 8%, and a widened anion gap occurred in 20%.

Group 3 had 16 patients, MHM negative and IRS2 negative. Mean atrophic nuclei was 2.8, with a mean IRS2 value of −1.67. Only one patient had superior lateral ventricle enlargement (6.1%). PAH was seen in no patients, while the anion gap widened in 33%.

Group 4 only had eight cases with MHM negative and IRS2 positive. Atrophic nuclei were 1.16, the lowest of all measured groups, with a mean IRS2 of 1.14. No superior lateral ventricle enlargement, PAH or widened anion gap was noted.

6.9.6 DISCUSSION

As we have discussed in detail, the MHM patients will have suppression of translocases and/or closed VDAC, as shown by elevated tubulins, use of itraconazole or reactive exposure to actinomycetes. An open VDAC is required to deliver pyruvate across the outer mitochondrial membrane. If pyruvate cannot get into the mitochondria, there will be no additional ATP. If enhanced glycolysis due to IRS2 positivity is present, an additional influx of glucose enters the cell for conversion by cytosolic aerobic glycolysis to lactic acid. Lactic acid is then exported outside the cell, contributing to metabolic acidosis.

The combination of metabolic hypometabolism and IRS2+ results suggests a proliferative mechanism for enhanced grey matter nuclear atrophy in our cases. However, we see that in the absence of translocases due to molecular hypometabolism, there is the effect of an increase in glucose delivery, flooding the cytosol without any transport of breakdown products of glycolysis into mitochondria. When converted to lactic acid, this excessive pyruvate will contribute to systemic metabolic acidosis and neuronal injury to grey matter nuclei and cortical grey and fomenting underlying PAH.

Note that PAH was defined by finding elevated levels of tricuspid regurgitation on baseline echocardiogram with a value for tricuspid regurgitation exceeding 2.5 meters per second and assuming right atrial pressure was 5 mm Hg. As noted previously, the measurement of tricuspid regurgitation was not a requirement for the performance of GENIE, and not all cases had echocardiogram testing done. Validation will need a larger trial.

Interestingly, measurement of anion gap was not required for the performance of transcriptomic testing but was frequently submitted with additional clinical materials by physicians.

Only upon reviewing Group 4 do we see that the absence of MHM and the presence of IRS2 positivity result in essentially an ablation of metabolic complications related to the interaction of inflammatory genes, ribosomal genes and nuclear-coded mitochondrial genes with metabolism.

If we do not have excessive glucose inputs due to IRS2 negativity, but MHM is present, the metabolic complications of metabolic acidosis and PAH are less severe.

6.10 CONCLUSIONS

The complexity of cellular use of glucose includes diverting metabolites from glycolysis, interaction with inflammatory mediators, aerobic glycolysis and biosynthetic pathways used to make needed nucleotides, lipids, amino acids and intermediates. Differential gene activation/suppression influences the metabolic stress response elements. Both metabolic and inflammatory systems interact to maintain cell viability, energy conservation and cell proliferation.

When systems go awry, for example when an imbalance of glycosylation genes OGT and OGA persists beyond recovery from stressors such as trauma, ischemia or infection, an acute response can be converted into a chronic disease, such as insulin resistance.

MHM is such a process. When chronic fatigue, as part of a multisystem, multi-symptom illness, becomes entrenched, possibly after exposure to ribotoxins, especially those made by actinomycetes, we now know to look for adaptive, survival-based abnormalities in ribosomal genes, translocases and ATP synthases, among others.

Compared with control data sets, we see a group of patients here showing a correlation of MHM+/IRS2 (+) with worsening end-organ injury in untreated Stage 1 CIRS patients. There is a widened anion gap, consistent with metabolic acidosis. There is an increased percentage of cases in this group with atrophic grey matter nuclei or enlarged superior lateral ventricle enlargement, as shown by NeuroQuant®. PAH is far more common in this group compared with MHM + / (–) IRS2; MHM (–) / (–) IRS2; and MHM (–) / IRS2 (+).

When evaluated by published metabolic literature, these data are consistent with the adverse effects of proliferative physiology, which has its roots in aerobic glycolysis. In turn, aerobic glycolysis requires compartmentalization of glucose metabolism. A closed VDAC hastens the process. Patients found by transcriptomic testing showing MHM+/IRS2 (+) may well benefit from additional testing by NeuroQuant®, a comprehensive metabolic panel to determine anion gap, and echocardiogram. If available, flow cytometry for CD4+CD25++ cells and CD4+CD25++CD127–/lo is recommended.

While proliferative physiology, a systemic process, is required for acute host defenses, persistent proliferative states are manifestly not healthy when the host has MHM. The host response once again becomes the enemy. As long as standard CIRS treatment protocols are followed carefully and in order, without omissions, salutary benefits, including repair of CNS injury, can reasonably be expected.

Weaknesses of this study include missing data, as not all transcriptomic patients had echocardiograms, NeuroQuant® and comprehensive metabolic panel performed. As such, a prospective study will be necessary. Further, the absence of T-reg assays leaves a hole in analysis, as the proliferative model would predict marked T-reg deficiency in Group 1, with steadily increasing numbers through Group 4 (Table 6.1).

TABLE 6.1

Stage 1 of Treatment

	MHM+IRS2+	MHM+IRS2–	MHM–IRS2–	MHM–IRS2+	Controls
N	62	26	16	8	15
Atrophic nuclei/6	4.1	3.0	2.8	1.2	1.4
SLV increase	16.1	7.6	6.1	0	0
Mean IRS2	1.78	–0.97	–1.67	1.14	1.33
Anion gap >12	85	20	33[a]	0	1
PASP increase	80	8	0[a]	0	0

[a] N < 4.

Potential conflict of interest: Dr. Shoemaker holds an interest in ProgeneDx, a company that sells GENIE tests.

BIBLIOGRAPHY

1. Lunt, Sophia Y., and Matthew G. Vander Heiden. "Aerobic Glycolysis: Meeting the Metabolic Requirements of Cell Proliferation." *Annual Review of Cell and Developmental Biology* 27, no. 1 (2011): 441–64. https://doi.org/10.1146/annurev-cellbio-092910-154237.
2. Shoemaker, Ryan. "RNA-Seq on Patients With Chronic Inflammatory Response Syndrome (CIRS) Treated With Vasoactive Intestinal Peptide (VIP) Shows a Shift in Metabolic State and Innate Immune Functions That Coincide With Healing." *Medical Research Archives* 4, no. 7 (2016). https://doi.org/10.18103/mra.v4i7.862.
3. Ryan, James C., Qingzhong Wu, and Ritchie C. Shoemaker. "Transcriptomic Signatures in Whole Blood of Patients Who Acquire a Chronic Inflammatory Response Syndrome (CIRS) Following an Exposure to the Marine Toxin Ciguatoxin." *BMC Medical Genomics* 8, no. 1 (2015): 1–12. https://doi.org/10.1186/s12920-015-0089-x.
4. Shoemaker, Ritchie C., Dennis House, and James C. Ryan. "Vasoactive Intestinal Polypeptide (VIP) Corrects Chronic Inflammatory Response Syndrome (CIRS) Acquired Following Exposure to Water-Damaged Buildings." *Health* 5, no. 3 (2013): 396–401. https://doi.org/10.4236/health.2013.53053.
5. Fukuda, Keiji, Stephen E. Strauss, Ian Hickie, Michael C. Sharpe, James G. Dobbins, and Anthony Komaroff. "The Chronic Fatigue Syndrome." *Journal of Chronic Fatigue Syndrome* 1, no. 2 (1995): 67–84. https://doi.org/10.1300/j092v01n02_06.
6. Jason, Leonard A., Madison Sunnquist, Abigail Brown, Julia L. Newton, Elin Bolle Strand, and Suzanne D. Vernon. "Chronic Fatigue Syndrome Versus Systemic Exertion Intolerance Disease." *Fatigue: Biomedicine, Health & Behavior* 3, no. 3 (2015): 127–41. https://doi.org/10.1080/21641846.2015.1051291.
7. Shoemaker, R., S. McMahon, and M. Dooley. " Diagnostic Process for CIRS: A Consensus Statement Report of the Consensus Committee of Surviving Mold." *IMR* 4, no. 5 (2018): 1–47.
8. Shi, Xinying, Prashant K. Khade, Karissa Y. Sanbonmatsu, and Simpson Joseph. "Functional Role of the Sarcin–Ricin Loop of the 23S Rrna in the Elongation Cycle of Protein Synthesis." *Journal of Molecular Biology* 419, nos. 3–4 (2012): 125–38. https://doi.org/10.1016/j.jmb.2012.03.016.
9. Prasun, Pankaj. "Mitochondrial Genetics." *Mitochondrial Medicine*, 2019, 7–9. https://doi.org/10.1016/b978-0-12-817006-9.00003-4.
10. Grevel, Alexander, and Thomas Becker. "Porins as Helpers in Mitochondrial Protein Translocation." *Biological Chemistry* 401, nos. 6–7 (2020): 699–708. https://doi.org/10.1515/hsz-2019-0438.
11. Ellenrieder, Lars, Martin P. Dieterle, Kim Nguyen Doan, Christoph U. Mårtensson, Alessia Floerchinger, María Luisa Campo, Nikolaus Pfanner, and Thomas Becker. "Dual Role of Mitochondrial Porin in Metabolite Transport Across the Outer Membrane and Protein Transfer to the Inner Membrane." *Molecular Cell* 73, no. 5 (2019): 1056–65. https://doi.org/10.1016/j.molcel.2018.12.014.
12. Krimmer, Thomas, Doron Rapaport, Michael T. Ryan, Chris Meisinger, C. Kenneth Kassenbrock, Elizabeth Blachly-Dyson, Michael Forte, M. G. Douglas, W. Neupert, F. E. Nargang, and N. Pfanner. "Biogenesis of Porin of the Outer Mitochondrial Membrane Involves an Import Pathway Via Receptors and the General Import Pore of the Tom Complex." *Journal of Cell Biology* 152, no. 2 (2001): 289–300. https://doi.org/10.1083/jcb.152.2.289.
13. Potter, Michelle, Emma Newport, and Karl J. Morten. "The Warburg Effect: 80 Years On." *Biochemical Society Transactions* 44, no. 5 (2016): 1499–505. https://doi.org/10.1042/bst20160094.
14. Burns, Jorge, and Gina Manda. "Metabolic Pathways of the Warburg Effect in Health and Disease: Perspectives of Choice, Chain or Chance." *International Journal of Molecular Sciences* 18, no. 12 (2017): 2755. https://doi.org/10.3390/ijms18122755.
15. Shoshan-Barmatz, Varda, Edna Nahon-Crystal, Anna Shteinfer-Kuzmine, and Rajeev Gupta. "VDAC1, Mitochondrial Dysfunction, and Alzheimer's Disease." *Pharmacological Research* 131 (2018): 87–101. https://doi.org/10.1016/j.phrs.2018.03.010.
16. Manczak, M., and P. H. Reddy. "Abnormal Interaction of VDAC1 With Amyloid Beta and Phosphorylated Tau Causes Mitochondrial Dysfunction in Alzheimer's Disease." *Human Molecular Genetics* 21, no. 23 (2012): 5131–46. https://doi.org/10.1093/hmg/dds360.
17. Manczak, Maria, and P. Hemachandra Reddy. "RNA Silencing of Genes Involved in Alzheimer's Disease Enhances Mitochondrial Function and Synaptic Activity."

18. Reddy, P. Hemachandra. "Is the Mitochondrial Outermembrane Protein VDAC1 Therapeutic Target for Alzheimer's Disease?" *Biochimica et Biophysica Acta (BBA) - Molecular Basis of Disease* 1832, no. 1 (2013): 67–75. https://doi.org/10.1016/j.bbadis.2012.09.003.

19. Smilansky, Angela, Liron Dangoor, Itay Nakdimon, Danya Ben-Hail, Dario Mizrachi, and Varda Shoshan-Barmatz. "The Voltage-Dependent Anion Channel 1 Mediates Amyloid β Toxicity and Represents a Potential Target for Alzheimer Disease Therapy." *Journal of Biological Chemistry* 290, no. 52 (2015): 30670–83. https://doi.org/10.1074/jbc.m115.691493.

20. van der Poll, Tom, Frank L. van de Veerdonk, Brendon P. Scicluna, and Mihai G. Netea. "The Immunopathology of Sepsis and Potential Therapeutic Targets." *Nature Reviews Immunology* 17, no. 7 (2017): 407–20. https://doi.org/10.1038/nri.2017.36.

21. Shoemaker, Ritchie C., Dennis House, and James C. Ryan. "Structural Brain Abnormalities in Patients With Inflammatory Illness Acquired Following Exposure to Water-Damaged Buildings: A Volumetric MRI Study Using NeuroQuant®." *Neurotoxicology and Teratology* 45 (2014): 18–26. https://doi.org/10.1016/j.ntt.2014.06.004.

22. Shoemaker, R., S. McMahon, and J. Ryan. "Reduction in Forebrain Parenchymal and Cortical Grey Matter Swelling Across Treatment Groups in Patients With Inflammatory Illness Acquired Following Exposure to Water-Damaged Buildings." *Journal of Neuroscience and Clinical Research* 1 (2016): 1–4.

23. Shoemaker, Ritchie. "Intranasal VIP Safely Restores Volume to Multiple Grey Matter Nuclei in Patients With CIRS." *Internal Medicine Review* 3, no. 4 (2017): 1–14. https://doi.org/10.18103/imr.v3i4.412.

24. Shoemaker, R., and J. Ryan. A Gene Primer for Health Care Providers: The Genomics of CIRS and Associated Molecular Pathways: Interpreting the Transcriptomics Results. *Ebook*, 2018.

25. Vander Heiden, Matthew G., Lewis C. Cantley, and Craig B. Thompson. "Understanding the Warburg Effect: The Metabolic Requirements of Cell Proliferation." *Science* 324, no. 5930 (2009): 1029–33. https://doi.org/10.1126/science.1160809.

26. van Beek, Hans. "Faculty Opinions Recommendation of Genome-Scale Metabolic Modeling Elucidates the Role of Proliferative Adaptation in Causing the Warburg Effect." *Faculty Opinions – Post-Publication Peer Review of the Biomedical Literature*, 2011. https://doi.org/10.3410/f.13357132.14726450.

27. César Rosa, José, and Marcelo de Cerqueira César. "Role of Hexokinase and VDAC in Neurological Disorders." *Current Molecular Pharmacology* 9, no. 4 (2016): 320–31. https://doi.org/10.2174/1874467209666160112123036.

28. Kuehn, Bridget M. "In Alzheimer Research, Glucose Metabolism Moves to Center Stage." *JAMA* 323, no. 4 (2020): 297. https://doi.org/10.1001/jama.2019.20939.

29. Wu, Long, Xin Zhang, and Liqin Zhao. "Human ApoE Isoforms Differentially Modulate Brain Glucose and Ketone Body Metabolism: Implications for Alzheimer's Disease Risk Reduction and Early Intervention." *The Journal of Neuroscience* 38, no. 30 (2018): 6665–81. https://doi.org/10.1523/jneurosci.2262-17.2018.

30. Ryan, John J., and Stephen L. Archer. "Emerging Concepts in the Molecular Basis of Pulmonary Arterial Hypertension." *Circulation* 131, no. 19 (2015): 1691–702. https://doi.org/10.1161/circulationaha.114.006979.

31. Archer, Stephen L., Yong-Hu Fang, John J. Ryan, and Lin Piao. "Metabolism and Bioenergetics in the Right Ventricle and Pulmonary Vasculature in Pulmonary Hypertension." *Pulmonary Circulation* 3, no. 1 (2013): 144–52. https://doi.org/10.4103/2045-8932.109960.

32. Paulin, Roxane, and Evangelos D. Michelakis. "The Metabolic Theory of Pulmonary Arterial Hypertension." *Circulation Research* 115, no. 1 (2014): 148–64. https://doi.org/10.1161/circresaha.115.301130.

33. Dromparis, Peter, Gopinath Sutendra, and Evangelos D. Michelakis. "The Role of Mitochondria in Pulmonary Vascular Remodeling." *Journal of Molecular Medicine* 88, no. 10 (2010): 1003–10. https://doi.org/10.1007/s00109-010-0670-x.

34. Tuder, Rubin M., Laura A. Davis, and Brian B. Graham. "Targeting Energetic Metabolism." *American Journal of Respiratory and Critical Care Medicine* 185, no. 3 (2012): 260–66. https://doi.org/10.1164/rccm.201108-1536pp.

35. Shoshan-Barmatz, Varda, Nurit Keinan, and Hilal Zaid. "Uncovering the Role of VDAC in the Regulation of Cell Life and Death." *Journal of Bioenergetics and Biomembranes* 40, no. 3 (2008): 183–91. https://doi.org/10.1007/s10863-008-9147-9.

36. Heslop, K. A., A. Rovini, E. G. Hunt, D. Fang, M. E. Morris, C. F. Christie, M. B. Gooz, D. N. DeHart, Y. Dang, J. J. Lemasters, and E. N. Maldonado. "JNK Activation and Translocation to Mitochondria Mediates Mitochondrial Dysfunction and Cell Death Induced by VDAC Opening and Sorafenib in Hepatocarcinoma Cells." *Biochemical Pharmacology* 171 (2020): 113728. https://doi.org/10.1016/j.bcp.2019.113728.

37. Andersson, M. A., R. Mikkola, R. M. Kroppenstedt, F. A. Rainey, J. Peltola, J. Helin, K. Sivonen, and M. S. Salkinoja-Salonen. "The Mitochondrial Toxin Produced by Streptomyces Griseus Strains Isolated From an Indoor Environment is Valinomycin." *Applied and Environmental Microbiology* 64, no. 12 (1998): 4767–73. https://doi.org/10.1128/aem.64.12.4767-4773.1998.

38. DeHart, David N., John J. Lemasters, and Eduardo N. Maldonado. "Erastin-Like Anti-Warburg Agents Prevent Mitochondrial Depolarization Induced by Free Tubulin and Decrease Lactate Formation in Cancer Cells." *Slas Discovery: Advancing the Science of Drug Discovery* 23, no. 1 (2017): 23–33. https://doi.org/10.1177/2472555217731556.

39. Azoulay-Zohar, Heftsi, Adrian Israelson, Salah Abu-Hamad, and Varda Shoshan-Barmatz. "In Self-Defence: Hexokinase Promotes Voltage-Dependent Anion Channel Closure and Prevents Mitochondria-Mediated Apoptotic Cell Death." *Biochemical Journal* 377, no. 2 (2004): 347–55. https://doi.org/10.1042/bj20031465.

40. "Simultaneous Targeting of NPC1 and VDAC1 by Itraconazole Leads to Synergistic Inhibition of Mtor Signaling and Angiogenesis." n.d. https://doi.org/10.1021/acschembio.6b00849.s003.

41. Head, Sarah A., Wei Shi, Liang Zhao, Kirill Gorshkov, Kalyan Pasunooti, Yue Chen, Zhiyou Deng, R. J. Li, J. S. Shim, W. Tan, and T. Hartung. "Antifungal Drug Itraconazole Targets VDAC1 to Modulate the AMPK/Mtor Signaling Axis in Endothelial Cells." *Proceedings of the National Academy of Sciences* 112, no. 52 (2015): E7276–85. https://doi.org/10.1073/pnas.1512867112.

42. Puurand, Marju, Kersti Tepp, Natalja Timohhina, Jekaterina Aid, Igor Shevchuk, Vladimir Chekulayev, and Tuuli Kaambre. "Tubulin βII and βIII Isoforms as the Regulators of VDAC Channel Permeability in Health and Disease." *Cells* 8, no. 3 (2019): 239. https://doi.org/10.3390/cells8030239.

43. Wang, Hai, Can Liu, Yongxin Zhao, and Ge Gao. "Mitochondria Regulation in Ferroptosis." *European Journal of Cell Biology* 99, no. 1 (2020): 151058. https://doi.org/10.1016/j.ejcb.2019.151058.

44. Zhou, Hui-Ren, Kaiyu He, Jeff Landgraf, Xiao Pan, and James Pestka. "Direct Activation of Ribosome-Associated Double-Stranded RNA-Dependent Protein Kinase (PKR) by Deoxynivalenol, Anisomycin and Ricin: A New Model for Ribotoxic Stress Response Induction." *Toxins* 6, no. 12 (2014): 3406–25. https://doi.org/10.3390/toxins6123406.

45. Cargnello, Marie, and Philippe P. Roux. "Activation and Function of the Mapks and Their Substrates, the MAPK-Activated Protein Kinases." *Microbiology and Molecular Biology Reviews* 76, no. 2 (2012): 496–96. https://doi.org/10.1128/mmbr.00013-12.

46. Shoemaker, R., and D. Lark. "HERTSMI-2 and ERMI: "Correlating Human Health Risk with Mold Specific QPCR in Water-Damaged Buildings"." In *#658 Proceedings of the 14th International Conference on Indoor Air Quality and Climate, International Society for Indoor Air Quality and Climate*, Ghent, 2016.

47. Oliveira, Joana Moitinho, Sandra A. Rebuffat, Rosa Gasa, and Ramon Gomis. "Targeting Type 2 Diabetes: Lessons From a Knockout Model of Insulin Receptor Substrate 2." *Canadian Journal of Physiology and Pharmacology* 92, no. 8 (2014): 613–20. https://doi.org/10.1139/cjpp-2014-0114.

48. Long, Yun Chau, Zhiyong Cheng, Kyle D. Copps, and Morris F. White. "Insulin Receptor Substrates IRS1 and IRS2 Coordinate Skeletal Muscle Growth and Metabolism Via the AKT and AMPK Pathways." *Molecular and Cellular Biology* 31, no. 3 (2011): 430–41. https://doi.org/10.1128/mcb.00983-10.

49. Schmitz-Peiffer, Carsten, and Jonathan Whitehead. "IRS-1 Regulation in Health and Disease." *IUBMB Life (International Union of Biochemistry and Molecular Biology: Life)* 55, no. 7 (2003): 367–74. https://doi.org/10.1080/1521654031000138569.

50. Benzi, L., P. Cecchetti, A. M. Ciccarone, A. Nardone, A. Nardone, E. Merola, R. Maggiorelli, F. Campi, G. Di Cianni, and R. Navalesi. "Inhibition of Endosomal Acidification in Normal Cells Mimics the Derangements of Cellular Insulin and Insulin-Receptor Metabolism Observed in Non-Insulin-Dependent Diabetes Mellitus." *Metabolism* 46, no. 11 (1997): 1259–65. https://doi.org/10.1016/s0026-0495(97)90227-4.

51. Desbuguois, B. "Role of Acidic Subcellular Compartments in the Degradation of Internalized Insulin and in the Recycling of the Internalized Insulin Receptor in Liver Cells: In Vivo and In Vitro Studies." *Diabetes Metab* 18 (1992): 104–12.

52. Benzi, L., A. M. Ciccarone, P. Cecchetti, G. DiCianni, F. Caricato, L. Trincavelli, L. Volpe, and R. Navalesi. "Intracellular Hyperinsulinism: A Metabolic Characteristic of Obesity With and Without Type 2 Diabetes." *Diabetes Research and Clinical Practice* 46, no. 3 (1999): 231–37. https://doi.org/10.1016/s0168-8227(99)00100-x.

53. Culley, Miranda K., and Stephen Y. Chan. "Mitochondrial Metabolism in Pulmonary Hypertension: Beyond Mountains There Are Mountains." *Journal of Clinical Investigation* 128, no. 9 (2018): 3704–15. https://doi.org/10.1172/jci120847.

54. Liu, Pengfei, Yue Gu, Jie Luo, Peng Ye, Yaguo Zheng, Wande Yu, and Shaoliang Chen. "Inhibition of SRC Activation Reverses Pulmonary Vascular Remodeling in Experimental Pulmonary Arterial Hypertension Via AKT/MTOR/HIF-1 Signaling Pathway." *Experimental Cell Research* 380, no. 1 (2019): 36–46. https://doi.org/10.1016/j.yexcr.2019.02.022.

55. Ryan, John J., and Stephen L. Archer. "The Right Ventricle in Pulmonary Arterial Hypertension." *Circulation Research* 115, no. 1 (2014): 176–88. https://doi.org/10.1161/circresaha.113.301129.

56. Gomez-Arroyo, Jose, Shiro Mizuno, Karol Szczepanek, Benjamin Van Tassell, Ramesh Natarajan, Cristobal G. dos Remedios, Jennifer I. Drake, et al. "Metabolic Gene Remodeling and Mitochondrial Dysfunction in Failing Right Ventricular Hypertrophy Secondary to Pulmonary Arterial Hypertension." *Circulation: Heart Failure* 6, no. 1 (2013): 136–44. https://doi.org/10.1161/circheartfailure.111.966127.

57. Gabriel, Sarah Sharon, and Axel Kallies. "Sugars and Fat - A Healthy Way to Generate Functional Regulatory T Cells." *European Journal of Immunology* 46, no. 12 (2016): 2705–9. https://doi.org/10.1002/eji.201646663.

58. Thenappan, Thenappan, Mark L. Ormiston, John J. Ryan, and Stephen L. Archer. "Pulmonary Arterial Hypertension: Pathogenesis and Clinical Management." *BMJ*, 2018. https://doi.org/10.1136/bmj.j5492.

59. Mukhopadhyay, Rupak, Jie Jia, Abul Arif, Partho Sarothi Ray, and Paul L. Fox. "The Gait System: A Gatekeeper of Inflammatory Gene Expression." *Trends in Biochemical Sciences* 34, no. 7 (2009): 324–31. https://doi.org/10.1016/j.tibs.2009.03.004.

60. Arif, Abul, Peng Yao, Fulvia Terenzi, Jie Jia, Partho Sarothi Ray, and Paul L. Fox. "The Gait Translational Control System." *WIREs RNA* 9, no. 2 (2017): e1441. https://doi.org/10.1002/wrna.1441.

61. Arif, Abul, Piyali Chatterjee, Robyn A. Moodt, and Paul L. Fox. "Heterotrimeric Gait Complex Drives Transcript-Selective Translation Inhibition in Murine Macrophages." *Molecular and Cellular Biology* 32, no. 24 (2012): 5046–55. https://doi.org/10.1128/mcb.01168-12.

62. Stienstra, Rinke, Romana T. Netea-Maier, Niels P. Riksen, Leo A. B. Joosten, and Mihai G. Netea. "Specific and Complex Reprogramming of Cellular Metabolism in Myeloid Cells During Innate Immune Responses." *Cell Metabolism* 26, no. 1 (2017): 142–56. https://doi.org/10.1016/j.cmet.2017.06.001.

63. Chang, Chih-Hao, Jonathan D. Curtis, Leonard B. Maggi, Brandon Faubert, Alejandro V. Villarino, David O'Sullivan, Stanley Ching-Cheng Huang, G. J. Van Der Windt, J. Blagih, J. Qiu, and J. D. Weber. "Posttranscriptional Control of T Cell Effector Function by Aerobic Glycolysis." *Cell* 153, no. 6 (2013): 1239–51. https://doi.org/10.1016/j.cell.2013.05.016.

64. Gumaa, K. A., and Patricia McLean. "The Pentose Phosphate Pathway of Glucose Metabolism. Enzyme Profiles and Transient and Steady-State Content of Intermediates of Alternative Pathways of Glucose Metabolism in Krebs Ascites Cells." *Biochemical Journal* 115, no. 5 (1969): 1009–29. https://doi.org/10.1042/bj1151009.

65. Araujo, Lindsey, Phillip Khim, Haik Mkhikian, Christie-Lynn Mortales, and Michael Demetriou. "Glycolysis and Glutaminolysis Cooperatively Control T Cell Function by Limiting Metabolite Supply to N-Glycosylation." *eLife* 6 (2017). https://doi.org/10.7554/elife.21330.

66. Chatham, John C., Laszlo G. Nöt, Norbert Fülöp, and Richard B. Marchase. "Hexosamine Biosynthesis and Protein O-Glycosylation." *Shock* 29, no. 4 (2008): 431–40. https://doi.org/10.1097/shk.0b013e3181598bad.

67. Teo, Chin Fen, Edith E. Wollaston-Hayden, and Lance Wells. "Hexosamine Flux, the O-Glcnac Modification, and the Development of Insulin Resistance in Adipocytes." *Molecular and Cellular Endocrinology* 318, nos. 1–2 (2010): 44–53. https://doi.org/10.1016/j.mce.2009.09.022.

68. Özcan, Sabire, Sreenath S. Andrali, and Jamie E. L. Cantrell. "Modulation of Transcription Factor Function by O-Glcnac Modification." *Biochimica et Biophysica Acta (BBA) - Gene Regulatory Mechanisms* 1799, nos. 5–6 (2010): 353–64. https://doi.org/10.1016/j.bbagrm.2010.02.005.

69. Park, Seung Yoon, Jiwon Ryu, and Wan Lee. "O-Glcnac Modification on IRS-1 and AKT2 by Pugnac Inhibits Their Phosphorylation and Induces Insulin Resistance in Rat Primary Adipocytes." *Experimental & Molecular Medicine* 37, no. 3 (2005): 220–29. https://doi.org/10.1038/emm.2005.30.

70. Vosseller, Keith, Lance Wells, M. Daniel Lane, and Gerald W. Hart. "Elevated Nucleocytoplasmic Glycosylation by O-Glcnac Results in Insulin Resistance Associated with Defects in Akt Activation in 3T3-L1 Adipocytes." *Proceedings of the National Academy of Sciences* 99, no. 8 (2002): 5313–18. https://doi.org/10.1073/pnas.072072399.

71. Kamemura, Kazuo, and Gerald W. Hart. "Dynamic Interplay Between O-Glycosylation and O-Phosphorylation of Nucleocytoplasmic Proteins: A New Paradigm for Metabolic Control of Signal Transduction and Transcription." *Progress in Nucleic Acid Research and Molecular Biology*, 2003, 107–36. https://doi.org/10.1016/s0079-6603(03)01004-3.

72. Lim, Jae-Min, Edith E. Wollaston-Hayden, Chin Fen Teo, Dorothy Hausman, and Lance Wells. "Quantitative Secretome and Glycome of Primary Human Adipocytes During Insulin Resistance." *Clinical Proteomics* 11, no. 1 (2014): 1–23. https://doi.org/10.1186/1559-0275-11-20.

73. Buse, Maria G. "Hexosamines, Insulin Resistance, and the Complications of Diabetes: Current Status." *American Journal of Physiology-Endocrinology and Metabolism* 290, no. 1 (2006). https://doi.org/10.1152/ajpendo.00329.2005.

74. Charbonnier, Louis-Marie, Ye Cui, Emmanuel Stephen-Victor, Hani Harb, David Lopez, Jack J. Bleesing, Maria I. Garcia-Lloret, K. Chen, A. Ozen, P. Carmeliet, and M. O. Li. "Functional Reprogramming of Regulatory T Cells in the Absence of Foxp3." *Nature Immunology* 20, no. 9 (2019): 1208–19. https://doi.org/10.1038/s41590-019-0442-x.

75. Díaz-García, Carlos Manlio, Rebecca Mongeon, Carolina Lahmann, Dorothy Koveal, Hannah Zucker, and Gary Yellen. "Neuronal Stimulation Triggers Neuronal Glycolysis and Not Lactate Uptake." *Cell Metabolism* 26, no. 2 (2017): 361–74. https://doi.org/10.1016/j.cmet.2017.06.021.

76. Yellen, Gary. "Fueling Thought: Management of Glycolysis and Oxidative Phosphorylation in Neuronal Metabolism." *Journal of Cell Biology* 217, no. 7 (2018): 2235–46. https://doi.org/10.1083/jcb.201803152.

77. Tyssowski, Kelsey M., Nicholas R. DeStefino, Jin-Hyung Cho, Carissa J. Dunn, Robert G. Poston, Crista E. Carty, Richard D. Jones, S. M. Chang, P. Romeo, M. K. Wurzelmann, and J. M. Ward. "Different Neuronal Activity Patterns Induce Different Gene Expression Programs." *Neuron* 98, no. 3 (2018): 530–46. https://doi.org/10.1016/j.neuron.2018.04.001.

78. Díaz-García, Carlos Manlio, and Gary Yellen. "Neurons Rely on Glucose Rather Than Astrocytic Lactate During Stimulation." *Journal of Neuroscience Research* 97, no. 8 (2018): 883–89. https://doi.org/10.1002/jnr.24374.

79. Fu, Wen, and Jack H. Jhamandas. "Role of Astrocytic Glycolytic Metabolism in Alzheimer's Disease Pathogenesis." *Biogerontology* 15, no. 6 (2014): 579–86. https://doi.org/10.1007/s10522-014-9525-0.

80. Kalsbeek, Martin J. T., Laurie Mulder, and Chun-Xia Yi. "Microglia Energy Metabolism in Metabolic Disorder." *Molecular and Cellular Endocrinology* 438 (2016): 27–35. https://doi.org/10.1016/j.mce.2016.09.028.

81. Ashrafi, Ghazaleh, and Timothy A. Ryan. "Glucose Metabolism in Nerve Terminals." *Current Opinion in Neurobiology* 45 (2017): 156–61. https://doi.org/10.1016/j.conb.2017.03.007.

82. Falkowska, Anna, Izabela Gutowska, Marta Goschorska, Przemysław Nowacki, Dariusz Chlubek, and Irena Baranowska-Bosiacka. "Energy Metabolism of the Brain, Including the Cooperation Between Astrocytes and Neurons, Especially in the Context of Glycogen Metabolism." *International Journal of Molecular Sciences* 16, no. 11 (2015): 25959–81. https://doi.org/10.3390/ijms161125939.

7 Urinary Mycotoxin Testing
An Understanding of Its Use in the Evaluation of Human Health

Ritchie Shoemaker, David Lark and April Vukelic

CONTENTS

7.1 INTRODUCTION

There are multiple definitions of mycotoxins. Simple approaches such as "secondary metabolites of fungi that can injure humans and other animals" omit potentially pathogenic compounds or fungal elements, including beta glucans, hemolysins, mannans and spirocyclic drimanes. Defining mycotoxins as "toxic substances made by fungi" would include other secondary metabolites like antibiotics and immune suppressants. The main role of mycotoxins is to enhance the efficiency of predation on plants,[1] not acting as offensive or defensive functions, as is oft pontificated.

These attempts at defining mycotoxins fail to address the problem of including a mechanism of injury or toxicity in vivo. Consideration of route of exposure such as ingestion of mycotoxins or skin exposure versus inhalation brings about additional confounders. Assessing inhalation exposure injury stemming from exposure to mycotoxins in vitro ignores (i) protective host mechanisms, including antigen presentation; (ii) loss of regulatory control of immune responses; and in the case of water-damaged buildings (WDB), (iii) eliminates the role of inflammatory responses, which taken as a whole, has been called chronic inflammatory response syndrome (CIRS) since 2010. CIRS shows innate immune activation following exposure to a diverse series of immunogenic effectors, including over 30 published effectors found inside WDB.

As we have seen,[2] omitting consideration of differential gene activation following exposure to mycotoxins ignores the main mechanism of mycotoxin injury to people, namely, ribotoxin and ribosomal inhibitory protein attack on ribosomal production (including initiation, elongation and termination) of protein.[3]

A more detailed definition of mycotoxins, yet one that is still incomplete, focuses more on the role of mycotoxins in plants:[4]

DOI: 10.1201/b23304-8

Mycotoxins are toxic secondary metabolic products of molds present on almost all agricultural commodities worldwide. Unlike primary metabolites (sugars, amino acids, and other substances), secondary metabolites are not essential in the normal metabolic function of the fungus. Other known secondary metabolites are phytotoxins and antibiotics.

Currently, there are around 400 mycotoxins reported. These compounds occur under natural conditions in feed as well as in food. Mycotoxins include aflatoxins, trichothecenes, fumonisins, zearalenone, ochratoxin, and ergot alkaloids. Different strains of fungi produce mycotoxins, and each strain can produce more than one mycotoxin.

Each plant can be affected by more than one fungus, and each fungus can produce more than one mycotoxin. Consequently, there is a high probability that many mycotoxins are present in one feed ingredient, thus increasing the chances of interaction between mycotoxins and synergistic effects, which are of great concern in livestock health and productivity. Synergistic effects occur when the combined effects of two mycotoxins (even at low levels) are greater than individual effects of each toxin alone.

Given that mycotoxins in feed and food are metabolized (in stomach, gut and liver) to make new metabolites, we must expand our consideration of the adverse effects of ingestion to include consumption of and endogenous production of metabolites from parent mycotoxins. These compounds can stay in the blood for variable amounts of time before appearing in the urine, as enterohepatic recirculation can greatly reduce fecal excretion.[5] Urinary excretion of mycotoxins and metabolites has become the main source of information regarding dietary exposure and metabolism, with robust literature on findings of mycotoxins in the urine of cases and controls.

We will review pertinent literature regarding mycotoxins in food and mycotoxins found in the urine in control populations to understand the firm stance of the Centers for Disease Control and Prevention (CDC) against the use of urinary mycotoxin testing as an indication for use of antifungals.[6] The CDC acknowledges that healthy controls can have urinary mycotoxins and their metabolites.

Consider a functional definition of mycotoxins as different from the preceding one:

Mycotoxins are products of fungal metabolism in which secondary metabolites are manufactured in response to environmental stimuli that turn on mycotoxin synthetic gene clusters in the fungi, so they can make products that can be directly injurious to animals and people, and indirectly by adversely affecting protein production by impairing the function of the sarcin-ricin loop in ribosomes and mitoribosomes, and mitochondrial function by interfering with nuclear-encoded mitochondrial gene function.

We cannot limit our discussion to naturally occurring mycotoxins as the main source of adverse human health effects. Fungi live in ecosystems where many bacteria and actinobacteria co-exist.[7] Actinobacteria ("actinos") are adept at making toxic compounds and manufacturing ribotoxins that co-occur with mycotoxins. Actinobacteria are richly endowed with gene sequences to make a host of bioactive compounds,[8] including antibiotics, anti-virals, anti-parasites and immune suppressants.

We need to separate toxins made by actinobacteria from endotoxins and fungal mycotoxins if we are going to impute adverse human health effects to mycotoxins when we think about biological exposures.

7.2   DIETARY MYCOTOXINS

For our discussion herein, we will be looking at three main categories of mycotoxins commonly ingested. Trichothecenes include some of the "dreaded" toxins made by some *Stachybotrys* spp. However, trichothecenes also come from *Aspergillus* species.[9] Trichothecenes are widely known, with type A and B toxins described. These compounds share unique structures, which in turn, create a lack of specificity when measured using enzyme-linked immunosorbent analysis (ELISA). Deoxynivalenol (DON) is a by-product of fungal gene activation in that DON will induce the production of peroxidases that block the generation of hydrogen peroxide by a plant when the

Aspergillus species eat the plant.[1] The idea that fungi make mycotoxins as a defensive mechanism or as an offensive weapon to kill other fungi is not well supported.

The second category of mycotoxins of concern is ochratoxins. Ochratoxins have notoriety in the medical literature for their ability to cause renal injury, called Balkan nephropathy. The scientists named the condition after the geographic region of its discovery, but renal injury from ochratoxin is rare in the United States.

The third group of mycotoxins of focus is aflatoxins. Several species of *Aspergillus*, especially *A. flavus*, make aflatoxins. Aflatoxins have a reputation for causing human health effects, including liver damage and possibly cancer. However, when we discuss mycotoxins and prevention of mycotoxin injury following ingestion, it appears, at least in pigs, that supplementation of protein in the diet, to include glutamic acid in small amounts (possibly as low as 5 mg daily) every week, can prevent mycotoxin injury.

Trichothecenes are associated with satratoxins and roridins. Also, *Wallemia* sp. (and *Aspergillus* sp.) is associated with sterigmatocystin (STC) production. *Chaetomium* spp. has its own toxins, including chaetoglobosins.

7.3 CIRS IS NOT AN ALLERGY

Before it became known that "mold illness" was caused by inflammation, some defense consultants suggested that the WDB-illness was simply an allergy. Indeed, some people have allergies to mold, and hypersensitivity pneumonitis can occur following exposure to thermophilic actinobacteria.

Allergy comes from excessive antibody responses to exposure. Removing the patient from the allergen will resolve allergy symptoms. CIRS symptoms do not resolve with mere removal from exposure. High levels of IgE are typically found in an allergy, but seldom do we see high IgE in CIRS. Defective antigen presentation occurs in CIRS. Proteomic findings seen in CIRS but not in an allergy include excessive levels of cytokines, split products of complement activation, transforming growth factor (TGF)β-1, and an increased relative risk for a limited number of HLA haplotypes.

However, as the inexorable march of science has shown, we now know that ribotoxins commonly initiate genomic injuries in CIRS. These are compounds made by one-celled microbes, including fungi, bacteria and actinobacteria, that stop or reduce normal protein synthesis by disrupting an evolutionarily conserved structural element on ribosomes called the sarcin-ricin loop (SRL). Ribotoxins initiate the cascades of inflammatory events seen in CIRS. The fact that the differential gene activation seen in CIRS comes from biowarfare among one-celled creatures that began four billion years ago is stunning.[10]

Negligent maintenance or construction defects do not cause allergy, but they do cause chronic inflammatory response syndrome from water-damaged buildings (CIRS-WDB). Landlords might have to pay for causing injury to a tenant if they were negligent in providing a safe indoor environment if the problem is CIRS. Convincing a jury that the problem was just allergy can shield the landlord from paying for their negligence.

Additional insight into CIRS-WDB comes from multiple published, peer-reviewed case/control studies involving over 5000 patients. Four of these elements (not including visual contrast sensitivity testing) form the accepted case definition of "mold illness" promulgated by the US Government Accountability Office (US GAO) in 2008.[11] There is no mention of urinary mycotoxins in that federal publication. Prospective, double-blinded, placebo-controlled clinical trials were also published to confirm that the causation of CIRS and treatment benefit are not random.[5, 12]

Additional biomarkers come from NeuroQuant®, a Food and Drug Administration (FDA)-cleared software program added to brain magnetic resonance imaging (MRI), which shows a distinctive fingerprint in CIRS-WDB patients.[13] Correction of the inflammation that causes the illness can result in correction of NeuroQuant® deficits as symptoms abate, demonstrating that the neurologic and cognitive abnormalities seen in CIRS can be reversed.[14] Inflammation causes neurologic injury, and reduction of inflammation is the appropriate treatment.

A subset of patients with CIRS-WDB have an excessive amount of gray matter nuclear atrophy shown in published studies to respond to published treatment protocols and the use of vasoactive intestinal polypeptide.[15] Since this study's publication in 2017, no other subsequent studies using other modalities have successfully shown gray matter nuclear atrophy correction. There was no correlation between sequential mycotoxin testing and the improvement of brain volumes.

Other objective biomarkers typified in CIRS patients include pulmonary hypertension at rest, but more commonly after exercise. The tricuspid regurgitation (TR) velocity, measured in meters per second, is elevated. Four times the square of TR added to right atrial pressure will exceed 30 as a cutoff separating normal pulmonary artery pressure from acquired pulmonary hypertension.

$$PASP = 4(V_{TR})^{2^2} + RAP$$

In a stress echo, measured by achievement of a pulse rate greater than 90% of predicted, we see a rise greater than 8 mm of mercury (Hg) in patients with acquired pulmonary hypertension.[16] Sequential mycotoxin testing in urine does not correlate with improvement of pulmonary hypertension.

Maximal oxygen consumption exercise, called VO_2 max, can be greatly diminished in patients with CIRS-WDB. Correction of inflammation results in improvement of VO_2 max. Sequential mycotoxin testing in urine does not correlate with improvement of VO_2 max.

The greatest progress in looking at definable, objective biomarkers for CIRS[17] and CIRS-WDB comes from transcriptomics.[2, 3] Transcriptomics shows differences in gene activity in cases compared with controls and patients observed prospectively. When combined with NeuroQuant® studies showing resolution of gray matter nuclear atrophy and/or reduction of the enlarged forebrain parenchyma and/or cortical gray, these transcriptomics studies give us a new basis for understanding neuronal injury and repair. Sequential mycotoxin testing in urine does not correlate with the improvement of transcriptomics.

A disproportionate increase in activation of coagulation genes in CIRS, together with β-tubulin genes, demonstrates the marked correlation of a subset of CIRS cases with enhanced gray matter nuclear atrophy. These findings support the vascular hypothesis of dementia.[18–20] A small number of patients with coagulation gene excess activation returned to baseline cognitive state with correction of transcriptomics.

7.4 FAULTY GEFFCKEN DEFENSES

There is confirmation of causation of mold-related illness and correction with treatment protocols published repeatedly. The *Geffcken defense* demanded that evidence of mycotoxins in patient tissues be identical to mycotoxins found in a given building to which the affected patient was exposed. Unfortunately, identifying mycotoxins accurately in a room is compromised even if mycotoxins could be found accurately in tissue. However, that was the legal statute until 2006 in the United States. Sequential assessment of urinary mycotoxins could have provided cover for Geffcken-type arguments in court had urinary measurements ever been shown in the published literature to correlate with exposure.

When *Geffcken* and allergy defenses did not win cases very often, new legal arguments from defense interests claimed that the illness seen in patients from WDB was simply due to mycotoxin *ingestion* (or skin absorption). The idea of ingestion creating illness was supported largely by a study from Russia in 1947 reporting horses dying after eating hay contaminated by *Stachybotrys* sp. The study was inherently flawed, with very little objective data to support it, and had little success.

In the mid-2000s, a new concept arose as advocated by several physicians from the Mayo Clinic in Rochester, Minnesota. These physicians believed that fungi growing in sinuses were a marker for chronic rhinosinusitis, and that nasal cultures could demonstrate the fungi.[20–22] Chronic rhinosinusitis is an inflammatory condition in which eosinophilic basic protein actually causes a runny nose. An important paper from the German literature showed that fungi are indeed found in nearly everyone's nose, with cases of chronic rhinosinusitis having 2.3 species of fungi, but controls had 3.1 species.[23] The association of enhanced mycotoxin production with water activity (Aw) bears consideration. While variable water activities are associated with the growth of fungal species, production of mycotoxins commonly occurs at the higher Aw of 0.98 for ochratoxins, 0.93 for fumonisins and 0.90 for DON.[24] These values of Aw are not found on mucous membranes in humans, especially in the nose. These data rule out the possibility of intranasal production of mycotoxins.

In 2009, a pathologist named Dennis Hooper published a paper[25] showing that patients exposed to WDB had putative evidence of mycotoxin carriage that could be detected using an ELISA technique in urine. Notwithstanding the lack of precision of ELISA analyses, as they are non-specific, laboratories started selling tests for mycotoxins found in urine.

The paper referred to a control group but omitted specific (i) control group demographics and (ii) building testing that confirmed microbial amplification. The absence of reliable control data from Hooper's laboratory and other urinary mycotoxin vendors remains a problem. If one claims causation of illness, there need to be prospective studies demonstrating acquisition of illness. If one relies on only a case/control study, there must be a transparent association in which abnormalities of exposed patients are different from abnormalities in non-exposed patients derived following transparent and thorough differential diagnosis. The scientific concept is simple: No controls, no conclusions.

An explanation for finding mycotoxins in urine was that fungi growing in the nose made toxins. The use of antifungal nasal sprays began to rise in 2014 and 2015. By 2016, it was found that extensive acquisition of antifungal resistance occurred in fungi and bacteria, apparently through the mechanism of horizontal gene transfer (personal communication, MicrobiologyDx, 8/2016).

The alarming feature of the new-found antibiotic resistance in bacteria was resistance to (i) vancomycin, an antibiotic necessary for dangerously ill septic patients, as well as (ii) gentamicin, an aminoglycoside, emerged in a group of organisms called coagulase negative staphylococci. Multiply antibiotic resistant coagulase negative staphylococci (MARCoNS) let us trace the development of vancomycin and gentamicin resistance back to physicians who used antifungals. Now that the antifungal resistance has spread (likely through plasmid exchange and free DNA transfer), the genes for fungal resistance are not just found in antifungal users but have spread rapidly in the MARCoNS population. MARCoNS are prolific exchangers of DNA and antibiotic resistance factors with other one-celled creatures. We need to look at the experience with *Staphylococcus aureus*, a coagulase positive staphylococcus, in the 1970s to 1980s to suspect that the reservoir of resistance to penicillin was in MARCoNS.

7.5 MYCOTOXINS IN FOOD PRODUCTION

Fungi are ubiquitous in nature and food. Moist food, especially starches, will support fungal growth in a few days. Dry foods will take longer to spoil, but fungal presence in foods of all types creates human and animal health problems. Predictably, toxigenic fungi are also found routinely in food supplies worldwide. The absence of massive numbers of cases of mycotoxicosis suggests that the role of foods is minimal. Nevertheless, when we hear experts telling us to avoid coffee, mushrooms, wine, cheeses, bread and more because of the toxicity of fungi found in these foods, as shown by finding mycotoxins in urine, we do not see epidemiologic confirmation of such advice.

The source of mycotoxins in food comes from three categories of pre-harvest, post-harvest and warehouse-based growth. The foods involved are diverse, but colonization of foods is primarily due to only several genera of fungi. These are *Aspergillus*, *Fusarium* and *Penicillium*, with *Stachybotrys* less common but still an important contaminant. *Fusarium* species come from corn products. In food manufacturing, from warehouse to table, attempts to destroy mycotoxins by food processing are an ongoing challenge. Mycotoxins are resistant to most physical methods of destruction. The sheer volume of foodstuffs complicates detection.[26]

The concerns about health effects caused by ingestion of mycotoxin-contaminated food have weighed into in vitro studies, but confirmation of the same abnormalities is rare in vivo. These problems can include autoimmunity, allergy, congenital disabilities, cancers and mutagenesis.[27] The most important mycotoxins for consideration are aflatoxins, ochratoxins, zearalenone, patulin and trichothecenes. This latter group includes DON, metabolites of DON, T2 toxin and satratoxin. Zearalenone is important for estrogenic effects. Additional human health concerns include renal dysfunction due to ochratoxin A exposure and the largely uninvestigated field of chronic low-level, long-term exposure to not just a single group of mycotoxins but multiple mycotoxins.[28]

There are *Aspergillus* species that make ochratoxin found in food and WDB, but none of those fungi commonly are seen in the top ten species associated with adverse human health effects. Similarly, *Stachybotrys*, one of the top five species most pathogenic for human hosts, is associated with the significant appearance of parent trichothecenes and their metabolites in the urine of healthy patients. Interestingly, aflatoxin (which derives its name from *Aspergillus flavus*) rarely appears in the top ten fungi most commonly associated with human illness. The only thing one can tell from urinary mycotoxin testing is whether the patient has eaten warehoused foods in the last 60 days.[6]

Patulin is an interesting toxin found in fruit juices, especially in apple and grape juice, and stone fruits, including apricots, peaches and plums. Patulin rarely is found in intact fruit, but any fruit with a damaged surface is susceptible to fungal infestation. Patulin is in almost all apple juice. There is no convincing evidence that patulin from apple juice ingestion causes illness. Perhaps, clues to the relative absence of adverse human health effects from ingested mycotoxins come from the findings that patulin, for example, is rapidly destroyed before leaving the stomach, resulting in a residual of less than 3%.[27]

Much of the concern about food contamination with mycotoxins has given rise to odd dietary alterations and claims of enhanced safety of mycotoxin-free foods. As much as 50% of human daily intake of ochratoxin and its metabolites is due to its direct consumption in cereals or grains, but the remainder will be due to the consumption of animals after they eat contaminated feed. The list of common food sources of ochratoxins includes corn, rice, wheat, barley, oats, rye, sorghum, millet, wine, beer, raisins, wine, wine vinegar, coffee and pork. Ochratoxin A (OTA) occurs in cheese and meat products, dried and smoked fish, soybeans, garbanzo beans, nuts and dried fruits.

The analysis problem for ochratoxin is complex, usually requiring high-performance liquid chromatography (HPLC) and mass spectrometry (MS) to separate the molecule of ochratoxin A from its 18 known congeners, which have a variable half-life in blood, ranging up to 60 days.[27] With so many metabolites of ochratoxin A, with some lasting for several months in blood, where are the billions of people suffering worldwide from ochratoxin A-associated nephropathy? The risks of OTA appear to be over-stated.

Concerning cancer causation, aflatoxin (AFB1), especially when associated with hepatitis B virus, is widely reported to be associated with hepatic cell carcinoma. The marker for the breakdown product of aflatoxin is AFB1-N7-guanine adduct, which enters the urine.[26] Laboratories considered to be expert in analyzing urine for mycotoxins should look for this one marker of cancer causation from aflatoxins.

7.6 FARM-BASED PREVENTION

The detoxification of aflatoxins is accomplished internally by an enzyme, glutathione S-transferase (GST), which will bind to an ingested metabolite of aflatoxin and then combine with glutathione, detoxifying the compound. GST is ancient and evolutionarily conserved, with a complex genome in plants.[9] T2 toxin and DON will induce activation of groups of the GST genome. Of interest is the existence of gene super-families for GST in honeybees and Drosophila[29] and human GST polymorphisms that can increase sporadic colorectal cancer risk in Caucasians.[30]

Regarding sources of T-2 toxins globally, the natural occurrence of host genera *Fusarium* or *Sporotrichioides* has been reported in Asia, Africa, South America, Europe and North America. Predominant genera that make other trichothecenes include *Stachybotrys*, *Trichoderma* and *Trichothecium*. All these sources of T-2 will be detected similarly using an ELISA assay.[27] We note that the main production of mycotoxins is associated with the greatest water content before and immediately after harvest. Once food materials dry out, mycotoxin production declines in step with reduction of Aw.

DON and its metabolites are the most prevalent trichothecenes found in food. DON exists with its metabolites together with T-2 toxin and nivalenol. DON is easily separated from other trichothecenes in urine. However, only a few commercial laboratories will perform this standard assay. Given the disparity of known effects of trichothecenes compared with the known ribotoxin effect, there is an absence of the fundamental mechanism of molecular hypometabolism with a poly-ribosomal breakdown in mammalian cell lines following exposure delineation of trichothecene.

A problem faced by microbiologists is how to separate direct ribosomal injury from DON versus indirect injury from ribotoxins or ribosomal inhibitory proteins. The ribotoxic stress response manifests by immunotoxicity, causing enhanced activation of mitogen-activated protein kinases (MAPK), which can be a marker for exposure to trichothecenes.

Three papers from the Scientific Observing and Experimental Station of Animal Nutrition and Feed Science in South Central China[31–33] bear significant weight in assessing host factors protecting piglets from ingested mycotoxin injury. DON damage in groups of piglets by measurements of oxidative parameters occurred in the first study,[31] including catalase, malic dialdehyde, nitric oxide, peroxide levels in the blood; total antioxidant capacity; d-lactate, and amino acids. Glutamic acid prevented harm from DON in terms of catalase, peroxide, dialdehyde, lactate (NB: a marker for molecular hypometabolism) and nitric acid.

DON diminished villus height in jejunum and ileum, but the villus height increased in glutamic acid–fed piglets. Glutamic acid also blocked increased lymphocytes caused by DON and protected goblet cells. Interestingly, the DON-induced ribotoxic stress response indicator genes were activated in DON-fed pigs and reduced protein synthesis. Protein reduction did not occur in pigs fed with the combination of DON and 2% glutamic acid.

The second study[32] used the same control and experimental designs. This time, glutamic acid prevented decreased weight gain caused by mycotoxins.

The final study[33] used nuclear magnetic resonance to show additional benefits of glutamic acid in DON-challenged piglets. Here, the authors showed additional manifestations of protection; namely, glutamic acid treatment corrected DON-driven high levels of low-density lipoprotein (LDL) cholesterol and lowered high-density lipoprotein (HDL) and corrected elevated levels of alanine, arginine, acetate, glycoprotein, trimethylamine-N-oxide, glycine, lactate, urea and glutamate/creatinine ratio. Further, glutamic acid increased superoxide dismutase and glutathione peroxidase. The authors conclude that glutamic acid can repair injuries associated with oxidative stress and disturbances of energy and amino acid metabolism induced by DON.

Remember that glutamate consists of two forms. One is L-glutamate, and the other is D-glutamate or MSG. We are not speaking of MSG. Glutamate occurs in proteins and peptides, and virtually every food contains some glutamate. Superimposing aflatoxicosis on areas of protein-calorie malnutrition, we see an association between adequate food ingestion and dramatically reduced mycotoxicosis from food. This association suggests that something found in food has much to do with protection from mycotoxin injury. Protein-rich foods, including meat, eggs, poultry, milk, cheese and fish, are major components of glutamate in the diet.

Of interest is the three-dimensional structure of glutamate, because it has an amino group in the middle of the chain of five carbons with a carbocyclic acid moiety found on either end. At acid pH, one hydrogen lost from a hydroxyl group balances as a zwitterion with an NH_3 replacing an NH_2. At the pH in the stomach, there can be production of a single positive charge, with the amino group becoming an ammonium group and with each hydroxyl group losing an electron. This molecular dipole could create a mechanism for binding the anion rings of mycotoxins by the cation found in glutamate at gastric pH. This is how cholestyramine binds a variety of mycotoxins.[41,42]

Given that at least 25% of foods are contaminated with mycotoxins worldwide, we would expect anywhere between one and a half and two billion individuals to be sickened if this were a simple linear expression of causation with exposure resulting in illness. The absence of two billion sick people suggests strongly that the model used for excessive mycotoxin pathogenicity is flawed.

Host factor analysis is potentially flawed, as rarely mentioned fungi may be confounders. Such is the case with sterigmatocystin (STC) in foodstuffs. STC from *Wallemia sebi* occurs in grains, corn, bread, cheese, spices, beans, soybeans, pistachios, animal feed and silage.[34]

We can use urine levels to implicate ochratoxin A in cancer. In a Turkish population,[35] hydroxy-deoxyguanosine and malondialdehyde correlated with ochratoxin A. The advantage of finding specific urinary markers with MS is that there are 18 different metabolites known for ochratoxin A.

7.7   DIETARY PROTECTION FACTORS

The patulin degradation showed 94% disappearance from the blood within 2 minutes of ingestion.[35] Further confirmation of the disintegration of patulin comes from studies in rats.[36] Isolated rat stomachs had a luminal application of patulin with the rapid emergence of mycotoxin into the stomach itself. Concentrations of 350 mg per liter and 3.5 mg per liter were tested, with mycotoxins appearing almost instantly with both the high and low doses. The residual toxin was 3% and 0.06% in gastric tissue, respectively. This disintegration of 8400 μg and 700 μg, respectively, was partly due to intracellular glutathione (GHS). The massive dose of patulin did reduce the GHS content by 87% in controls.

Dietary supplementation of animal feed with organic activated bentonite, a clay product, and humic acid polymer has shown benefit in vitro,[37] confirmed by binding of ochratoxin and zearalenone by both bentonite and humic acids, with binding exceeding 96% of the total burden. These products *did not* demonstrate benefit from the reduction in *inflammatory biomarkers* acquired following exposure to the interior environment of WDB. The ability of these compounds to adsorb toxins but not to prevent disease suggested that ingestion and gastrointestinal exposure to mycotoxins is *not* the relevant causative feature of CIRS-WDB.

Other dietary strategies[38] tested for the ability to prevent toxic effects of ingested mycotoxins include antioxidants (selenium, vitamins, pro-vitamins), bacteria and yeast, and food components including fructose, aspartame, chlorophyll and phenols, together with biological binding agents, hydrated sodium, calcium, aluminosilicate, bentonites, zeolites and activated carbons. While these dietary strategies provide promise, the discrepancy between in vitro and in vivo studies is difficult to reconcile. These additional dietary compounds just do not work to prevent CIRS-WDB, so once again, the problem is not mycotoxin ingestion.

Additional efforts to use microbiologicals for deactivating mycotoxins show some initial promise. A *Eubacterium* sp. (BBSH 797), isolated from a cow's rumen, showed the ability to deactivate trichothecenes. Also, a novel yeast strain, *Trichosporon mycotoxinivorans*, was isolated and characterized as degrading ochratoxin A and zearalenone.[39]

In a study showing promise,[40] 32 separate strains of *Rhodococcus* were degraded to aflatoxin B-1, zearalenone, fumonisins B-1, T-2 toxin and ochratoxin A. In addition, *Rhodococcus* species could protect against injury from multi-mycotoxin exposure. While this was a promising study in 2013, no *Rhodococcus* strains are available as commercially available probiotics. The effects of biotransformation include acetylation, glycosylation, ring cleavage, hydrolysis, deamination and decarboxylation. These promising solutions have not been tested in humans yet.

Trichosporon, a yeast isolated from the hindgut of the termite[41] *Mastotermes darwiniensis*, shows promise to detoxify ochratoxin A.[41] *Trichosporon* may be used in clinical trials to deactivate mycotoxins in animal feeds.

In tests performed in lambs, injected aflatoxin localized in the liver, nasal olfactory mucosa, nasopharynx, esophagus, larynx, trachea, bronchi and conjunctiva. The nasal mucosa was the most active in forming DNA-bound aflatoxin metabolites. When incubated with reduced glutathione, a drastic decrease in active DNA binding occurred without adding glutathione transferase (GST).[42]

Experiments on chickens fed ochratoxin A[43] provided an additional approach to preventing mycotoxin-induced injury in animals. There was a marked reduction of the relative weight of immune organs (bursa of Fabricius and spleen) when chickens consumed ochratoxin-contaminated diets of up to 1.5 mg/kg for 3 weeks. In a follow-up experiment on phagocytic function and lymphoprolif-erative response,[44] silymarin, vitamin E and antioxidants in chicken feed prevented ochratoxin-induced immunotoxicity. There is no indication of benefit in humans.

The mechanism of DON-induced proinflammatory gene expression[45] appears in humans and animals to involve activation of constitutive protein kinases on the damaged ribosome and autophagy of the endoplasmic reticulum stress response. DON induced activation of MAPKs in the known ribotoxic stress response. Pathological abnormalities in chronic low-dose exposure included anorexia, impaired weight gain, growth hormone dysregulation, high-dose exposure-evoked gas-troenteritis, vomiting and a shock-like syndrome. DON evokes a ribotoxin stress response in mono-nuclear phagocytes, contributing to acute and chronic toxic effects in vivo.

Early work in this field from Pestka[46] has shown that the mechanism of ribotoxic stress response involves double-stranded RNA activated protein kinase (PKR) as well as hematopoietic cell kinases (Hck). Inhibitors in gene silencing studies have revealed that PKR plays a role in DON-induced gene expression and apoptosis. Continuing his studies, Pestka has investigated the role of trichot-hecenes[47] in white blood cells. His laboratory has found that monocytes, macrophages, and T- and B-lymphocytes are cellular targets of DON and trichothecenes. Even at low dose concentrations, exposure reflected upregulation, both transcriptionally and post-transcriptionally, of cytokines, chemokines, and inflammatory genes. High concentrations of exposure bring about apoptosis of leukocytes. Again, Pestka discusses the ribotoxic stress response, binding to ribosomes and rapidly activating MAPKs. The immune events in CIRS-WDB are unrelated to ingestion but are genomic and transcriptomic abnormalities induced by toxin and/or ribotoxin exposure.

Experience with DON inoculation[46] showed a whole series of gene activation in the MAPK fam-ily. For example, tyrosine phosphorylation of hematopoietic cell kinase (Hck) was detected within 1 to 5 minutes after addition of toxin, with this gene activation suppressed by incubation with inhibi-tors of the family of tyrosine kinase.

Investigating the source of apoptosis has shown that BAK, a pro-apoptotic Bcl-2 family protein, is expressed in many tissues.[48] Bcl-2 proteins regulate apoptosis as well as autophagy. When acti-vation of apoptosis occurred following treatment with nigericin, a ribosomal toxin, both transient and stable overexpression of various forms of BAK exerted a protective role, but it did not inhibit the extent of nigericin-mediated activation of caspase-3. This study strengthens the link between exposure to ribotoxins and induction of apoptosis.

7.8   MYCOTOXIN ANALYSIS

Mycotoxins are toxic fungal secondary metabolites that frequently contaminate food and animal feed worldwide and represent a major safety hazard. To estimate human exposure arising from con-taminated food, so-called biomarker approaches developed as a complementary biomonitoring tool besides traditional food analysis.[49–59] The first methods are radio-immunoassays, ELISA and liquid chromatography (LC), developed in the late 1980s and early 1990s to detect carcinogenic aflatoxins.

Since 2010, there has been a clear trend towards developing and applying multianalyte methods based on LC/electrospray ionization/tandem MS. With these advanced methods, traces of myco-toxins and the relevant breakdown and conjugation products can be quantified simultaneously in human urine as so-called biomarkers and can be used to precisely describe the real exposure, toxi-cokinetics and bioavailability of the toxins present.

Special attention is paid to the main challenges when analyzing these toxic food contaminants in urine, i.e., very low analyte concentrations, appropriate sample preparation, matrix effects and a lack of authentic, nuclear magnetic resonance (NMR)-confirmed calibrants and reference materi-als. Traditionally, mycotoxin testing used ELISA technology, which relies on antibodies, some-times monoclonal but more often polyclonal. Among all published immunological-based methods, these ELISAs were the most commonly used for mycotoxin determination. ELISA provides rapid screening, with many kits commercially available for detecting and quantifying major mycotoxins, including aflatoxins (AFs), AFM1, OTA, ZEA (zearalenone), DON, fumonisins and T-2 toxin.

ELISA methods have been validated in various food matrices by urine only in a few instances. The principle of ELISA is based on the competitive interactions between mycotoxins (acting as an antigen) and assigned antibodies labeled with toxin–enzyme conjugate for many binding sites. The amount of antibody-bound toxin–enzyme conjugate will determine the level of color development. This technique provides a rapid, specific and relatively simple method for analyzing mycotoxins.

However, ELISA has certain disadvantages, including potential cross-reactivity, dependent on antibody specificity. In addition, the kit detects only a single mycotoxin for one-time use; thus, it can be costly and impracticable if one needs to test samples contaminated with multiple mycotoxins. Moreover, the manufacturer specifies each test kit for a set matrix. While some third-party validations, e.g., by AOAC, have been done for some mycotoxin ELISA kits, the validations used specific toxins at specific contamination levels. Therefore, the kit is not valid for all food matrices and contamination levels, let alone human samples like blood and urine. Even when used in their appropriate settings, the manufacturers of these kits recommend that positive ELISA results be confirmed by a suitable chromatographic method, especially when used in a matrix not specified by the manufacturer.

Alternatively, lateral flow devices (LFD) are a single-step test that includes a negative control line and the sample lines on the same strip. A lateral flow test can provide semi-quantitative results in less than 10 min and requires no specialized equipment. A lateral flow test consists of a conjugate pad, a porous membrane and an absorbent pad, and a competitive immunoassay that uses labeled antibody acts as a signal reagent. This device has also recently been coupled with spectrometric readers to provide quantitative results. LFDs are commercially available for detecting AFs, DON, T-2 toxin, OTA and ZEA. However, their applications in the field are limited. There are numerous problems associated with the sensitivity, reliability of different matrices and costs.

Another simplified system comprises flow-through membranes, which utilize the same basic principle as LFD but may not yield accurate results near the detection limit. Flow-through immuno-assays screen OTA in green and roasted coffee, AFB1 in nuts, and ZEA in cereals and feed samples. Although many different rapid strip tests detect major mycotoxins in different food commodities, they are not common due to sensitivity, cost and accuracy issues.

Chromatography is the most commonly used method for mycotoxin analysis in food and feed. The earliest chromatographic method was thin layer chromatography (TLC), which is still used as a rapid screening method for certain mycotoxins by visual assessment or instrumental densitom-etry. However, current trends in mycotoxin analysis in food focus on applying robust, fast, easy to use, and cheap technologies that can detect and quantify various mycotoxins with high sensitivity and selectivity in a single run. Many chromatographic methods were developed, such as HPLC coupled with ultraviolet (UV), diode array (DAD), fluorescence (FLD) or MS detectors, and ultra high-performance chromatography (UHPLC or UPLC) with reduced column packing material. Additionally, gas chromatography (GC) coupled with electron capture (ECD), flame ionization (FID) or MS detectors identified and quantitated volatile mycotoxins. Due to most mycotoxins' low volatility and high polarity, GC analysis often requires a derivatization step. Therefore, this method is rare in mycotoxin analysis with the advance of coupling liquid chromatography techniques to MS (e.g., LC-MS; LC-MS/MS).

Apart from the advantages of the conventional HPLC methods mentioned earlier, MS offers several distinct advantages over all-LC methods for mycotoxin analysis in food. The mass spectrometer works by ionizing the molecules and sorting and identifying them based on their mass-to-charge ratio (m/z). MS offers higher sensitivity, selectivity and chemical structural information by the molecular identity of the analyte based on m/z, providing the mass spectrum as an ideal confirmatory technique. MS detection reduces time by eliminating error-prone sample derivatization and clean-up steps needed for fluorescence enhancement. Different MS interfaces and analyzers have been used, such as atmospheric pressure chemical ionization (APCI), electrospray ionization (ESI) and atmospheric pressure photoionization (APPI). In addition, there are many types of mass analyzers, such as quadrupole, time-of-flight (TOF), ion-trap and Fourier transform-ion cyclotron resonance (FT-ICR). ESI, triple quadrupole and TOF have been used extensively for mycotoxin analysis. Although the early applications of MS were for the analysis of single mycotoxins, the technique can now simultaneously quantify many hundreds of mycotoxins and their metabolites in a single run, making it the current method of choice for detecting multiple mycotoxins in a wide variety of foods.

Since the arrival of modern HPLC-MS/MS (liquid chromatography-tandem mass spectroscopy) and GC-MS/MS (gas chromatography-tandem mass spectroscopy) instruments, multi-analyte methods for mycotoxin determination have become available. However, these are not without substantial cost, with most mycotoxin determination in urine performed recently by LC-MS/MS. However, a major challenge in urine mycotoxin analysis is the extremely low analyte concentrations present following dietary exposure.

Thus, effective, specific, sensitive and accurate methods for mycotoxin detection in urine require appropriate sample preparation protocols to accomplish the desired sensitivity while obtaining acceptable limits of detection (LODs) and quantitation (LOQs). Most of the methods available in the literature come from traditional extraction techniques such as liquid/liquid extraction (LLE) or solid/liquid extraction (SLE), which have several disadvantages, mainly the high solvent volumes, high amounts of sample and the long times required for the analysis. In recent years, method simplification and miniaturization have been the most important trend in sample preparation, allowing low sample and solvent volume, fast analysis and greater efficiency.

Method validation by laboratories undertaking mycotoxin analysis should follow the guidelines established by the EU and other regulatory bodies, including the determination of linearity, matrix effect (ME), LODs, LOQs, recoveries, repeatability (intra-day precision) and reproducibility (inter-day precision).

Of utmost importance are calibration curves for all mycotoxins analyzed. They must be constructed from standard solutions (external calibrators) and in the matrix (matrix-matched calibrations). Matrix-matched calibration curves use blank urine samples spiked with standardized mycotoxins before and after extraction if used. There are limits to the range of these standard curves, and LOQ should also be validated.

A final cautionary note about validating analytical methods for mycotoxins is that reliance on avoidance of foods likely to contain mycotoxins or their metabolites is no guarantee that the urine obtained from "control" subjects will be a genuine baseline. Therefore, screening and analysis of the analytes of interest are prudent, because mycotoxin-producing molds may contaminate numerous agricultural commodities before harvest or in storage. Naturally occurring mycotoxins appear to cause a wide array of adverse health effects. Measuring urinary mycotoxin levels is a means of assessing an individual's exposure, but developing sensitive and accurate analytical methods for detecting mycotoxins and their metabolites in urine samples is challenging. Urinary mycotoxins are present in low pg/ml concentrations, and other endogenous metabolites can obscure the chromatographic identification of their metabolites.

As a result of the advent of the latest generation of high-performance LC-MS/MS instruments, there is a clear trend towards developing and applying multianalyte methods in mycotoxin biomarkers. Sophisticated sample clean-up approaches with subsequent separation by LC and detection using triple-quadrupole analyzers coupled via an ESI interface purify analytes. However, the latest studies have also successfully applied the so-called "dilute and shoot" approach by omitting any clean-up step.

A major challenge in mycotoxin biomarker research is the extremely low analyte concentrations present in biological fluids following dietary exposure. Hence, appropriate sample preparation protocols are crucial to obtain acceptable LODs. Detection is hampered by the great chemical diversity of analytes typically included in multi-biomarker methods. This issue becomes even more complex once polar conjugate inclusions such as glucuronides disappear during common clean-up approaches like solid-phase extraction (SPE) or immunoaffinity chromatography (IAC) procedures.

7.9 MYCOTOXIN TESTING FROM THE LITERATURE

MS is the state-of-the-art method[54] for testing mycotoxins, including aflatoxin, ochratoxin and trichothecenes. GC and LC liquid mechanisms, while regarded as accurate and precise, may show extreme and variable sensitivity due to different biological characteristics of mycotoxins, matrices and instruments. LC-MS response can be different depending on ionization techniques used. If fluorescence or UV absorbance makes quantitative measurements, LC-MS is a confirmatory technique.

If toxins are not volatile, LC-MS is uniquely able to render quantitative and qualitative results accurately. These problems are multiplied by attempts at determining mycotoxins in food, given the extreme variability of food matrices. Specific ionization interfaces are needed to reduce matrix effects and ion suppression.

Given the concerns about the health effects of mycotoxins in food and feed, risk assessment of mycotoxin contamination for both humans and animals requires clear identification and reliable quantitation in diversified matrices.[60] With MS emerging in the 1970s, we now are seeing a variety of hyphenated techniques that combine chromatography with MS. Indeed, LC-MS, or better still, LC-MS/MS, has become a routine technique.

The challenge of detecting multiple mycotoxins, as are commonly seen in the same sample, requires advanced techniques for each diagnostic run. LC-MS/MS can measure different levels of mycotoxins and their metabolites, both free and masked. Newer techniques will likely emerge as multi-dimensional chromatography-MS, capillary electrophoresis-MS and surface plasmon resonance array-MS have become available. The cost of the new advanced techniques will continue to be a factor.

With the enhanced multi-class mycotoxin analysis in food, environmental and biological matrices, and LC-MS/MS, detecting mycotoxins has become increasingly precise. However, this technical advance raises a curious condition, in that the presence or absence of molds is less frequently identified and correlated with mycotoxin presence.[61] Mycotoxins seldom develop alone. Co-occurrence of mycotoxins creates a real problem for assessing dose–response relationships, not to mention genetic susceptibility such that the mere presence of multiple mycotoxins should be considered a risk factor. However, the risk itself is not adequate to conclude the causation of illness.

A simple question for governing bodies regarding food safety is how one device can provide results that will be sensitive and specific for the wide variety of chemical structures in mycotoxin analysis.[62] An additional challenge remains that the heterogeneity of foods demands multiple analytical methods simultaneously, permitting rapid and inexpensive analysis. Ongoing problems include a proper collection of representative samples, avoiding secondary contamination after collection, the performance of emerging analytical methods, including immunochemical techniques, with validation of methods for those involved with enforcement of standards in regulatory affairs, and finally, limitations of current methods.

Gerding performed a study in Germany to confirm the precision of increasingly sophisticated MS techniques.[63] The study recorded food surveys with the food frequencies questionnaire followed by LC-MS/MS assessment of urinary biomarkers. The authors looked for 23 different urinary biomarkers, including trichothecenes (especially DON and its metabolites), T-2 toxin, HT-2 toxin, aflatoxins and aflatoxin metabolites, ochratoxin A, ochratoxin alpha and others. In 87% of samples, one or more in a group of six mycotoxins and urinary metabolites was detected in a single occurrence. Only DON and its metabolites were detectable in quantifiable amounts. There was no statistical significance in correlating staple food intake with urinary biomarker concentration. This important study supports the commonality of daily exposure of healthy patients to mycotoxins, with such mycotoxins being identifiable in urine. The study could not control for a variety of metabolic modifications together with metabolites to provide statistical surety of exposure.

A longer-term trial of measurement of urinary biomarkers for aflatoxins in Brazil confirmed these findings.[64] Sixteen volunteers, 14–55 years old, collected first-morning urine four times every 3 months from June 2011 to March 2012. Of these samples, 61% showed aflatoxin M-1. None of the urine samples indicated residues of aflatoxin metabolites. There was no GST evaluation. There were no differences in aflatoxin measurement over the four seasons of the study. Sophisticated measurement of urinary biomarkers shows little or no relationship to the development of adverse human health effects.

In a study from Spain,[65] human urine samples received an analysis for 15 mycotoxins and metabolites using a new multi-mycotoxin GC-MS/MS method following salting-out LLE. Fifty-four urine samples from healthy children and adults in Valencia were analyzed for mycotoxins and normalized by simultaneous creatinine measurement. Thirty-seven of the 54 samples showed quantifiable values of mycotoxins, finding H-2 toxin, nivalenol and DON. The co-occurrence of these contaminates happened in 20.4% of samples. Two of nine exposed children had levels of DON in urine exceeding international levels without adverse health effects.

7.10   URINARY MYCOTOXINS IN HUMAN HEALTH

In one of the few studies performed looking at occupational exposure of mill workers, an experimental design was adequate to sort out occupational exposure to mycotoxins from diet from three different grain mills in Germany, with matched controls having parallel analysis.[66] Mycotoxins tested by urinary measurements were citrinin, DON, ochratoxin A and zearalenone. Immunoaffinity columns and LLE (ochratoxin) were employed for urine sample clean-up prior to liquid chromatography with tandem mass spectrometry (LC-MS/MS) or by HPLC. Mycotoxin metabolites analyzed included DON-1, ochratoxin alpha, dihydrocitrinone, and alpha- and beta-zearalenone. Urine samples were positive in both groups for citrinin, DON, ochratoxin and zearalenone. DON had the highest concentration in both groups, followed by ochratoxin. Mean biomarker levels in urine from mill workers' controls were not significantly different, so levels of mycotoxins in urine reflected dietary exposure.

An ongoing problem in measuring urinary mycotoxins is the possible confounder created by exposure to multiple mycotoxins. In a study in South Africa of food and first-morning urine, sophisticated LC-MS evaluation[67] was able to show a correlation of food consumption with presence in morning urine of fumonisins, DON, zearalenone and ochratoxin A. This paper demonstrates the value of multi-biomarker measurements in detecting exposures in populations exposed to multiple mycotoxins.

This study assessed sample preparation procedures for evaluating mycotoxins in foods and urine, comparing dispersive liquid-liquid microextraction and salting-out LLE of ten fumonisins; mycotoxins and metabolites in urine were compared.[55, 68] Under optimal extraction techniques, salting-out LLEs showed better accuracy in precision than dispersive liquid-liquid microextraction. Based on these preliminary results, a multi-biomarker method was initiated based on salting-out LLE followed by GC and tandem MS. The method resulted in low detection limits and quantitation down to 0.12 and 0.25 µg per liter, respectively.

A follow-up paper[55] from the same group looked at quantitative LC-MS/MS measurement of 11 mycotoxins (aflatoxin, ochratoxin and others in human urine). Using dispersive liquid-liquid microextraction methods on ten urine samples from healthy volunteers showed the presence of mycotoxins in low concentration.

Ongoing enhancements of LC-MS/MS technology are reported in this study from China, looking at zearalenone and its metabolites in urine. Researchers collected 301 urine samples from healthy volunteers of all ages in China, with 71% of all samples positive for zearalenone and metabolites.[69]

Another study, one of the few that still use ELISA kits to assay for aflatoxins[70], compared urinary aflatoxin measurements in 84 individuals in Nigeria's rural and semi-urban community. Ninety-nine percent of urine samples had detectable aflatoxin. Levels were higher in the semi-urban population than in the rural population. Still, there was no significant difference in mean urinary aflatoxin levels in males and females compared among children, adolescents and adults.

One of the few studies comparing mycotoxins found in urine with those in dust had 21 cases who worked in a bread dough factory compared with 19 individuals who were controls. There were no reports of illness in either group.[71]

In workers, DON and ochratoxin were the most prevalent biomarkers, found in 66% and 90% of participants. In controls, researchers found ochratoxin in 68%, with DON in 58%. DON was the mycotoxin measured in the highest amounts in settled dust samples. Workers in both groups were exposed to several mycotoxins simultaneously, but there was no difference in urine findings between cases and controls. There was no evidence that exposure in the workplace contributed to adverse health effects. However, the workers did have higher contact with flour dust, which revealed higher exposure to DON. It becomes problematic to institute risk management when the selected biomarker of mycotoxins in urine has no relationship to illness in studies performed with control groups and exposed workers alike.

The BIOMYCO study from Belgium was a human biomonitoring study of multiple mycotoxins in urine.[71] A metabolite of DON, deoxynivalenol-15-glucuronide, was the main DON biomarker found in every sample. Researchers detected DON itself in 70% of children and 30% of adults. They found ochratoxin in 51% of children and 35% of adults. No symptoms were presented that correlate with those amounts.

An interesting study from the UK assessment of DON in an elderly cohort[72] had 20 patients over 65 reporting urine findings on two consecutive days. The authors detected levels in 90% of elderly men and women on both days. Dietary assessment of DON suggested only 10% of the elderly exceeded the maximum provisional tolerated daily intake for DON. There was no data on health or illness in these patients.

A study without human health assessments looked at the occupational exposure of forklift drivers at waste management facilities and the toxicity of dust collected from filters mounted inside forklifts.[73] Mycotoxin analyses were performed using LC-MS/MS methods. For cytotoxicity, a filter extract was analyzed using MTT cell culture. *Aspergillus* species were the predominant organism detected, but no mycotoxins were detected in aqueous filter extracts, although those same extracts were either highly toxic or moderately toxic in cell culture. What in this mixture of dust material, besides mycotoxins, created the cellular injury? Did the forklift drivers have evidence of illness? Those questions remain unanswered.

In an approach to gliotoxin, the authors[74] discuss gliotoxin isolated from *Trichoderma* species as an antibiotic substance involved in the biological control of plant pathogenic fungi. Gliotoxin may be a defense molecule thought to have a role in aspergillosis and is used in *Trichoderma*-based bio-fungicides. Gliotoxin has medicinal properties as a potential diagnostic marker and is important in biological crop protection. Gliotoxin has a critical role in pathobiology for *Aspergillus fumigatus*. It modulates the immune response and induces apoptosis in different cell types.[75].

With the focus on the gene clusters of *Aspergillus fumigatus* for gliotoxin biosynthesis, several important metabolites produced by the gliotoxin biosynthetic pathway were identified.[76] These metabolites influence either gliotoxin or specific reactions within the pathway. The activity of gliotoxin against animal cells and fungi is mediated via interference with redox hemostasis. Glutamic acid could oppose gliotoxins in animals.

One study[77] from Germany specifically focuses on citrinin, looking at urine samples from a group of 50 healthy adults (27 females, 23 males). Citrinin and its metabolite occurred in over 80% of all urine samples of healthy people.

An important study[78] looked at piglets fed with *Fusarium* toxin–contaminated maize. The presence of mycotoxins found in blood, liquor and urine was assessed with LC-MS/MS, and a variety of levels of dietary contamination were tested during 29 days of treatment. Concentrations of zearalenone and DON and their metabolites were analyzed. Researchers detected all analytes in urine in significantly higher concentrations than in serum and liquor. The toxin intake for bodyweight 3–4 hours before slaughter correlated with the sum of DON metabolites and zearalenone in all three specimens.

Finding ochratoxin in the blood of healthy human patients is not unusual. In a patient study in Tunisia,[79] 107 blood samples from healthy subjects underwent analysis using HPLC measurements. The healthy patients had evidence of ochratoxin. The highest ochratoxin plasma levels were found mostly in summer. Ochratoxin levels in populations showed variations from year to year, but intra-individual repetition showed no specific trend. Health status did not correlate with ochratoxin in human plasma.

In a study in the Balkans,[80] researchers identified variations of ochratoxin A in healthy populations. Ochratoxin was measured in 983 samples using the HPLC technique with fluorescent detection. Samples containing ochratoxin above the detection level were found in populations from all Croatian cities at all collecting periods. The highest levels of ochratoxin were in June. While the levels of ochratoxin found in Croatia were lower than in other European countries, the study shows that healthy populations of Croatia received exposure to low but seasonally/regionally variable amounts of ochratoxin. Nine hundred and eighty-three samples are the largest study seen in the preparation of this review. The study showed no evidence of adverse effects from elevated ochratoxin in blood.

7.10.1   Control Studies

Twenty-one studies covered 2756 controls, from children to adults, from North and South America, Europe, Asia and Africa. One study showed positive urine mycotoxins in 60% of 15 patients; one showed 66% of 19 patients, with the rest showing 80–100% positive.

Of specialized groups, there were 11 studies covering 421 controls. The lowest percentage positive was 38% in Egyptian children, 48% each for nursing mothers and infants, with the rest being >75% to 100%.

7.11   THE URINARY MYCOTOXIN HYPOTHESIS AND JUNK SCIENCE

A fundamental question for those health care providers who feel that (i) the presence of urinary mycotoxins define a new illness and (ii) the use of antifungals will treat the illness is, "What does exposure to mycotoxins mean?" If one breathes in mycotoxins, an immune response is adequate to generate the potential inflammatory responses in 24% of the population. All, however, are at risk for a positive urine mycotoxin test.[25] How does one assign the weight of causation to a biomarker that does not separate cases from controls? Or, are we simply looking at dietary sources of mycotoxins? If so, what is the value of doing urinary testing to diagnose sick people?

As discussed in the preceding section, a high percentage of control patients show mycotoxins in urine. We saw that not only will trichothecenes, aflatoxin and ochratoxin routinely appear in the urine of controls, but their metabolites will as well. Newer techniques like MS readily determine these metabolites. However, ELISA testing is fundamentally flawed in that there will be a variety of compounds with similar but not identical structures, called epitopes, to the quested mycotoxins found in urine. Testing for metabolites of mycotoxins, which one would expect to be mandatory under standard uses of ELISA, would skew, as these epitopes would give the false appearance of significance in the urine. Since metabolites are not reported by two commercial urine mycotoxin test labs in the United States, what criteria assist us in ruling out a positive test by the presence of a benign metabolite?

An even greater challenge is: What did mycotoxins do on the way through the human body, perhaps through the gastrointestinal tract or the respiratory tract, to get to the urine? Did they set off an immune response, creating CIRS, or did they break down into benign metabolites and undergo elimination?

The peer-reviewed literature supporting the use of antifungals and urinary mycotoxins is not non-existent but certainly is far less robust than what we would expect over the past 10 years from proponents of the idea trying to establish its validity.

We look for a distinct method section in any published paper. The first paper advocating ELISA methods for mycotoxins in urine was published in 2009 by Dennis Hooper and David Straus. This paper appeared in the *International Journal of Molecular Sciences* with a PubMed citation.[25] We see an abstract introduction, results (methods are not in a specific section), and a conclusion without a stand-alone discussion (there is a section called "preparation and evaluation of specimens for mycotoxin detection"). The paper presents urinary findings for ochratoxin, aflatoxin and trichothecenes without discussing metabolites. There is no discussion of any of the known congeners for ochratoxins or discussion of epitopes confounding ELISA results found in cases.

The author notes that the experimental design allows them to derive *qualitative* results but not *quantitative* results. The results claimed that spiked samples confirmed the antibody procedure's ability to detect increasing amounts of toxin. How was this possible if the method was not *quantitative*?

Of vital importance in any test considered for public use is to compare (i) known cases with (ii) defined controls. Hooper and Straus use no case or control definition and do not attempt to present a transparent differential diagnosis. The only control is a "negative control group," determined by absent or low mycotoxin levels. One wonders if controls were named simply due to a negative test, because the world's literature we looked at had no control groups less than 38% positive, with most over 80–90%. The paper is silent regarding this concern.

Since people exposed to WDB must fulfill four layers of case definition to be called a case, we would expect some algorithm on how controls were shown *not to be exposed*. Specimens from patients with no known toxic mold exposures received testing to develop a reference data set for a control group. There is no table presenting methods used to show the absence of microbial amplification in buildings for each control or the presence of amplification for each case.

The author omits human health data regarding the case samples other than "symptoms acknowledged by physicians as being related to mycotoxin mold exposure in and out." The lack of a clear case definition is an egregious error. Symptoms alone are never adequate to make a diagnosis without (i) differential diagnosis and (ii) satisfaction of a case definition. It is clear from 25 years of work in the chronic inflammatory response world that the symptoms cited, including asthma, memory loss, fatigue, headache, muscle pain and weakness, are not specific to WDB exposure. Indeed, these are a small portion of the 37 symptoms found in over 30% of CIRS cases, as evidenced by published literature beginning in 1997. There is no discussion of the validity of symptoms selected by authors for applicability to case definition.

There is no discussion of known biomarkers, well established in peer-reviewed literature, including the US Government Accountability Office (GAO) study of 2008, but more importantly, published in thousands of cases compared with hundreds of controls beginning in 1998. These publications failed to cite this important paper. Bias, as shown by deliberate omission, has no basis in science.

The author has acknowledged that the ELISA mycotoxin detection antibodies employed were not monoclonal. Mycotoxin detection used "specific polyclonal antibodies" for aflatoxins, monoclonal antibodies ochratoxin A (congener not specified), and roridin antibodies for trichothecenes. We cannot ignore metabolites as possible confounders. The size of the study is inadequate to compare with MS and LC. There is inadequate information on the control group. Based on the data presented in the prior section, the likelihood of finding 55 consecutive control patients in Texas without mycotoxins in urine *approaches the number of (1/2) to the 55th power*. We may conclude that the likelihood that this control group is reliable is not supported.

The next paper, by Joseph Brewer and Dennis Hooper, again with a PubMed citation in 2013,[81] reported the detection of mycotoxins in patients with chronic fatigue syndrome (CFS). Ten of 104 cases had building samples with no results reported. This published paper presents a case/control study involving hundreds of patients, in which biomarkers for CIRS-WDB were presented.[15] A previously published diagnostic and treatment protocol added vasoactive intestinal polypeptide (VIP) to enhance patient recovery. As seen in the first paper, there are no published data references. The authors use a published case definition of CFS from Fukuda but provide no objective biomarkers.

As previously reported, urinary mycotoxin testing falsely claimed to compare cases with healthy controls. Dr. Brewer identified these controls for the first time as 28 males and 27 females, aged

18–72 years. These were from diverse geographical areas and resided in various areas of the United States. Researchers asked control subjects about complaints and/or symptoms related to "mold exposure," but none appeared in a standard data table. One assumes that the controls had exposure to foods, and airborne mold spores could occur in their daily activity. As referenced earlier, these groups, who nearly always have mycotoxins in urine, are found to have trivial levels at best.

There was no delineation of any environmental sampling used to confirm the potential for exposure as required by the US GAO Report of 2008. They do not discuss cases or controls for exposure to WDB with musty smells, visible mold, or DNA sampling to delineate species in genus or fungi present. Without documenting the potential or absence of potential for cases and controls, respectively, one cannot draw conclusions about exposure. Once again, the testing was for the urine mycotoxins aflatoxin, ochratoxin and macrocyclic trichothecene. Note that the antibodies used in Hooper's 2009 paper were the antibodies satratoxin and roridin. Extrapolation from these two to DON and others cannot be justified, even though there is possible cross-reactivity from zearalenone and DON confounding diagnosis for satratoxins

Urine was sent in a non-refrigerated container and analyzed at some time after receipt. There is no documentation on the stability of clinical samples by whatever delivery method (not sent on dry ice, not sent on wet ice, not sent overnight).

The statistics presented ignore metabolites and ignore other types of macrocyclic trichothecenes. The only documentation of qualitative results is in cases published by Hooper in 2009, and yet in 2013, the authors now claim ELISA data to be both quantitative and specific. Methods do not disclose the source of conversion of the ELISA from qualitative to quantitative. We find the controls used are the same 55 patients without mycotoxins in urine. The same argument of lack of credibility for this finding applies.

Brewer states, "The environmental histories of these patients for positive exposure to WDB many with visible mold and over 90% of these illnesses tested included residential and workplace." This data was not in the paper.

Additionally, this paper quotes the Mitochondrial Disease Foundation as a significant reference. "Mitochondrial deficiency" is claimed to be the underlying factor causing manifestations including autoimmune disorders, chronic fatigue, neurodegenerative disorders including amyotrophic lateral sclerosis, multiple sclerosis, Parkinson's disease, depression, psychiatric disorders and glycogen disorders. There is no basis presented for these claims.

Of CFS patients, "a majority had prior exposure to WDB," when data on 10 out of 104 were alluded to, and fewer than 5 had any data. Even with impeccable lab results from ELISA and standard differential diagnosis, there is no basis to ascribe significance to urine mycotoxin testing.

REFERENCES

1. Audenaert, Kris, Adriaan Vanheule, Monica Höfte, and Geert Haesaert. "Deoxynivalenol: A Major Player in the Multifaceted Response of Fusarium to Its Environment." Toxins 6, no. 1 (2013): 1–19. https://doi.org/10.3390/toxins6010001.
2. Shoemaker, Ryan. "RNA-Seq on Patients With Chronic Inflammatory Response Syndrome (CIRS) Treated With Vasoactive Intestinal Peptide (VIP) Shows a Shift in Metabolic State and Innate Immune Functions That Coincide With Healing." *Medical Research Archives* 4, no. 7 (2016). https://doi.org/10.18103/mra.v4i7.862.
3. Shoemaker, R., and J. Ryan. "A Gene Primer for Health Care Providers: The Genomics of CIRS and Associated Molecular Pathways: Interpreting the Transcriptomics Results." *Ebook*, 2018.
4. "Mycotoxins.info." Biomin. Accessed August 21, 2019. http://www.mycotoxins.info/.
5. Shoemaker, R. "Residential and Recreational Acquisition of Possible Estuarine Associated Syndrome: A New approach to Successful Diagnosis and Therapy, Environmental Health Perspectives, Special CDC Pfiesteria Supplement §." 2001.
6. Kawamoto, M., and E. Page. "Notes From the Field: Use of Unvalidated Urine Mycotoxin Tests for the Clinical Diagnosis of Illness." *Morb Mort Wkly Rep* 64, no. 6 (2014): 157–58.

7. Järvi, K., A. Hyvärinen, M. Täubel, A. M. Karvonen, M. Turunen, K. Jalkanen, R. Patovirta, T. Syrjänen, J. Pirinen, H. Salonen, and A. Nevalainen. "Microbial Growth in Building Material Samples and Occupants' Health in Severely Moisture-Damaged Homes." *Indoor Air* 28, no. 2 (2017): 287–97. https://doi.org/10.1111/ina.12440.

8. Arakawa, Kenji. "Manipulation of Metabolic Pathways Controlled by Signaling Molecules, Inducers of Antibiotic Production, for Genome Mining in Streptomyces Spp." *Antonie van Leeuwenhoek* 111, no. 5 (2018): 743–51. https://doi.org/10.1007/s10482-018-1052-6.

9. Wahibah, Ninik Nihayatul, Tomokazu Tsutsui, Daisuke Tamaoki, Kazuhiro Sato, and Takumi Nishiuchi. "Expression of Barley Glutathione S-Transferase13 Gene Reduces Accumulation of Reactive Oxygen Species by Trichothecenes and Paraquat in Arabidopsis Plants." *Plant Biotechnology* 35, no. 1 (2018): 71–79. https://doi.org/10.5511/plantbiotechnology.18.0205a.

10. Shoemaker, R., K. Johnson, M. Dooley, L. Jim, Y. Berry, and J. Ryan. "Diagnostic Process for Chronic Inflammatory Response Syndrome (CIRS): A Consensus Statement Report of the Consensus Committee of Surviving Mold." *Internal Medicine Review*, May 2018.

11. US GAO. Indoor Mold: Better Coordination of Research on Health Effects and More Consistent Guidance Would Improve Federal Efforts §, 2008.

12. Shoemaker, Ritchie C., and Dennis E. House. "Sick Building Syndrome (SBS) and Exposure to Water-Damaged Buildings: Time Series Study, Clinical Trial and Mechanisms." *Neurotoxicology and Teratology* 28, no. 5 (2006): 573–88. https://doi.org/10.1016/j.ntt.2006.07.003.

13. Shoemaker, Ritchie C., Dennis House, and James C. Ryan. "Structural Brain Abnormalities in Patients With Inflammatory Illness Acquired Following Exposure to Water-Damaged Buildings: A Volumetric MRI Study Using NeuroQuant®." *Neurotoxicology and Teratology* 45 (2014): 18–26. https://doi.org/10.1016/j.ntt.2014.06.004.

14. Shoemaker, R., S. McMahon, and J. Ryan. "Reduction in Forebrain Parenchymal and Cortical Grey Matter Swelling Across Treatment Groups in Patients With Inflammatory Illness Acquired Following Exposure to Water-Damaged Buildings." *Journal of Neuroscience and Clinical Research* 1, no. 1 (2016): 1–4.

15. Shoemaker, Ritchie. "Intranasal VIP Safely Restores Volume to Multiple Grey Matter Nuclei in Patients With CIRS." *Internal Medicine Review* 3, no. 4 (2017). https://doi.org/10.18103/imr.v3i4.412.

16. Shoemaker, Ritchie C., Dennis House, and James C. Ryan. "Vasoactive Intestinal Polypeptide (VIP) Corrects Chronic Inflammatory Response Syndrome (CIRS) Acquired Following Exposure to Water-Damaged Buildings." Health 5, no. 3 (2013): 396–401. https://doi.org/10.4236/health.2013.53053.

17. Ryan, James C., Qingzhong Wu, and Ritchie C Shoemaker. "Transcriptomic Signatures in Whole Blood of Patients Who Acquire a Chronic Inflammatory Response Syndrome (CIRS) Following an Exposure to the Marine Toxin Ciguatoxin." *BMC Medical Genomics* 8, no. 1 (2015): 1–12. https://doi.org/10.1186/s12920-015-0089-x.

18. Cortes-Canteli, Marta, Justin Paul, Erin H. Norris, Robert Bronstein, Hyung Jin Ahn, Daria Zamolodchikov, Shivaprasad Bhuvanendran, Katherine M. Fenz, and Sidney Strickland. "Fibrinogen and β-Amyloid Association Alters Thrombosis and Fibrinolysis: A Possible Contributing Factor to Alzheimer's Disease." *Neuron* 66, no. 5 (2010): 695–709. https://doi.org/10.1016/j.neuron.2010.05.014.

19. Zamolodchikov, Daria, and Sidney Strickland. "A Possible New Role for AB in Vascular and Inflammatory Dysfunction in Alzheimer's Disease." *Thrombosis Research* 141, Suppl. 2 (2016): S59–61. https://doi.org/10.1016/s0049-3848(16)30367-x.

20. Ahn, Hyung J., Zu-Lin Chen, Daria Zamolodchikov, Erin H. Norris, and Sidney Strickland. "Interactions of β-Amyloid Peptide With Fibrinogen and Coagulation Factor XII May Contribute to Alzheimer's Disease." *Current Opinion in Hematology* 24, no. 5 (2017): 427–31. https://doi.org/10.1097/moh.0000000000000368.

21. Ponikau, Jens U., David A. Sherris, Amy Weaver, and Hirohito Kita. "Treatment of Chronic Rhinosinusitis With Intranasal Amphotericin b: A Randomized, Placebo-Controlled, Double-Blind Pilot Trial." *Journal of Allergy and Clinical Immunology* 115, no. 1 (2005): 125–31. https://doi.org/10.1016/j.jaci.2004.09.037.

22. Ebbens, Fenna A., and Wytske J. Fokkens. "The Mold Conundrum in Chronic Rhinosinusitis: Where Do We Stand Today?" *Current Allergy and Asthma Reports* 8, no. 2 (2008): 93–101. https://doi.org/10.1007/s11882-008-0018-6.

23. Fokkens, Wytske J., Cornelis van Drunen, Christos Georgalas, and Fenna Ebbens. "Role of Fungi in Pathogenesis of Chronic Rhinosinusitis." *Current Opinion in Otolaryngology & Head & Neck Surgery* 20, no. 1 (2012): 19–23. https://doi.org/10.1097/moo.0b013e32834e9084.

24. Braun, H. "Incidence and Detection of Fungi and Eosinophilic Granulocytes in Chronic Rhinosinusitis." *Laryngorhinootologie* (2003): 330–40.

25. Hooper, Dennis, Vincent Bolton, Frederick Guilford, and David Straus. "Mycotoxin Detection in Human Samples From Patients Exposed to Environmental Molds." *International Journal of Molecular Sciences* 10, no. 4 (2009): 1465–75. https://doi.org/10.3390/ijms10041465.

26. Institute of Food Technologists. "Updates on the Science of Fungal Toxins." *Food Science* 71, no. 5 (2006). https://doi.org/doi:10.1111/j.1750-3841.2006.00052.

27. Bosco, Francesca, and Chiara Molle. "Mycotoxins in Food." *Food Industrial Processes - Methods and Equipment*, 2012. https://doi.org/10.5772/33061.

28. Wallin, S., L. Gambacorta, N. Kotova, E. Warensjö Lemming, C. Nälsén, M. Solfrizzo, and M. Olsen. "Biomonitoring of Concurrent Mycotoxin Exposure Among Adults in Sweden Through Urinary Multi-Biomarker Analysis." *Food and Chemical Toxicology: An International Journal Published for the British Industrial Biological Research Association*. U.S. National Library of Medicine, September 2015. https://www.ncbi.nlm.nih.gov/pubmed/26070503.

29. Tu, Chen-Pei D., and Bünyamin Akgül. "Drosophila Glutathione s-Transferases." *Methods in Enzymology* (2005): 204–26. https://doi.org/10.1016/s0076-6879(05)01013-x.

30. Gao, Yong, Yunfei Cao, Aihua Tan, Cun Liao, Zengnan Mo, and Feng Gao. "Glutathione S–Transferase M1 Polymorphism and Sporadic Colorectal Cancer Risk: An Updating Meta-Analysis and Huge Review of 36 Case-Control Studies." *Annals of Epidemiology* 20, no. 2 (2010): 108–21. https://doi.org/10.1016/j.annepidem.2009.10.003.

31. Wu, Miaomiao, Hao Xiao, Wenkai Ren, Jie Yin, Bie Tan, Gang Liu, Lili Li, Charles Martin Nyachoti, Xia Xiong, and Guoyao Wu. "Therapeutic Effects of Glutamic Acid in Piglets Challenged With Deoxynivalenol." *PLoS One* 9, no. 7 (2014): e100591. https://doi.org/10.1371/journal.pone.0100591.

32. Duan, Jielin, Jie Yin, Miaomiao Wu, Peng Liao, Dun Deng, Gang Liu, Qingqi Wen, Y. Liu, and X. Wu. "Dietary Glutamate Supplementation Ameliorates Mycotoxin-Induced Abnormalities in the Intestinal Structure and Expression of Amino Acid Transporters in Young Pigs." *PLoS One* 9, no. 11 (2014): e112357. https://doi.org/10.1371/journal.pone.0112357.

33. Wu, Miaomiao, Hao Xiao, Wenkai Ren, Jie Yin, Jiayu Hu, Jielin Duan, Gang Liu, B. Tan, X. Xiong, A. O. Oso, and O. Adeola. "An NMR-Based Metabolomic Approach to Investigate the Effects of Supplementation With Glutamic Acid in Piglets Challenged With Deoxynivalenol." *PLoS One* 9, no. 12 (2014): e113687. https://doi.org/10.1371/journal.pone.0113687.

34. Veršilovskis, Aleksandrs, and Sarah De Saeger. "Sterigmatocystin: Occurrence in Foodstuffs and Analytical Methods - An Overview." *Molecular Nutrition & Food Research* 54, no. 1 (2009): 136–47. https://doi.org/10.1002/mnfr.200900345.

35. Ates, Ilker, Ozge Cemiloglu Ulker, Cigdem Akdemir, and Asuman Karakaya. "Correlation of Ochratoxin a Exposure to Urinary Levels of 8-Hydroxydeoxyguanosine and Malondialdehyde in a Turkish Population." *Bulletin of Environmental Contamination and Toxicology* 86, no. 3 (2011): 258–62. https://doi.org/10.1007/s00128-011-0225-z.

36. Rychlik, Michael. "Rapid Degradation of the Mycotoxin Patulin in Man Quantified by Stable Isotope Dilution Assays." *Food Additives and Contaminants* 20, no. 9 (2003): 829–37. https://doi.org/10.1080/0265203031000152424.

37. Santos, R. R., S. Vermeulen, A. Haritova, and J. Fink-Gremmels. "Isotherm Modeling of Organic Activated Bentonite and Humic Acid Polymer Used as Mycotoxin Adsorbents." *Food Additives & Contaminants: Part A* 28, no. 11 (2011): 1578–89. https://doi.org/10.1080/19440049.2011.595014.

38. Galvano, Fabio, Andrea Piva, Alberto Ritieni, and Giacomo Galvano. "Dietary Strategies to Counteract the Effects of Mycotoxins: A Review." *Journal of Food Protection* 64, no. 1 (2001): 120–31. https://doi.org/10.4315/0362-028x-64.1.120.

39. Schatzmayr, Gerd, Florian Zehner, Martin Täubel, Dian Schatzmayr, Alfred Klimitsch, Andreas Paul Loibner, and Eva Maria Binder. "Microbiologicals for Deactivating Mycotoxins." *Molecular Nutrition & Food Research* 50, no. 6 (2006): 543–51. https://doi.org/10.1002/mnfr.200500181.

40. Cserháti, M., B. Kriszt, Cs. Krifaton, S. Szoboszlay, J. Háhn, S. Z. Tóth, I. Nagy, and J. Kukolya. "Mycotoxin-Degradation Profile of Rhodococcus Strains." *International Journal of Food Microbiology* 166, no. 1 (2013): 176–85. https://doi.org/10.1016/j.ijfoodmicro.2013.06.002.

41. Molnar, Orsolya, Gerd Schatzmayr, Elisabeth Fuchs, and Hansjoerg Prillinger. "Trichosporon Mycotoxinivorans Sp. Nov., a New Yeast Species Useful in Biological Detoxification of Various Mycotoxins." *Systematic and Applied Microbiology* 27, no. 6 (2004): 661–71. https://doi.org/10.1078/0723202042369947.

42. Larsson, Pia, Lief Busk, and Hans Tjälve. "Hepatic and Extrahepatic Bioactivation and GSH Conjugation of Aflatoxin B1 in Sheep." *Carcinogenesis* 15, no. 5 (1994): 947–55. https://doi.org/10.1093/carcin/15.5.947.

43. Hassan, Zahoor Ul, Muhammad Zargham Khan, Muhammad Kashif Saleemi, Ahrar Khan, Ijaz Javed, and Mnaza Noreen. "Immunological Responses of Male White Leghorn Chicks Kept on Ochratoxin a (Ota)-Contaminated Feed." *Journal of Immunotoxicology* 9, no. 1 (2011): 56–63. https://doi.org/10.3109 /1547691x.2011.627393.

44. Khatoon, Aisha, Muhammad Zargham Khan, Ahrar Khan, Muhammad Kashif Saleemi, and Ijaz Javed. "Amelioration of Ochratoxin A-Induced Immunotoxic Effects by Silymarin and Vitamin E in White Leghorn Cockerels." *Journal of Immunotoxicology* 10, no. 1 (2012): 25–31. https://doi.org/10.3109 /1547691x.2012.686533.

45. Pestka, James J. "Deoxynivalenol-Induced Proinflammatory Gene Expression: Mechanisms and Pathological Sequelae." *Toxins* 2, no. 6 (2010): 1300–1317. https://doi.org/10.3390/toxins2061300.

46. Zhou, Hui-Ren, Qunshan Jia, and James J. Pestka. "Ribotoxic Stress Response to the Trichothecene Deoxynivalenol in the Macrophage Involves the Src Family Kinase Hck." *Toxicological Sciences* 85, no. 2 (2005): 916–26. https://doi.org/10.1093/toxsci/kfi146.

47. Pestka, J. J. "Mechanisms of Deoxynivalenol-Induced Gene Expression and Apoptosis." *Food Additives & Contaminants: Part A* 25, no. 9 (2008): 1128–40. https://doi.org/10.1080/02652030802056626.

48. Lim, Junghyun, Yunsu Lee, Hyun-Wook Kim, Im Joo Rhyu, Myung Sook Oh, Moussa B. H. Youdim, Zhenyu Yue, and Young J. Oh. "Nigericin-Induced Impairment of Autophagic Flux in Neuronal Cells is Inhibited by Overexpression of Bak." *Journal of Biological Chemistry* 287, no. 28 (2012): 23271–82. https://doi.org/10.1074/jbc.m112.364281.

49. "Mycotoxin Test Kits: Fast & Reliable Mycotoxin Detection." *Romer Labs.* Accessed September 28, 2019. https://www.romerlabs.com/en/products/test-kits/mycotoxin-test-kits/.

50. Alshannaq, Ahmad, and Jae-Hyuk Yu. "Occurrence, Toxicity, and Analysis of Major Mycotoxins in Food." *International Journal of Environmental Research and Public Health MDPI,* June 13, 2017. https://www.ncbi.nlm.nih.gov/pmc/articles/PMC5486318/.

51. "A Brand-New Urine Test for Mycotoxin Exposure." Accessed March 23, 2022. https://www.greatpl ainslaboratory.com/upcoming-webinars/2017/8/31/gpl-mycotox-a-brand-new-urine-test-for-mycotoxin -exposure. Great Plains Lab, n.d.

52. Zöllner, P, J. Jodlbauer, M. Kleinova, H. Kahlbacher, T. Kuhn, W. Hochsteiner, and W. Lindner. "Concentration Levels of Zearalenone and Its Metabolites in Urine, Muscle Tissue, and Liver Samples of Pigs Fed With Mycotoxin-Contaminated Oats." *Journal of Agricultural and Food Chemistry.* U.S. National Library of Medicine. Accessed September 28, 2019. https://pubmed.ncbi.nlm.nih.gov /11958611/.

53. van Bennekom, E. O., L. Brouwer, E. H. M. Laurant, H. Hooijerink, and M. W. F. Nielen. "Confirmatory Analysis Method for Zeranol, Its Metabolites and Related Mycotoxins in Urine by Liquid Chromatography-Negative Ion Electrospray Tandem Mass Spectrometry." *Analytica Chimica Acta.* Elsevier, October 12, 2002. https://www.sciencedirect.com/science/article/pii/S0003267002009753.

54. Warth, Benedikt, Michael Sulyok, Philipp Fruhmann, Hannes Mikula, Franz Berthiller, Rainer Schuhmacher, Christian Hametner, W. A. Abia, G. Adam, J. Fröhlich, and R. Krska. "Development and Validation of a Rapid Multi-Biomarker Liquid Chromatography/Tandem Mass Spectrometry Method to Assess Human Exposure to Mycotoxins." *Rapid Communications in Mass Spectrometry* 26, no. 13 (2012): 1533–40. https://doi.org/10.1002/rcm.6255.

55. Escrivá, Laura, Lara Manyes, Guillermina Font, and Houda Berrada. "Mycotoxin Analysis of Human Urine by LC-MS/MS: A Comparative Extraction Study." *MDPI: Multidisciplinary Digital Publishing Institute,* October 19, 2017. https://www.mdpi.com/2072-6651/9/10/330/html.

56. "Comprehensive Reviews in Food … - Wiley Online Library." Accessed September 7, 2019. https://ift .onlinelibrary.wiley.com/doi/10.1111/1541-4337.12412.

57. "Urine as a Biomarkers of Exposure to Fusarium Mycotoxins." Food Standards Agency. Accessed September 7, 2019. https://www.food.gov.uk/research/research-projects/urine-as-a-biomarkers-of -exposure-to-fusarium-mycotoxins.

58. Ahn, J., D. Kim, H. Kim, and K.Y. Jahng. Quantitative Determination of Mycotoxins in Urine by LC-MS/MS, January 1, 1970. https://pubag.nal.usda.gov/catalog/2380339.

59. Ali, Nurshad, Meinolf Blaszkewicz, M. Manirujjaman, and Gisela H. Degen. "Biomonitoring of Concurrent Exposure to Ochratoxin A and Citrinin in Pregnant Women in Bangladesh." *Mycotoxin Research* 32, no. 3 (2016): 163–72. https://doi.org/10.1007/s12550-016-0251-0.

60. Capriotti, Anna Laura, Giuseppe Caruso, Chiara Cavaliere, Patrizia Foglia, Roberto Samperi, and Aldo Laganà. "Multiclass Mycotoxin Analysis in Food, Environmental and Biological Matrices With Chromatography/Mass Spectrometry." *Mass Spectrometry Reviews* 31, no. 4 (2011): 466–503. https:// doi.org/10.1002/mas.20351.

61. Li, Peiwu, Zhaowei Zhang, Xiaofeng Hu, and Qi Zhang. "Advanced Hyphenated Chromatographic-Mass Spectrometry in Mycotoxin Determination: Current Status and Prospects." *Mass Spectrometry Reviews* 32, no. 6 (2013): 420–52. https://doi.org/10.1002/mas.21377.

62. Köppen, Robert, Matthias Koch, David Siegel, Stefan Merkel, Ronald Maul, and Irene Nehls. "Determination of Mycotoxins in Foods: Current State of Analytical Methods and Limitations." *Applied Microbiology and Biotechnology* 86, no. 6 (2010): 1595–612. https://doi.org/10.1007/s00253-010-2535-1.

63. Gerding, Johannes, Benedikt Cramer, and Hans-Ulrich Humpf. "Determination of Mycotoxin Exposure in Germany Using an LC-Ms/MS Multibiomarker Approach." *Molecular Nutrition & Food Research* 58, no. 12 (2014): 2358–68. https://doi.org/10.1002/mnfr.201400406.

64. Jager, Alessandra, Fernando Tonin, Pollyana Souto, Rafaela Privatti, and Carlos Oliveira. "Determination of Urinary Biomarkers for Assessment of Short-Term Human Exposure to Aflatoxins in São Paulo, Brazil." *Toxins* 6, no. 7 (2014): 1996–2007. https://doi.org/10.3390/toxins6071996.

65. Rodríguez-Carrasco, Yelko, Juan Carlos Moltó, Jordi Mañes, and Houda Berrada. "Exposure Assessment Approach Through Mycotoxin/Creatinine Ratio Evaluation in Urine by GC–MS/MS." *Food and Chemical Toxicology* 72 (2014): 69–75. https://doi.org/10.1016/j.fct.2014.07.014.

66. Föllmann, Wolfram, Nurshad Ali, Meinolf Blaszkewicz, and Gisela H. Degen. "Biomonitoring of Mycotoxins in Urine: Pilot Study in Mill Workers." *Journal of Toxicology and Environmental Health, Part A* 79, nos. 22–23 (2016): 1015–25. https://doi.org/10.1080/15287394.2016.1219540.

67. Shephard, Gordon S., Hester-Mari Burger, Lucia Gambacorta, Yun Yun Gong, Rudolf Krska, John P. Rheeder, Michele Solfrizzo, C. Srey, M. Sulyok, A. Visconti, and B. Warth. "Multiple Mycotoxin Exposure Determined by Urinary Biomarkers in Rural Subsistence Farmers in the Former Transkei, South Africa." *Food and Chemical Toxicology* 62 (2013): 217–25. https://doi.org/10.1016/j.fct.2013.08.040.

68. Rodríguez-Carrasco, Yelko, Juan Carlos Moltó, Jordi Mañes, and Houda Berrada. "Development of Microextraction Techniques in Combination With GC-MS/MS for the Determination of Mycotoxins and Metabolites in Human Urine." *Journal of Separation Science* 40, no. 7 (2017): 1572–82. https://doi.org/10.1002/jssc.201601131.

69. Li, Chenglong, Chunli Deng, Shuang Zhou, Yunfeng Zhao, Dan Wang, Xiaodan Wang, Yun Yun Gong, and Yongning Wu. "High-Throughput and Sensitive Determination of Urinary Zearalenone and Metabolites by UPLC-MS/MS and Its Application to a Human Exposure Study." *Analytical and Bioanalytical Chemistry* 410, no. 21 (2018): 5301–12. https://doi.org/10.1007/s00216-018-1186-4.

70. Ezekiel, Chibundu N., Oyetunde T. Oyeyemi, Oluwawapelumi A. Oyedele, Kolawole I. Ayeni, Ifeoluwa T. Oyeyemi, Williams Nabofa, Chinomso U. Nwozichi, and Adeyemi Dada. "Urinary Aflatoxin Exposure Monitoring in Rural and Semi-Urban Populations in Ogun State, Nigeria." *Food Additives & Contaminants: Part A* 35, no. 8 (2018): 1565–72. https://doi.org/10.1080/19440049.2018.1475752.

71. Viegas, Susana, Ricardo Assunção, Carla Nunes, Bernd Osteresch, Magdalena Twarużek, Robert Kosicki, Jan Grajewski, C. Martins, P. Alvito, A. Almeida, and C. Viegas. "Exposure Assessment to Mycotoxins in a Portuguese Fresh Bread Dough Company by Using a Multi-Biomarker Approach." *Toxins* 10, no. 9 (2018): 342. https://doi.org/10.3390/toxins10090342.

72. Papageorgiou, Maria, Liz Wells, Courtney Williams, Kay L.M. White, Barbara De Santis, Yunru Liu, Francesca Debegnach, B. Miano, G. Moretti, S. Greetham, and C. Brera. "Occurrence of Deoxynivalenol in an Elderly Cohort in the UK: A Biomonitoring Approach." *Food Additives & Contaminants: Part A* 35, no. 10 (2018): 2032–44. https://doi.org/10.1080/19440049.2018.1508890.

73. Viegas, Carla, Tiago Faria, Ana Cebola de Oliveira, Liliana Aranha Caetano, Elisabete Carolino, Anita Quintal-Gomes, Magdalena Twarużek, Robert Kosicki, Ewelina Soszczyńska, and Susana Viegas. "A New Approach to Assess Occupational Exposure to Airborne Fungal Contamination and Mycotoxins of Forklift Drivers in Waste Sorting Facilities." *Mycotoxin Research* 33, no. 4 (2017): 285–95. https://doi.org/10.1007/s12550-017-0288-8.

74. Scharf, Daniel H., Axel A. Brakhage, and Prasun K. Mukherjee. "Gliotoxin - Bane or Boon?" *Environmental Microbiology* 18, no. 4 (2015): 1096–109. https://doi.org/10.1111/1462-2920.13080.

75. Scharf, Daniel H., Thorsten Heinekamp, Nicole Remme, Peter Hortschansky, Axel A. Brakhage, and Christian Hertweck. "Biosynthesis and Function of Gliotoxin in Aspergillus Fumigatus." *Applied Microbiology and Biotechnology* 93, no. 2 (2011): 467–72. https://doi.org/10.1007/s00253-011-3689-1.

76. Dolan, Stephen K., Grainne O'Keeffe, Gary W. Jones, and Sean Doyle. "Resistance is Not Futile: Gliotoxin Biosynthesis, Functionality and Utility." *Trends in Microbiology* 23, no. 7 (2015): 419–28. https://doi.org/10.1016/j.tim.2015.02.005.

77. Ali, Nurshad, Meinolf Blaszkewicz, and Gisela H. Degen. "Occurrence of the Mycotoxin Citrinin and Its Metabolite Dihydrocitrinone in Urines of German Adults." *Archives of Toxicology* 89, no. 4 (2014): 573–78. https://doi.org/10.1007/s00204-014-1363-y.

78. Brezina, U., I. Rempe, S. Kersten, H. Valenta, H.-U. Humpf, and S. Dänicke. "Determination of Zearalenone, Deoxynivalenol and Metabolites in Bile of Piglets Fed Diets With Graded Levels of Fusarium Toxin Contaminated Maize." *World Mycotoxin Journal* 9, no. 2 (2016): 179–93. https://doi.org/10.3920/wmj2015.1902.

79. Karima, Hmaissia-Khlifa, Ghali Ridha, Aouni Zied, Mazigh Chekib, Machgoul Salem, and Hedhili Abderrazek. "Estimation of Ochratoxin A in Human Blood of Healthy Tunisian Population." *Experimental and Toxicologic Pathology* 62, no. 5 (2010): 539–42. https://doi.org/10.1016/j.etp.2009.07.005.

80. Peraica, Maja, Ana-Marija Domijan, Mirjana Matašin, Ana Lucić, Božica Radić, Frane Delaš, Martina Horvat, Ivanka Bosanac, Melita Balija, and Damir Grgičević. "Variations of Ochratoxin a Concentration in the Blood of Healthy Populations in Some Croatian Cities." *Archives of Toxicology* 75, no. 7 (2001): 410–14. https://doi.org/10.1007/s002040100258.

81. Brewer, Joseph, Jack Thrasher, David Straus, Roberta Madison, and Dennis Hooper. "Detection of Mycotoxins in Patients With Chronic Fatigue Syndrome." *Toxins* 5, no. 4 (2013): 605–17. https://doi.org/10.3390/toxins5040605.

8 Euthyroid Sick Syndrome, CIRS and Glyphosate Toxicity

Stephanie Seneff

CONTENTS

8.1 INTRODUCTION

Nonthyroidal illness syndrome (NTIS), also known as euthyroid sick syndrome, is a medical condition often associated with chronically ill patients. In this syndrome, thyroid hormone activity is deficient despite the fact that the thyroid appears to be functioning normally. A case study published in 2017 was based on nine patients in Finland with a history of mold exposure from water-damaged buildings who suffered from symptoms of chronic fatigue and cognitive impairment as a consequence. These patients were not responsive to thyroxine (T4) therapy, but all of them were successfully treated with triiodothyronine (T3)-based thyroid hormone, along with adrenal support with hydrocortisone and dehydroepiandrosterone (DHEA), nutritional supplementation and elimination of gluten-containing foods likely to be a source of mycotoxin.[1] The authors proposed that exposure to metabolites produced by toxigenic fungi can lead to an imbalance of many hormones, but particularly leading to symptoms of thyroid hormone deficiency, despite a healthy thyroid gland.

The system that regulates tissue levels of thyroid hormone is complex. T4 (L-thyroxine) is converted to T3 (triiodothyronine) by an enzyme named deiodinase 2 (DIO2) through removal of an outer ring iodide from T4. The enzyme DIO3, on the other hand, removes an inner ring iodide from T4, yielding reverse T3 (rT3), and it can also convert T3 to T2 (diiodothyronine) through the removal of an inner ring iodide from T3. Both rT3 and T2 are inactive. In fact, rT3 actually blocks the T3 receptors, preventing access by T3, an effect that actively suppresses thyroid signaling. The patients in the cited study all had a very low ratio of T3 to rT3, likely the primary cause of their hypothyroid symptoms. T3 is a potent stimulator of mitochondrial activity, both increasing the production of ATP and inducing mitochondrial biogenesis.[2] Therefore, it is not surprising that suppression of T3 leads to extreme fatigue and cognitive dysfunction. NTIS is a common phenomenon observed in critically ill patients in the intensive care unit. Low levels of free T3 are a strong predictor of poor outcome, along with elevated levels of rT3.[3] But, it is also a feature of many chronic diseases, especially when linked to mold exposures.

Chronic Inflammatory Response Syndrome (CIRS), also referred to as biotoxin illness or mold illness, is a term coined originally by Dr. Ritchie Shoemaker in the late 1990s.[4] It characterizes a syndrome that can become chronic following exposure to toxins produced by mold and other organisms present in a water-damaged building. It is in many ways similar to chronic fatigue syndrome and Lyme disease. It is characterized by persistent fatigue, weakness, flu-like symptoms, exhaustion and insomnia. There is often a diverse array of other symptoms such as joint pain, shortness of breath, a metallic taste in the mouth, headaches, dizziness, sensitivity to cold, blurred vision, etc. People suffering from CIRS are often overly sensitive to exposure to multiple environmental toxins.

In this chapter, an argument will be presented to show how glyphosate, the active ingredient in the pervasive herbicide Roundup, may be playing a critical role in promoting an increased risk to exposure to mycotoxins while at the same time inducing mitochondrial dysfunction that predisposes the patient to sensitivity to mold. It is proposed that mitochondrial dysfunction leads directly to CIRS and associated euthyroid sick syndrome, specifically through impairment of clathrin-based endocytosis of DIO3 in the liver. This results in excessive conversion of T4 to rT3 and of T3 to T2, maintaining low thyroid signaling despite a healthy thyroid gland.

8.2 MUCH OF THE ACTION IS IN THE LIVER

The word "aflatoxin" is an acronym formed from *Aspergillus FLAvus* TOXIN, and it characterizes a large class of toxic heterocyclic compounds produced by the mold species *A. flavus*. The liver is the primary detoxification organ in the body, and therefore, it carries the primary burden for clearance of aflatoxins and other toxic mycotoxins, which are common contaminants in nuts and grains. Cytochrome P450 (CYP) enzymes play a crucial role in detoxifying mycotoxins.[5] However, glyphosate suppresses the activity of liver CYP enzymes.[6] With CYP enzyme deficiency, aflatoxins are preferentially oxidized by epoxygenases to produce highly reactive aflatoxin epoxides that can cause DNA mutations leading to hepatic carcinoma.[7] These toxic epoxides are conjugated to reduced glutathione in the liver by glutathione-S-transferase, and this is a critical phase II detoxification mechanism.[5] Here too, glyphosate can be expected to interfere, because as we will see later, it induces oxidative stress in the liver, causing glutathione to be mainly in its oxidized (unavailable) form as glutathione disulfide (GSSG). Glyphosate also causes an upregulation of the enzyme gamma glutamyl transpeptidase (GGT), which breaks glutathione apart into its component amino acids.[8] Therefore, with insufficient supply of reduced glutathione and defective CYP enzyme activity, aflatoxins and other mycotoxins cause much more liver damage than would be the case without chronic glyphosate exposure.

Both glyphosate and aflatoxins are linked to liver fibrosis and hepatocellular carcinoma. A study on humans suffering from fatty liver disease found significantly higher levels of glyphosate in the urine of patients compared with controls, as well as significantly higher levels of urinary glyphosate in more advanced cases with extensive liver fibrosis compared with less advanced cases.[9] A rat study that involved exposing rats to doses of Roundup that were below regulatory limits also demonstrated evidence of fatty liver disease in exposed rats compared with controls.[10]

A meta-analysis found that a significant increase in the risk of liver cirrhosis is associated with aflatoxin exposure (unadjusted odds ratio of 3.35).[11] A study focused on carriers of hepatitis B virus found a much shorter time interval to a diagnosis of cirrhosis and hepatocarcinoma in participants with high serum levels of aflatoxin B ($p < 0.0001$).

The liver is the primary organ involved in the peripheral conversion of T4 into its metabolites, T3, rT3 and T2. Patients with liver cirrhosis typically have low serum levels of T3 and elevated levels of rT3, along with a normal level of thyroid stimulating hormone.[12] This likely reflects upregulation of DIO3 in the liver in response to manifest liver disease. As we will show in more detail later in this chapter, a likely source of this imbalance is the influx of macrophages into the liver in response to inflammation, and a defective capability of those macrophages to endocytose DIO3. Liver fibrosis results in increased stiffness of the extracellular matrix, and this causes a phenomenon called "frustrated endocytosis" in the invasive macrophages. Clathrin-mediated endocytosis is the mechanism by which DIO3 is removed from the extracellular space. If this process is impeded, DIO3 remains exposed in the plasma membrane of cells, where it can freely convert external T4 into rT3 and convert T3 into T2, resulting in the observed serum imbalance in cirrhosis patients.

8.3   GLYPHOSATE AND FUNGI

Not only is glyphosate widely used as an herbicide on crops such as corn, soy, canola and sugar beets that have been genetically engineered to resist it, but it is also routinely used on wheat, oats and barley crops as a desiccant just before harvest, particularly in northern climates where application can induce ripening before frost sets in. Glyphosate has been shown to predispose exposed crop plants to damage from multiple pathogens. The mechanisms include disruption of the rhizosphere microbial balance, restriction of the availability of minerals to crops through its action as a strong chelator, and interfering with innate physiological defenses of the plants due to blockage of the shikimate pathway.[13] Glyphosate-based herbicides can also enhance the population or the virulence of pathogenic species in the soil, especially when these species possess genes for enzymes that can fully metabolize glyphosate, giving them a strong advantage over other species.

Many species of fungi can use glyphosate as a source of both nutrients and energy. In particular, there are certain fungal strains that are being exploited for their ability to degrade glyphosate for applications in soil remediation.[14] A study involving two nontoxic strains of *Aspergillus oryzae* demonstrated that these fungi were able to use glyphosate as a sole source of nitrogen or as a sole source of phosphorus. More than half of the glyphosate present in a soil microcosm assay was eliminated after just 15 days of incubation with these species. The authors advocated for their potential use as bioremediation agents.[15, 16] While this is encouraging news for the removal of glyphosate, what is likely to happen in reality is that virulent strains of fungus able to metabolize glyphosate thrive among glyphosate-exposed crops and produce metabolites that are toxic to humans consuming the foods derived from those crops.

Grains such as corn, wheat and barley are often contaminated with mold, especially Fusarium. A disease called Fusarium head blight (FHB) is widespread among cereal crops in the western Canadian Prairies. A study examining potential factors increasing risk in wheat and barley crops in eastern Saskatchewan found that glyphosate usage, along with reduced tillage, tended to result in an increase in the presence of two pathogenic species of Fusarium, *Fusarium avenaceum* and *Fusarium graminearum*, associated with the disease.[17]

Among the many genera that produce mycotoxins, Fusarium fungi are the most widespread in cereal-growing areas of the planet. Some of the toxic metabolites they produce include zearalenone (ZEA), fumonisins, moniliformin and trichothecenes. ZEA has strong estrogenic activity, giving it the potential to stimulate the growth of human breast cancer cells, and fumonisins are also cancer-promoting metabolites. Trichothecenes have toxic effects in the gut and the skin, and they can destroy red blood cells. The health of livestock depends critically on maintaining low levels of mycotoxins in their feed.[18]

8.4   MYCOTOXINS, GLYPHOSATE AND MITOCHONDRIA

It is widely accepted that a key mechanism of toxicity of mycotoxins is through oxidative stress leading to mitochondrial damage. As early as 1970, a study involving isolated liver mitochondria obtained from rats demonstrated impairment in oxidative phosphorylation following exposure of the mitochondria to ochratoxin A (OTA) or its common metabolite.[19] OTA is commonly produced by multiple species of mold, including *Aspergillus ochraceus*, *A. carbonarius*, *A. niger* and *Penicillium verrucosum*, and it is a widespread contaminant in cereal grains, dried fruits, wine and coffee. Other mycotoxins that cause mitochondrial dysfunction include citrinin, aflatoxin and T-2 toxin. In fact, it has recently been argued that these mycotoxins might be promising compounds for chemotherapy in cancer.[20]

Aflatoxin B is a common mycotoxin produced by pathogenic Aspergillus species that is especially damaging to DNA. It can be detoxified in the liver through a hydroxylation step followed by glutathionylation, but this depends on adequate supplies of glutathione in the liver.[21]

Aflatoxin B can cause significant liver damage to exposed individuals. It gets metabolized in the liver through epoxidation into a highly reactive molecule that is a well-established carcinogen, causing genetic mutations in mitochondrial DNA. However, if there is sufficient glutathione in the reduced form in the liver mitochondria, glutathione-S-transferase can be invoked to glutathionylate the carcinogen, converting it to a water-soluble molecule that can be excreted through the urine.[22] Ochratoxin A has been found to suppress enzymes that are specifically involved in the de novo synthesis of glutathione, and it was suggested that this could be its primary mechanism of toxicity.[23]

Many plants, including maize, wheat, barley, chickpeas and sugarcane, express glutathione-S-transferase activity, and so it is possible that they could detoxify aflatoxins through the same process that takes place in exposed humans, removing the toxin a priori from food sources. Plants also produce CYP enzymes that could convert mycotoxins to less toxic forms, but plant CYP enzymes, like liver CYPs, are suppressed by glyphosate.[24] Even the aflatoxin-producing fungi themselves express glutathione-S-transferase, which suggests that an adequate supply of sulfur to maintain high levels of glutathione could reduce mycotoxin levels expressed by the fungi.[22]

Glyphosate has been shown to induce oxidative stress in both plants and animals, which results in glutathione oxidation to glutathione disulfide (GSSG), a glutathione dimer that cannot be used for glutathionylation. In an experiment involving exposing pea plants to glyphosate, it was demonstrated that glyphosate induced an increase in the oxidized form of glutathione (GSSG) relative to the total glutathione pool. By 2 days after glyphosate had been applied to the leaves of the plants, oxidized glutathione content in the leaves had doubled.[25] The authors hypothesized that this was due to oxidative stress induced by glyphosate. A study on rice leaves exposed to glyphosate used a proteomic approach to demonstrate clearly that glyphosate caused oxidative stress in the rice leaves. Several antioxidant enzymes were upregulated, including ascorbate peroxidase, glutathione-S-transferase, peroxiredoxin and superoxide dismutase, among others. Furthermore, there was peroxidation and destruction of lipids in the rice leaves through the generation of reactive oxygen species.[26]

Glyphosate similarly causes oxidative stress in exposed animals. For example, in a study on rats exposed to Roundup, a glyphosate-based herbicide, at sublethal concentrations, it was demonstrated through increased levels of lipid peroxidation that the liver suffered from oxidative stress, and glutathione levels were depleted as well.[27] Glyphosate's induction of oxidative stress not only depletes glutathione but also has the potential to directly cause DNA damage to the mitochondria, leading to impaired mitochondrial function. Glyphosate is therefore likely synergistically toxic with mycotoxins, both by impairing the detoxification process for mycotoxin clearance in food crops and exposed humans, and by itself contributing additional damage to the mitochondria.

Many studies have provided direct evidence of damage to mitochondrial function by glyphosate or its formulations. An in vitro study on human semen exposed to a low dose of Roundup (1 mg/liter) showed that Roundup impaired sperm motility after just 1 hour, and this was associated with impaired mitochondrial function.[28] Roundup has been shown experimentally to inhibit both succinate dehydrogenase and cytochrome C reductase, two enzymes that play a crucial role in mitochondrial oxidative phosphorylation.[29] Succinate dehydrogenase is the primary enzyme in Complex II, and cytochrome C reductase is crucial in Complex III. Succinate dehydrogenase is the only enzyme that is involved in both the citric acid cycle and oxidative phosphorylation. Low levels of glyphosate-based formulations have been shown to induce cell death in human umbilical, embryonic and placental cells, attributed to suppression of succinate dehydrogenase.[30] Exposure of mitochondria in vitro to glyphosate demonstrated that glyphosate increased permeability of the membrane to both protons and calcium, and this would also disturb mitochondrial function.[31]

Multiple studies have shown that glyphosate induces excessive calcium uptake by several different cell types, through the accumulation of excess glutamate in the extracellular space, and that this induces neuroexcitotoxicity in the hipppocampus.[32–34] Glutamate neurotoxicity is triggered by massive calcium influx following overstimulation of NMDA receptors. Mitochondria sequester excess calcium, and this causes mitochondrial depolarization. The reduced membrane potential opens up the permeability transition pore, further collapsing the potential. Uncoupling of electron transfer from ATP synthesis results in the abundant release of reactive oxygen species, with subsequent injury to the mitochondria.[35]

8.5   AN ESSENTIAL ROLE FOR NEUTROPHILS

Granulocytes are a class of white blood cells, also called polymorphonuclear leukocytes (PMNs), that includes neutrophils, eosinophils, basophils and mast cells. The nomenclature reflects their content of many large cytoplasmic granules containing antimicrobial proteins, acid hydrolases, lysozyme and DIO3. They also have enzymes that produce various reactive oxygen and nitrogen species. All of these tools are very effective for controlling invasive species such as fungi. Neutrophils in particular play a powerful role in controlling a fungus infection.[36]

The enzyme complex NADPH oxidase is released by neutrophils following activation, and the resulting "respiratory burst" produces an abundance of superoxide. At the same time, iNOS (inducible nitric oxide synthase) releases nitric oxide, and the superoxide reacts with nitric oxide to produce the extremely reactive molecule peroxynitrite ($ONOO^-$), a powerful agent for clearing the invasive fungus.

8.6   INTERLEUKIN-6 DRIVES INFLAMMATION

Increased production of inflammatory cytokines, especially interleukin 6 (IL-6), is a hallmark of the acute phase of NTIS.[37] In cells grown in culture, exposure to IL-6 suppressed active T3 generation by DIO1 and DIO2, while increasing activity of DIO3 to inactivate T4 and T3. This effect was prevented by the addition of N-acetylcysteine (NAC) to the culture medium.[38] It was determined that NAC supplementation restored intracellular glutathione concentrations, which prevented the inhibitory effect of IL-6. The authors proposed that the response to IL-6 depletes glutathione stores through its induction of oxidative stress. It can also be concluded that thyroid hormone homeostasis is tightly regulated by glutathione availability in the mitochondria. When glutathione levels are depleted, a process ensues that prevents uptake of thyroid hormone, perhaps in order to protect the mitochondria from oxidative damage by suppressing their activity. But, this leaves the patient with a feeling of extreme fatigue. A schematic of the process by which overproduction of IL-6 due to mycotoxins working together with chronic glyphosate exposure leads to euthyroid sick syndrome is presented in Figure 8.1.[38]

8.7   GRANULE RELEASE BY NEUTROPHILS

Systemic candidiasis is most commonly caused by the commensal yeast *Candida albicans*. It has emerged as the leading cause of bloodstream infections in immune-compromised hospital patients in the United States.[39] Aspergillus infections in the lungs are also a common development among immune-compromised people.[40] It is increasingly becoming apparent that granulocytes, and most especially neutrophils, play a significant role in controlling fungal infections.[41, 42] The degranulation of their cytoplasmic granules is critical for fighting off the infection.

A G-protein coupled receptor for IL-8, known as CXC chemokine receptor 1 (CXCR1), is highly induced in kidneys infected with *Candida albicans*.[41] CXCR1−/− mice were more susceptible to kidney failure following Candida exposure due to impaired release of granules by neutrophils. Humans with a defective mutant form of CXCR1 also show increased susceptibility to candidiasis.

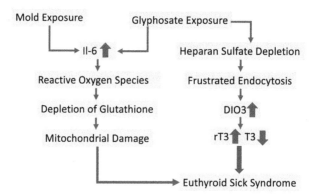

FIGURE 8.1 Proposed mechanism for the effects of IL-6 and glyphosate, resulting in euthyroid sick syndrome.

These observations suggest that CXCR1 signaling induces granule release by neutrophils, and that granule release is essential for clearing the fungus infection.

Among many other proteins, granulocytes also contain DIO3 within their granules, and it is released upon activation by stressors such as an infection.[43] Interestingly, it is unclear whether the importance of DIO3 expression is due to suppression of thyroid hormone signaling or to the supply of iodide to the extracellular milieu after it is detached from thyroid hormones. It is probable that the two aspects are closely intertwined.

8.8   CLATHRIN-COATED PITS AND DIO3

Clathrin-mediated endocytosis (CME) is a mechanism by which cells absorb a number of different metabolites, hormones and proteins through inward budding of the plasma membrane. Clathrin is a specialized protein that forms a mesh along the internal side of the plasma membrane, causing an indentation to form. A clathrin-coated pit eventually buds off the membrane and is internalized as a vesicle, encased in the clathrin–protein complex. The entire process is mediated by receptors on the surface of the cell. Following internalization, the vesicle merges with an early endosome, and the receptor then recycles back to the membrane.

ATP is required for the internalization of clathrin-coated pits. When cellular ATP is depleted, these pits remain in an open state at the cell surface and cannot be internalized.[44] It follows that mitochondrial dysfunction, such as that induced by mycotoxins, impairs CME. Depletion of membrane cholesterol also blocks CME.[45]

The term "frustrated" endocytosis was first coined in the 1970s when investigators found that neutrophils or macrophages grown in culture on a glass coverslip were unable to complete the process of CME.[46] A phagocytic cup would spread out on the glass, but the budding pit could not be internalized as a vesicle. Further research determined that the impaired endocytosis could be attributed to the fact that the glass surface was very stiff. Later, it was found that frustrated endocytosis was not limited to cells grown in culture. In fact, a stiff collagen matrix could cause cells to adhere to the matrix through integrin binding at sites where clathrin-coated pits are forming. The excessive stiffness of the collagen matrix could then, through this mechanism, impede CME.

Frustrated endocytosis may be a mechanism by which DIO3 becomes overactive in converting T4 to rT3 and converting T3 to T2. Unlike DIO1 and DIO2, DIO3 is an integral membrane protein.[47] Because it is located extracellularly, DIO3 has ready access to circulating thyroid hormones and can therefore rapidly inactivate T4 and T3 while it is in the membrane.[48] DIO3 is internalized via CME into early endosomes and then continuously recycled back to the membrane. If CME is impaired due to frustrated endocytosis, DIO3 will stay for a longer period of time at the membrane, actively converting T4 to rT3 and interfering with thyroid hormone signaling.

8.9 HEPARAN SULFATE AND FIBROSIS

Hepatic stellate cells are the primary cells that produce fibrotic liver. Stellate cells become activated following liver injury, and in the activated state, they proliferate and evolve into myofibroblasts that produce and deposit abundant collagen fibers, eventually leading to the scar tissue defining liver fibrosis.[49] The signaling that controls their behavior in the activated state depends on growth factors such as fibroblast growth factor (FGF) that adhere to heparan sulfate proteoglycans via integrins.[50]

Perlecan is a basement membrane–type heparan sulfate proteoglycan that is highly expressed in necrotic areas of damaged liver by both activated stellate cells and endothelial cells.[51] Under stress conditions, both the enzymes that synthesize heparan sulfate and the enzymes that degrade it (e.g., heparinase) are sharply upregulated. My hypothesis is that the heparan sulfate fragments that are dislodged from the matrix by heparinase are taken up by stellate cells, macrophages, endothelial cells and other cell types via endocytosis, along with any signaling molecules such as growth factors that adhere to the heparan sulfate. Heparan sulfate chains are taken up into the lysosomes, where they are completely degraded in a process that involves at least seven different enzymes.[52] This releases free sulfate to support ionic buffering of the acidic environment of the lysosome, essential for breaking down and recycling cellular debris. The debris includes damaged mitochondria. The importance of heparan sulfate metabolism for mitochondrial health becomes apparent by considering the severely disturbed mitochondria associated with the group of devastating genetic diseases called lysosomal storage disorders.[53] There are six different lysosomal sulfatases that detach sulfate from heparan sulfate, and deficiencies in these lead to severe lysosomal storage disease, with impaired lysosomal function and a pathological cascade outside the lysosomes.[54]

The signaling molecules originally trapped by the heparan sulfate in the membrane emerge at the endosomal stage and migrate to the nucleus of the cell to influence metabolic policy, promoting growth, proliferation and build-up of the collagen basement membrane and its attached perlecan heparan sulfate proteoglycans.

Frustrated endocytosis occurs when the cells adhere to a basement membrane that is too stiff. A major controlling factor in stiffness is the amount of heparan sulfate adhering to the collagen matrix.[55] When there is an abundance of cellular debris from dead and dying hepatic cells, the macrophages need to endocytose excessive amounts of heparan sulfate to support lysosomal clearance of the debris. If synthesis can't keep up with the loss, the matrix becomes too stiff, and large clathrin plaques accumulate on the adherent cells. This impedes CME in stellate cells and immune cells, resulting in high activity of DIO3, with quantities of rT3 being released into circulation and causing systemic thyroid hormone deficiency. Interestingly, T3 inhibits the differentiation of monocytes into macrophages.[56] Upregulation of DIO3 may therefore also be important for inhibiting T3 in order to induce monocyte maturation into macrophages under inflammatory conditions.

8.10 PUTTING IT ALL TOGETHER

We are now prepared to connect the dots to explain how glutathione deficiency combined with chronic hepatic exposures to toxins and toxic chemicals drives the excess production of rT3 and the resulting condition of hypothyroidism associated with a perfectly functioning thyroid gland in NTIS. Glutathione plays a central role in maintaining healthy mitochondria through its role as an antioxidant. But, it also plays another not so well recognized role of providing the raw materials to sustain massive production of heparan sulfate. In the presence of stressors, hepatocytes release glutathione along with GGT, the enzyme needed to separate it into its component amino acids: Glycine, glutamate and cysteine. Elevated GGT is a strong risk factor not only for liver disease but also for atherosclerosis, heart failure, arterial stiffness and plaque, and gestational diabetes, among others.[57] Glutathione is most likely a storage form of sulfur that can be used to refurbish heparan sulfate supplies under multiple stress conditions.

Cysteine plays an essential role as a precursor to hydrogen sulfide gas, which is produced from cysteine either enzymatically, via cystathionine gamma lyase and cystathionine beta synthase,[58] or nonenzymatically in the presence of reactive oxygen species, vitamin B6 and iron.[59] Glycine and glutamate are the precursors needed to synthesize the pyrrole ring of heme, and heme synthesis becomes important both to sequester iron and to serve as a catalyst for the enzymes that oxidize H_2S to sulfate and thiosulfate. Ultimately, it's sulfate deficiency that interferes with the ability to maintain adequate supplies of heparan sulfate in the face of the upregulation of heparanase in association with developing liver fibrosis.[60] Fragmented heparan sulfate proteoglycans are taken up by the macrophages, because they will use them as a source of sulfate for acid buffering in the lysosomes in order to clear cellular debris from dead and dying cells.

It now becomes apparent that the body has developed an elegant solution for blocking CME by macrophages when heparan sulfate is deficient. It is the heparan sulfate bound to the membrane-attached proteins in a cell that facilitates signal transfer from multiple signaling molecules regulating growth and repair. The main constituents of the fibrotic liver tissue are collagen VI and perlecan, a heparan sulfate proteoglycan. Studies have shown that stripping away the perlecan results in increased stiffness,[55] and as we've seen, a stiff matrix interferes with CME in the adhering macrophages.

During the process of resolving an inflammatory state associated with healing from injury, macrophages transition from an M1 (proinflammatory) to an M2 (anti-inflammatory) type. Enzymes involved in synthesizing heparan sulfate are sharply upregulated in the M2 state, and M2 macrophages are characterized by a much greater abundance of heparan sulfate in their membranes.[61] For as long as heparan sulfate supplies are inadequate, the macrophages stay in the M1 state, and inflammation continues unabated. Not only does this depend on the oxidation of H_2S to produce sulfate in the mitochondria, but it also depends on the further step of converting sulfate to the universal sulfate donor PAPS (phosphoadenosine phosphosulfate). PAPS synthase consumes one ATP molecule as the substrate for PAPS and another ATP molecule to provide energy for the reaction. When ATP is deficient due to mitochondrial dysfunction, it becomes difficult to maintain adequate sulfate levels in the glycocalyx. FGF signaling is upregulated in the absence of sulfated heparan sulfate proteoglycans, which can be induced by inhibiting PAPS synthetase.[62]

I hypothesize that a shortage of sulfate needed to synthesize heparan sulfate keeps macrophages in the M1 state and sustains chronic inflammation. And ultimately, this can be traced back to a shortage of glutathione and impaired synthesis of sulfate and PAPS from H_2S. It has been argued that glyphosate disrupts the supply of sulfate to the glycocalyx, through several mechanisms, and that this is a major factor in many diseases.[63, 64]

Remarkably, T3 suppresses the synthesis of cystathionine gamma lyase in the liver, thus suppressing H_2S synthesis.[65] This could justify increased synthesis of DIO3 by activated stellate cells. When combined with frustrated endocytosis, reflecting heparan sulfate deficiency, decreasing the supply of T3 through overproduction of rT3 serves the need to induce H_2S synthesis. This makes sense, because the H_2S can be converted to sulfate by macrophages and by stellate cells. Ultimately, heparan sulfate supplied as perlecan by the stellate cells will reduce the stiffness of the matrix and allow the macrophages to endocytose cellular debris and begin the recovery process. But, only if the enzymes involved have not been disabled by toxic exposures.

8.11 THERAPIES FOR NTIS

Given the premise in this chapter that glyphosate severely disrupts the liver's ability to detoxify mycotoxins, it becomes compelling that one of the most important steps one can take towards healing from NTIS is to adopt a strictly certified organic diet. This is a natural way to reduce not only glyphosate exposure but also mycotoxin exposure, because glyphosate increases the likelihood that mycotoxins will be present in the food sources. Obviously, it is also expedient to avoid eating foods such as seeds, nuts and grains that are most likely to be contaminated with mycotoxins. And, it is essential to identify any environmental exposures to mold due to a water-damaged building either at home or in the office, and to find a way to ameliorate those exposures. Furthermore, a residence adjacent to a farm where glyphosate is heavily used is also going to pose major risk – moving to a new residence may be the only option in such cases.

Beyond this, glutathione stands out as a major nutrient that plays a central role in the pathology of NTIS. Too little liver glutathione or a high ratio of GSSG to GSH is a major driver behind the disease process. Studies have found benefit in treatment with either N-acetyl cysteine (NAC) or liposomal glutathione. An in vitro study that involved exposing human mononucleocytes to ochratoxin A demonstrated oxidative stress and DNA strand breaks following exposure. Importantly, they showed that pretreatment with NAC ameliorated the effect.[66]

Remarkably, NTIS occurs in 30% to 90% of patients with acute myocardial infarction. A randomized prospective multi-center study based in Brazil involved 67 consecutive patients admitted into a hospital following a myocardial infarction.[67] The patients were randomized to receive a NAC supplement or a placebo. The baseline serum rT3 levels in both treatment and placebo groups were elevated three- to fourfold compared with healthy subjects. However, the serum levels of rT3 fell over time in the treatment group but remained high in the placebo group. The mean serum level after 5 days of rT3 was 29 ng/dL in the treatment group compared with 50 ng/dL in the placebo group ($p = 0.003$). Serum antioxidant defenses were also restored almost to the level of controls in the treated group compared with the placebo group.

As I mentioned earlier, some mycotoxins can suppress the enzymes that synthesize glutathione. In this case, cysteine supplementation may not be sufficient. Glutathione is synthesized in the liver from its amino acid precursors, but if the enzymes that synthesize it are defective, it might be necessary to provide a supplement that contains the entire glutathione molecule rather than its individual components. Glutathione can be a very useful supplement for people suffering from mold exposure. However, it needs to be given in such a way so as to prevent the breakdown of orally delivered glutathione into its component amino acids by the digestive system. Some options are to administer reduced glutathione (GSH) in an intravenous, nebulized, transdermal, oral liposomal, or nasal form.[23]

There are other steps that can be taken to improve dietary choices by selecting foods that are rich in sulfur as well as foods that are rich in polyphenols, flavonoids and terpenoids – complex organic molecules produced by colorful fruits and vegetables that act as antioxidants. Vegetable-based sources of sulfur include onions, garlic and cruciferous vegetables. Seafood, cheese, eggs and meats are all good animal-based sources of sulfur. Animal-based foods are better sources in general of the sulfur-containing amino acids compared with plants.

8.12 CHAPTER SUMMARY

In summary, this chapter has proposed that there is synergistic toxicity between glyphosate and mycotoxins, specifically with respect to the development of euthyroid sick syndrome, also known as nonthyroidal illness syndrome (NTIS). Mycotoxins and glyphosate are both known to cause mitochondrial dysfunction through oxidative stress, DNA damage and depletion of glutathione supplies, especially in the liver. In NTIS, DIO3 is sharply upregulated in the liver, and this leads to the overproduction of rT3, which enters the circulation and blocks the receptor response to T3 systemically, leading to symptoms of extreme fatigue due to a suppression of mitochondrial activity. Glutathione deficiency in the liver plays a central role in the disease process through two distinct mechanisms – impaired antioxidant defenses and impaired supply of heparan sulfate to the matrix proteins in the liver. A stiff basement membrane leads to a pathology called frustrated clathrin-based endocytosis, which results in excessive activity of DIO3 and resulting overproduction of rT3. Invasive macrophages are unable to mature from an M1 to an M2 state, and this becomes a state of chronic inflammation and associated disease symptoms.

REFERENCES

1. Somppi, T. L. 2017. Non-thyroidal illness syndrome in patients exposed to indoor air dampness microbiota treated successfully with triiodothyronine. *Frontiers in Immunology* 8:919.
2. Cioffi, F., R. Senese, A. Lanni, and F. Goglia. 2013. Thyroid hormones and mitochondria: With a brief look at derivatives and analogues. *Molecular and Cellular Endocrinology* 379, nos. 1–2:51–61. https://pubmed.ncbi.nlm.nih.gov/23769708/.
3. Gutch, M., S. Kumar, and K. K. Gupta. 2018. Prognostic value of thyroid profile in critical care condition. *Indian Journal of Endocrinology and Metabolism* 22, no. 3:387–391. https://www.ncbi.nlm.nih.gov/pmc/articles/PMC6063192/.
4. Shoemaker, R. C., A. Heyman, A. Mancia, and J. C. Ryan. 2017. Inflammation induced chronic fatiguing illnesses: A steady march towards understanding mechanisms and identifying new biomarkers and therapies. *Internal Medicine Review* 3, no. 11:1–29.
5. Wild, C. P., and Y. Y. Gong. 2010. Mycotoxins and human disease: A largely ignored global health issue. *Carcinogenesis* 31, no. 11:71–82. https://pubmed.ncbi.nlm.nih.gov/19875698/.
6. Hietanen, E., K. Linnainmaa, and H. Vainio. 1983. Effects of phenoxyherbicides and glyphosate on the hepatic and intestinal biotransformation activities in the rat. *Acta Pharmacol Toxicol (Copenh)* 53, no. 2:103–112. https://pubmed.ncbi.nlm.nih.gov/6624478/.
7. McCullough, A. K., and R. S. Lloyd. 2019. Mechanisms underlying aflatoxin-associated mutagenesis implications in carcinogenesis. *DNA Repair (Amst)* 77:76–86. https://pubmed.ncbi.nlm.nih.gov/30897375/.
8. Jasper, R., G. O.Locatelli, C. Pilati, and C. Locatelli. 2012. Evaluation of biochemical, hematological and oxidative parameters in mice exposed to the herbicide glyphosate-Roundup®. *Interdisciplinary Toxicology* 5(3):133–140. https://www.ncbi.nlm.nih.gov/pmc/articles/PMC3600513/.
9. Mills, P. J., C. Caussy, and R. Loomba. 2020. Glyphosate excretion is associated with steatohepatitis and advanced liver fibrosis in patients with fatty liver disease. *Clinical Gastroenterology and Hepatology* 18, no. 3:741–743. https://pubmed.ncbi.nlm.nih.gov/30954713/.
10. Mesnage, R., G. Renney, G.-E. Séralini, M. Ward, and M. N. Antoniou. 2017. Multiomics reveal non-alcoholic fatty liver disease in rats following chronic exposure to an ultra-low dose of Roundup herbicide. *Science Report* 7:39328. https://www.nature.com/articles/srep39328.
11. Makuria, A. N., M. N. Routledge, Y. Y. Gong, and M. Sisay. 2020. Aflatoxins as a risk factor for liver cirrhosis: A systematic review and meta-analysis. *BMC Pharmacology and Toxicology* 21:39. https://bmcpharmacoltoxicol.biomedcentral.com/articles/10.1186/s40360-020-00420-7.
12. Punekar, P., A. K. Sharma, and A. Jain. 2018. A study of thyroid dysfunction in cirrhosis of liver and correlation with severity of liver disease. *Indian Journal of Endocrinology and Metabolism* 22, no. 5:645–650. https://pubmed.ncbi.nlm.nih.gov/30294575/.
13. Martinez, D. A., U. E. Loening, and M. C. Graham. 2018. Impacts of glyphosate-based herbicides on disease resistance and health of crops: A review. *Environmental Sciences Europe* 30, no. 1:2. https://enveurope.springeropen.com/articles/10.1186/s12302-018-0131-7.
14. Romero, M. C., E. H. Reinoso, M. Kiernan, and S. Córdoba. 2004. Biodegradation of glyphosate by wild yeasts. *Revista Mexicana de Micologa* 19:46–50.
15. Carranza, C. S., C. L. Barberis, S. M. Chiacchiera, and C. E. Magnoli. 2017. Assessment of growth of *Aspergillus* spp. from agricultural soils in the presence of glyphosate. *Revista Argentina de Microbiología* 49(4):384–393.
16. Carranza, C. S., J. P. Regñicoli, M. E. Aluffi, N. Benito, S. M. Chiacchiera, C. L. Barberis, and C. E. Magnoli. 2019. Glyphosate in vitro removal and tolerance by *Aspergillus oryzae* in soil microcosms. *International Journal of Environmental Science and Technology* 16:7673–7682. https://link.springer.com/article/10.1007/s13762-019-02347-x.
17. Fernandez, M. R., R. P. Zentner, P. Basnyat, D. Gehl, F. Selles, and D. Huber. 2009. Glyphosate associations with cereal diseases caused by *Fusarium* spp. in the Canadian Prairies. *European Journal of Agronomy* 31, no. 3:133–143. https://www.sciencedirect.com/science/article/abs/pii/S1161030109000689.
18. Nesic, K., S. Ivanovic, and V. Nesic. 2014. Fusarial toxins: Secondary metabolites of Fusarium fungi. *Reviews of Environmental Contamination and Toxicology* 228:101–120. https://link.springer.com/chapter/10.1007/978-3-319-01619-1 5.
19. Moore, J. H., and B. Truelove. 1970. Ochratoxin A: Inhibition of mitochondrial respiration. *Science* 168:1102–1103.
20. Islam, M. T., S. K. Mishra, S. Tripathi, M. V. O. B. de Alencar, J. M. D. C. e Sousa, H. M. L. Rolim, M. D. G. F. de Medeiros, P. M. P. Ferreira, R. Rouf, S. J. Uddin, and M. S. Mubarak. 2018. Mycotoxin-assisted

mitochondrial dysfunction and cytotoxicity: Unexploited tools against proliferative disorders. *IUBMB* 70(11):1084–1092. https://pubmed.ncbi.nlm.nih.gov/30180298/.

21. Heidtmann-Bemvenuti, R., G. L. Mendes, P. T. Scaglioni, E. Badiale-Furlong, and L. A. Souza-Soares. 2011. Biochemistry and metabolism of mycotoxins: A review. *African Journal of Food Science* 5(16):861–869.

22. Ziglari, T., and A. Allameh. 2013. Chapter 13: The significance of glutathione conjugation in afla-toxin metabolism 2. In *Aflatoxins - Recent Advances and Future Prospects*, edited by Mehdi Razzaghi-Abyaneh. Intech Open. https://www.intechopen.com/books/aflatoxins-recent-advances-and-future-prospects/the-significance-of-glutathione-conjugation-in-aflatoxin-metabolism.

23. Guilford, F. T., and J. Hope. 2014. Deficient glutathione in the pathophysiology of mycotoxin-related illness. *Toxins (Basel)* 6, no. 2:608–623. https://pubmed.ncbi.nlm.nih.gov/24517907/.

24. Lamb, D. C., D. E. Kelly, S. Z. Hanley, Z. Mehmood, and S. L. Kelly. 1998. Glyphosate is an inhibitor of plant cytochrome P450: Functional expression of *Thlaspi arvensae* cytochrome P45071b1/reductase fusion protein in *Escherichia coli. Biochemical and Biophysical Research Communications* 244:110–114. https://pubmed.ncbi.nlm.nih.gov/9514851/.

25. Miteva, L. P. E., S. V. Ivanov, and V. S. Alexieva. 2010. Alterations in glutathione pool and some related enzymes in leaves and roots of pea plants treated with the herbicide glyphosate. *Russian Journal of Plant Physiology* 57, no. 1:131–136. https://link.springer.com/article/10.1134/S1021443710010188.

26. Ahsan, N., D.-G. Lee, K.-W. Lee, I. Alam, and S.-H. Lee. 2009. Glyphosate-induced oxidative stress in rice leaves revealed by proteomic approach. *Plant Physiology and Biochemistry* 46, no. 12:1062–1070. https://pubmed.ncbi.nlm.nih.gov/18755596/.

27. El-Shenaway, N. S. 2009. Oxidative stress responses of rats exposed to roundup and its active ingredient glyphosate. *Environmental Toxicology and Pharmacology* 28, no. 3:379–85. https://pubmed.ncbi.nlm.nih.gov/21784030/.

28. Anifandis, G., G. Amiridis, K. Dafopoulos, A. Daponte, E. Dovolou, E. Gavriil, V. Gorgogietas, E. Kachpani, Z. Mamuris, C. I. Messini, and K. Vassiou. 2018. The in vitro impact of the herbicide roundup on human sperm motility and sperm mitochondria. *Toxics* 6:2. https://www.ncbi.nlm.nih.gov/pmc/articles/PMC5874775/.

29. Peixoto, F. 2005. Comparative effects of the roundup and glyphosate on mitochondrial oxidative phosphorylation. *Chemosphere* 61, no. 8:1115–1122. https://pubmed.ncbi.nlm.nih.gov/16263381/.

30. Benachour, N., and G.-E. Seralini. 2009. Glyphosate formulations induce apoptosis and necrosis in human umbilical, embryonic, and placental cells. *Chemical Research in Toxicology* 22, no. 1:97–105. https://pubmed.ncbi.nlm.nih.gov/19105591/.

31. Olorunsogo, O. O. 1990. Modification of the transport of protons and Ca^{2+} ions across mitochondrial coupling membrane by N-(phosphonomethyl)glycine. *Toxicology* 61:205–209. https://pubmed.ncbi.nlm.nih.gov/2157305/.

32. Cattani, D., V. L. de Liz Oliveira Cavalli, C. E. Heinz Rieg, J. T. Domingues, T. Dal-Cim, C. I. Tasca, F. R. M. B. Silva, and A. Zamoner. 2014. Mechanisms underlying the neurotoxicity induced by glyphosate-based herbicide in immature rat hippocampus: Involvement of glutamate excitotoxicity. *Toxicology* 320:34–45. https://www.sciencedirect.com/science/article/pii/S0300483X14000493.

33. Cattani, D., P. A. Cesconetto, M. K. Tavaresa, E. B. Parisotto, P. A. De Oliveira, C. E. H. Rieg, M. C. Leite, R. D. S. Prediger, N. C. Wendt, G. Razzera, and D. Wilhelm Filho. 2017. Developmental exposure to glyphosate-based herbicide and depressive-like behavior in adult offspring: Implication of gluta-mate excitotoxicity and oxidative stress. *Toxicology* 387:67–80. https://www.sciencedirect.com/science/article/pii/S0300483X17301683.

34. Rueda-Ruzafa, L., F. Cruz, P. Roman, and D. Cardona. 2019. Gut microbiota and neurological effects of glyphosate. *Neurotoxicology* 75:1–8. https://pubmed.ncbi.nlm.nih.gov/31442459/.

35. Schinder, A. F., E. C. Olson, N. C. Spitzer, and M. Montal. 1996. Mitochondrial dysfunction is a primary event in glutamate neurotoxicity. *Journal of Neuroscience* 16, no. 19:6125–6133. https://www.ncbi.nlm.nih.gov/pmc/articles/PMC6579180/.

36. Kullberg, B. J., M. G. Netea, A. G. Vonk, and J. W. M. van der Meer. 1999. Modulation of neutrophil function in host defense against disseminated *Candida albicans* infection in mice. *FEMS Immunology & Medical Microbiology* 26, nos. 3–4:299–307. https://pubmed.ncbi.nlm.nih.gov/10575142/.

37. Tanaka, T., M. Narazaki, and T. Kishimoto. 2014. L-6 in inflammation, immunity, and disease. *Cold Springs Harbor Perspectives in Biology* 6:a016295. https://pubmed.ncbi.nlm.nih.gov/25190079/.

38. Wajner, S. M., I. M. Goemann, A. L. Bueno, and P. R. Larsen. And IL-6 promotes nonthyroidal illness syndrome by blocking thyroxine activation while promoting thyroid hormone inactivation in human cells. *The Journal of Clinical Investigation* 121, no. 5:1834–1845. https://pubmed.ncbi.nlm.nih.gov/21540553/.

39. Magill, S. S., J. R. Edwards, W. Bamberg, Z. G. Beldavs, G. Dumyati, M. A. Kainer, R. Lynfield, M. Maloney, L. McAllister-Hollod, J. Nadle, and S. M. Ray. 2014. Multistate point-prevalence survey of health care-associated infections. *The New England Journal of Medicine* 370:1198–1208. https://www.nejm.org/doi/full/10.1056/NEJMoa1306801.

40. Margalit, A., and K. Kavanagh. 2015. The innate immune response to *Aspergillus fumigatus* at the alveolar surface *FEMS Microbiology Reviews* 39, no. 5:670687. https://pubmed.ncbi.nlm.nih.gov/25934117/.

41. Swamydas, M., J. L. Gao, T. J. Break, M. D. Johnson, M. Jaeger, C. A. Rodriguez, J. K. Lim, N. M. Green, A. L. Collar, B. G. Fischer, and C. C. Lee. 2016. CXCR1-mediated neutrophil degranulation and fungal killing promote Candida clearance and host survival. *Science Translational Medicine* 8, no. 322:322ra10. https://pubmed.ncbi.nlm.nih.gov/26791948/.

42. Desai, J. V., and M. S. Lionakis. 2018. The role of neutrophils in host defense against invasive fungal infections. *Current Clinical Microbiology Reports* 5, no. 3:181–189. https://link.springer.com/article/10.1007/s40588-018-0098-6.

43. Boelen, A., J. Boorsma, J. Kwakkel, C. W. Wieland, R. Renckens, T. J. Visser, E. Fliers, and W. M. Wiersinga. 2008. Type 3 deiodinase is highly expressed in infiltrating neutrophilic granulocytes in response to acute bacterial infection. *Thyroid* 18, no. 10:1095–1103. https://pubmed.ncbi.nlm.nih.gov/18816180/.

44. Schmid, S. L., and L. L. Carter. 1990. ATP is required for receptor-mediated endocytosis in intact cells. *Journal of Cell Biology* 111:2307–2318. https://www.ncbi.nlm.nih.gov/pmc/articles/PMC2116413/.

45. Wu, X., X. Zhao, L. Baylor, S. Kaushal, and E. Eisenberg. Clathrin exchange during clathrin-mediated endocytosis. *The Journal of Cell Biology* 155, no. 2:291–300. https://www.ncbi.nlm.nih.gov/pmc/articles/PMC2198830/.

46. Baschieri, F., K. Porshneva, and G. Montagnac. 2020. Frustrated clathrin-mediated endocytosis causes and possible functions. *Journal of Cell Science* 133:jcs240861. https://jcs.biologists.org/content/133/11/jcs240861.

47. Bianco, A. C., and R. R. da Conceição. 2018. The deiodinase trio and thyroid hormone signaling. *Methods in Molocular Biology* 1801:67–83. https://www.ncbi.nlm.nih.gov/pmc/articles/PMC6668716/.

48. Baqui, M., D. Botero, B. Gereben, Cyntia Curcio, John W. Harney, Domenico Salvatore, Kenji Sorimachi, P. Reed Larsen, and Antonio C. Bianco. 2003. Human type 3 iodothyronine selenodeiodinase is located in the plasma membrane and undergoes rapid internalization to endosomes. *The Journal of Biological Chemistry* 278, no. 2:1206–1211. https://pubmed.ncbi.nlm.nih.gov/12419801/.

49. Gao, R., and D. R. Brigstock. 2004. Connective tissue growth factor (CCN2) induces adhesion of rat activated hepatic stellate cells by binding of its C-terminal domain to integrin alphavbeta3 and heparan sulfate proteoglycan. *Journal of Biological Chemistry* 279:88488855. https://www.jbc.org/article/S0021-9258(17)47786-6/fulltext.

50. Schumacher, J. D., and G. L. Guo. 2016. Regulation of hepatic stellate cells and fibrogenesis by fibroblast growth factors. *BioMed Research International* 2016:8323747. https://pubmed.ncbi.nlm.nih.gov/27699175/.

51. Gallai, M., I. Kovalszky, T. Knittel, K. Neubauer, T. Armbrust, and G. Ramadori. 1996. Expression of extracellular matrix proteoglycans perlecan and decorin in carbon-tetrachloride-injured rat liver and in isolated liver cells. *The American Journal of Pathology* 148, no. 5:1463–1471. https://pubmed.ncbi.nlm.nih.gov/8623917/.

52. Veraldi, N., N. Zouggari, and A. de Agostini. 2020. The challenge of modulating heparan sulfate turnover by multitarget heparin derivatives. *Molecules* 25:390. https://pubmed.ncbi.nlm.nih.gov/31963505/.

53. Pshezhetsky, A. V. 2015. Crosstalk between 2 organelles: Lysosomal storage of heparan sulfate causes mitochondrial defects and neuronal death in mucopolysaccharidosis III type C. *Rare Diseases* 3, no. 1:e1049793. https://pubmed.ncbi.nlm.nih.gov/26459666/.

54. Kowalewski, B., W. C. Lamanna, R. Lawrence, M. Damme, S. Stroobants, M. Padva, I. Kalus, M. A. Frese, T. Lübke, R. Lüllmann-Rauch, and R. D'Hooge. 2012. Arylsulfatase G inactivation causes loss of heparan sulfate 3-O-sulfatase activity and mucopolysaccharidosis in mice. *Proceedings of the National Academy of Sciences USA* 109, no. 26:1031010315. https://www.pnas.org/content/109/26/10310.

55. Wilusz, R. E., E. Defrate, and F. Guilak. 2012. A biomechanical role for perlecan in the pericellular matrix of articular cartilage. *Matrix Biology* 31, no. 6:320–327. https://pubmed.ncbi.nlm.nih.gov/22659389/.

56. Perrotta, C., M. Buldorini, E. Assi, D. Cazzato, C. de Palma, E. Clementi, and D. Cervia. 2014. The thyroid hormone triiodothyronine controls macrophage maturation and functions protective role during inflammation. *The American Journal of Pathology* 184, no. 1. https://www.sciencedirect.com/science/article/pii/S0002944013006846.

57. Koenig, G., and S. Seneff. 2015. Gamma-glutamyltransferase: A predictive biomarker of cellular anti-oxidant inadequacy and disease risk. *Disease Markers* 2015:818570. https://pubmed.ncbi.nlm.nih.gov/26543300/.

58. Renga, B. 2011. Hydrogen sulfide generation in mammals: The molecular biology of cystathionine beta synthase (CBS) and cystathionine--lyase (CSE). *Inflammation & Allergy – Drug Targets* 10, no. 2:85–91. https://pubmed.ncbi.nlm.nih.gov/21275900/.

59. Yang, J., P. Minkler, D. Grove, R. Wang, B. Willard, R. Dweik, and C. Hine. 2019. Non-enzymatic hydrogen sulfide production from cysteine in blood is catalyzed by iron and vitamin B6. *Communications Biology* 2:194. https://www.nature.com/articles/s42003-019-0431-5.

60. Secchi, M. F., M. Crescenzi, V. Masola, F. P. Russo, A. Floreani, and M. Onisto. 2017. Heparanase and macrophage interplay in the onset of liver fibrosis. *Scientific Reports* 7:14956. https://www.nature.com/articles/s41598-017-14946-0.

61. Swart, M., and L. Troeberg. 2019. Effect of polarization and chronic inflammation on macrophage expression of heparan sulfate proteoglycans and biosynthesis enzymes. *Journal of Histochemistry & Cytochemistry* 67, no. 1:9–27. https://pubmed.ncbi.nlm.nih.gov/30205019/.

62. Jung, S. H., H. C. Lee, D.-M. Yu, B. C. Kim, S. M. Park, Y. S. Lee, H. J. Park, Young-Gyu Ko, and J. S. Lee. 2016. Heparan sulfation is essential for the prevention of cellular senescence. *Cell Death and Differentiation* 23:417–429. https://www.nature.com/articles/cdd2015107.

63. Seneff, S., N. J. Causton, G. L. Nigh, G. Koenig, and D. Avalon. 2017. Can glyphosates disruption of the gut microbiome and induction of sulfate deficiency explain the epidemic in gout and associated diseases in the industrialized world? *Journal of Biological Physics and Chemistry* 17:53–76. https://www.amsi.ge/jbpc/21717/17-2-abs-2.htm.

64. Seneff, S. and G Nigh. 2019. Sulfate's critical role for maintaining exclusion zone water: Dietary factors leading to deficiencies. *Water* 11:22–42. https://waterjournal.org/current-volume/seneff-summary/.

65. Hine, C., H.-J. Kim, Y. Zhu, E. Harputlugil, A. Longchamp, M. S. Matos, P. Ramadoss, K. Bauerle, L. Brace, J. M. Asara, and C. K. Ozaki. 2017. Hypothalamic-pituitary axis regulates hydrogen sulfide production. *Cell Metabolism* 25, no. 6:1320-1333.e5. https://pubmed.ncbi.nlm.nih.gov/28591635/.

66. Liu, J., Y. Wang, J. Cui, L. Xing, H. Shen, S. Wu, H. Lian, J. Wang, X. Yan, and X. Zhang. 2012. Ochratoxin A induces oxidative DNA damage and G1 phase arrest in human peripheral blood mononuclear cells in vitro. *Toxicology Letters* 211, no. 2:164–171. https://pubmed.ncbi.nlm.nih.gov/22498431/.

67. Vidart, J., S. M. Wajner, R. S. Leite, A. Manica, B. D. Schaan, P. R. Larsen, and A. L. Maia. 2014. N-acetylcysteine administration prevents nonthyroidal illness syndrome in patients with acute myocardial infarction: A randomized clinical trial. *The Journal of Clinical Endocrinology & Metabolism* 99, no. 12:4537–4545. https://pubmed.ncbi.nlm.nih.gov/25148231/.

9 Are Water-Damaged Buildings Safe?
The Literature Speaks

Scott W. McMahon

CONTENTS

9.1 INTRODUCTION

It is a foregone conclusion that chronic exposure to mold in the interior of water-damaged buildings (WDB) is associated with adverse human health effects. About this, there is absolutely no controversy, and literally hundreds of epidemiological articles bear the proof. Where some disagree is whether chronic exposure to the interior of WDB can cause multisystem illness. Is inhalation a primary route of exposure? Can such inhaled exposures trigger illness outside the domains of allergy, infection and direct toxicities? Some say mold can only cause illness in these three realms. Others believe exposure to indoor mold and dampness causes non-allergic (innate) immune responses. What answers does the medical literature provide?

The short, and overwhelmingly supported, answer is YES; exposure in WDB is causative of several respiratory/immunological issues and associated with a wide variety of human health effects, including a whole host of multisystem health issues. Inhalation is the primary route of exposure. Most of the accompanying symptoms appear to be triggered, in whole or in part, by abnormalities seen in innate immune system functioning.

This chapter will examine the literature in two epochs. The first deals with publications up through 2010, while the second discusses later works, including the findings of a systematic review of all peer-reviewed epidemiological articles published between 2011 and 2018 referencing chronic indoor microbial growth/dampness exposure and human health effects.

9.2 EARLY LITERATURE

Peer-reviewed reports linking indoor mold, dampness and other amplified microbial growth with adverse human health effects have been accumulating for over 50 years.[1] Localized skin growth/infections, allergic manifestations, exacerbation of attacks and causation of asthma are well supported. IgE-mediated allergies (Type I hypersensitivity reactions) have been clearly documented. Invasive infection, primarily in the immune-compromised, has been proven beyond all doubt.

DOI: 10.1201/b23304-10

During this same time period, research was undertaken studying non-allergic-mediated immune responses, gastrointestinal distresses, neurological changes, cognitive losses, pulmonary hemorrhages, ophthalmologic issues, difficult-to-diagnose dermatologic lesions, generalized symptoms such as headaches, fatigue and sleep problems, and more. Some evidence was found supporting each of these system abnormalities and symptom constellations. The sheer number of studies performed was lower than with asthma and allergy patients. Less was known during this period about the innate immune system and its global immunologic functions.

The medical literature during this time period falls roughly into three categories. The first group has been called "naysayer" literature and is written to declare the position that exposure to inhaled mycotoxins from indoor sources is unlikely to cause significant human illness. The second listing, dubbed "summary" literature, comes from systematic reviews, meta-analyses and other articles objectively attempting to summarize the literature. The third portion could be called "yaysayer" literature supporting the idea that chronic exposure to inhaled air from WDB causes illness via infection, allergy, direct toxicity and other mechanisms too.

9.3   NAYSAYER LITERATURE BEFORE 2011

Looking first at the naysayer work, there is a stunning paucity in the medical literature of peer-reviewed articles that show no associations between the aforementioned exposures and adverse human health effects. Presumably, there is so little data because one is attempting to demonstrate that multisystem mold-based illness does not exist or cannot exist. What little literature has been published generally falls into two categories. The first attempts to diminish or neutralize previously published epidemiological articles by discrediting one or more studies' methodologies. The second approach is the use of a negative argument. This refers to stating than an outcome is impossible, or very unlikely to happen, under less than extraordinary circumstances. An example of a negative argument would be to say that a human without a spaceship could not live in the outer space existing between the earth and the moon. It is seemingly and logically very difficult to generate data about an event that purportedly does not exist. Hence, these articles add no new human data, and this makes proving the negative argument very difficult.

Those who posit that chronic exposure to indoor mold cannot, or is very unlikely to, cause multisystem illness, or illness beyond traditional allergies, infection and direct toxicity, have a difficult time proving their argument. The very nature of a negative argument, the attempt to show that an entity cannot exist, is very challenging to substantiate. How does one prove that something cannot exist when finding even one positive example invalidates the entire negative argument? Literally tens of thousands of patients with multisystem illness after WDB exposure have been described in this early literature. Since one could not ethically prove experimentally that such an outcome could not exist, alternate methods were undertaken. While difficult to achieve, endeavors to prove the negative argument have been undertaken. The initial attempt to confirm the negative argument regarding mold is discussed in great detail in Chapter 12, Legal and Ethical Considerations in Mold, Mycotoxins, CIRS and Building Biology.

The thrust of that article,[2] published in 2002 by the American College of Occupational and Environmental Medicine (ACOEM 2002), was a mathematical proof developed using rodent data to show it was very unlikely that sufficient mycotoxin could accumulate in a room with amplified mold growth to cause a human to have multisystem illness from direct toxicity. Though this proof only discussed direct toxicity, non-critical thinkers may automatically assume that chronic indoor mold exposure cannot cause multisystem illness. As noted later, this conclusion is contrary to a near consensus of the literature. As we all learned in high school Geometry or other critical thinking classes, a mathematical proof must 1) identify its assumptions and 2) contain no mathematical errors. A single faulty assumption or a single math error would invalidate the entire proof, all its conclusions and any other articles that based their conclusions on that proof.

While the logical approach taken in this proof appeared sound, the constants employed were repeatedly low estimates (by several magnitudes of order), and at least nine assumptions were incorrect. An example of a low estimate occurred when evaluating half-lives of mycotoxins in the human body. Estimates were used suggesting hours or days before toxins would be metabolized or eliminated. In 2005, published data showed half-lives of mycotoxins of[3] up to 26 years in mice brains! Another faulty constant was obtained by using spore trap testing to estimate the number of *Stachybotrys chartarum* spores in a water-damaged room when it was known industry-wide by mold testers that spore trap sampling often completely missed *Stachybotrys* spores even when large amounts of *Stachybotrys* were found by other testing methods in the same room. The effect of fragments[4, 5] was also ignored using this sampling technique. One faulty assumption required that ingestion, not inhalation, of mycotoxins was the primary source of toxin entry, while the proof also evaluated direct toxicity from mycotoxins alone as the only potential cause of illness. Yaysayer and summary literature documented that inhalation is the primary portal for damage, which can be caused by mycotoxins, bacterial endotoxins and numerous other inflammagenic classes of substances found in excess as a result of microbial amplification in a WDB. Berndston (2016)[6] provided a table of 30 classes of such substances, and mycotoxins occupy only one class. These same documents also demonstrate non-allergy-mediated immune system responses, and more specifically, innate immune system derangements, occurring as a result of chronic inhalation of air from the interior of WDB.

Much, if not all, of the naysayer literature is built upon the chassis of the ACOEM 2002 flawed mathematical proof and former position statement. Two examples would be the American Academy of Allergy, Asthma, and Immunology's (AAAAI 2006) former position statement[7] and the position statement of the American College of Medical Toxicology.[8]

The other strategy employed was to nullify the literature that supported the positive argument: That chronic exposure to the interior of WDB with their obligatorily amplified microbial growth caused multisystem illness and illness outside of allergy, infection and direct toxicity. These negative articles looked at the methods of peer-reviewed published works that defined associations between chronic inhaled mold exposure and various symptoms, then leveled criticisms at the methodology in an attempt to discredit the article and hence, its conclusions.

One example[9] would be Terr (2009), which claimed as non-controversial that "The evidence from such [case and epidemiologic] reports and studies is overwhelmingly that human mycotoxicity arises almost exclusively through ingestion" and that "There are three well-documented pathogenic mechanisms [for human illness from molds] … These are infection, allergy, and toxicity." Terr offered no references for such astounding statements except a single citation for pulmonary mycotoxicosis and another for organic dust toxic syndrome. Indeed, though published in 2009, there are only two citations from 2007 and two from 2006. The 2008 Government Accountability Office (GAO) report[10] on mold is not cited. This GAO review suggested that inhalation was the most likely means of exposure and that non-allergic immune responses appeared to be at play. It criticized the AAAAI 2006 position statement, which Terr cited, for ignoring such immune derangements, as Terr also did. Terr went on to cite the ACOEM 2002 study saying, "based on experimental data in mice, make it extremely unlikely that toxic concentrations would occur within buildings."

The Terr paper then attempted to discredit four previously peer-reviewed studies,[11–14] which quantified cognitive losses through neuropsychological testing.

> These studies of toxic encephalopathy from exposure to inhaled mould spores lack credible evidence for such an association in large part because of patient selection bias. Neuropsychological data are necessarily subjective in nature. Comparison groups lack validity, being based instead on either estimates of pre-morbid intelligence or normative data. Most importantly, none of these published studies provide measurements of mycotoxin exposure. Thus, there is no credible evidence in these reports that abnormal psychologic testing indicates mycotoxic encephalopathy.

In five sentences, the author twice stated there was no credible evidence linking mycotoxins to cognitive loss, described objective neuropsychological testing as "necessarily subjective," criticized pre-morbid estimates of intelligence (based on pre-morbid academic and career achievement), criticized comparing scores with widely accepted and published norms, and criticized studies without publication of mycotoxin exposure levels, all without a single study cited. Ironically, the ACOEM 2002 report, upon which Terr relied heavily, as the backbone of its data, cited rodent studies, five acute toxicity and one chronic toxicity, most of which did not report mycotoxin exposure levels.

Another example of such an article[15] was written by Chang and Gershwin (2005). Titled "Mold hysteria: Origin of the hoax," this article discussed the authors' opinions about Sick Building Syndrome (SBS) and indoor mold exposure as its possible causation. Without a supporting reference, the authors described "environmentally induced adverse effects fall into several broad categories, including allergic, infectious, toxic and psychogenic." The article discussed SBS briefly and segued into a pejorative discussion of "toxic mold syndrome," a term used by legal professionals, laypersons and the press. The article is then subtitled "The truth about mold" and states regarding visible mold that:

> Just because something in the environment looks "bad" does not mean that it is necessarily bad for one's health. The reason this point must be addressed is because many of the judgments in mold related litigation cases are rendered based on appearances and emotion, with no consideration of the scientific evidence available.

Contrary to this "unscientific" (and unsupported) statement, The Centers for Disease Control and Prevention (CDC) in guidance documents[16] has declared that if mold is visible or can be smelled, it should be remediated without the need for commercial testing, and the Environmental Protection Agency (EPA) stated in its guidance documents that remediators should wear personal protective equipment similar to a full body Hazmat suit. The GAO 2008 report[10] also stated that the presence of visible mold OR musty odors has been used as evidence of abnormal amounts of mold growth in many scientific papers.

One other unifying theme of the naysayer articles is that they typically fail to present any new data. For instance, the ACOEM 2002 article presents a mathematical model. It is, for all intents and purposes, a hypothesis, and without any new data to validate it. The Scientific Method demands that predictions should be made from such a hypothesis, and those predictions need to be tested, in order to test the hypothesis' veracity. To date, to this author's understanding, such testing has never been performed, and such data does not exist. Therefore, it would be scientifically inappropriate to hang one's proverbial hat upon the hypothesis presented in the ACOEM 2002 report.

The goal of outlining a few of the naysayer studies is to highlight that it is very difficult to prove a negative argument. That negative, which naysayer literature has attempted to prove, is that chronic exposure to the interior of WDB and the amplified microbes (molds, bacteria and *Actinomycetes*), as well as the toxic and immunogenic particles they create, are very unlikely to cause adverse human health effects. Without performing direct experimentation with humans, which would be considered unethical, both the naysayers and the yaysayers must rely on epidemiological studies in humans and controlled experiments in animals with the hope of extrapolating the latter results to humans. There are comparatively few naysayer reports; they tend to cite each other, creating a circular argument, and they use, as a central dogma, the ACOEM 2002 flawed and untested mathematical hypothesis.

9.4 SUMMARY LITERATURE BEFORE 2011

Since the vast majority of the epidemiological mold literature before 2011 supported mold causing adverse human health effects, it should be no surprise that the systematic reviews and meta-analyses of the day also supported the same. The literature then was mostly focused on respiratory system issues such as bronchitis, asthma, manifestation of allergies, etc. Occasional studies evaluated other systems and while mostly supportive, did not generate systematic reviews or meta-analyses for these other systems. One paper[17] published by Fisk (2007) performed a quantitative meta-analysis of dampness or mold and a number of respiratory symptoms. Antova (2008) reported a pooling of data[18] from

12 cross-sectional studies representing over 58,000 children aged 6–12 years. "Positive associations between exposure to mould and children's respiratory health were seen with considerable consistency across studies and across outcomes." Fisk (2010) evaluated for the first time a quantitative meta-analysis of dampness or mold and respiratory infections,[19] also yielding positive associations.

In 2004, the Institute of Medicine of the National Academy of Science (IOM) published its review of the literature.[20]. It "found sufficient evidence to document an association between qualitatively assessed indoor dampness or mold and upper respiratory tract symptoms, cough, wheeze, and asthma symptoms in sensitized persons." In 2008, the United States GAO published its report on indoor mold,[10] reviewing governmental grants, guidance documents and 20 review articles in the peer-reviewed literature. This report discussed non-allergy mediated immune responses, offered a three-tiered algorithm, or case definition, for determining whether mold exposure was causative of a person's illness and directly criticized one review article[7] for failing to mention non-allergic-mediated immune abnormalities as a potential cause of symptoms. This report recognized the IOM's findings regarding respiratory symptoms, noted there were reports of mold associations with non-respiratory symptoms and stated more evidence needed to be gathered.

The World Health Organization (WHO) published an updated treatise on indoor mold[21] in 2009. This report echoed the IOM and GAO reports regarding respiratory symptoms and repeatedly discussed non-allergic-mediated immune system effects caused by chronic inhalation exposure to molds. The following quotes emphasize this paper's position:

Mechanisms of injury include exposure to B-glucans, toxins, spores, cell fragments and chemicals followed by immune stimulation, suppression and autoimmunity as well as neurotoxic effects.

Introduction, page 5.

Fungal (1→3)-β-D-glucans are non-allergenic, water-insoluble structural cell-wall components of most fungi ... and may account for up to 60% of the dry weight of the cell wall of fungi ... (1→3)-β-D-glucans have immunomodulating properties and may affect respiratory health.

Chapter 2, page 17.

The variety of respiratory symptoms and disease observed in damp and moldy indoor environments suggests that the airways are the primary route of entry for agents.

Chapter 4, page 84.d.

In damp buildings, people are exposed to constantly changing concentrations of different microbial species, their spores, metabolites and components, and other compounds in indoor air, including chemical emissions from building materials. This complex mixture of exposures inevitably leads to interactions, which affects outcomes in different situations. Furthermore, the effects of microorganisms, microbial substances or dampness – related chemical compounds seen in experimental animals, or cells often result from exposures that are orders of magnitude higher than the average doses that reach the human lungs under normal conditions in indoor air. Nevertheless, the surface doses within the lungs of patients with respiratory conditions can vary a thousand-fold, due to uneven particle deposition (Phalen et al., 2006),[22] thus resulting in even larger maximal surface doses in human lungs than in those used in experimental toxicological studies. Moreover, many other factors, such as exercise, can result in larger-than-average doses in the human lung.

Chapter 4, page 85.a.

Many of the health effects may result from recurrent activation of immune defense, leading to *exaggerated* immune responses and prolonged production of inflammatory mediators. Over production of these compounds damages the surrounding tissue and may manifest itself as chronic inflammation and inflammation-related diseases.

Chapter 4, page 85.b

In 2010, the Policyholders of America (POA) commissioned a panel of chronic inflammatory response syndrome (CIRS) expert physicians, an expert industrial hygienist and an expert mycologist to review the literature and produce a position paper.[23]. This peer-reviewed report cited over 600 unique references, represented over 40,000 patients in the peer-reviewed literature from 14 countries and strongly supported the connection between CIRS and chronic exposure to the interior of WDBs linked to the development or exacerbation of multisystem symptoms.

9.5   YAYSAYER LITERATURE BEFORE 2011

In 1997, Shoemaker published his findings of a multisystem illness caused by exposure to *Pfiesteria* sp.,[24] or dinoflagellates, found in overabundance at the time in the Chesapeake Bay. Some *Pfiesteria* made a toxin, fish ate the dinoflagellates and their toxin, people ate the fish and became ill. Shoemaker made the serendipitous observation that not only did treating these patients' secretory diarrhea with cholestyramine (CSM) make their loose stools disappear, but most or all of the other multisystem symptoms also unexpectedly improved or resolved with only CSM therapy. Over subsequent years, he noted other patients with a similar set of symptoms as a result of Lyme disease,[25] ciguatoxin ingestion,[26] inhalation and/or swimming around cyanobacteria blooms and chronic exposure to WDB.[27]

Shoemaker and Hudnell developed the first biomarker for this illness, reporting decreased VCS (visual contrast sensitivity).[28] Early on, this closely related group of illnesses was thought to be solely caused by biologically produced toxins.[29]. As more biomarkers were established, it became clear that an innate immune component[30] was also in play. The illness was eventually dubbed CIRS or chronic inflammatory response syndrome.[31] Regardless of trigger, be it *Pfiesteria*, *Ciguatera*, Lyme disease, exposure to cyanobacteria or chronic exposure to WDB,[32] patients developed a multisystem, multi-symptom illness with numerous abnormal biomarkers. The underlying pathology involved chronic innate immune system activation coupled with an HLA-inherited genetic hole in antigen presentation leading to chronic innate immune system dysregulation, noted by decreased levels of VIP and MSH (vasoactive intestinal polypeptide and α-melanocyte stimulating hormone) and increased levels of pro-inflammatory cytokines TGF-β1, MMP-9 and C4a (human transforming growth factor - beta1, matrix metalloproteinase-9 and the split product of complement protein C4, respectively).[31]

Shoemaker also developed a treatment protocol and tested it with two blinded, placebo-controlled trials.[33, 34] In addition, three studies have been published reviewing NeuroQuant® (NQ), a volumetric advanced technique brain magnetic resonance imaging (MRI),[35–37] and another involving the transcriptomics[32] of CIRS. The GAO proposed a diagnostic algorithm for mold-based illnesses[10] in 2008, which paralleled the case definition proposed by Shoemaker 2 years earlier. Alternative and summary diagnostic criteria[38, 39] were published in 2017 and 2018, respectively.

Animal studies prior to 2011 demonstrated a host of findings. Numerous studies showed pulmonary damage[40–51] as a result of exposure to mycotoxins, bacterial endotoxin and lipopeptides from *Mycoplasma* in mice, rats and fetal rabbits. Brains of mice and rats,[52–56] and the blood–brain barrier,[57] were also injured.

Study across species of the innate immune system registered responses too. Toll-like receptors (TLRs) assisted in identifying foreign particles[58] such as fungal fragments. Inhaled bacterial, fungal and *Actinomycetes* fragments and products were inflammagenic.[59] In rats, β-glucan exposure led to increased lung inflammatory markers.[60] C-type lectins responded to fungal exposures.[61–63] Dectin-1and non-Toll-like receptors (PRRs or pattern recognition receptors) were involved with detecting fungal exposure.[64, 65] Roda (2020) demonstrated that human bone marrow progenitor cells were nearly four times more sensitive than their mouse counterparts, affecting CFU-GM (myeloid) and BFU-E (erythroid) lineages more than DVU-E colonies.

Synergism between secondary metabolic products of *Actinomycetes* and mycotoxins was demonstrated in mice,[66–68] affecting cytokine production, cytotoxicity and macrophage function.

Synergy between products from *Actinomycetes* and bacterial endotoxin[69, 70] has also been established, affecting TLRs 2 and 4, cytokine and chemokine production, 4-MyD88-dependent and independent signaling, and apoptosis[71, 72] (via differential gene induction). Synergy appeared between vomitoxin and lipopolysaccharide[73] and other bacterial and fungal product combinations[74] in mice macrophages too. Inflammatory responses to fungi, *Actinomycetes* and bacteria[75-79] were additionally shown.

Nikulin (1997) subjected mice to six repeated courses of low levels of spores over 3 weeks,[80] roughly equivalent to 18 months of human life. Inflammatory responses were noted from mice exposed to non-toxin-forming spores and toxin-forming spores alike, though the responses were greater with the former exposure. Rand et al. showed in numerous studies[42, 45, 47, 48, 50, 79, 154] pathogenicity of exposure to at least nine different mycotoxins and also non-toxin-forming spores.[81] This was a crucial understanding documented by Nikulin, Rand and Flemming[81]. Both toxins and non-toxic substances from inhaled fungi caused inflammatory responses.

Human health studies before 2011 also built a framework for understanding multisystem illness resulting from chronic inhalation of substances produced in WDB. Immune system studies suggested the pathophysiology of non-allergic, innate-mediated immune-related illness. The outline of innate immune responses was postulated by Janeway[82] in 1989. Foreign antigen enters the body and its PAMPs (pattern-associated molecular patterns) or the host's DAMPS (either danger- or damage-associated molecular patterns) are detected either in cells (MHC-I, MHC-II) or extracellularly (PRRs). Foreign particles are marked for destruction via innate immune pathways, and antigen presentation occurs to initiate antibody release or preparation of new antibody creation.

Jiang et al. (2006) gave an overview of cellular immunity.[83] Gonzalez-Rey (2007) provided a summary of immune tolerance and highlighted the central roles of the anti-inflammatory neuroimmunoregulatory peptides VIP and MSH.[84] MSH worked in part through regulation of auto-immune regulating T_{reg} cells and also had inhibitory action on synthesis and release of pro-inflammatory cytokines.[85, 86]. Mannose-based molecular patterns (fungal origin) trigger the arachidonic acid pathway of inflammation.[87] TGF-β1, PRRs, antigen presentation cells (APCs), inflammatory and other aspects of innate immunity were all functioning in the lung,[88] where microbial fragments and fine and ultrafine particulates often end their journey. MyD88 signaling in lungs helped define early immune responses to *Aspergillus*[89, 90] with Toll receptors and through MAPK (mitogen-activated protein kinases) pathways. TLR 9 detects *A. fumigatus* intracellularly.[91] Dectin-1 receptors on neutrophils, dendritic cells, eosinophils and macrophages detected β-glucans.[92] Complement factors were involved in the development of asthma[93, 94] and chronic obstructive pulmonary disease in some cases. Complement activation with increased cytokines led to MMP-9 release[95] in neutrophils and eosinophils.[96] Complement C3a receptors existed in the pituitary and could modulate hormone release involved in inflammation control.[97] Pestka et al. (2008) reviewed compounds causing biological effects from WDB.[98] Trichothecenes could interfere with dendritic cell maturation and function.[99] T-2 toxin affected differentiation of monocytes.[100] Each of these activated innate immune pathways is independent of antibody production.

The pathophysiology of CIRS is explained in greater detail in Chapter 4, "Pediatric Chronic Inflammatory Response Syndrome." The central understanding is that patients have an HLA-predicated genetic hole in antigen presentation, which disables the adaptive immune system from entering the fight for certain antigens obtained through inspiring air chronically in WDB. As such, chronic inhalation of inflammagenic and toxic substances (microbially created toxins are inflammagenic too) leads to chronic activation of the earlier described and other innate immune pathways with little help from the adaptive immune system. Chronic innate activation likely causes elevated levels of VIP and MSH initially, then decreased levels as the body's compensations cannot keep up with the continual challenges to the innate immune pathways. As the VIP and/or MSH levels decrease, so does the body's ability to counterbalance the chronic innate immune activation, there is chronic pro-inflammatory cytokine overproduction, and chronic systemic innate inflammation reigns. Measuring erythrocyte sedimentation rates (ESR) and C-reactive protein (CRP) levels demonstrates elevation in about 10% of patients, as these tests are better to measure the inflammatory response of an engaged adaptive immune system. Markers of the innate immune system, such as TGF-β1, MMP-9 and C4a, must be evaluated, as CIRS is an innate immune system in dysregulation.

Symptoms come through capillary hypoperfusion[39] attack on the hypothalamic–pituitary–end organ axes and blood–brain barrier breaches, allowing excess inflammatory cytokines and if present, neuropathic mycotoxins., into the protected space of brain parenchyma. Fallout from these mechanisms of injury explains nearly every consequence seen in CIRS patients at a macroscopic level.

Other studies before 2011 show that chronic exposure to inhaled contents of WDB leads to pulmonary,[14, 93, 94, 101–104] general,[105–107] cognitive (with autonomic and growth hormone issues)[11, 12, 14, 108–114] and hypothalamic problems.[115] Indeed, mycotoxins have been studied, and used, for military purposes (biological warfare).[116–119]

Shoemaker et al. (2010) cited 17 studies (pages 95–97) from 14 countries, including 40,365 cases with mold-based illness, showing single and multisystem illness after chronic inhalation in WDB. In addition to the IOM, GAO and WHO papers, Shoemaker also cited numerous U.S. governmental papers and guidance documents and the same from other governments around the world. Examples from the Canadian Ministry of Health,[120] the CDC,[101, 121–127] the EPA,[128] National Institute for Occupational Safety and Health (NIOSH)[129–134] and the NIEHS[135–141] (National Institute of Environmental Health Sciences) are cited. The messages sent by these documents varied, but major themes were apparent:

1) Chronic indoor mold exposures are inimical to human health.
2) Inhalation, not ingestion, is the primary mode of entry.
3) If one sees mold, or smells mold, there *is* mold, and one needs to remediate the space or move, regardless of mold species.
4) Proper remediation requires personal protective equipment consistent with Hazmat protection, eliminating the cause of water intrusion and removal of all affected paper-based building materials in a contained fashion.
5) Chronic indoor mold exposure is related to a number of symptoms, including respiratory effects, headaches, sore throat, fatigue and more.

That was the state of the medical literature prior to 2011.

9.6 LITERATURE FROM 2011 TO THE PRESENT

This section of the literature is dominated by epidemiological studies with considerably more emphasis on reports evaluating diverse systems beyond the respiratory tract. While Caillaud (2018) declared there was both sufficient evidence of a causal relationship for asthma development and exacerbation as well as sufficient evidence of an association with allergic rhinitis,[142] one systematic review examined all peer-reviewed epidemiological articles published between 2011 and 2018 referencing indoor dampness/microbial growth and adverse human health effects. In all, 114 of the 116 articles meeting these criteria were examined. Of these 114 studies, 98.2% (112) of the peer-reviewed published epidemiological articles demonstrated findings supporting the concept that chronic exposure to the inhaled air of WDB was associated with single and multisystem illness in humans.[143] Only two studies (1.8%) found no associations or evidence supporting mold causing human maladies. This review included over 273,000 subjects from over 30 countries and 5 continents.

Quantifiable associations were found in 99 of the 112 articles. OR (odds ratio) and RR (relative risk) were calculated for various indicators of dampness or mold and differing symptoms or illnesses and reported at three different thresholds. The three groups included associations of OR or

RR ≥2.0, ≥1.5 and ≥1.25, and all with 95% confidence. In sum, the number of associations with OR or RR ≥2.0 was 251, found in 79 articles; there were 384 associations ≥1.5, in 98 studies, and 460 associations with OR or RR ≥1.25, in 99 articles. The other 13 supportive articles did not include sufficient data to calculate OR. Only two reports showed no associations.

The same study gave significant evidence suggesting that chronic inhaled mold exposure could cause multisystem illness. The respiratory system was the most frequently studied aspect of human health. It was evaluated in 102 studies, with 100 (98.0%) reinforcing chronic exposure to WDB causing illness in this system. The immune system, or illness with an immune component, was studied in 62 articles, with 60 (96.8%) supporting. The general, or constitutional, system was evaluated 24 times. Symptoms such as fatigue, headaches and sleep disturbances fall into this system. All 24 reports (100%) endorsed increased general symptoms as a result of chronic exposure to the interior of WDB. Cognitive decline was reviewed in 16 articles, with 100% finding supportive evidence. All musculoskeletal (7), ophthalmic (16), gastrointestinal (9), neurologic (10), otolaryngology (2), mental health (5) and neonatal/pregnancy related studies (3) demonstrated evidence supporting exposure to dampness and/or mold leading to abnormalities in those systems. Finally, 14 of 15 (93.3%) dermatologic studies also found evidence of the same conclusion.

One study[144] from this group stands out as exemplary. This NIOSH article compared two high schools in different cities. The first was evaluated pre-Katrina in New Orleans, Louisiana. The authors' intent was to evaluate another school in the same vicinity, but Hurricane Katrina hit, and no suitable non-water-damaged control school could be found locally. The investigators then chose a control school in Cincinnati, Ohio.

Thorough environmental evaluation was undertaken at both schools, including visual inspection and sampling with spore trap analysis, bulk and swab testing, and ERMI (Environmental Relative Moldiness Index). All modalities of evaluation demonstrated that the New Orleans school was heavily water-damaged and visibly moldy, while the Cincinnati school had minimal water damage.

A medical team evaluated 95 staff of the highly water-damaged school and 110 from the other. Symptoms reviewed fell into four systems, namely, dermatologic, general, neurobehavioral and respiratory (further subdivided into upper and lower respiratory). VCS testing was also performed, gathering objective evidence of visual contrast function. The investigators found a statistically significant increase in 18 of 22 health symptoms covering all 4 systems and also discovered statistically significantly decreased VCS in all 5 columns of the test in the staff of the water-damaged New Orleans school. This study validated the previous findings of Shoemaker.

Shifting to imaging, NeuroQuant® (NQ) is an advanced technique for brain MRI, which automatically segments and calculates a volume for individual paired brain structures. NQ performs in 10 minutes of computer time what a skilled neuroradiologist could do in 100 hours. NQ allows a look at what disease does in brains at an earlier and more subtle level.

Three studies have looked at CIRS and NQ. The first[35] defined a pattern of subtle but structural brain damage occurring in subjects with CIRS due to chronic exposure to WDB. The pattern in adults showed increased forebrain parenchyma (FP), cortical gray (CG) and globus pallidum volumes with a decrease in caudate nucleus (CN) volumes. Of note, the FP and CG contribute roughly 50% of one's total brain volume. The authors theorized microinterstitial edema (due to inflammation) as the cause for enlarged volumes and neuronal death or dendritic pruning of the CN resulting in atrophy. The second study[36] confirmed the pattern (although pallidum involvement was significantly weaker and is not used as a marker any more), defined a pattern for subjects with structural brain damage due to CIRS caused by Lyme disease (enlarged right thalamus and decreased putamen) and documented FP, CG and pallidum volumes returning to control values in subjects who underwent therapy using all but the last step of the Shoemaker Protocol. The third article[37] provided more evidence for the Shoemaker Protocol returning pre-treatment enlarged volumes to control values, touched on multi-nuclear atrophy and demonstrated that usage of intranasal VIP may reduce (or correct) the degree of CN atrophy and multi-nuclear atrophy too.

One transcriptomics study[32] (Shoemaker 2015) looked at CIRS caused by ciguatoxin poisoning. *Ciguatera* is a toxin-producing dinoflagellate that causes CIRS, typically obtained after eating piscivorous reef fish which themselves dieted upon *Ciguatera*. The syndrome is almost indistinguishable from CIRS caused by chronic exposure to WDB, much as the common cold can be triggered by numerous different viruses. This report noted abnormal activity at the sarcin-ricin loop (SRL), an extremely highly conserved segment in ribosomes.[145] Binding at the SRL leads to cleavage of the 23S portion (prokaryotes) and the 28S portion (eukaryotes) of the large ribosomal subunits. Ricin is produced by castor beans. Sarcin and other rRNA endonucleases (all mycotoxins) are noted to bind here too.[146–148] This cleavage essentially stops protein production at this ribosome and eventually leads to apoptosis.

Transcriptomic data[149] revealed a hypometabolic state in the cells of untreated CIRS subjects, evidenced by downregulation of ribosomal activity, mitoribosomal protein assembly, nuclear-encoded protein production affecting mitochondria, and manufacture of transport proteins that allow nuclear-encoded proteins, built in the cytosol, to cross the outer and inner mitochondrial membranes for use in energy production. These four levels of downregulation lead to decreased cellular energy production and global energy deficiency for a human, dubbed "molecular hypometabolism." Untreated CIRS patients show a predilection for glycolysis, even when adequate oxygen is available. This is proliferative physiology, also seen in some cancers. Molecular hypometabolism, with or without proliferative physiology, is likely the primary mechanism for chronic fatigue in mold-related illness.

One study, from the German Society of Hygiene, Environmental Medicine and Preventative Medicine (Hurrass et al., 2017),[150] published more conservative findings. The authors evaluated individual systems and found little supportive evidence for multisystem illness. There are some problems with this study, however. In contrast to Dooley (2020),[143] which undertook a comprehensive literature review, in the German study, no fewer than 80 of the 241 citations were published in German. The literature used was not all-inclusive but rather, appeared selected. For instance, the report stated: "To date, there have been no systematic investigations or case descriptions that provide evidence of, or suggest an association between, indoor moisture damage or mould and gastrointestinal or renal disease," whereas Dooley (2020) cited eight different epidemiological articles referencing associations between gastrointestinal symptoms and exposure to indoor moisture/mold. The German paper reviewed a half dozen articles on cognitive issues. One was the previously discussed AAAAI 2006 former position statement[7] built upon the flawed hypothesis of the ACOEM 2002 report.[2] Three others were papers from before 2006, which offered no new data but merely criticized the methods of other studies that showed cognitive decline in objective neuropsychological testing after mold exposure.[151–153] The authors cited only one of the 10 articles cited in this chapter and published before 2011, and none of the 16 published after 2011, that offered data supporting cognitive decline. Just 1 out of 26 of these articles offering evidence in favor of cognitive decline after chronic exposure to WDB was cited and summarily dismissed.

It is not clear why the authors of the German Society of Hygiene, Environmental Medicine and Preventative Medicine study chose and excluded the articles they did. However, there was one quote that might explain: "The specialist literature does not point to a consistent causal relationship between indoor toxin levels and neurotoxic effects." The key phrase is "relationship between indoor toxin levels," indicating these authors believe cognitive decline might only occur as a result of direct toxicity. It is a re-iteration of the false assumption behind the mathematical proof[4] in ACOEM 2002. Further, this study was clearly an exception compared with the robust data since 2011, and before, which supported single-system and multisystem illness in humans after exposure to amplified indoor microbial growth/dampness. The report did indicate that evidence for non-IgE (allergy)-mediated immune responses existed. CIRS is predicated upon non-IgE-mediated immune responses.

One final report, discussed in Dooley 2020, was published by Harding et al. in 2019. This study repeatedly exposed mice to known doses of toxic and non-toxic mold spores and found activation in both groups of a central neural immune response with concomitant cognitive and emotional dysfunction. Their research confirmed the previous work of Rand[42, 154] that innate immune system activation is a mechanism of chronic exposure to both toxin-forming and non-toxigenic mold species. Specifically, Harding showed innate immune system activation in the central nervous system with both cognitive and behavioral abnormalities with a non-toxic basis. These are also seen in CIRS patients.

9.7 CONCLUSIONS

The listed references of data for this chapter go back to 1985, when Schoental[100] evaluated behavioral changes related to mycotoxin exposure. The majority of the cited studies are from 2000 and later. Significant questions have been answered by these studies. Can chronic exposure to indoor microbial growth/dampness *cause* single-system illness? Yes, asthma and IgE-mediated allergies (type I hypersensitivity) can be caused by exposure to indoor molds. IgE-mediated allergic bronchopulmonary Aspergillosis (ABPA) and hypersensitivity pneumonitis (or HP, a non-IgE-mediated type III or type IV hypersensitivity reaction) are caused by mold exposures. Can chronic exposure to indoor microbial growth/dampness lead to single-system illness? Yes. The amount of evidence is not as large as for the respiratory illnesses, but the number of supportive studies continues to mount, demonstrating that chronic indoor microbial growth/dampness is associated with cognitive deficits, neurological changes, gastrointestinal symptoms, dermatological problems, ophthalmologic irregularities and general system abnormalities such as fatigue, headaches, sleep disturbances, flu-like symptoms and more.

Is inhalation, ingestion or dermal contact the primary portal of entry for secondary metabolic products? Wannemaker[116] showed that inhalation is clearly the most dangerous entry point, with LD_{50} levels 4–20 times lower through inhalation than through other entrance points. Over 80 human health studies from before 2011 are cited in this chapter, and another 112 reports from 2011 on are cited in the Dooley 2020 systematic review, all demonstrating human illness acquisition from chronic exposure to air in WDB. Indeed, every study from the systematic review evaluated inhalation, not ingestion! However, there is a paucity of literature linking human illness to low levels of ingested microbial toxins. The ACOEM 2002 report[2] insisted ingestion must be primary, but the same 196 studies mentioned immediately before argue against ingestion being primary and place inhalation as the dominant entry source in humans.

Is there an identifiable multisystem illness that is caused by chronic exposure to indoor microbial growth/dampness? Yes, Shoemaker defined this illness and called it CIRS, reflecting the immune system's response to chronic exposure. He has published 37 reproducible symptoms,[23,26,27,38,39] recurrent physical findings,[38,39] 10 diagnostic biomarkers,[28,29,30,31,33] reproducible structural brain abnormalities on NQ,[35,36,37] and a treatment protocol that has been tested through two double-blinded placebo-controlled trials,[33,34] and has transcriptomic findings elucidating intracellular causes of fatigue[149] already published. Incidentally, all CIRS patients show symptom and objective evidence of immune system dysfunction, while nearly all demonstrate endocrine system dysfunction and neurological damage in the form of toxic encephalopathy, cognitive decline and/or cognitive changes.

Can chronic inhaled mold exposure cause illness outside of allergies, infection and direct toxicity? Yes, as evidenced by much data and many summary articles declaring that immune mechanisms beyond allergy can be triggered by mold exposure. CIRS is caused by a dysregulation of the innate immune system, typically predisposed by an HLA-inherited hole in antigen presentation precluding adequate adaptive immune response as a result of chronic innate immune challenges. CIRS is not an allergic response but is most definitely an illness affecting the innate immune system.

Is illness that develops after chronic exposure primarily toxin based or immune based? The ACOEM 2002[2] attempted to mathematically prove that it was very unlikely that sufficient mycotoxin could accumulate in an indoor space to cause serious human illness. The proof contained several flawed physiologic assumptions and used several constants at inaccurately low levels by several orders of magnitude each. Some of the errors were avoidable, as published information regarding constants was available at the time; other constants were found and published by 2005. Regardless, even a single error invalidated the proof and its negative conclusions. In addition, other reports were built on the chassis of this proof, such as the AAAAI 2006 former position statement[7] and the ACMT position statement,[8] invalidating their conclusions also. A considerable number of animal and *in vitro* human studies cited here suggest that direct toxicity of toxins plays a role, but the established pathophysiology appears to be primarily immune related, with at least five of the diagnostic tests for CIRS reflecting derangements in the innate immune system. The answer for now is that chronic exposure to toxins, inflammagens and microbes found in WDB causes a combination of toxic and immune-related damage, and further study will be required to parse out the individual contributions. Transcriptomic studies and improving the sensitivity of mycotoxin assays from human and air samples may pave the way for more complete understanding.

REFERENCES

1. Stoll A, Hofmann A. The Ergot alkaloids. In: Manske RHF, ed. *The Alkaloids*. Vol. VIII. New York, NY: Academic Press, Inc. 1965:725–83.
2. Hardin B, Kelman B, Saxon A. Adverse human health effects associated with molds in the indoor environment. *J Occup Environ Med*. 2003;45(5):470–478. 19.
3. Sanchez-Ramos J. *Brain's DNA Repair Response to Neurotoxicants*. Tampa University, Florida. Annual report. 1 Jul 2004–30 Jun 2005. Available at: http://www.dtic.mil/dtic/tr/fulltext/u2/a452374.pdf
4. Górny RL, Reponen T, Willeke K, Schmechel D, Robine E, Boissier M, Grinshpun SA. Fungal fragments as indoor air biocontaminants. *Appl Environ Microbiol*. 2002 Jul;68(7):3522–31.
5. Cho S-H, Seo S-C, Schemechel D, Grinshpun SA, Reponen T. Aerodynamic characteristics and respiratory deposition of fungal fragments. *Atmos Environ*. 2005;39:5454–5465.
6. Berndtson K, McMahon S, Ackerley M, Rapaport S, Gupta S, Shoemaker R. Medically sound investigation and remediation of water-damaged buildings in cases of chronic inflammatory response syndrome. 1/1/2020. January 19, 2016. Available at: https://www.survivingmold.com/docs/MEDICAL_CONSENSUS_1_19_2016_INDOOR_AIR_KB_FINAL.pdf
7. Bush RK, Portnoy JM, Saxon A, Terr AI, Wood RA. The medical effects of mold exposure. *J Allergy Clin Immunol*. 2006;117:326–333.
8. Sudakin D, Kurt T. *ACMT Position Statements: Institute of Medicine Report on Damp Indoor Spaces and Health*. 2006. Available at: https://www.acmt.net/cgi/page.cgi/_zine.html/Position_Statements/Institute_of_Medicine_Report_on_Damp_Indoor_Spaces_and_Health
9. Terr AI. Sick Building Syndrome: is mold the cause? *Med Mycol*. 2009;47(Supp 1):S217–S22.
10. *GAO Report to the Chairman, Committee on Health, Education, Labor and Pensions, U.S. Senate, Indoor Mold*. 2008.
11. Baldo JV, Ahmad L, Ruff R. Neuropsychological performance of patients following mold exposure. *Appl Neuropsychol*. 2002;9(4):193–202.
12. Crago BR, Gray MR, Nelson LA, Davis M, Arnold L, Thrasher JD. Psychological, neuropsychological, and electro-cortical effects of mixed mold exposure. *Arch Environ Health*. 2004;58(8):452–462.
13. Campbell AW, Thrasher JD, Madison RA et al. Neural antibodies and neurophysiologic abnormalities in patients exposed to molds in water-damaged buildings. *Arch Environ Health*. 2003;58:464–474.
14. Kilburn KH. Indoor mold exposure associated with neurobehavioral and pulmonary impairment: a preliminary report. *Arch Environ Health*. 2003;58:390–8.
15. Chang C, Gershwin ME. Mold hysteria: Origin of the hoax. *Clin Dev Immunol*. 2005;1(2):151–8.
16. Basic facts about mold and Dampness. CDC. Available at: https://www.cdc.gov/mold/faqs.htm#:~:text=If%20you%20can%20see%20or,present%2C%20you%20should%20remove%20it.
17. Mudarri D, Fisk WJ. Public health and economic impact of dampness and mold. *Indoor Air* 2007:17(3):226–235.
18. Antova T, Pattenden S, Brunekreef B, Heinrich J, Rudnai P, Forastiere F, Luttman-Gibson H, Grize L, Katsnelson B, Moshammer H, Nikiforov B, Slachtova H, Slotova K, Zlotkowska T, Fletcher T. Exposure to indoor mould and children's respiratory health in the PATY study. *J Epidemiol Community Health*. 2008;62(8):708–714.
19. Fisk WJ, Eliseeva EA, Mendell MJ. Association of residential dampness and mold with respiratory tract infections and bronchitis: A meta-analysis. *Environ Health*. 2010;9:72.

20. Clark N, Amman HM, Brunekreef B, et al. Damp Indoor spaces and Health. In: *Medicine Io*, Washington, DC: National Academy Press. 2004.
21. Afshari A, Anderson HR, Cohen A, et al. *World Health Organization Guidelines for Indoor Air Quality: Dampness and Mould. WHO Guidelines for Indoor Air Quality*. 2009.
22. Phalen RF, Oldham MJ, Nel AE. Tracheobronchial particle dose considerations for in vitro toxicology studies. *Toxicol Sci.* 2006;92(1):126–132.
23. Shoemaker RC, McMahon SW, Thrasher JD, Grimes C. Research committee report on diagnosis and treatment of chronic inflammatory response syndrome caused by exposure to the interior environment of water-damaged buildings. *Policyholders Am.* 2010;27:1–161.
24. Shoemaker R. Diagnosis of Pfiesteria-human illness syndrome. *Md Med J.* 1997;46(10):521–523.
25. Shoemaker R, Giclas P, Crowder C, House D. Complement split products C3a and C4a are early markers of acute Lyme disease in tick bite patients in the United States. *Int Arch Allergy Immunol.* 2008;146:255–261.
26. Shoemaker R, House D, Ryan J. Defining the neurotoxin derived illness chronic ciguatera using markers of chronic systemic inflammatory disturbances: A case/control study. *Neurotoxicol Teratol.* 2010;32(6):633–639.
27. Shoemaker RC, House DE. A time-series study of sick building syndrome: chronic, biotoxin-associated illness from exposure to water-damaged buildings. *Neurotoxicol Teratol.* 2005;27(1):29–46.
28. Shoemaker R, Hudnell K. Possible estuary-associated syndrome: Symptoms, vision, and treatment. *Environ Health Perspect.* 2001;109(5):539–545.
29. Shoemaker R. Linkage disequilibrium in alleles of HLA DR: differential association with susceptibility to chronic illness following exposure to biologically produced neurotoxins. American Society of Microbiology (conference peer review), 2003.
30. Shoemaker R, Maizel M. Innate immunity, MR spectroscopy, HLA DR, TGF beta-1, VIP and capillary hypoperfusion define acute and chronic human illness acquired following exposure to water-damaged buildings. International Healthy Buildings (conference peer review), 2008.
31. Shoemaker R, House D, Ryan J. Vasoactive intestinal polypeptide (VIP) corrects chronic inflammatory response syndrome (CIRS) acquired following exposure to water-damaged buildings. *Health.* 2013;3:396–401.
32. Ryan J, Wu Q, Shoemaker R. Transcriptomic signatures in whole blood of patients who acquire CIRS following an exposure to the marine toxin ciguatoxin. *BMC Med Genomics.* 2015;8:15.
33. Shoemaker R. Residential and recreational acquisition of possible estuary-associated syndrome: A new approach to successful diagnosis and treatment. *Environ Health Perspect.* 2001;109(Supplement 5):791–796.
34. Shoemaker RC, House D. Sick building syndrome (SBS) and exposure to water-damaged buildings: Time series study, clinical trial and mechanisms. *Neurotoxicol Teratol.* 2006;28(5):573–588.
35. Shoemaker R, House D, Ryan J. Structural brain abnormalities in patients with inflammatory illness acquired following exposure to water damaged buildings a volumetric MRI study using NeuroQuant. *Neurotoxicol Teratol.* 2014;45:18–26.
36. McMahon SW, Shoemaker RC, Ryan, JC. Reduction in forebrain parenchymal and cortical grey matter swelling across treatment groups in patients with inflammatory illness acquired following exposure to water-damaged buildings. *J Neurosci Clin Res.* 2016;1(1):1–4.
37. Shoemaker R, Katz D, Ackerley M, Rapaport S, McMahon S, Berndtson K, Ryan J. 2017;3(4):1–14.
38. McMahon SW. An evaluation of alternate means to diagnose chronic inflammatory response syndrome and determine prevalence. *Med Res Arch.* March 2017;5(3):1–18.
39. Shoemaker R, Johnson K, Jim L, Berry Y, Dooley M, Ryan J, McMahon S. Diagnostic process for chronic inflammatory response syndrome (CIRS): A consensus statement report of the consensus committee of Surviving Mold. *Intern Med Rev.* 2018;4(5):1–47.
40. Islam Z, Harkema JR, Pestka JJ. Satratoxin G from the black mold Stachybotrys chartarum evokes olfactory sensory loss and inflammation in the murine nose and brain. *Environ Health Perspect.* 2006;224:1099–1107.
41. Pieckova E, Hurbankova M, Cerna S, Pivovarova Z, Kovacikova Z. Pulmonary cytotoxicity of secondary metabolites of Stachybotrys chartarum (EHRENB.) Hughes. *Ann Agric Environ Med.* 2006;13:259–62.
42. Rand TG, Mahoney M, White K, Oulton M. Microanatomical changes in alveolar type II cells in juvenile mice. *Toxicol Sci.* 2002;65:239–45.
43. Rao CY, Brain JD Burge HA. Reduction of pulmonary toxicity of Stachybotrys chartarum spores by methanol extraction of mycotoxins. *Appl Environ Microbiol.* 2000; 66(7):2817–2821.

44. Creasia DA, Thurman JD, Jones J, Nealley ML, York CG, Wannemacher RW, Bunner DL. Acute inhalation toxicity of T-2 mycotoxin in mice. *Fundam Appl Toxicol.* 1987;8:230–235.

45. Yike I, Rand TG, Dearborn DG. Acute inflammatory responses to Stachybotrys chartarum in the lungs of infant rats: time course and possible mechanisms. *Toxicol Sci.* 2005;84(2):407–417.

46. Medvedev AE, Kopydlowski KM, Vogel SN. Inhibition of lipopolysaccharide induced signal transduction in endotoxin-tolerized mouse macrophages: Dysregulation of cytokine, chemokine, and Toll-like receptor 2 and 4 gene expression. *J Immunol.* 2000;164(11):5564–5574.

47. Rand TG, Flemming J, Miller JD, Womiloju TO. Comparison of inflammatory responses in mouse lungs exposed to atranones A and C from Stachybotrys chartarum. *J Toxicol Environ Health.* 2006;69:1–13.

48. Rand TG, Giles S, Flemming J, Miller JD, Puniani E. Inflammatory and cytotoxic responses in mouse lungs exposed to purified toxins from building isolated Penicillium brevicompactum dierckx and P. chrysogenum thom. *Toxicol Sci.* 2005;87(1):213–222.

49. Rao CY, Burge HA, Brain JD. The time course of responses to intratracheally instilled toxic Stachybotrys chartarum spores in rats. *Mycopathologia.* 2000;149:27–34.

50. Mason CD, Rand TG, Oulton M, MacDonald JM, Scott JE. Effects of Stachybotrys chartarum (atra) conidia and isolated toxin on lung surfactant production and homeostasis. *Natural Toxins.* 1998;6:27–33.

51. Shimizu T, Kida Y, Kuwano K. Mycoplasma pneumoniae-derived lipopeptides induce acute inflammatory responses in the lungs of mice. *Infect Immun.* 2008;76(1):270–277.

52. Martin LJ, Doebler JA, Anthony A. Scanning cytophotometric analysis of brain neuronal nuclear chromatin changes in acute T-2 toxin-treated rats. *Toxicol Appl Pharmacol.* 1986;85(2):207–214.

53. Martin LJ, Morse JD, Anthony A. Quantitative cytophotometric analysis of brain neuronal RNA and protein changes in acute T-2 mycotoxin poisoned rats. *Toxicon.* 1986;24(9):933–941.

54. Sava V, Velasquez A, Reunova O, Sanchez-Ramos J. Acute ochratoxin neurotoxicity: kinetics of distribution of the toxin, indices of oxidative stress and DNA repair activities in mouse brain. Accepted Abstract for Platform Presentation Society for Neuroscience, Annual Meeting, Washington, DC, November 2005.

55. Bergmann F, Yagen B, Jarvis BB. The toxicity of macrocyclic trichothecenes administered directly into the rat brain. *Toxicon.* 1992;30(10):1291–1294.

56. Donohue M, Wei W, Wu J, Zawia NH, Hud N, De Jesus V, Schmechel D, Hettick JM, Beezhold DH, Vesper S. Characterization of nigerlysin C, hemolysin produced by Aspergillus niger, and effect on mouse neuronal cells *in vitro. Toxicology.* 2006;219:150–155.

57. Wang J, Fitzpatrick DW, Wilson JR. Effect of T-2 toxin on blood-brain barrier permeability monoamine oxidase activity and protein synthesis in rats. *Food Chem Toxicol.* 1998;36(11):955–961.

58. Netea MG, Van der Meer JWM, Sutmuller RP, Adema GJ, Kullberg BJ. From the Th1/Th2 paradigm towards a Toll-like receptor/T-helper bias. *Antimicrob Agents Chemother.* 2005;49(10):3991–3996.

59. Huttunen K, Hyvarinen A, Nevalainen A, Komulainen H, Hirvonen MR. Production of proinflammatory mediators by indoor air bacteria and fungal spores in mouse and human cell lines. *Environ Health Perspect.* 2003;111:85–92.

60. Young SH, Roberts JR, Antonini JM. Pulmonary exposure to 1, 3-beta-glucan alters adaptive immune responses in rats. *Inhal Toxicol.* 2006;18(11):865–874.

61. Endo Y, Takahashi M, Fujita T. Lectin complement system and pattern recognition. *Immunobiology.* 2006;211(4):283–293.

62. Zhu Y, Ng PM, Wang L, Ho B, Ding JL. Diversity in lectins enables immune recognition and differentiation of wide spectrum of pathogens. *Int Immunol.* 2006;18(12):1671–1680.

63. Robinson MJ, Sancho D, Slack EC, LeibundGut-Landmann S, Reis e Sousa C. Myeloid C-type lectins in innate immunity. *Nat Immunol.* 2006;7(12):1258–1264.

64. Brown GD. Dectin-1: a signaling non-TLR pattern-recognition receptor. *Nat Rev Immunol.* 2006;6:33–43.

65. Taylor PR, Tsoni SV, Willment JA, Dennehy KM, Rosas M, Findon H, Haynes K, Steele C, Botto M, Gordon S, Brown GD. Dectin-1 is required for beta-glucan recognition and control of fungal infection. *Nat Immunol.* 2007;8(1):31–38.

66. Penttinen P, Pelkonen J, Huttunen K, Hirvonen MR. Co-cultivation of Streptomyces with Streptomyces californicus and Stachybotrys chartarum stimulates the production of cytostatic compound(s) with immunotoxic properties. *Toxicol Appl Pharmacol.* 2006;217:342–351.

67. Huttunen K, Pelkonen J, Nielsen KF, Nuutinen U, Jussila J, Hirvonen MR. Synergistic interaction in simultaneous exposure to Streptomyces californicus and Stachybotrys chartarum. *Environ Health Perspect.* 2004;112(4):659–665.

68. Murtoniemi T, Penttinen P, Nevalainen A, Hirvonen MR. Effects of microbial cocultivation on inflammatory and cytotoxic potential of spores. *Inhal Toxicol.* 2005;17(12):681–693.

69. Zughaier SM, Zimmer SM, Datta A, Carlson RW, Stephens DS. Differential induction of the Toll-like receptor 4-MyD88-dependent and independent signaling pathways by endotoxins. *Infect Immun.* 2006;74(5):3077.

70. Medvedev AE, Lentschat A, Wahl LM, Golenbock DT, Vogel SN. Dysregulation of LPS-induced Toll-like receptor 4-MyD88 complex formation and IL-1 receptorassociated kinase 1 activation in endotoxin-tolerant cells. *J Immunol.* 2002;169(9):5209–5216.

71. Islam Z, King LE, Fraker PJ, Pestka JJ. Differential induction of glucocorticoid-dependent apoptosis in murine lymphoid subpopulations in vivo following co-exposure to lipopolysaccharide and vomitoxin (deoxynivalenol). *Toxicol Appl Pharmacol.* 2003;182(2):69–99.

72. Islam Z, Pestka JJ. Role of IL-1beta in endotoxin potentiation of deoxynivalenol-induced corticosterone response and leukocyte apoptosis in mice. *Toxicol Sci.* 2003;74(1):93–102.

73. Zhou HR, Harkema JR, Hotchkiss JA, Yan D, Roth RA, Pestka JJ. Lipopolysaccharide and the trichothecene vomitoxin (deoxynivalenol) synergistically induce apoptosis in murine lymphoid organs. *Toxicol Sci.* 2000;53(2):253–263.

74. Hirvonen MR, Huttunen K, Roponen M. Bacterial strains from moldy buildings are highly potent inducers of inflammatory and cytotoxic effects. *Indoor Air.* 2005;15(Suppl 9):65–70.

75. Romani L. Immunity to fungal infections. *Nat Rev Immunol.* 2004;4:11–23.

76. Vesper SJ, Vesper MJ. Possible role of fungal hemolysins in sick building syndrome. *Adv Appl Microbiol.* 2004;55:191–213.

77. Jussila JJ. *Inflammatory responses in mice after intratracheal instillation of microbes isolated from moldy buildings.* PhD dissertation 01/24/03 National Public Health Institute, Finland.

78. Huang H, Ostroff G, Lee C, Wang J, Specht C, Levitz S. Distinct patterns of dendritic cell cytokine release stimulated by fungal B-glucans and toll-like receptor agonists. *Infect Immun.* 2009;77:1744–1781.

79. Miller JD, Sund M, Gilyan A, Roy J, Rand TG. Inflammation-associated gene transcription and expression in mouse lungs induced by low molecular weight compound from fungi from the built environment. *Chem-Biol Interact.* 2009;183(1):113–124.

80. Nikulin M, Reijula K, Jarvis BB, Veijalainen P, Hintikka EL. Effects of intranasal exposure to spores of Stachybotrys atra in mice. *Fundam Appl Toxicol.* 1997;35:182–188.

81. Flemming J, Hudson B, Rand TG. Comparison of inflammatory and cytotoxic lung responses in mice after intrathecal exposure to two different Stachybotrys chartarum strains. *Toxicol Sci.* 2004;78:267–75.

82. Janeway CA. Approaching the asymptote? Evolution and Revolution in immunology. *Cold Spring Harb Symp Quant Biol.* 1989;54:1–13.

83. Jiang H, Chess L. Regulation of immune responses by T cells. *N Engl J Med.* 2006;354:1166–1176.

84. Gonzalez-Rey E, Chorny A, Delgado M. Regulation of immune tolerance by anti-inflammatory neuropeptides. *Nat Rev Immunol.* 2007;7:52–63.

85. Mastronardi C, Srivastava V, Yu W, Les Dees W, McCann S. Lipopolysaccharide induced leptin synthesis and release are differentially controlled by alpha-melanocyte stimulating hormone. *Neuroimmunomodulation.* 2005;3:182–8.

86. Brzoska T, Luger T, Maaser C, Abels C, Bohm M. Melanocyte-stimulating hormone and related tripeptides: Biochemistry, anti-inflammatory and protective effects in vitro and in vivo, and future perspectives for the treatment of immune-mediated inflammatory diseases. *Endocr Rev.* 2008;5:581–602.

87. Valera I, Vigo AG, Alonso S, Barbolla L, Crespo MS, Fernandez N. Peptidoglycan and mannose-based molecular patterns trigger the arachidonic acid cascade in human polymorphonuclear leukocytes. *J Leukoc Biol.* 2007;81(4):925–933.

88. Holt PG, Strickland DH, Wikstrom ME, Jahnsen FL. Regulation of immunological homeostasis in the respiratory tract. *Immunology.* 2008;8:142–152.

89. Bretz C, Gersuk G, Knoblaugh S, Chaudhary N, Randolph-Habecker J, Hackman RC, Staab J, Marr KA. MyD88 signaling contributes to early pulmonary responses to Aspergillus fumigatus. *Infect Immun.* 2008;76:952–958.

90. Dubourdeau M, Athman R, Ballov V, Huerre M, Chignard M, Philpott D, Latge J, Ibrahim-Granet O. Aspergillus fumigatus induces innate immune responses in alveolar macrophages through the MAPK pathway independently of TLR2 and TLR4. *J Immunol.* 2006;6:3994–4001.

91. Ramirez-Ortiz ZG, Specht CA, Wang JP, Lee CK, Bartholomeu DC, Gazzinelli RT, Levitz SM. Toll-like receptor 9-dependent immune activation by unmethylated CpG motifs in Aspergillus fumigatus DNA. *Infect Immun.* 2008;76:2123–2129.

92. Willment JA, Marshall AS, Reid DM, Williams DL, Wong SY, Gordon S, Brown GD. The human beta-glucan receptor is widely expressed and functionally equivalent to murine dectin-1 on primary cells. *Eur J Immunol.* 2005;35(5):1539–1547.

93. Marc MM, Korosec P, Kosnick M, Kern I, Flezar M, Suskovic S, Sorli J. Complement factors C3a, C4a, and C5a in chronic obstructive pulmonary disease and asthma. *Am J Respir Cell Mol Biol.* 2004;31:31-33.

94. Kohl J, Baelder R, Lewkowich IP, Pandey MK, Hawlisch H, Wang L, Best J, Herman NS, Sproles AA, Zwirner J, Whirsett JA, Gerard C, Sfyroera G, Lambris JD, Wills-Karp M. A regulatory role for the C5a anaphylatoxins in type 2 immunity in asthma. *J Clin Investig.* 2006;116(3):783–796.

95. Takafugi S, Ishida A, Miyakuni T, Nakagawa T. Matrix metalloproteinase-9 release from human leukocytes. *J Investig Aller Clin Immunol.* 2003;13:50–5.

96. DiScipio R, Schraufstatter I, Sikora L, Zuraw B, Sriramarao P. C5a mediates secretion and activation of matrix metalloproteinase 9 from human eosinophils and neutrophils. *Int Immunopharmacol.* 2006;7:1109–18.

97. Francis K, Lewis BM, Akatsu H, Monk PN, Cain SA, Scanlon MF, Morgan BP, Ham J, Gasque P. Complement C3a receptors in the pituitary gland: A novel pathway by which an innate immune molecule releases hormones involved in the control of inflammation. *FASEB J.* 2003;17:2266–2268.

98. Pestka JJ, Yike I, Dearborn DG, Ward MDW, Harkema JR. Stachybotrys chartarum, trichothecene mycotoxins and damp building-related illness: new insights into a public health enigma. *Toxicol Sci.* 2008;104:4–26.

99. Hymery N, Sibiril Y, Parent-Massin D. In vitro effects of trichothecenes on human dendritic cells. *Toxicol in Vitro.* 2006;6:899–909.

100. Hymery N, Leon K, Carpentier F, Jung J, Parent-Massin D. T-2 toxin inhibits the differentiation of human monocytes into dendritic cells and macrophages. *Toxicol in Vitro.* 2009;3:509–19.

101. Dangman KH, Bracker AL, Storey E. Work-related asthma in teachers in Connecticut schools with chronic water damage and fungal growth. *Connecticut Med.* 2005;69:9–17.

102. Vesper SJ, Vesper MJ. Stachylysin may be a cause of hemorrhaging in humans exposed to Stachybotrys chartarum. *Infect Immun.* 2002;70(4):2065–2069.

103. Pei L, Shan S, Sun X. Effects of injuries pulmonary arterial endothelial cell induced by endotoxin on proliferation of pulmonary artery smooth muscle cells and interference effect of bone morphogenetic protein-2. *Zhonghua Yi Xue Za Zhi.* 2008;88(1):40–5.

104. Hodgson MJ, Morey P, Leung WY, Morrow L, Miller D, Jarvis BB, Robbins H, Halsey JF, Storey E. Building-associated pulmonary disease from exposure to Stachybotrys chartarum and Aspergillus versicolor. *J Occup Environ Med.* 1998;40(3):241–249.

105. Jarvis BB, Miller JD. Mycotoxins as harmful indoor air contaminants. *Appl Microbiol Biotechnol.* 2005;66(4):367–372.

106. Johanning E, Biagini R, Hull D. Health and immunology study following exposure to toxigenic fungi (Stachybotrys chartarum) in a water-damaged office environment. *Int Arch Occup Environ Health.* 1996;68:207–218.

107. Brasel T, Campbell A, Demers R, Ferguson B, Fink J, Vojdani A, Wilson S, Straus D. Detection of trichothecene mycotoxins in sera from individuals exposed to Stachybotrys chartarum in indoor environments. *Arch Environ Health.* 2004;59:317–23.

108. Anyanwu EC, Kanu I, Nwachukwu NC, Saleh MA. Chronic environmental exposure to Alternaria tenuis may manifest symptoms of neuropsychological illnesses: A study of 12 cases. *J Appl Sci Environ Mgt.* 2005;9(3):45–51.

109. Schoental R. Fusarial mycotoxins and behaviour: possible implications for psychiatric disorder. *Br J Psychiatry.* 1985;146:115–119.

110. Empting LD. Neurologic and neuropsychiatric syndrome features of mold and mycotoxins exposure. *Toxicol Indust Health.* 2009;25:81.

111. Gordon KE, Masotti RE, Waddell WR. Tremorgenic encephalopathy: a role of mycotoxins in the production of CNS disease in humans? *Can J Neurol Sci.* 1993;20:237–239.

112. Gordon WA, Cantor JB, Johanning E, Charatz H, Ashman TA, Breeze JL, Haddad L, Abramowitz S. Cognitive impairment associated with toxigenic fungal exposure: a replication and extension of previous findings. *Appl Neuropsychol.* 2004;11(2):65–74.

113. Dennis D, Robertson D, Curtis C, Black J. Fungal exposure endocrinopathy in sinusitis with growth hormone deficiency. *Toxicol Indust Health.* 2009;25:669–80.

114. Rea WJ, Didriksen N, Simon TR, Pan Y, Fenyves EJ, Griffiths B. Effects of toxic exposure to molds and mycotoxins in building-related illnesses. *Arch Environ Health.* 2003;58(7):399–405.

115. Taylor MJ, Smart RA, Sharma RP. Relationship of the hypothalamic-pituitary-adrenal axis with chemically induced immunomodulation. I. Stress-like response after exposure to T-2 toxin. *Toxicology.* 1989;56(2):179–195.

116. Wannemacher RW, Wiener SL. *Trichothecene Mycotoxins. Textbook of Military Medicine: Medical Aspects of Chemical and Biological Warfare*: Chapter 34.

117. Casadevall A, Pirofski LA. The weapon potential of human pathogenic fungi. *Med Mycol.* 2006;44:689–696.

118. Sidell FR, Takafuji ET, Franz DR. Medical aspects of chemical and biological warfare. *NLM Unique ID.* 1997: 9709389.

119. Desjardins AE. Trichothecenes: from yellow rain to green wheat. *ASM News.* 2003;69(4):182–185.

120. Minister of Health. Residential indoor air quality guideline for moulds. *Canada Gazette Part I.* 2007–03–31;141(13):1–2.

121. Chew GL, Wilson J, Rabito FA, Grimdley F, Iqbal S, Reponen T, Muilenberg ML, Thorne PS, Dearborn DG, Morley RL. Mold and endotoxin levels in the aftermath of hurricane Katrina: a pilot of homes in New Orleans undergoing renovation. *Environ Health Perspect.* 2006;114:1883–1889.

122. Redd SC. *State of the Science on Molds and Human Health. Statement for the Record Before the Subcommittees on Oversight and Investigations and Housing and Community Opportunity - Committee on Financial Services, United States House of Representatives.* 2002:1–10.

123. Rao CY, Riggs MA, Chew GL, Muilenburg ML, Thorne PS, Van Sickle D, Dunn KH, Brown C. Characterization of airborne molds, endotoxins, and glucans in homes in New Orleans after Hurricanes Katrina and Rita. *Appl Environ Microbiol.* 2007;73(5):1630–1634.

124. Verhoeff AP, Burge HA. Health risk assessment of fungi in home environments. *Ann Allergy Asthma Immunol.* 1997;78:544–556.

125. Gent JF, Ren P, Belanger K, Triche E, Bracken MB, Holford TR, Leaderer BP. Levels of household mold associated with respiratory symptoms in the first year of life in a cohort at risk for asthma. *Environ Health Perspect.* 2002;110(12):A781–A786.

126. Solomon GM, Hjelmroos-Koski M, Rotkin-Ellman M, Hammond SK. Airborne mold and endotoxin concentrations in New Orleans, Louisiana, after flooding, October through November 2005. *Environ Health Perspect* 2006;114(9):1381–1386.

127. Brandt M, Burkhart J, Burton NC, Cox-Ganser J, Damon S, Falk H, Fridkin S, Garbe P, Kreiss K, McGeehin M, Morgan J, Page E, Rao C, Redd S, Sinks T, Trout D, Wallingford KM, Warnock D, Weissman DN. Mold prevention strategies and possible health effects in the aftermath of Hurricanes Katrina and Rita. *CDC.* October 2005:1–45.

128. Mendell MJ, Cozen M, Lei-Gomez Q, Brightman HS, Erdmann CA, Girman JR, Womble SE. Indicators of moisture and ventilation system contamination in U.S. office buildings as risk factors for respiratory and mucous membrane symptoms: analyses of the EPA BASE data. *J Occup Environ Hyg.* 2006;3(5):225–233.

129. Park JH, Cox-Ganser JM, Kreiss K, White SK, Rao CY. Hydrophilic fungi and ergosterol associated with respiratory illness in a water-damaged building. *Environ Health Perspect.* 2008;116(1):45–50.

130. Park JH, Schleiff PL, Attfield MD, Cox-Ganser JM, Kreiss K. Building-related respiratory symptoms can be predicted with semi-quantitative indices of exposure to dampness and mold. *Indoor Air.* 2004;14:425–433.

131. Park JH, Cox-Ganser J, Rao C, Kreiss K. Fungal and endotoxin measurements in dust associated with respiratory symptoms in a water-damaged office building. *Indoor Air.* 2006;16(3):192–203.

132. Rao CY, Cox-Ganser JM, Chew GL, Doekes G, White S. Use of surrogate markers of biological agents in air and settled dust samples to evaluate a water-damaged hospital. *Indoor Air.* 2005;15(Suppl 9):89–97.

133. Cox-Ganser JM, White SK, Jones R, Hilsbos K, Storey E, Enright PL, Rao CY, Kreiss K. Respiratory morbidity in office workers in a water-damaged building. *Environ Health Perspect.* 2005;113(4):485–490.

134. Sorenson WG. Fungal spores: hazardous to health? *Environ Health Perspect.* 1999;107(3) Supplement 3:469–472.

135. Weinhold B. A spreading concern on inhalational health effects of mold. *Environ Health Perspect.* 2007;115(6):A300–A305.

136. Wu F, Jacobs D, Mitchell C, Miller D, Karol MH. Improving indoor environmental quality for public health: Impediments and policy recommendations. *Environ Health Perspect.* 2007;115(6):953–957.

137. Mitchell CS, Zhang J, Sigsgaard T, Jantunen M, Lioy PJ, Samson R, Karol MH. Current state of the science: Health effects and indoor environmental quality. *Environ Health Perspect.* 2007;115(6):958–964.

138. Loftness V, Hakkinen B, Adan O, Nevalainen A. Elements that contribute to healthy building design. *Environ Health Perspect.* 2007;115(6):965–970.

139. Wu F, Takaro TK. Childhood asthma and environmental interventions. *Environ Health Perspect.* 2007; 115(6):971–975.

140. Jacobs DE, Kelly T, Sobolewski J. Linking public health, housing and indoor environmental policy: Successes and challenges at local and federal agencies in the United States. *Environ Health Perspect.* 2007;115(6):976–981.
141. Adan OCG, Ng-A-Tham J, Hanke W, Sigsgaard T, van de Hazel P, Wu F. In search of a common European approach to a healthy indoor environment. *Environ Health Perspect.* 2007;115(6):983–988.
142. Caillaud D, Leynaert B, Keirsbulck M, Nadif R. Indoor mould exposure, asthma and rhinitis:findings from systematic reviews and recent longitudinal studies. *Eur Resp Rev.* 2018;27(148).
143. Dooley M, McMahon SW. A comprehensive review of mold research literature from 2011–2018. *Intern Med Rev.* 2020;3(1):1–39.
144. Thomas G, Burton NC, Mueller C, Page E, Vesper S. Comparison of work-related symptoms and visual contrast sensitivity between employees at a severely water-damaged school and a school without significant water damage. *Am J Ind Med.* 2012;55(9):844–854.
145. Shi X, Khade PK, Sanbonmatsu KY, Joseph S. Functional role of the sarcin-ricin loop of the 23S rRNA in the elongation cycle of protein synthesis. *J Mol Biol.* 2012;419(3–4):125–138.
146. Pérez-Cañadillas JM, Santoro J, Campos-Olivas R, Lacadena J, Martínez-del-Pozo A, Gavilanes JG, Rico M, Bruix M. The highly refined solution structure of the cytotoxic ribonuclease α-sarcin reveals the structural requirements for substrate recognition and ribonucleolytic activity. *J Mol Biol.* 2000;299(4):1061–1073.
147. Yang X, Moffat K. Insights into specificity of cleavage and mechanism of cell entry from the crystal structure of the highly specific Aspergillus ribotoxin, restrictocin. *Structure.* 1996;4(7):837–852.
148. Viegas A, Herrero-Galán E, Oñaderra M, Macedo AL, Bruix M. Solution structure of hirsutellin A - new insights into the active site and interacting interfaces of ribotoxins. *FEBS J.* 2009;276(8):2381–2390.
149. Shoemaker RC. Metabolism, molecular hypometabolism and inflammation: Complications of proliferative physiology include metabolic acidosis, pulmonary hypertension, Treg cell deficiency, insulin resistance and neuronal injury. *Trends Diabetes Metab.* 2020;3:1–15.
150. Hurrass J, Heinzow B, Aurbach U, et al. Medical diagnostics for indoor mold exposure. *Int J Hyg Environ Health.* 2017;220(2 Pt B):305–328.
151. Khalili B, Montanaro MT, Bardana EJ. Inhalational mold toxicity: fact or fiction? A clinical review of 50 cases. *Ann Allergy Asthma Immunol.* 2005;95:239–246.
152. Chapman JA, Terr AI, Jacobs RL, Charlesworth EN, Bardana EJ. Toxic mold: phantom risk vs science. *Ann Allergy Asthma Immunol.* 2003;91:222–232.
153. Lees-Haley PR. Toxic mold and mycotoxins in neurotoxicity cases: Stachybotrys, Fusarium, Trichoderma, Aspergillus, Penicillium, Cladosporium, Alternaria, Trichothecenes. *Psychol Rep.* 2003;93:561–584.
154. Rand TG, White K, Logan A, Gregory L. Histological, immunohistochemical and morphometric changes in lung tissue in juvenile mice experimentally exposed to Stachybotrys chartarum spores. *Mycopathlogia* 2003:156(2):119–131.

10 Guidelines for Public Policy Considerations in Building Standards

Safe Buildings Are a Human Right

Ritchie Shoemaker, David Lark and April Vukelic

CONTENTS

10.1 WHAT IS A WATER-DAMAGED BUILDING?

Exposure to damp indoor environments is not healthy for anyone. Furthermore, if one is ill with Chronic Inflammatory Response Syndrome (CIRS), removal from exposure is the priority. These water-damaged buildings (WDBs) are everywhere. The most neglected expense for the health of buildings is maintenance. These buildings are bought, sold and rented to unwitting tenants every day. WDBs could be someone's place of work, grocery store, school, university or government building. WDBs may pass inspections, be "up to code" and receive "passable" spore counts. However, public policies and standard practices do not protect those genetically vulnerable to biotoxins. With sequential gene activation, one can see that these buildings are the causation of illness. To people with CIRS, these buildings may be as inaccessible as stairs to someone in a wheelchair.

DOI: 10.1201/b23304-11

As many as 50% of our public buildings are water damaged. What makes WDBs unsafe is the growth of a group of single-cell microbes. These microbes produce compounds that can cause inflammation (called inflammagens). Some of these may be toxins made by bacteria (endotoxins or exotoxins), fungi (mycotoxins), mycobacteria (mycolactones) and actinobacteria. In addition, tiny cell wall fragments of fungi (beta glucans and mannans) and fungal and bacterial enzymes/proteins (hemolysins, spirocyclic drimanes, and proteinases) cause inflammation. We have not yet adequately defined a pathogenic role for microbial volatile organic compounds (mVOCs), but consensus opinion supports mVOCs having some role in creating adverse human health effects. Each of these non-living elements acts synergistically, one with another.

Remember that musty smells, usually stemming from geosmin made by actinobacteria and occasionally by bacteria, are often used to support a diagnosis of a *mold* problem. The use of accurate mold-specific quantitative polymerase chain reaction (QPCR) testing is readily and inexpensively available.

Unfortunately, some practitioners still think that air sampling has a role in the medical workup of CIRS patients. The use of air samples for diagnosis is nearly worthless because sampling air for spores, at least 3 microns in diameter or greater, ignores *99.8% of the total* amount of fragments that cause inflammatory responses! These fragments are so small that they pass through the spore trap devices. Spore trapping, then, cannot possibly be used to look for disease-causing inflammation. Do not forget that exposure to small particles, which are merely *biochemicals*, means that most bad actors in WDBs are *not alive*. Killing spores does not remediate a damp home.

Spore sampling is still widely used, even though it provides flawed information. Even worse than wrong-headed data generated by spore traps is the problem that occurs when people *believe that spore trapping makes sense* and that spore count results indicate something real in nature. Of note:

1. Air samples performed for only 5 or 10 minutes in a single-center location in a room do not tell us what happened to bacteria or fungal spores that have *settled* out before the sampling.
2. Air samples do not tell us what particulates were missed by sampling in the center of a room and not in boundary layers on the bottom and sides of a room.
3. Air samples do not separate benign species from pathogenic species of *Aspergillus* and *Penicillium* (spore counts combine these two very large genera as Asp/Pen).
4. They rarely show the presence of heavier particulates such as those made by *Stachybotrys*.
5. They will never show the presence of xerophilic organisms such as *Wallemia sebi*.
6. Without repetition of air sampling findings, multiple times per day in a given room for multiple days per week, multiple weeks per month and multiple months per year, the World Health Organization has declared that air sampling is of *no benefit*.

One reason for the commonality of microbial findings in WDBs being similar across the states and worldwide is that the indoor ecosystem of a wet building is uniquely similar in all climates. There rarely is any wind indoors. There certainly is not any rain or frozen precipitation. There is only a narrow range of temperature in an occupied building and only limited diversity of visiting or exotic organisms. Often, there will be limited movement of fixed objects in a room, setting up areas of reduced ventilation ("still air"). Not to mention floors and ceilings, fixed walls create boundary layers of air and particulates.

MSQPCR (mold-specific QPCR) is a marker of different species of filamentous fungi found inside homes, both water-damaged and not. The fungal DNA present *tells us much about the water activity* found inside the building. The Environmental Protection Agency (EPA)-developed ERMI (Environmental Relative Moldiness Index) aims to quantify an index of microbial contamination in a building from the assessment of MSQPCR measured on dust samples. Initially done on vacuumed samples, ERMI uses electrostatic cloth wipe (Swiffer) samplings. Both Swiffer and vacuum methods bear comparable validity.

Proper ERMI testing demands the proper use of high-quality probes and primers for detection and reporting. Laboratories that license the ERMI technology from the EPA must show accurate and ongoing quality control. Never send a sample off to a laboratory that does not have ongoing EPA licensing, as errors routinely occur with faulty use of primers or inexpensive, inadequate reagents. If an MSQPCR laboratory does not disclose its quality control methods over the phone, do not use its services.

The Health Effects Roster of Type Specific (Formers) of Mycotoxins and Inflammagens, Version II (HERTSMI-2) is a laboratory test far more useful than ERMI. HERTSMI-2 is more accurate than ERMI in measuring the risk of recrudescence with re-exposure of CIRS patients to WDB. HERTSMI-2 is now in broader use since its inception in 2011. Its accuracy sorts health abnormalities associated with exposure into five species of fungi in WDB:

1. These "span the globe" of water activity (Aw) from the driest to the wettest organisms.
2. The test shows the overwhelming increase in CIRS when these specified organisms exist.

By relying on the correlation of spore equivalents/mg dust with the risk of acquiring adverse human health effects, we finally have a measure that predicts degrees of safety for over 95% of CIRS patients entering schools, workplaces and residences. One can always calculate a HERTSMI with the data from an ERMI. Greg Weatherman states that ERMI may be used in forensic data and provide critical information about the source of exposure.

The scoring system for HERTSMI-2 weighs the severity of contamination from 0 to 10 points for given organisms. When we sort these organisms by Aw, we find that the drier-loving species of *Wallemia* and *Aspergillus penicillioides* are routinely found at Aw of 0.65–0.8 but are rare in air samples. The common *Aspergillus versicolor*, usually found in higher Aw of 0.8 to 0.9, is reported by ERMI but is never reported at the species level by spore traps. *Chaetomium* and *Stachybotrys* reflect environmental conditions with an Aw of 0.9–1.0 and are detected infrequently in air samples using spore traps.

A word regarding dust collection: When using electrostatic cloths (like Swiffer), a single, new pad per sample is best. Put a glove on the left hand and wipe in one direction, either left to right or right to left. Use one cloth for all the sampling. Sample dust on high, undisturbed areas like curios and entertainment centers. Do not use windowsills or "public" areas, like hallways. Avoid shoes on closet floors, but closet shelves are fair game. Avoid bathrooms because of the role of water saturation following showers or bathing. If there is evidence of obvious microbial growth, resist the temptation to wipe it, as sampling the black patch on the bedroom wall, for example, will skew the sample to render results less reliable. If there is a crawl space, a sump pump, a basement or an indoor spa, or areas in bathrooms that have hampered airflow with inadequate exhaust, be sure to test for endotoxins with the same sample used for HERTSMI-2. Testing for the presence of *actinobacteria* species is of tremendous value, especially when *Aspergillus penicillioides* or *Wallemia* are predominant. Actinobacteria may grow in wetter environments but are more common in drier indoor spaces. They also prefer alkaline surfaces like concrete that remain chronically damp.

We have seen that the causation of illness from WDBs is multi-factorial. We cannot just rely on fungal DNA. The question is, "Can we identify a single source of causation of human illness from WDBs?" *The answer is no.*

Countless different measurements, mostly not available, are needed for 100% certainty. One such example is spirocyclic drimanes, known to cause inflammation but for which there is no commercial test available. We are less able to measure beta glucans and mannans. Moreover, microbial VOCs show great potential as a biomarker for water damage. However, human health effects data associated with mVOC exposure is not confirmed. Please note that transcriptomics is bringing us closer to understanding causation. Differential gene activation can tell us if it is likely that reactivity to mycotoxins, actinobacteria or endotoxins has occurred.

Not everyone exposed becomes ill. Furthermore, more curiously, people with successful treatment will relapse through re-exposure. What is our protective antibody arm of the immune system doing? Could antigen detection and antigen presentation *both* be defective?

Inflammation sets off more inflammation, uncontrolled like a runaway freight train without brakes. This inflammatory cascade causes changes in gene activation, which are the fundamental source of CIRS.

10.2 WATER ACTIVITY

It is a basic tenet of real estate that landlords, building owners/sellers and construction companies are responsible for providing a safe indoor environment. When an outdoor deck collapses, for example, throwing a group of wedding guests into a creek, an injured guest might claim that negligent construction caused a personal loss, pain and suffering. The exchange of money might not make a person whole again, but the idea of compensation for caused injury applies. Who is negligent if water intrusion gives rise to the growth of one-celled organisms that then cause inflammation and a multisystem, multi-symptom illness? Who pays the plaintiff when causation of personal injury receives confirmation in court?

When water enters an enclosed space, and that space stays wet for as little as 48 hours, microbial growth will occur. While bacteria might be the first colonizers, fungi are not far behind. Precisely which microbes grow is entirely dependent on the availability of moisture. We call this availability of water or water activity "Aw." Aw of 1.0 (or 100% relative humidity) is open water compared with the water vapor pressure above the water. Bacteria and "wet" fungi, like *Chaetomium* and *Stachybotrys*, need a minimum Aw of >0.9 (>90% relative humidity) to grow. "Medium-wet" filamentous fungi, like *Aspergillus versicolor*, need Aw of 0.8–0.9 to grow. "Drier" fungal organisms, including *Aspergillus penicillioides*, need a minimum Aw of 0.58–0.8 to grow. The dry (xerophilic) fungi, especially *Wallemia sebi*, like a range of Aw that can go as low as 0.55 to 0.75 to grow.

The availability of water has relevance for all involved in the WDB field. Consider nasal mucus. It is full of water, yet mucus prevents the growth of the vast percentage of potential pathogens that land in the nose during breathing. Why does not every germ in the nose cause infection? Because the water needed for the growth of bacteria and fungi *is not bioavailable*. The mucopolysaccharide matrix prevents the water from nourishing fungi, for example. In the end, it is irrelevant whether fungi are in nasal secretions. They will not make toxins or secondary metabolites without available water.

Cases of fungal sinusitis have 2.4 species of fungi cultured in mucus in their noses, but controls have 3.1 species cultured. In a classic German report from 2003, 87% of all cases had positive cultures, but 91.3% of controls also had positive cultures. Because "fungi can be identified in almost everybody's nose … when inhaled, these airborne fungi are only 'in transit' through the nose. Positive fungal cultures from nasal secretions have to be considered normal findings."

If we only assay dust found in a WDB for fungal DNA, the presence of indicator fungal DNA tells us a lot about the building ecology described by Aw. By looking at indicator DNA, we can get a solid idea of what is abnormal in the ecology of a WDB that is making people sick.

Perhaps the most important organisms found in WDB are *actinobacteria*. Not fungi, not mold, black molds and toxic black molds, but these filamentous bacteria in clinical dust samples may be the most significant players in adverse human health effects. If we add assays for endotoxins and actinobacteria to assays of fungal DNA, we can obtain a robust picture of the harmful microbes in a WDB.

10.3 HOW DOES WATER GET INSIDE? THE VALUE OF VIGILANT MAINTENANCE OF THE BUILDING ENVELOPE

10.3.1 ROOFS

How many thousands of nails are required to shingle a 3000 square foot roof (4 nails/shingle in low wind areas; 320 nails per 100 square feet)? If 1 in 100 nail heads are exposed, that means 10 exposed per 300 square feet. Not much room for error! Remember, it takes fewer than ten exposed nail heads to create a significant risk for a leak. Get out the binoculars and look for exposed nail heads peeking out from under the shingles, reflecting light on a sunny day. Flat roofs with membranes have a limited shelf-life because it only takes a pinhole defect and gravity for water to enter a building.

"Boots" woven under shingles around the ventilation pipes take moisture out of bathrooms and exhaust to the outside world. The cheap ones might last 10 years until they leak. Newer boots are rated at 50 years (with 20 nights of 40 mph winds per year) but cost three times as much as the cheaper boots. Take a trip to the attic. Look at the attic side of the boots. Are there any moisture stains? Make sure all vent pipes go through the roof deck too.

Look at ventilating soffits inside the attic and outside. Is air flowing as expected through the soffit and out the ridge vent? Is there daylight between the edge of the roof and the chimney stack? If daylight is visible, there will be water coming down the outside of the chimney into the home. Time to flash and counter-flash. Or, how about the chimney that is off-center in a gable end of a house? Water coming down from the higher-pitched areas will flow against the flashing around the chimney. Use a mini-roof ("cricket") to deflect water away from the pocket created by siding touching flashing.

Snow dogs will help prevent ice dams but will eventually leak. Inspect the snow dogs and the attic below where ice dams might form. Look for discolored insulation.

10.3.2 Windows

Windows are complicated to install. It is common in new construction to find moisture from leaking windows in wall cavities below windowsills. New construction ends up being far riskier for hidden defects than older construction. The reason might not be apparent. It can take a year or two to recognize construction problems and microbial growth. WDBs usually have moisture intrusion over time as various defects become apparent.

10.3.3 Doors

Improper door installation causes leaks from above and below. Every year, it is necessary to caulk inset fanlights over doors. Inspect doors for warps, swelling and leaks.

10.3.4 Gutters

Gutter inspection and maintenance are crucial. If an overhanging tree is present, the obstruction problem is essentially guaranteed. As the gutter continues to fill with debris, the water has to go somewhere. It will usually overflow the front or the back. If there is a slight backward pitch of the gutter, water will impact against the fascia board. If this wide flat board is not tight, there is free entry for water behind the fascia into the attic or inside the cladding. Once inside the attic, water can then run downhill, sometimes going a very long way along a rafter. When water meets a drop-off point, maybe just a bow of the wood or a protruding nailhead, gravity will direct the water downwards. Homes with blocked gutters can show leaks 40 feet away on the opposite side of the attic.

10.3.5 Siding (Cladding)

Any siding materials can leak. Brick, stone, wood, vinyl, concrete, block and stucco are just a barrier. Wind-driven water can track uphill under the edges of siding through nail holes and cracks. Inadequate seals around fake stucco often invite water intrusion. If porous oriented strand board (OSB) protects the stud walls underneath the cladding inside the house, the water coming from seal leaks is an invitation to microbial growth. OSB acts as a nurturing sponge of life for microbes. Significantly, mold and bacteria will rapidly grow through the 4' by 8' wood particle-chip-glue sheet, leading to microbial growth on *both sides* of the OSB. If OSB remains wet and fungi digest the cellulose, it does not take too long before additional water is dumped into a wall cavity, creating potential problems. As particulates from microbial growth go airborne, even in wall cavities, they can find their way into the home traveling on air flowing around switch plates, receptacles, defective drywall joints or even nails used to hang pictures. Actinobacteria get through interior walls more often than fungi, but bacteria are the swiftest to penetrate.

The same moisture penetration problem applies to *exterior masonry walls* because there is a space behind bricks or stone in which air circulates. Bricks and stone are both porous, which means moisture that hits the outside of the brick can migrate through to the inner surface. Once inside, water will drain downward. At the bottom of the exterior wall, there should be an opening called a "weep hole" that will let water leave the inner space and not create microbial growth between the brick and plywood or OSB.

10.3.6 Vinyl Siding

Vinyl siding is inexpensive, goes up quickly, and comes in many colors. It is no surprise that we have so many vinyl-sided homes in the United States. While the vinyl itself is impervious to the inflow of outside water, the junctions between pieces of vinyl or areas around vinyl nails create potential portals for water intrusion. Wind makes gaps in vinyl walls!

The green material growing on exterior walls is not mold but *algae*. The algal growth can be so profuse that a mat of algae may form in corners. Under the mat, there can be an air space between overlapping pieces of siding that lets water wick underneath. Attempts to clean siding can create new problems. Power washing will remove algae but may cause water intrusion inside the building envelope.

10.3.7 Crawl Spaces

Basements and crawl spaces are sources of microbial growth found in 95% of homes with subterranean features. Having a walkout basement is no guarantee of safety, because the inground side of a walkout basement is subject to additional water pressure that can create a wet wall. Water pressure will overcome any temporary barrier created by tar solutions or fancy paints designed to be waterproof.

Many people with a walkout basement dig trenches on the inground side approximately 3–4 feet deep and install perforated pipe covered by pebbles to create a "French drain." At the corners of the building, pipes form a right angle to direct groundwater away from the building. The pipes extend beyond the downhill side of the house. When homeowners perform this kind of preventive maintenance, they are surprised by how much water comes out of the drainpipes.

Some people install sump pumps to fix moisture problems created by subterranean structures. Using a chiseled notch or trench, cut into the concrete slab of the floor that leads to the sump pump, and then, the pump will move the water somewhere, hopefully outside of the basement. This approach sounds pretty good, except when we recognize that the water that has just come in and is in a trench creates a microclimate of elevated Aw that is perfect for bacterial growth. Sump pumps themselves almost guarantee a source of bacterial colonization and endotoxins. A better solution is not to have a basement!

In Maryland, basements are uncommon, unlike crawl spaces. Usually three–four cinder blocks high, crawls are the standard approach to lower-cost new home construction. A finished crawl space will often have several vents installed every 8–12 feet. When the hot moist air hits the cool air over the exposed soil in the crawl (usually about 54 degrees), the condensation has nearly the effect of rain. The excessive moisture from the earth below provides a continuous source of moisture to nourish micro-organisms growing in soil. Do not be confused by the dry appearance of the soil in a crawl space: It just means that soil water has evaporated over time. More is on the way from deeper soils.

Condition or seal off the crawl spaces to reduce moisture from soil or the sidewalls from entering the air in the crawl. By putting 20–28-gauge plastic (pond liners are best) and then folding the edges of the liner upwards so that the liner can be attached to the board (sill plate) sitting on top of the foundation, we can create a water intrusion barrier that works. Meanwhile, any water coming from the earth remains under plastic. There is no excess moisture on the floor side of the liner available to nourish microbes that might be living opportunistically in the crawl space. The vents are sealed shut.

This conditioning idea sounds radical. Traditionally, crawl spaces have vents. Newer building practices opt for ventless crawl spaces. Nevertheless, the moisture problems continue. Conditioning is defeated when heating, ventilation, and air conditioning (HVAC) systems pump warm or cool air into the crawlspace and create a temperature gradient. Now, we are creating the opportunity to mix indoor moisture with a sealed crawl space, thereby defeating the purpose of a moisture-tight chamber.

If there is a basement or a crawl space, use expandable foam to seal any holes in the subfloor. It is incredible how much air can come through small openings around pipes. Such spray foams will release VOCs, so seal well before occupying the building.

10.3.8   INTERNAL SOURCES

Internal sources of moisture are easy to overlook. Outside humidity is a problem in tropical regions. Two choices exist to prevent exposure. The first involves matching the tonnage of HVAC equipment to the volume of a building. The second approach is to increase ventilation. In the United States, buildings often use HVAC to safeguard homes from tropical fungi (especially *A. penicillioides*).

10.3.9   COOKING

Cooking creates the most significant source of moisture on the first floor of most homes, with bathrooms creating the source of moisture most commonly on the second floor.

Assume, of course, that there are no sliding glass doors that leak, no skylights that leak, no elaborate roof structures with valleys and pitches that are impossible to close off, and no flat roofs that will predictably leak. These are all standard practices in the suburban blight of so-called McMansions.

10.3.10   HUMAN SOURCES

Human sources of moisture, such as breathing, also contribute to water availability inside the home. Leaking shower pipes are notorious for having small pinhole leaks above the sweat joint where a copper supply tube meets a plastic or PVC junction. These pinhole leaks are rarely visible in the bathroom side of a wall cavity, but if there is a closet that abuts the back of the wall cavity, that is where moisture will accumulate, and mold will grow. If the closet is closed most of the time, expect to find *A. penicillioides*. *A. penicillioides* does not like to be ventilated. It is present in bathroom vanities, behind refrigerators, at the end of hallways with poor ventilation or in closets. Reduced ventilation can cause shoes in a closet to grow mold. *A. penicillioides* is also found on carpets, soft furnishings and drapes.

10.3.11   DECKS

Adding decks makes for enjoyable living. However, screwing the deck ribbon board into the foundation board of the home without ensuring adequate flashing can cause water coming off the deck understructure to enter the foundation. Consider well-graded patios made from pavers as a durable alternative to decks.

10.3.12   STILTS

A unique circumstance applies to coastal living. There is a financial benefit to building homes on elevated pilings, usually 8–10 feet off the sand, to avoid flood damage. For some people, this 10-foot high space, the size of the footprint of the building, is too tempting. Just look at this ground-floor bonus room! This enclosed area is an outdoor fungal growth chamber sitting outside the entry door. Every time one goes in or out, a vortex of unhealthy air enters the living space. Do not make extra storage space or living space by sacrificing health.

10.4 SEQUENTIAL ACTIVATION OF INNATE IMMUNE EFFECTS (SAIIE): DEFINING CAUSATION

An adaptation of the treatment protocol permits a diagnostic, prospective re-exposure trial. Called Sequential Activation of Innate Immune Effects (SAIIE), this protocol demonstrates causation. As opposed to a case/control study, which lets us conclude an association of exposure with symptoms, VCS deficits, proteomics or transcriptomic abnormalities, a prospective study design can confirm the presence of the epidemiologic concept of risk and causation.

Perform an SAIIE trial on a known patient who meets the GAO case definition and use the Shoemaker Protocol to correct symptoms, VCS and proteomics. Before starting, we know that the building suspected of making the patient ill is contaminated. We will also know that the building where the patient is staying is safe (using ERMI or HERTSMI-2).

Obtain informed consent and start the first step after RX 1 (after CSM (AC1), usually beginning on Friday). Record symptoms, VCS and selected labs (C4a, MMP-9, leptin, vascular endothelial growth factor, and von Willebrand's profile). Stop all CIRS medications. The patient does not enter the suspect building for 3 days after being exposed to "the ubiquitous fungi of the world." On Monday morning, having completed the prospective trial of no known exposure to a WDB, record symptoms, VCS and repeat labs. This step, called Home Off CSM (HOC), ends with the blood draws on Monday.

The patient then enters the suspect building each day for 3 days, with study measures performed daily. Symptoms, VCS and labs are performed on Tuesday AM, showing us what happened on day 1 of re-exposure (Building Off CSM (BOC-1), Tuesday). The patient re-enters the building. Symptoms, VCS and labs are performed on Wednesday, telling us what happened on day 2 of exposure (BOC-2). The patient returns to the WDB a third time, with symptoms, VCS and labs done on Thursday (BOC-3), showing us what happened on Wednesday, day 3. If the building is causative, by BOC-3, VCS will fall, symptoms will increase to approximately 95% of initial levels; labs will show distinctive profiles sorted by day of trial. Because the lab changes are stereotyped, according to known physiology, apply a scoring system to quantitate recrudescence of symptoms and recrudescence of objective parameters.

As an aside, this protocol readily shows the absence of validity for alternative hypotheses regarding causation, such as the presence of mycotoxins in urine reflecting fungal infection, for example. SAIIE certainly answers an employer's or school's question, "How do you know you are getting sick here?" The SAIIE is an antidote to the willful ignorance of employers responsible for WDBs.

10.5 PERSPECTIVE ON THE TREATMENT OF WDB

The treatment protocol begins with the one step that has been called *hardest of all*: removal from exposure. Removal from exposure can mean moving away from a school, workplace or residence. It can also mean removing particulates from the air and eliminating inflammagen reservoirs. Remediation of a building can be expensive. Alternatively, correction of particulate reservoirs can be agonizingly obsessive, especially with incomplete remediation. The advantage of clearing the air and reservoirs of particulates is that we are not talking about burning a house down or leaving all possessions, walking out with the clothes on one's back. One needs to correct the source of inhalation of particulates and eliminate all potential sources of contamination. However, it may be necessary to abandon the home and virtually all possessions under certain conditions. This decision can depend upon the home's value, remediation cost, genetic susceptibility, expression of biomarkers and severity of continued symptoms.

Here are a few remediation concepts. Follow the ABCs: *A*bate the water intrusion. *B*uilding materials that are contaminated must be removed (or be encapsulated if structurally irreplaceable). One must *C*lean reservoirs of contamination from possessions, air, walls, floors and ceilings. Every room must be cleaned in a given building if air from one room could get into another. Even though many individuals will not be affected by CIRS, cleaning must be performed, assuming that all who enter the rooms in the future are CIRS patients. Finally, if a remediator does not use HERTSMI-2, one cannot presume the building is safe for a CIRS patient to re-occupy.

By taking another look at the section on WDB definition, we can look at our checklist of what is present and not present. In other words, it is a checklist of safe and unsafe features of a house. We know that there is no such thing as a safe basement, even though people do all they can to make such structures safe. A dedicated air purifier should run continuously in the basement. We look for maintenance of ambient humidity to be less than 55%. Sometimes, that will require using a dehumidifier with a pump to push the water outside.

To prevent exposure, one can use the "three machines" approach. This approach will employ an air sanitizer as the "heavy lifter." The author has no conflicts of interest to disclose in this regard but does use Air Oasis devices as an air sanitizer of choice. A paper from 2019 showed iAdaptAir corrected transcriptomic abnormalities in a CIRS case without causing adverse changes in a control patient.

The second machine is a HEPA filter. HEPA means high-efficiency particulate air. It involves passing air in an indoor environment through a filter that is 0.3 microns in diameter. Use HEPA filters on each floor of a building. The crawl space or the basement should have a HEPA unit that does not move to the main house. Moving the HEPA units about every 12 hours helps deal with the boundary layer problem. Finally, with an Air Oasis sanitizer, particulates in the air become heavy enough to fall to the floor. We must have a mechanism to vacuum these particulates up and remove them from the indoor space. So, the three machines are an air sanitizer, a HEPA filter and a HEPA vacuum cleaner.

10.6 TRANSCRIPTOMICS

In the annals of medical history, some advances have changed both the art and the science of the practice of medicine. Here are a few we learned about in high school. Edward Jenner worked to prevent smallpox by inoculation with cowpox. Sterilization from Joseph Lister also comes to mind. There was Louis Pasteur and the germ theory. Robert Koch with his proof of microbiologic causation, not to mention Semmelweis with his insights into the prevention of childbed fever and maternal/fetal loss, was a revered pioneer. Technical advances included radiation for X-ray machines, with computed tomography (CT) and MRI scans in succession. Indeed, automated blood chemistries, not to mention advances in the development of antibiotics, beginning with penicillin and sulfa and extending to the modern armamentarium of effective oral and parenteral bacteria-killers, were significant achievements. The new T-cell cancer therapies may soon be next.

However, even these revolutionary advances pale compared with work done in the early 2000s in the Human Genome Project. While Watson and Crick get credit for discovering DNA, it was the ability to identify individual genes that has heralded the advances we now see. Who knew that there would only be 50,000 genes: 20,000 protein-coding and 30,000 non-protein-coding? There is much complexity in protein interaction and the diversity of diseases, which have roots in genes and gene activity. Objectively, 50,000 seems like a small number.

The initial $3–5 billion spent to sequence the human genome seemed like an overwhelming hurdle that practitioners would have to clear before manipulation of gene activity came to primary care. In just 10 years, however, automated sequencing devices brought next-generation sequencing and RNA Seq into practice, resulting in the entire human genome sequencing presently costing $5000, not $5 billion. What an achievement!

10.7   FOR THE FUTURE

There is no limit to the questions raised by the transcriptomic findings accumulated to date. Sometimes, the more essential features of a new paradigm are not simply what is true but what was incorrect about older ideas. As we return to Aldous Huxley telling us "the key to understanding is casting out false knowledge," it appears we are "casting out" every day. Let us not forget that only a few ideas in the sciences survive the passage of time.

Simple acts of "casting out" in the domain of transcriptomics let us see that viral reactivation is not likely to be a root cause of chronic fatigue syndrome, despite antibody testing that appears significant. Another is the diagnosis of "mycotoxin illness," already exposed earlier as flawed. With the ability to define the expected differential gene activation associated with mycotoxin exposure from the literature, we can determine what is likely associated with pathologic changes after mycotoxin exposure and what is not. Remember that in CIRS-WDB, we see suspected endotoxin effects in over 50% of cases, closely followed by suspected incidence due to actinobacteria. Mycotoxin findings are a distant third.

We must also consider the role of several compensatory metabolic mechanisms due to hypometabolism. If mitochondrial injury from a ribotoxin attack on mitochondrial ribosomes (mitoribosomes) is present, the cell will not shuttle its usual amount of the fuel source pyruvate, created by glycolysis, into mitochondria. Excess pyruvate not taken into the mitochondria would otherwise convert to lactic acid, an intracellular poison. How does the cell avoid dying from lactic acid? It reduces glycolysis. Curiously, in the presence of interferon-gamma, one of the enzymes that do the work in glycolysis (GAPDH) also interacts with ribosomal protein L13a and a transfer RNA (EPRS) to form a protein complex called GAIT. The GAIT complex will bind to a specific set of messenger RNA in the cell to curb inflammation.

We are building a database to show what role the insulin receptor has in hypometabolism. We have exciting findings on insulin receptor substrate-2(IRS-2). The data show great promise.

The sustained finding of genes that contribute to defective apoptosis also holds great promise. We see one particular gene repeatedly in patients with abnormalities in the caspase-driven mechanism of programmed cell death. If the dying cell, programmed to be lysed by natural killer cells and cytotoxic T cells, fails to safely "package" intracellular materials that are intensely inflammogenic before lysis, damage will occur. If cellular contents, especially DNA, are released freely into circulation, we will have an endogenous source of inflammatory response. As Pogo told us, "We have met the enemy, and he is us."

Upcoming investigations are focused on the correlation of abnormal NeuroQuant findings with early dementia. We hope to bridge the gap between unknown gene activity in brain tissue and known activity in blood cells by looking at tau in spinal fluid and simultaneous transcriptomics. We cannot use brain tissue for gene expression studies. However, we may have a biomarker in blood to correlate with NeuroQuant abnormalities and cognitive decline, as one of the genes on our GENIE was overexpressed in CIRS patients and found in beta-amyloid plaques. The commonly found differential activation of coagulation genes responsive to vasoactive intestinal peptide (VIP) provides another reachable window for intervention.

10.8   SUMMARY

The story of CIRS could fit into Thomas Kuhn's *Structure of a Scientific Revolution*. What began as an *anomaly*, an isolated observation of fish kills and human illness from exposure to *Pfiesteria*, a dinoflagellate, has expanded over the past 23 years to an integrated *paradigm* of an entirely new illness concept that for the first time provides a supported, evidence-based explanation for countless chronic fatiguing illnesses. There may be no "modern illness" paradigm with more supporting biomarkers than CIRS: Beginning with exposure assessments, especially the use of HERTSMI-2 for CIRS-WDB, cluster analysis of symptoms, and labs ranging to proteomics and transcriptomics.

Including volumetric studies of brain injury, stress echocardiogram measurements and VO_2 max, the diagnosis and treatment have support from association studies, prospective re-exposure trials using a published protocol (SAIIE) and randomized clinical trials. Published protocols have corrected proteomics, transcriptomics and grey matter nuclear atrophy.

This density of objective biomarkers confirms diagnosis and treatment, backed by nearly 40 published papers and clinical use by thousands of physicians. As the research on CIRS continues to expand, CIRS may provide the basis to look for new approaches to inflammatory illnesses of our era, especially atherosclerosis, obesity, diabetes and chronic pain.

Hope now rests on hard clinical trials that show us how to help those trapped by WDB, among other causes of CIRS. The answers to the causes of chronic fatigue are apparent. Effective gene-based therapies also are apparent. Now that the magic of transcriptomics and differential gene activation is available, we no longer have to guess about treatment. In data, we will find our answers for today's hope and tomorrow's standard of care.

Unfortunately, patients who return to health will need to establish a life outside of all exposure. The reality is that their homes, work and school must remain pristine for the rest of their lives to maintain health. The social implications are profound but are part of the only known path back to the restoration of health. With the significant evidence for CIRS, public policy must catch up with cutting-edge medical developments. We must ensure that the 24% of the population susceptible to WDB can exercise their right to live, work and go to school in safe buildings.

BIBLIOGRAPHY

Bouquet, J., et al. "Longitudinal Transcriptome Analysis Reveals a Sustained Differential Gene Expression Signature in Patients Treated for Acute Lyme Disease." *MBio*, vol. 7, no. 1, 2016, https://doi.org/10.1128/mbio.00100-16.

Johansson, E., et al. "Streptomycetes in House Dust: Associations with Housing Characteristics and Endotoxin." *Indoor Air*, vol. 21, no. 4, 2011, pp. 300–310, https://doi.org/10.1111/j.1600-0668.2010.00702.x.

Kawamoto, M., and E. Page. "Notes from the Field: Use of Unvalidated Urine Mycotoxin Tests for the Clinical Diagnosis of Illness." *MMWR*, vol. 64, no. 6, 2014, pp. 157–158.

Keller, B. A., et al. "Inability of Myalgic Encephalomyelitis/Chronic Fatigue Syndrome Patients to Reproduce VO2peak Indicates Functional Impairment." *J Trans Med*, vol. 12, no. 1, 2014, p. 104, https://doi.org/10.1186/1479-5876-12-104.

McMahon, S., et al. "Reduction in Forebrain Parenchymal and Cortical Grey Matter Swelling Across Treatment Groups in Patients with Inflammatory Illness Acquired Following Exposure to Water-Damaged Buildings." *J Neurosci Clin Res.*, vol. 1, no. 1, ser. 1-11, 2016, pp. 1–11.

Mcmahon, S. "Pediatrics Norms for Visual Contrast Sensitivity Using an APT VCS Tester." *Med Res Arch*, vol. 5, no. 5, 2017, https://doi.org/10.18103/mra.v5i5.1295.

Park, J.-H. "Mold Exposure and Respiratory Health in Damp Indoor Environments." *Front Biosci*, vol. E3, no. 2, 2011, pp. 757–771, https://doi.org/10.2741/e284.

Pitt, J. I., and A. D. Hocking. "Influence of Solute and Hydrogen Ion Concentration on the Water Relations of Some Xerophilic Fungi." *J Gen Microbiol*, vol. 101, no. 1, 1977, pp. 35–40, https://doi.org/10.1099/00221287-101-1-35.

Richardson, M. "World Health Organization Guidelines for Indoor Air Quality: Dampness and Mould." *WHO Guidelines for Indoor Air Quality*, 2009.

Ryan, J. C., et al. "Transcriptomic Signatures in Whole Blood of Patients Who Acquire a Chronic Inflammatory Response Syndrome (CIRS) Following an Exposure to the Marine Toxin Ciguatoxin." *BMC Med Genom*, vol. 8, no. 1, 2015, https://doi.org/10.1186/s12920-015-0089-x.

Shoemaker, R., et al. "Medically Sound Investigation and Remediation of Water-Damaged Buildings in Cases of CIRS-WDB." Part 1. 10/15. www.survivingmold.com. Accessed 23 July 2017.

Shoemaker, R., Lark, D., Bennert, J. Clinical effects of air purification on transcriptomic profiles from two asymptomatic subjects. *Conference proceedings; Mold Congress,* Fort Lauderdale, Florida, 16 January 2019.

Shoemaker, R. "Sick Building Syndrome in Water Damaged Buildings: Generalization of the Chronic Biotoxin Associated Illness Paradigm to Indoor Toxigenic Fungi. Bioaerosols, Fungi, Bacteria, Mycotoxins and Human Health." *Bioaerosols, Fungi, Bacteria, Mycotoxins and Human Health: Patho-Physiology, Clinical Effects, Exposure Assessment, Prevention and Control in Indoor Environments and Work.* Fungal Research Group Foundation, Inc, 2006, pp. 52–63.

Shoemaker, R. "Research Committee Report on Diagnosis and Treatment of Chronic Inflammatory Response Syndrome Caused by Exposure to the Interior Environment of Water-Damaged Buildings." *Policyholders Am*, 2010.

Shoemaker, R., and J. Ryan. "RNA-Seq on Patients with Chronic Inflammatory Response Syndrome (CIRS) Treated with Vasoactive Intestinal Peptide (VIP) Shows a Shift in Metabolic State and Innate Immune Functions That Coincide with Healing." *Med Res Arch*, vol. 4, no. 7, 2016, https://doi.org/10.18103/mra.v4i7.862.

Shoemaker, R. MARCoNS monsters, antifungals, and grey matter atrophy. *Conference proceedings; Surviving Mold,* Salisbury, MD, 4 May 2018.

Shoemaker, R. C., et al. "Vasoactive Intestinal Polypeptide (VIP) Corrects Chronic Inflammatory Response Syndrome (CIRS) Acquired Following Exposure to Water-Damaged Buildings." *Health*, vol. 5, no. 3, 2013, pp. 396–401, https://doi.org/10.4236/health.2013.53053.

Shoemaker, R. C., et al. "Structural Brain Abnormalities in Patients with Inflammatory Illness Acquired Following Exposure to Water-Damaged Buildings: A Volumetric MRI Study Using NeuroQuant®." *Neurotoxicol Teratol*, vol. 45, 2014, pp. 18–26, https://doi.org/10.1016/j.ntt.2014.06.004.

Shoemaker, R., et al. "Chronic Fatiguing Illnesses: Entering the Era of New Biomarkers and Therapies." *Intern Med Rev*, vol. 3, no. 10, 2017, https://doi.org/10.18103/imr.v3i10.585.

Shoemaker, R. "Intranasal VIP Safely Restores Volume to Multiple Grey Matter Nuclei in Patients with CIRS." *Intern Med Rev*, vol. 3, no. 4, 2017, https://doi.org/10.18103/imr.v3i4.412.

Stammberger, B. "Incidence and Detection of Fungi and Eosinophilic Granulocytes in Chronic Rhinosinusitis." *Laryngorhinootologie*, vol. 82, Accessed 2003, pp. 330–340.

11 Building Science and Human Health

Larry Schwartz and April Vukelic

CONTENTS

11.1 WHAT IS A WATER-DAMAGED BUILDING?

As many as 50% of our public buildings are water damaged.[1] Water damage insurance claims are the second most frequent in the United States for houses and apartments. According to a recent survey by Chubb, internal water damage accounts for 45% of all interior property damage, happening more often than fire or burglary. However, fewer than 20% of homeowners say they have implemented even one preventative measure.[2] Almost 40% of all homeowners said that they had experienced loss from water damage. About 93% of all water damage is preventable.[3]

The July 2019 Townsend Letter, written by Dr. Richie Shoemaker, David Lark, CIEC (Council-Certified Indoor Environmental Consultant), and James Ryan, PhD, describes a water-damaged building and how exposure to it can affect human health. According to the Townsend Letter,

> What makes water-damaged buildings unsafe is the growth of a group of single-cell microbes invariably found in water-damaged buildings that make specific compounds that can cause inflammation (inflammagens), or toxins made by bacteria (endotoxins or exotoxins), fungi (mycotoxins), mycobacteria (mycolactones) and actinobacteria. Add to the rogues' gallery of en-suite bad actors the very cell wall fragments of fungi (beta-glucans and mannans), fungal and bacterial enzymes/proteins (hemolysins, spirocyclic drimanes, and proteinases), not to mention the result of each of these non-living elements acting synergistically, one with another.[4]

DOI: 10.1201/b23304-12

TABLE 11.1
Range of Toxins, Inflammagens, and Microbes Found in WDBs

Mycotoxins	Gram-negative bacteria	Hemolysins
Bioaerosols	Gram-positive bacteria	Proteinases
Cell fragments	Actinobacteria	Chitinases
Cell wall components	Nocardia	Siderophores
Hyphal fragments	Mycobacteria	Microbial VOCs
Conidia	Protozoa	Building material VOCs
Beta-glucans	Chlamydia	Coarse particulates
Mannans	Mycoplasma	Fine particulates
Spirocyclic drimanes	Endotoxins	Ultrafine particulates
Inorganic xenobiotics	Lipopolysaccharides	Nano-sized particulates

Source: https://www.survivingmold.com/docs/CONSENSUS_FINAL_IEP_SM_07_13_16.pdf

Moreover, "when water enters an enclosed space, and that space stays wet for as little as 48 hours, there will be microbial growth."[6] While bacteria might be the first colonizers, fungi are not far behind. Precisely which microbes grow is completely dependent on the availability of moisture. We call this availability of water or water activity (Aw). An Aw of 1.0 (or 100% relative humidity, RH) is open water compared with the water vapor pressure above the water. Bacteria and "wet" fungi like *Chaetomium* and *Stachybotrys* need a minimum Aw of >90% to grow. "Medium-wet" filamentous fungi, like *Aspergillus versicolor*, need an Aw of 0.8–0.9. "Drier" fungal organisms, including *Aspergillus penicillioides*, need a minimum Aw of 0.58–0.8. The dry (xerophilic) fungi, especially *Wallemia sebi*, appear in a range of Aw that can go as low as 0.55–0.75.[4] A xerophile (from Greek *xēros* "dry" and *philos* "loving") is a "xerotolerant" organism that can grow and reproduce in low water availability.

The article states that "perhaps the most important organisms found in WDB are *actinobacteria*. No, not fungi, not mold, not black molds, not toxic black molds, but these filamentous bacteria are only recently becoming recognized in clinical dust samples as major players in adverse human health effects."[4,5] (Table 11.1).

Microscopic forces cause these chemicals and extracellular material to emit ultrafine and nanosize droplets and particles into the air. These droplets and particles then attach to dust, interior structures and personal property, where they dry. They become dry contaminants if they are not alive and are not mold.[6] As these organisms grow, they and the chemicals they produce land on dust and interior surfaces. Afterward, these contaminants are disturbed, become airborne and cause symptoms in chronic inflammatory response syndrome (CIRS) patients.

Dr. Ritchie Shoemaker and David Lark, CIEC studied more than 800 CIRS patients. They found a high correlation between concentration levels of specific mold species, as found in Environmental Relative Moldiness Index (ERMI) laboratory results and Health Effects Roster of Type-Specific Formers of Mycotoxins and Inflammagens – 2nd Version (HERTSMI-2) testing, and patient relapse rates when entering their homes.[7]

11.2   PHYSICAL PROPERTIES OF WATER

Water is Earth's most prevalent compound, and according to the United States Geological Society (USGS), it covers about 71% of the Earth's surface.[8] In the temperature ranges that occur on Earth, water exists in four distinct phases: solid, liquid, gaseous vapor and steam. When water is in the liquid, vapor and steam phases, it needs a force to move it from one place to another. Understanding the ways that cause water to move is necessary to understand how water damage occurs:[9] Water moves from higher to lower pressure. So, a leak in a pressurized pipe will release much more water than a drain line, for example.

Water runs downhill due to gravity, but water wicks upward into porous materials because of capillary action – water wicks up the bottom and sides of building materials. Water will not move downward until droplets are large enough for gravity to overcome intermolecular forces.

Water vapor follows airflow. Dry or damp air may enter the home from outdoors because of air pressure differentials. Water migrates through materials by diffusion and enters them in the form of vapor. Vapor may enter an area without anything feeling damp. The vapor goes from areas of high pressure to lower pressure, wet to dry, and hot to cold. Water converts from liquid to gas (evaporation) and gas to liquid (condensation). Water evaporates faster from solid materials than from porous materials and condenses on cooler surfaces.[10, 11]

11.3   REMEDIATION

Water damage is of primary concern. It may originate from outside or inside the home. Therefore, we need to inspect, evaluate, control and maintain acceptable moisture levels in the home. It is imperative to remedy all current and past water sources and causes of contamination before remediation takes place. Contractors should follow Institute of Inspection Cleaning and Restoration Certification (IICRC) standards, emphasizing removal. Although optimal, complete removal of water-damaged material may not be possible, often due to structural concerns.

Many contractors use biocides to eliminate active growth. Biocides are ineffective because dead or alive, contaminants may cause symptoms in CIRS patients. These fragments may reach the lungs more quickly due to their small size. The best method of microbial cleanup is to use safe surfactants with no fragrances or outgassing chemicals to remove the contamination. Chemicals and fragrances alone may trigger symptoms in a CIRS patient. Compressed air is helpful for rough surfaces like concrete blocks and unfinished wood.

Carpet may be impossible to restore and will act as a reservoir for future contamination. Remove all carpets in containment, so that there is minimal disturbance of dust.

Small-particle remediation is a cornerstone of cleaning and comes from cleanroom technology and methods. High-efficiency particulate air (HEPA) filtration and physical wiping remove small particles. Misting can also be a good tool for *cleaning* small particles. By contrast, fogging to *kill* microorganisms is ineffective. HEPA vacuums are important for initial cleaning. The vacuum may repel some small particles by way of an electrostatic charge. Consequently, damp wiping with detergent and disposable microfiber cloths is helpful. Dispose of the cloth, and do not cross-contaminate the clean water (no "double-dipping"). Wiping with 5–10% ethyl alcohol removes soap film. The last cleaning step is final wiping with a disposable, dry electrostatic cloth. Use painter's tape as a test of how clean the surface is. If the painter's tape sticks, the surface is clean. If it does not stick, there is still residue or dirt.[12]

For those with CIRS, the surfaces of a structure and its contents may need to be cleaned following a special protocol to remove the dried contaminants. Perform this work with proper safe containments and personal protective gear, including HEPA face masks. The workplaces need to have proper air treatments, such as negative air pressure and filtration.

Porous materials will continue to act as a reservoir for illness in the CIRS patient. These materials need to be removed from the home or thrown away. If the patient fails to clean or remove contents from water-damaged buildings, they may not improve clinically. Sorting through and discarding contents is usually a stressful task for the client. Sometimes, it is best for them to put their items in storage until the remediation is complete and they have pursued medical treatment. It will be easier to make decisions and have perspective after treatment for CIRS.

11.4   CONSIDERATIONS REGARDING THE INDOOR ENVIRONMENTAL INVESTIGATION

The indoor environmental investigation starts with a comprehensive interview with the building occupant and a questionnaire or an in-person or video interview. Each interview details the building history and the client's basic medical history.

Obtain answers to questions such as the age of the building, the years the client has lived in it, the presence of mold/water damage in a home inspection, fires or structural damage, and the handling of each event. Ask about the surrounding neighborhood, especially regarding drainage issues and floods. Take a history of when and how the onset of CIRS symptoms began. Are the clients taking medical binders, for how long, and are they effective? Ask where the client feels better or worse inside the home. Do they feel better in other environments or outdoors? Are there issues in the workplace, schools or vehicles? Our investigations may be on-site or virtual. If virtual, assist the client in getting on-site help locally and acquire instruments, if needed, to perform some tasks themselves.

We understand that at least 24% of the population is vulnerable to CIRS, as defined by Dr. Ritchie Shoemaker. The mechanism of this vulnerability is a defect in antigen presentation of the innate immune system, which prevents the body from making antibodies to remove the inflammatory compounds. CIRS will result in a multisystem, multi-symptom illness that does not resolve after removal of exposure. CIRS is not an allergy. Allergies will produce high IgE. In contrast, CIRS patients will have a cascade of abnormal physiology, including cytokine production, complement activation and molecular hypometabolism. If the client has CIRS, they should work with a Shoemaker-certified physician.

Because dose does not determine illness in CIRS patients, remediation is not possible in every building for every patient. Even with the best efforts, a sensitive patient may need to move. Patients may experience detrimental reactions to seemingly negligible amounts of inflammagens. Although not always possible, it is ideal for the patient to live elsewhere during remediation.

Outdoor air may influence indoor air quality. Below ground, air is mixed in the soil. Soil contains microbes from dead and decaying organic materials, rich in actinobacteria, endotoxins and mold species. It also contains xerophilic species, some of which produce virulent mycotoxins. Homes push air outside due to clothes dryers, bathroom fans and kitchen fans. Rising warm air, known as the "stack effect," means the home is always "sucking" in outdoor air. This air may enter the home above and below ground and contain inflammagens.

Educate the client on the organisms associated with water-damaged building materials, their metabolism and the production of mycotoxins during metabolism, and how they distribute in the air, on structures and personal property. Biological vectors need water to grow and dissolve a food source.[13]

Safestart offers a risk assessment analysis called the Mold Propensity Index (MPI) based on visual observations of multiple home and exterior areas. Safestart performs a risk calculation by applying experience-generated algorithms in functional areas plus the total building risk of occurring water and mold. The MPI may help pinpoint possible correction areas to help reverse the risk and determine whether the expense to fix is reasonable. A proper investigation includes considering roofing; exterior; interior; exterior drainage; foundation; plumbing, heating, ventilation and air conditioning (HVAC); and topography.[6]

In many cases, the indoor environmental professional (IEP) consults with the client regarding whether they should move or remediate. The client may need to find appropriate contractors to perform the work and treatments. The indoor air professional may assist in analyzing data leading to important decisions, review proposals and offer opinions on proposed work, and oversee the work. Genetics, biomarkers, transcriptomics, symptoms and finances contribute to deciding whether the client should stay or move. The client should factor their physician's medical opinion into the decision.

Client finances often dictate the limitations of our plan. A step-wise and sequenced approach may be necessary to gauge the plan's effectiveness. An IEP oversees post-treatment testing. Many clients postpone this until they see how they feel in the environment after the cleaning.

11.5   THE WATER-DAMAGE BUILDING INVESTIGATION

11.5.1   Roofing

Water runs off the roof more slowly with a low pitch as opposed to a high pitch. Steep roofs should have gutters and downspouts to catch and carry away water. Additional common issues are leaky "boots" under shingles around plumbing stacks, leaks around nails into the sheathing, and leaky flashing around chimney chases. Roof penetrations tend to leak after 10 years.

11.5.1.1   Flat Roofs

The lifetimes of flat roofs are shorter than those of steep roofs, as they do not dry as quickly. Built-up tar and paper, modified bitumen, ethylene propylene diene monomer (EPDM) rolled membrane, asphalt rolls and metal are flat roof materials. Each has potential problems, such as cracks and openings and how the material terminates at the perimeter, like termination bars on parapet walls. Take into consideration unsealed masonry parapet walls, coping application, missing grout between coping sections, or missing flashing. Flaws in any of these will allow water to penetrate the building. Leaking may occur when the surface pitch of drains is incorrect, drains are missing guards and debris builds up, or when the client neglects maintenance. The size and materials of the drainpipes and their installation may also cause a problem.

11.5.1.2   Steep Roofs

Shingles are composed of many different materials, such as asphalt, cedar and other wood, metal, ceramic and rolled materials. Each has a different lifetime. Wood shingles expand horizontally as much as 10% of their size when wet and may harbor fungi and moss. Shingles may not have an air gap underneath to help them dry, leading to a shorter life.

Modern roofing styles on larger homes depart from the inverted "V," using intersecting junctions of rooflines that create steep valleys. Water collects in these valleys and speeds down to a gutter or scupper. If the gutter design system is incorrect, the water overwhelms the system and runs over the top to the ground alongside building foundations. More valleys create more potential water damage.

Water may also collect behind chimney chases and penetrate spaces between flashing if there is no "cricket," a sloped drainage surface behind the chase. There may also be openings around penetrations through the roof, such as plumbing stacks, roof vent, and junctions where a roof meets a vertical wall (Figure 11.1, Figure 11.2, Figure 11.3, Figure 11.4 and Figure 11.5).

11.5.2   Attic Ventilation

This ventilation design allows air exchange in the attic with outdoor air. When air blows over the roofline, it pulls air out of the attic space from the higher upper vents. With a steep roof, the air removal comes from lower vents. This method often does not work well because the vent space

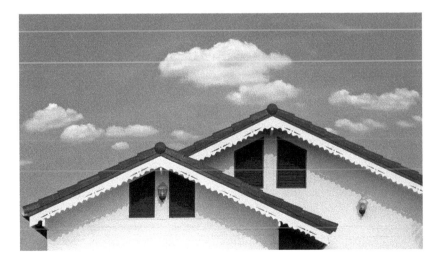

FIGURE 11.1   Medium-pitch roof.

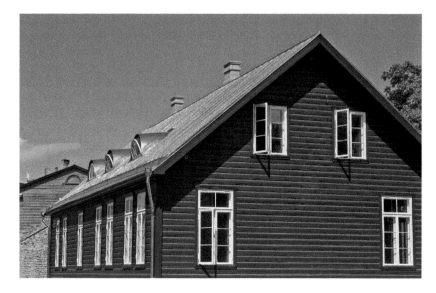

FIGURE 11.2 Steep roof.

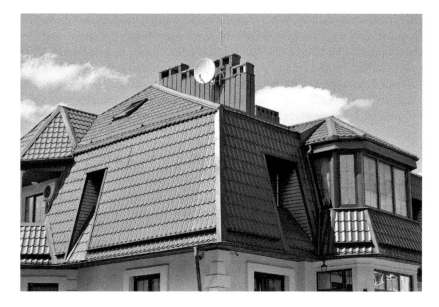

FIGURE 11.3 Mansard roof.

areas, as well as their ratios of higher and lower vents, were not designed properly or because of an improper ridge vent installation, and most commonly, insulation on the floor or the attic may cover the lower soffit vents in the eave areas.

Warmer house air is drawn up into the attic if this ventilation is not operating properly. Warm attic air is a problem in winter because winter air holds more moisture in it, and that moisture will then condense as water on wood surfaces. In late winter or spring, that condensation will allow mold growth.

With flat roofs, it is more complicated, as airflow in the tight attic space is reduced by height and insulation. Proper ventilation in these spaces is challenging (Figure 11.6, Figure 11.7, Figure 11.8, Figure 11.9 and Figure 11.10).

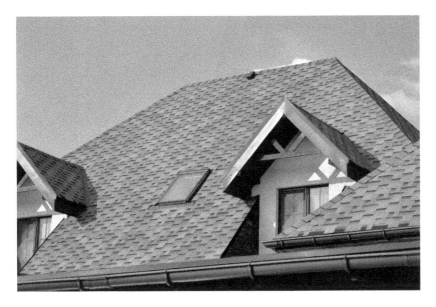

FIGURE 11.4   Hip roof.

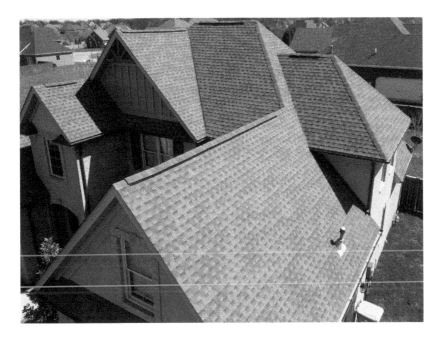

FIGURE 11.5   Roof valleys, which may overload gutters.

11.5.3   EXTERIOR DRAINAGE

Exterior drainage aims to move water from rain or other sources away from the building to prevent it from going down the foundation walls, where it may find ways to intrude into the building. The concerns that will create high-risk water intrusion include improper design, sizing, pitch and installation of gutters and downspouts, the condition of gutters and their connecting junctions, the extension of downspouts, the pitch of soils at the foundation, cracks in the foundation, as well as types of soils under and around the home (Figures 11.11–11.14).

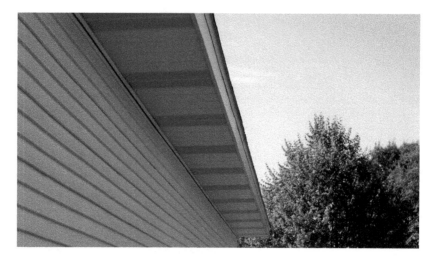

FIGURE 11.6 Soffit vents,

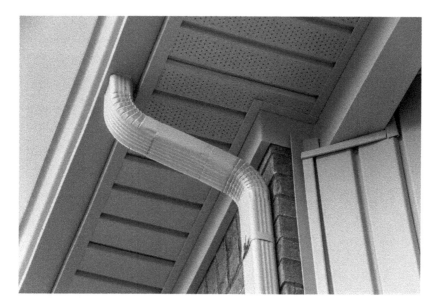

FIGURE 11.7 Soffit vents,

11.5.4 INTERIOR DRAINAGE

Depending on the home's age, there may or may not be a below-ground water drainage system around the perimeter of the foundation, which leads water into a basement pit containing a sump pump that pumps the water back outdoors, away from the foundation. Some basements may have an interior drainage system installed under the perimeter floor of the basement. Older homes often have a drain in the basement floor that goes into the sewer system. These may back up and cause flooding in the basement. Newer homes with basements may have overhead sewers to prevent this from happening. Newer homes might also have an ejector pit in the floor that pumps out the water collected from washing machines and category one or two water collections.[3]

There may be leakage at the junction of the floor and exterior walls or water from the high-water table under the basement floor, wicking through the floor onto its surface. Water can also come

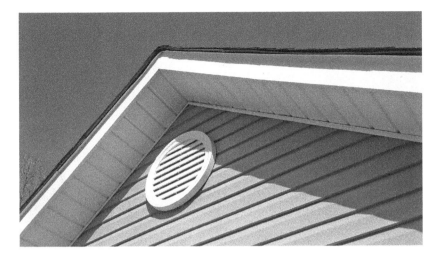

FIGURE 11.8 Gable vent.

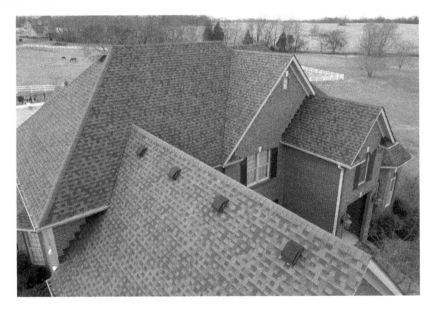

FIGURE 11.9 Mushroom vents.

through cracks in the foundation and from the base of window wells, and over the wall of the foundation (Figure 11.15)

11.5.5 CRAWL SPACES

High levels of water vapor and liquid water may come from the soil floor of the crawl space, even if covered with crushed stone or plastic sheeting. Because of high moisture levels in a crawl space, it is not unusual for condensation or mold to appear on the underside of the subfloor ceiling and supporting joists.

11.5.6 EXTERIOR

The exterior's primary source of water intrusion is around window junctions, doors and other penetrations in the exterior cladding. Commonly, this happens because windows are installed

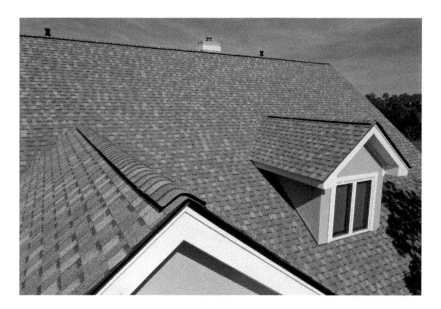

FIGURE 11.10   Ridge vents.

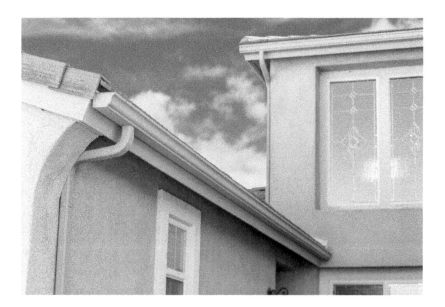

FIGURE 11.11   Extended gutter.

with an improper pitch and flashing. Hidden water coming into the building envelope may enter the space between the exterior and interior walls. Many surfaces will allow and create microbial growth.

Various cladding surfaces will allow moisture to diffuse through the materials into the building envelope and around material junctions. Without properly treated sheathing materials behind the cladding, they will permit moisture to wick through and support microbial growth. Some safer products include mold-proof drywall, mold-proof insulations, wood sheathing products with minimal formaldehyde outgassing, and products without volatile organic compounds (VOCs).

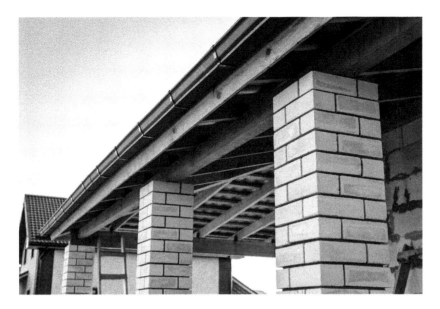

FIGURE 11.12   Extended gutter.

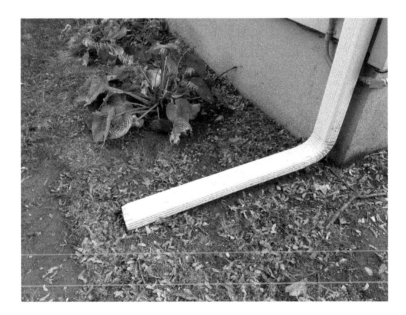

FIGURE 11.13   Long downspout to move water away from house.

11.5.7   PLUMBING

There are many potential water leak sources in plumbing. Plumbing includes both the supply-side and drainage. Much of the older plumbing in the United States is cast iron and in some cases, lead. Newer plumbing may include plastic supply lines and PVC drains. PVC drains may develop cracks and leaks around junctions with improper sealing.

Frozen and cracked spigots and broken pipes may all lead to water intrusion. It is not unusual for a cracked drainpipe to leak over a long time between the floor above and the ceiling below, allowing mold to grow in that space, which may not be easily detectable. Toilet wax ring seals shrink and crack, causing category one and two water to leak into the surrounding subfloor.

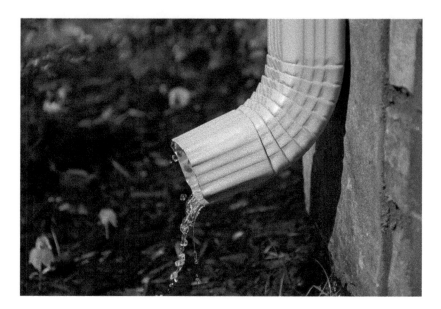

FIGURE 11.14   Short downspout too close to house.

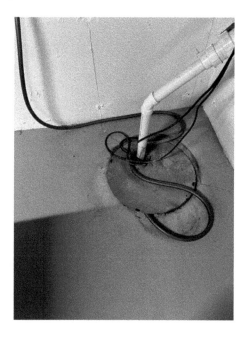

FIGURE 11.15   Sump pump pit.

Metal washers used in plumbing wear over time and create leaks. Water damage and mold are often seen inside vanities, underneath sinks and at junctions of supply lines behind shower stalls. Surround valves go to refrigerator icemakers, and supply lines go to toilets and sinks. Both of these can leak.

11.5.8   HEATING, VENTILATION AND AIR CONDITIONING (HVAC)

Humidifiers, air conditioning systems and dehumidifiers create and collect moisture when in operation. These units are attached to the return air plenum. They often leak into both the interior and the exterior of the air handler. Often, condensate drain lines create large amounts of mold on the interior surfaces. Condensate drain lines may empty onto the basement floor instead of into a drain, allowing the water to wick into surfaces and support microbial growth.

Clean the ducts with negative pressure control and minimal air velocity to create laminar flow. Replace flexible ductwork and internally lined ductwork. Avoid antimicrobial sprays for the same reasons we avoid biocides. Best practices avoid sealants and encapsulants, which may cause symptoms in sensitive patients.

Our bodies give off moisture. In fairly low ventilated buildings like homes, this adds to higher moisture levels. There is also a good deal of moisture generated in the air from cooking, bathing and showering. Most bathroom fans and vents above stoves and cooktops do not have the power to move heavy moisture outdoors (Figure 11.16, Figure 11.17, Figure 11.18).

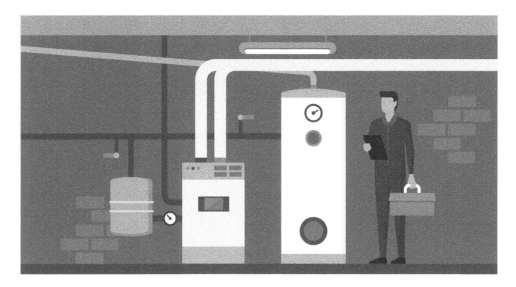

FIGURE 11.16 HVAC intake and exhaust.

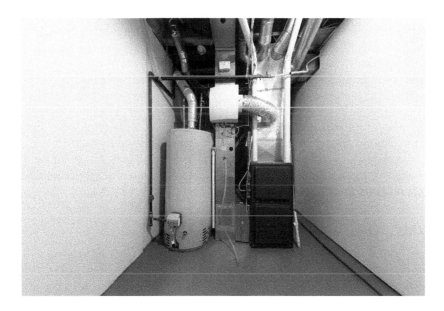

FIGURE 11.17 HVAC intake and exhaust.

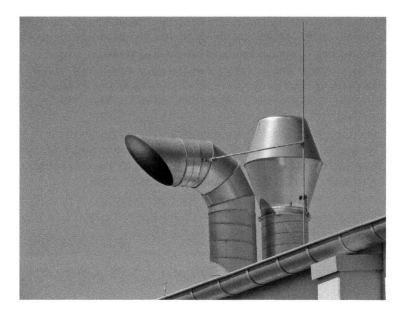

FIGURE 11.18   Exhaust points away from intake.

11.5.9   TOPOGRAPHY

Suppose the home is near the bottom of a hill or slope on one or more sides, close to a pond, lake or river. There is a higher risk of moisture levels in the soils, which will have a higher likelihood of getting through cracks and openings, and wicking or diffusing through foundations and cladding to get into the home's interior.

11.6   METHODS OF INVESTIGATION

With all the possible ways for water to enter a building, no wonder the World Health Organization says that 50% of all buildings have experienced water damage.[1] As far as buildings that have suffered water intrusion or creation, the author believes the percentage is substantially higher, based on his experiences and knowledge. There are often telltale clues of what is going on inside walls and spaces observed visually using a moisture meter, which will measure moisture levels and possible deformation of materials.

First, a good visual investigation looking for active or dried water stains is paramount. A flashlight held horizontally against a surface will highlight dried water stains on a surface that are otherwise almost invisible to the eye. This response needs to take place on every level of the home that we can access. An infrared imaging device is a great tool for identifying water and moisture. Along with knowledge of building science, this tool will help spot water/moisture in walls, ceilings and building materials with a certain intensity, size and location. One requires training in infrared technology to identify moisture content correctly. A meter to measure relative humidity and dew point temperatures is also helpful.

11.7   CORRECTIONS AND SOLUTIONS

One correction method deals with removing built-up contaminants on surfaces of the structure and personal property in the home. Another method deals with air purification, such as HEPA filtration. The last correction method deals with ventilation, defined as air changes between the outdoors and the interior. Install ventilation corrections to create positive air pressure. The corrections may range from reasonable to prohibitively expensive.

After performing an investigation and inspection as described earlier, an environmental professional must create a plan that eliminates the causes of the problems and states how to remove affected materials and contaminants safely. These protocols must also detail the safety measures of everyone involved.

The IEP also needs to outline a method of post-remediation verification and testing. When CIRS patients are involved, the IEP should minimize the use of chemicals. The IEP needs to discuss possible options with the client to meet their needs and achieve the best possible outcome. Furthermore, the environmental professional will offer guidance on monitoring and controlling moisture levels of water damage in the building or home and other methods to maintain safe indoor air quality for the future.

Potential Conflict of Interest: Larry Schwartz owns Safestart, which performs the Mold Propensity Index.

BIBLIOGRAPHY

1. Spengler, John, Lucas Neas, Satoshi Nakai, Douglas Dockery, Frank Speizer, James Ware, and Mark Raizenne. "Respiratory Symptoms and Housing Characteristics." *Indoor Air* 4, no. 2 (1994): 72–82. https://doi.org/10.1111/j.1600-0668.1994.t01-2-00002.x.
2. "Water Leaks in Your Home." *Chubb.* Accessed May 16, 2022. http://www.chubb.com/us-en/individuals-families/resources/5-questions-to-help-you-prevent-water-damage-in-your-home.html.
3. "Water Damage Statistics [2022]: Claim Data & Facts." Last Updated: December 9. iPropertyManagement.com, December 10, 2021. https://ipropertymanagement.com/research/water-damage-statistics.
4. "Moldy Buildings, CIRS, Sick People, and Damaged Brains, Part 1: Living in a Water-Damaged Building." *Townsend Letter*, December 11, 2019. https://www.townsendletter.com/article/432-moldy-buildings-cirs-mycotoxins-part-one/.
5. "SM-Aee Actino, Endotoxin, Ermi." *Envirobiomics*, April 22, 2022. https://www.envirobiomics.com/product/sm-aee-actino-endotoxin-ermi/.
6. "System and Method for Assessing Mold Risk Propensity and Dampness Index in Structure - Patent US-2008288224-A1 - Pubchem." National Center for Biotechnology Information. PubChem Compound Database. U.S. National Library of Medicine. Accessed May 16, 2022. https://pubchem.ncbi.nlm.nih.gov/patent/US-2008288224-A1.
7. "Hertsmi-2 and Ermi 5 22 2016 Correlating Human Health Risk with Mold ..." Accessed May 16, 2022. https://www.survivingmold.com/Publications/HERTSMI-2_AND_ERMI_5_22_2016_ _CORRELATING_HUMAN_HEALTH_RISK_WITH_MOLD_SPECIFIC_QPCR_IN_WATER _DAMAGED_BUILDINGS_CLEAN.pdf.
8. "How Much Water Is There on Earth? Completed." How Much Water is There on Earth? | U.S. Geological Survey. Accessed May 16, 2022. https://www.usgs.gov/special-topic/water-science-school/science/how-much-water-there-earth?qt-science_center_objects=0#qt-science_center_objects.
9. "IAQ: Moisture Control Guidance for Building Design, Construction and Maintenance." (2013).
10. Lstiburek, Joseph W., and John Carmody. *Moisture Control Handbook: Principles and Practices for Residential and Small Commercial Buildings.* New York: John Wiley & Sons, 1994.
11. says:, Adi Satria Pangestu, Caden Says: Rose Mendensia says: Bereket Says: Demarcus Cousins III says: Ace says: Mangale Pooja Suresh says, et al. "Biological Roles of Water: Why Is Water Necessary for Life?" *Science in the News*, September 26, 2019. http://sitn.hms.harvard.edu/uncategorized/2019/biological-roles-of-water-why-is-water-necessary-for-life/.
12. "Indoor Environmental Professional Panel of Surviving Mold Consensus ..." Accessed May 20, 2022. https://www.survivingmold.com/Publications/SM__2020_IEP_MICROBIAL_REMEDIATION_ DOCUMENT.pdf.
13. "Water, the Universal Solvent Completed." Water, the Universal Solvent | U.S. Geological Survey. Accessed May 16, 2022. https://www.usgs.gov/special-topic/water-science-school/science/water-universal-solvent?qt-science_center_objects=0#qt-science_center_objects.

12 Legal and Ethical Considerations in Mold, Mycotoxins, CIRS and Building Biology

Scott W. McMahon

CONTENTS

12.1 INTRODUCTION

The United States' legal system is the greatest method of Justice on Earth! That is what parents, schoolteachers and newscasts preached in the formative years. Though it is not obvious how one would substantiate such a dictum, Americans have incredible protections such as "innocent until proven guilty," "right to a speedy trial," "right to a trial by their peers," "right to an attorney even if a person cannot afford one," etc. There are negatives too, however. Prisons are filled with a disproportionate number of Black males, DNA evidence has overturned a sizable number of convictions associated with lengthy terms, and public defenders carry overwhelming caseloads, disallowing adequate preparation time and plea bargaining or losing for most of their usually impoverished clients. The system is not perfect, although millions of men and women dedicate their lives to making this system work. These include judges, lawyers, court reporters, bailiffs, clerks and many others. Of course, there is always the civil duty for the rest of U.S. citizens as potential jurors. This chapter stems from one non-legally trained person's observations and invites the reader into a closer look at the U.S. judicial system as it juxtaposes with indoor mold cases. This author has been retained as a medical expert by both plaintiffs and defenses in mold-based illness cases.

12.2 HISTORY

Starting at the beginning, it is well known that the American system of justice took its roots from England, and England's scheme grew from the Roman Empire. Significant legal advances were manifested through these. Many would be surprised to learn that some of the basics of Roman law, and hence the American code of justice, emanated from the Jewish law, specifically Torah,[1] as well as other Hebrew writings. From this literature come such concepts as "no man is above the law," "the rule of law," "freedom of speech," freedom of religion," "right to a fair trial" and "the punishment should fit the crime."

The Code of Hammurabi was written around 1754 BC,[2] or roughly 3800 years ago. It was a significant advancement, as it was the first written code dealing with both aristocrats and commoners. Torah is thought to have been written by Moses[3] around 1300 BC, though some scholars doubt his existence and his authorship – many date Torah's penning to near 600 BC (during the Jewish exile in Babylon). Torah consists of the history of humans from Divine Creation to the death of Moses (as the Israelites were preparing to inhabit the Land of Canaan) but also includes The Law, which the Israelites were to follow. Starting with the Ten Commandments and covering rules of worship, annual religious festivals, crime and punishment, accidents, cleanliness, dietary rules, and day-to-day relationships between man and wife, parents and children, masters and servants or slaves, locals and foreigners and more, Torah covered nearly every aspect of life.

Tertullian[4] and some Jewish scholars believe The Law was given to Adam and was passed down verbally through Adam's lineage and directly to Noah before finally being written. The Talmud holds that Noah was given seven laws, which included establishing courts of justice.[5] By the Jewish tradition, the Flood of Noah occurred around 2500 BC, or roughly 4500 years ago. Written accounts of a Flood exist as far back as the 19th century BC. If these dates are believed, the oral version of the Hebrew law could pre-date even the Code of Hammurabi.

While many do not believe in the actual existence of Adam, Noah or Moses, nonetheless, the writings exist, remain and speak for themselves. In Jewish law, a man could not be convicted of murder unless there were two or more eye-witnesses.[6] By the agreement of two or three witnesses, a matter regarding any crime was established.[7] In fact, one of the Ten Commandments dealt specifically with witnessing: "You shall not bear false witness against your neighbor."[8] Determining the truth, or what actually occurred, was a central focus in Hebrew judgments.

While The Law of the Jewish people was written, applied to all inhabitants and decided by judges through trials with witnesses, the Roman law took all these to higher levels. Starting with the Law of the Twelve Tables (c. 449 BC), Roman law emerged over a millennium, forming the basis of Eastern European and Western legal systems. Latin is still the language used for most of these concepts.

The Law of the Twelve Tables did not cover every offense possible, but it did create a method for expanding the law as need arose. Civil procedure was developed. The Tables were written down to allow consistency. Subsequent additions allowed differing levels of society to intermarry[9] (Lex Canuleia), access of plebians to the priesthood (Viri Sacris Faciundis)[10] and the beginnings of tort law (Lex Aquilia).[11]

Another significant advancement was the institution of a democratically elected body to make laws – the Senate. Parliaments and Congresses debating circumstances and writing laws around the world are extensions of the original Roman Senate.

The development of professional jurists to interpret and argue the law occurred in Rome. Some jurists authored lengthy books on law. One such 80-volume treatise prepared by Quintus Mucius Scaevola[12] became quite influential. Truth was still a central tenet, but procedure was making inroads. Much of the infrastructure of the American legal system can be found in the developing Roman code.

However, the American system of law was developed directly from the English system of Common Law, at least until the Revolutionary War. One of the greatest contributions of British law is the right to a trial by one's peers – a jury trial. While jury trials had been used by Egyptians, Greeks and Romans earlier, the Magna Carta, written in 1215 AD, cemented this right to all British peoples, effectively making every citizen "equal in the courtroom." Curiously, jury trials today typically, but not always, have 12 jurors, who must agree unanimously to convict a person of a crime. Under some circumstances, fewer than 12 may be sufficient to find in a personal injury trial that the defendant truly has injured the suing party. The number of 12 jurors was initially established by a Welsh king in 725 AD. This number is thought to emanate from the significance of the 12 disciples of Jesus Christ.[13] After one disciple betrayed him and died, another was chosen[14] specifically to maintain the number of inner circle witnesses at 12. That number of disciples likely represented the 12 tribes of Israel manifested by Jacob's 12 sons,[15] harkening back once again to Torah.

After American independence, the legal systems of the two nations (the United States and Britain) evolved and diverged significantly. Difference in governing structure shaped alterations in law. England is a monarchy, with Parliament making the laws for the nation, and limited judicial review exists. There is no constitutional document. The Founding Fathers of the United States, however, wrote the Constitution in 1789 and chose to divide power between states and the Federal Government. The latter is further subdivided into three branches, each with important powers but also with checks and balances to limit abuses. The Supreme Court interprets laws using the Constitution as its guide, though some justices evaluate that treatise literally, while others view it in more modern terms. Congress makes the federal laws. The Presidency signs or vetoes passed legislation. Congress can override a Presidential veto with a supermajority. Congress can amend the Constitution with a supermajority. The president can influence policy by executive orders and appointments.

States can pass their own laws and manage their own affairs independently, to a point. This includes civil and criminal trials. A supermajority of states can also amend the Constitution by calling for a Constitutional Convention. The Supreme Court can overturn any law passed by Congress or by any state. The president nominates both Federal judges and Supreme Court justices. The Senate approves or disapproves these jurists. It is a remarkable scheme envisioned by the Founding Fathers of America.

12.3   TRUTH VERSUS JUSTICE

One way in which today's courts differ from their historical roots is the pursuit of truth versus the pursuit of justice. Both these terms need defining.

One legal definition[16] of truth follows:

> **TRUTH**. The actual state of things. 2. In contracts, the parties are bound to toll the **truth** in their dealings, and a deviation from it will generally avoid the contract; Newl.

Justice is defined[17] legally as:

> **justice**. n. 1) fairness. 2) moral rightness. 3) a scheme or system of **law** in which every person receives his/her/its due from the system, including all rights, both natural and **legal**.

These two concepts are quite different. Truth is the actual state of things, but this can be distorted unintentionally, or intentionally, by witnesses' memories, perspectives, opinions, worldviews and even their personal agendas or biases. Courts have developed methods to attempt to determine whether a witness is offering truthful testimony. However, a credible witness with a wrong agenda can potentially speak distortions of the truth, and even lies, without the judge or jury being aware. This may be especially true with expert witnesses, as their testimony typically falls outside the realm of common knowledge for jurors and even jurists. Once the truth is ascertained, justice may be employed.

Justice, alternatively, is a concept based in fairness. Laws, case laws, legal precedents and appellate verdicts have shaped a system that is designed to be fair for every person in court. Victims have rights. Defendants and alleged criminals have rights. If these rights are maintained, it is presumed the trial was fair to plaintiffs and defendants regardless of the verdict. Procedures are developed to ensure the rights of all. Needless to say, there are limitations to this process, and justice can be subverted by the same things that sabotage truth. The truth might not be ascertained, yet justice may still be served. Justice is a constitutional right guaranteed to Americans. However, when the goal is to preserve each party's rights, seeking justice rather than truth may afford what some would consider an incorrect outcome. An innocent defendant may be found guilty and vice versa. If the proper procedures were followed, and each party given its full share of rights, justice will have been served even though the verdict may not be just from the point of view of truth.

One final consideration; as in every area of life, possessing vast resources allows one to obtain the absolute best legal representation. It would be difficult to argue that such an advantage does not dilute the principle of "every man equal in the courtroom." Racial and gender discrimination may occur. All systems run by humans, and dependent on humans, suffer from the frailties of imperfect and potentially even corrupt humans. Still, warts and all, the pursuit of truth, or justice, or even the American way, is maintained by the men and women who administer the American justice system, and the rights and protections therein, and arguably make it the greatest legal system on earth. While this discussion was not intended to be a comprehensive review of how U.S. jurisprudence was built, the takeaways are that the American legal system evolved from many cultures spanning thousands of years and that the chief aim is no longer the pursuit of truth but the pursuit of justice.

12.4   HISTORY OF MOLD IN THE COURTROOM

The first legal writings about mold are found, coincidentally enough, in the Hebrew Scriptures concerning The Law. Leviticus 13 and Leviticus 14 deal with "tzaraat" or "tzaraath," a Hebrew word with several renderings in English. The King James and New King James versions (NKJV) of the Christian Bible refer to this as a plague of leprosy and leprous plague, respectively. The New International Version renders this word as mold, and the Contemporary English Version calls it mildew. The two chapters refer to tzaraat of the human flesh, in clothing or fabric, and in the walls of a house. Leprosy affects human skin but not cloth or indoor building materials; therefore, these instances do not refer to the disease known as leprosy, or Hansen's disease.

Leviticus 14:33–53 articulate the then "best practices" of mold inspection and remediation of a moldy building. The edicts deal with inspection experts, cross-contamination, the technique of remediation, post-remediation expert evaluation and utter destruction of the home when mold recurs after remediation. Deuteronomy 28 offers a lengthy list of blessings[18] the Israelites would receive if the nation obeyed the Covenant to which they had agreed, followed by curses they would inure for failure to comply. Verse 22 (NKJV) adds among the curses, "The LORD will strike you with consumption, with fever, with inflammation, with severe burning fever, with the sword, with scorching and with mildew, they shall pursue you until you perish."

Not much was heard in courtrooms, or physician exam rooms, about mold and building structures for the next few millennia. Epidemics of ergotism killed thousands between the late 1500s and early 1900s.[19] In the early 20th Century, alimentary toxic aleukia (ATA) claimed the lives of nearly 100,000 Russians. Caused by a mycotoxin (T-2 toxin)[20] made by *Stachybotrys chartarum* and other molds, ATA destroyed the immune system, damaged the gut and caused rashes. It is commonly known that feeding on moldy alfalfa kills horses, though cows can eat the same foodstuffs with impunity. These examples are ingestion-related poisonings with mold and not building related.

Even though mold ingestion was known to cause illnesses, relatively massive quantities were required, and while epidemics did occur, they were not frequent. Several industrial and cultural changes have made inhalation the primary source of illness now. Once agrarian and outdoor peoples, the so-called developed world has moved indoors, averaging 22 hours a day[21] inside. Building materials rapidly shifted from plaster for walls and ceilings to cheaper and easier-to-use drywall[22] (gypsum board, sheetrock) after World War II. Plaster, with its higher pH, was relatively mold resistant, whereas drywall contained two paper layers made of cellulose, which molds devoured. Benomyl (benzimidazole), an anti-fungal, was introduced in 1968 as an agricultural product and then added to interior paints to inhibit mold growth. Significant fungal mutations followed, allowing some indoor molds to prosper.[23] Additionally, the Arab Oil Embargo of 1972–1973 changed American building design, affecting airflow through, and microbial competition in, newly built structures. As energy efficiency became king, the difference between the inside environment and the great outdoors was enlarged. These events set the stage for the inhaled mold epidemic and the accompanying lawsuits.

A few more historical facts are needed to understand where mold litigation is at now. The first related to Big Tobacco and the tobacco industry.

The Tobacco Master Settlement Agreement (MSA) was entered in November 1998, originally between the four largest United States tobacco companies (Philip Morris Inc., R. J. Reynolds, Brown & Williamson and Lorillard – the "original participating manufacturers", referred to as the "Majors") and the attorneys general of 46 states. The states settled their Medicaid lawsuits against the tobacco industry for recovery of their tobacco-related health-care costs.[1, 25] In exchange, the companies agreed to curtail or cease certain tobacco marketing practices, as well as to pay, in perpetuity, various annual payments to the states to compensate them for some of the medical costs of caring for persons with smoking-related illnesses. The money also funds a new anti-smoking advocacy group, called the Truth Initiative, that is responsible for such campaigns as Truth. The settlement also dissolved the tobacco industry groups Tobacco Institute, the Center for Indoor Air Research, and the Council for Tobacco Research. In the MSA, the original participating manufacturers (OPM) agreed to pay a minimum of $206 billion over the first 25 years of the agreement.[24]

Closing these Big Tobacco advocacy groups put some "tobacco experts," or those who would produce research and testify as experts in courts that tobacco was not harmful to humans, out of a job, or at least closed down that revenue stream. Some of these persons now reportedly testify for the defense in mold-based illness cases.

Around the same time, several high-profile mold events hit the news. In 1995, the CDC (Centers for Disease Control and Prevention) reported a number of infants dying from pulmonary hemorrhage related to inhalation of air with detected *Stachybotrys*.[25] The report was later retracted, though interestingly, pulmonary hemorrhage is seen routinely in rodent toxicity articles when their respiratory tracts are exposed to mold toxins. Erin Brockovich, made famous by the movie of the same name, testified before the California Legislature about the dangers of indoor mold in 2001 and sued in Superior Court over her own moldy house before settling. Melinda Ballard, in Texas in 2002, won $32.1 million initially after her 22-room mansion was found to be water damaged and moldy, shortly after moving in, and her family suffered significant health effects. One year later, Ed McMahon, of The Tonight Show, settled for $7.2 million after his mansion suffered water damage.[26] Other, less famous, multi-million-dollar cases were also settled.

Whether coordinated or acting independently, several industries with financial ties to this issue reacted. Insurance companies, with arguably the most to lose financially, added riders to their home and commercial policies excluding or limiting coverage to losses that were mold related. This occurred in most states to the point that several state legislatures have proposed or enacted law restricting insurance companies from including these limitations. Mold inspection and mold remediation companies proliferated. Some states required licensing of these environmental professionals. Educational companies developed to assist in training these same professionals. The construction industry created literature to inform contractors of the dangers of mold. Indoor hygienists and air quality specialists looked for guidelines for testing, remediation, post-remediation testing and safety suggestions. Researchers spent more time studying the effects of chronically inhaled mold on animals and humans. Hundreds of research articles demonstrated respiratory and other adverse human health effects from chronic inhalation of indoor mold, while two prominent medical societies published position statements only accepting respiratory problems. As detailed later, some suggested that the authors of these statements had conflicts of interest, as the majority testify as defense expert witnesses. The negative effect of these two statements on successful mold litigation cannot be overemphasized.

Some government and industry standards for determining when mold was excessive were created; others are still awaited. Standards exist to this day in many countries and used to exist in the United States; however, it appears that after litigation[27] over these standards, American institutions became reticent to publish such. Further, these standards usually require culturable mold testing techniques, whereas most American testing professionals use non-viable testing methods. The efforts of all these events have brought us to our current place.

12.5   MOLD IN THE COURTROOM TODAY

Every state and municipality passes its own laws, and each court jurisdiction is different. Attorneys are also unique, each bringing diverse experiences and strategies. Each case offers its own nuances. Some lawyers desire a comprehensive explanation of what is happening to their client in an expert witness report. Others, where their jurisdiction allows, prefer "trial by ambush," where as little as possible is disclosed before the actual trial. While there are a few "landmark" cases, such as *Federico v. Lincoln Military Housing, LLCs*, it is likely more instructional for medical and other lay readers to look at the court process as a whole than to look at individual cases. It is important to remember that whichever side legal people work for, they are just doing their job, trying to present the best case they can. Justice requires this.

The distinction between the pursuit of truth and the pursuit of justice becomes relevant. In a system where the determination of truth is of paramount importance, both plaintiffs and defense would ideally work toward the same goal, determining what actually happened. Once accomplished, then the chips would fall where they might, and appropriate damages would be assessed, or not. However, the American system of law is based on meting out justice. A primary principle is that the defense attorney is required to provide the best possible defense he or she can, regardless of their client's guilt or lack thereof. Indeed, the defense attorney is not even allowed to take guilt into consideration. As such, instead of attempting to expose the truth, which could be damaging for a defendant, said attorney is required to do everything legally and ethically in their power to have their client exonerated. It is particularly important to understand that this fact does not change no matter how guilty the client is. The defendant's barrister MUST provide as effective a defense as possible. If that attorney does not do so, they face the potential of disbarment and loss of personal livelihood.

This creates a potential for an inequity, from the point of view of truth, in mold cases. While procedures and codified law are intended to preserve the rights of all parties, the side with the greatest resources frequently prevails regardless of perceived fault. The plaintiff in a mold case frequently has lost their health, their job, their life savings, their home and often, their family. They pursue a personal injury case against an alleged perpetrator, typically a landlord, contractor or employer, or some combination of all, whom the plaintiff perceives to have caused, or allowed to continue, a moldy environment in their home or at work. The plaintiff and their doctor also have surmised that exposure to this water-damaged built environment has caused a loss of the plaintiff's personal health, and typically all the other losses. Sometimes, their children have become ill too. This is the plaintiff's last chance to regain any sense of wholeness.

Plaintiffs *always* feel they have been unjustly treated, and they are often quite emotional about the issues. They know winning money cannot replace their health deficits, but what else can they win back? Commonly, they feel they are "doing the right thing," as they believe that if the person, or company, they are suing loses badly enough, it will send a message to others in the field. In this manner, they believe they are helping others to avoid their own health fate. They frequently have few financial resources to fight this fight, as they have already "lost everything."

Contrast this scenario with typical defendants. Landlords are often owners of multiple apartment complexes and/or rental houses. Contractors usually have thriving businesses. Employers are typically doing well financially. They may be very ethical persons, or they may engage in numerous uninformed or even shady business and real estate maintenance practices. They almost always have insurance companies backing them, who are potentially on the hook for millions, or tens of millions, of dollars. This is almost assured, as plaintiffs' attorneys will rarely take a case if there is not someone with "deep pockets" involved. After all, what is the point of winning such a case if there is no one who can pay the damages?

Insurance companies are commonly multi-billion-dollar corporations that have the resources to hire teams of savvy lawyers and as many credible and experienced experts as are needed to win. They have a lot to lose if the verdict goes against the defendants they insure. The plaintiffs usually have barely enough in financial resources to get a case going, even on a contingency basis. This is another potential inequity and how it plays out. It is David versus Goliath, be it disability, Workman's Compensation or personal injury, in almost every case making it to court. Rest assured; Goliath is out to win by any (legal) means possible.

Personal injury lawsuits are not for the faint of heart, nor for those with tight resources. This is stated for those who are contemplating taking a legal action against another person or company. One may think one is in the right. One may very well be in the right. Proving that to a judge's or jury's satisfaction is a whole other story. Just getting to court can cost $30,000 or more in legal fees, expert witness costs, etc., and that is a contingency case. In mold cases, one cannot win without these elements. Litigation takes an enormous emotional toll on plaintiffs, too. So much of their hope is tied into winning. Cases can go on for 3–4 years. Most settle and never see the courtroom. Therefore, people should think very carefully before they file. The easiest way to lose a case is to have insufficient resources to see it to the end.

In the pursuit of justice and properly ensuring each party's rights, concepts such as truth, and simple terms like right and wrong, as understood by lay people, can be blurred, at least from the perspective of lay people. Lawyers, who are officers of the court, have their own language. Some of these seemingly simplistic terms have quite different and precise legal definitions, which might seem foreign to the Average Joe who never attended law school. Lay people are poorly prepared to understand what occurs in the courtroom and are typically at the mercy of their attorney. Again, the apparent inequity of hiring the best lawyer one can afford, with greatly depleted health and financial resources, versus the team of the region's best barristers is evident.

12.6 MOLD IN THE COURTROOM TODAY: EXPERT WITNESSES

Nowhere in the process is the potential for inequity greater than in the procurement and testimony of medical expert witnesses. By definition, expert witnesses possess knowledge that is unlikely common knowledge for judges or jurors. In the mold realm, this knowledge is highly scientific. While judges are typically quite intelligent and given some training in how to determine scientific matters and opposing views, most jurors are unlikely to have the basics of high-level scientific critical thinking. They are expected to discern the value of competing views when many do not understand the difference between anecdotal data and a randomized control trial with thousands of participants. How would jurors, in the position of deciding such cases, tell the difference between truth and an intentional bald-faced lie if it came from a corrupted expert? Since jurors do not possess the training, they must rely on factors such as likeability, credibility and their own gut feeling to determine the veracity of one expert over the other. The potential for a juror's individual biases could come into play here too.

The plaintiff's expert medical witness is typically also a treating physician for the plaintiff. They often have published in the area of mold medicine and read quite a few journal articles about the same. Usually, they have seen a considerable number of patients with mold-based illness, taught at mold-based illness conferences and developed some form of credential or certification in the mold-based illness field. This latter credential ensures they have been educated to some degree in the arena by those who possess even more knowledge. These experts have expert credentials in the mold-based illness discipline and commonly have testified before.

The defense expert witness routinely falls into one of two categories. The first group are local physicians, who often teach at a local medical school. They do not treat patients with mold-based illnesses. They have never written or spoken about mold-based illness subjects. Their knowledge of the subject appears to extend to a few "naysayer" articles. There are only a few such articles – a 2020 article calculated that the number of studies demonstrating mold-based illness from inhalation outweighed the articles against by 56 to 1 – and a much more in-depth discussion of the medical literature is found in Chapter 9, "Are Water-Damaged Buildings Safe?" It is hard to understand how these persons have developed sufficient expertise in the field to be considered experts.

The second group of defense experts often have long and illustrious resumes, typically having been tenured at prestigious medical schools. Their CVs will contain hundreds of published entries, but curiously, only one or two (<1%) in mold-based medicine. These persons may actually be the authors of the rarified naysayer literature. During their practice years, they did not see, treat or diagnose a sizable number of mold-based illness patients. It is also hard to understand how they can be considered experts based on their lack of experience. They are quite expensive and testify with tremendous authority and considerable frequency around the country. They are Goliaths.

Remembering that trials are about finding justice and balancing rights, the defense attorney is required to provide the best possible defense for their client. That often includes hiring the best defense expert(s) available. A medical expert's job is to assess the plaintiff, and any available medical records, in light of the available medical literature, and offer unbiased opinions about the plaintiff's history, physical exam findings, lab results and responses to therapy. Most experts will offer a differential diagnosis to explain certain symptoms. Typically, they will also offer their views on the medical literature regarding mold-based illnesses and causation of illness.

Plaintiff's experts usually view the medical literature regarding mold-based illness in a positive light. Defense expert witnesses know the naysayer literature and may or may not review the "yaysayer" literature at all. They suggest that such mold-based illnesses do not exist, even though there is a near-consensus in the medical literature to the contrary. Frequently, somatization or conversion disorders, both being psychiatric diagnoses, are suggested as causative of symptoms by defense experts. Reported physical exam findings are ignored or minimized, and these experts have rarely ever examined the plaintiff. Attempts are made to discredit objective laboratory testing. Successful treatment protocols are considered to be placebo effect.

One might ask how defense experts could opine that the medical literature does not support the existence of mold-based illnesses when "yaysayer" studies outnumber non-supporting articles[28] by 56 to 1. Several possibilities exist in solitude or in combination. Namely, 1) some of these experts were the authors of naysayer articles; 2) these experts may not have widely read the yaysayer studies; 3) they may be the equivalent of "flat-earthers" – persons who despite conclusive evidence still choose to believe the opposite of the scientific community; and 4) there may be biases in their approach that may be unintentional, but possibly, intentional. If an intentional bias included the willingness to "sell their opinions," that would be the equivalent of a false witness.

From personal conversations with more than a dozen lawyers regarding both criminal and personal injury cases, it seems there is a well-known but rarely spoken dark truth: Given enough money, one can always find a medical expert to support the defense's position. This author saw this firsthand in a murder trial many years ago. A wheelchair-bound pre-teen died of head injuries and characteristic bleeds in and around the brain, which are taught in medical schools as being caused by trauma. This author was involved because he was the treating physician for the child and received a phone call from the accused on the morning the child died. The defense produced a medical expert, who claimed the brain findings on autopsy could have been caused by pneumonia or even a chicken pox immunization the child received a week earlier. Even though there was no objective evidence that the child had pneumonia, this expert's testimony was smooth, assured, confident … and went against almost all of the published medical literature. But if such a person testified, and seemed credible, would a judge or jury be able to discern their deviation from what almost all physicians considered established truth? If such "experts" do exist, where their "opinions" can be bought and paid for, the following question must be raised: When the standard is to preserve one's rights, rather than discover the truth of the matter, do the financial inequalities between the parties afford additional opportunities to affect the outcome in Goliath's favor?

Interestingly, the yaysayer articles are almost always epidemiological studies demonstrating human data and statistically significant associations between indoor microbial growth or dampness and adverse human health effects. There are hundreds of such reports. These are the articles plaintiff's witnesses usually cite. The few naysayer articles most often have no human or animal data and spend most of their space criticizing the methods of a few peer-reviewed published yaysayer studies, attempting to cast doubt on all supportive articles. In medical lingo, without new data, these are merely "opinion pieces" and do not have much standing in the minds of those who see them as such. They rank low on the pyramid of evidence-based medicine. However, these are the articles most defense witnesses cite.

12.7   MOLD IN THE COURTROOM TODAY: ACOEM 2002

One especially important example of a naysayer article worth reviewing was published by the ACOEM (American College of Occupational and Environmental Medicine) in 2002. The ACOEM is a well-respected medical society whose members often work in occupational health. This 2002 article attempted to demonstrate by a mathematical proof that it was very unlikely, or by extension impossible, to amass sufficient mycotoxin from a single strain of mold inside a water-damaged building (WDB) to cause serious human illness. The authors created a mathematical model, which has never been tested. While scientifically, their conclusions amounted to no more than a hypothesis, the article became the position statement of the ACOEM until 2011, when a second article was published with similar verbiage. The 2011 article was on the ACOEM's website until late 2014 and then abruptly "sunsetted." At the time it was removed, 23 position statements of longer duration were still intact on the ACOEM's site. So, sunsetting was not performed because of age (more likely because the article was not consistent with what the scientific literature articulated). It reappeared in 2016, evidently due to a "beta site" error, and was removed immediately at the request of an Occupational Safety and Health Administration (OSHA)[29] official. The 2011 article cannot be found in the archives of the ACOEM's website, and they have not subsequently published another position statement.

The ACOEM 2002 article was fatally and fundamentally flawed by at least a dozen incorrect assumptions and questionable constants used in the calculations. As such, the mathematical proof had no validity, and its conclusions were equally invalid. The study was criticized publicly by a half dozen mold science leaders, an ACOEM member,[30] the *Wall Street Journal*[31] and a book[32] about "science for sale," titled *Bending Science: How Special Interests Corrupt Public Health Research*.

Even the ACOEM professional college itself came under fire and was portrayed by one scathing article[33] in the medical literature as being an advocate for various industries instead of a non-partial portrayer of scientific truth. Adding to the fire, internal e-mails from ACOEM decision makers, regarding the ACOEM 2002 paper before publication, were released on the internet, discussing the problems seen with the subsequently published paper. A position paper purportedly should summarize all aspects of the available science and offer best practices. The e-mail string suggested the paper deviated from the scientific understanding of many ACOEM members. Objectively, it is difficult to understand why a respected medical body would publish an untested hypothesis as its official position.

One of the main complaints of Dr. Craner's article[30], the *Wall Street Journal* and the book referenced here was the apparent conflicts of interest of the ACOEM 2002 paper's authors. These objectors noted that the authors performed significant legal work for the defense of mold cases, and this was not noted in the position piece. As such, someone reading the ACOEM 2002 report would not be aware that the authors could possess such a bias. Craner suggested the paper read like a mold defense expert witness's report. The LaDou[33] article, criticizing the ACOEM, accused the society itself of conflicts of interest in its dealings with multiple occupational industries. The quickly sunsetted ACOEM 2011 article got around the issue of potential conflicts of interest by not even reporting who the authors were.

Returning to the ACOEM 2002 article itself, as a hypothesis, predictions one could make from the mathematical model were never tested to this author's knowledge by either human or animal trials, and such predictions as one could make are contrary to the near-consensus of mold researchers. However, this article became the lynchpin upon which all subsequent naysayer articles hung their hats. Because this study supposedly "proved" indoor mold could not cause serious human health issues, the ACOEM 2002 report is the declared or undeclared assumption upon which every naysayer article this author has read has based its arguments. This study, or the other studies based upon its conclusions, is cited by every defense witness in the dozens of mold cases with which this author has been involved. Therefore, understanding the errors of the ACOEM 2002 study is necessary and critical.

There are a number of incorrect assumptions in the article. First and foremost, the assumption is that illness from a WDB could only occur from direct toxicity, infection and allergies, and no other mechanism was possible. Since allergies are usually not a serious health threat, and infections typically occur in relatively rare persons with immunodeficiencies, based on this incorrect assumption, if one could prove that sufficient mycotoxins could not be amassed to make humans seriously ill, that would constitute sufficient evidence by itself to demonstrate that humans could not get seriously sick from WDB. Second, the authors used only one species of mold, and its toxins, but there are hundreds of toxigenic mold species. Third, they assumed that acute toxicity *must* be worse than low-level, chronic exposure, even though there may be different mechanisms of action (also based on the first assumption). Fourth and fifth, they used *acute* exposure studies (in rodents) and correlated those with *chronic* exposure (in humans).

Sixth, the authors looked at intratracheal and intranasal injections of toxins in the rodents and correlated those with inhalation in humans. Seventh, they assumed incorrectly that chronic *non-allergic immune responses*, such as innate immune system–triggered inflammation, could not be triggered by mold exposure. Eighth, they assumed that evaluation of a single species of mold (*Stachybotrys chartarum*) correlated with exposure to the presence of multiple species of amplified mold often found in WDB. Ninth, they incorrectly assumed that molds are the only microbes that could be injurious in a WDB. This last point ignored amplified bacteria, their endotoxins and the contribution of *Actinomycetes*. Further, studies have shown synergy between toxins produced by molds with *Actinomycetes*[34,35,36] and *Actinomycetes* with bacterial endotoxins.[37,38] Some of the data contradicting these assumptions and calling constants used into question were available in 2002; some were not known until 4–5 years later. However, 20 years later, some defense expert witnesses still stand by this flawed report.

In performing the calculations, the authors of ACOEM 2002 made other mistakes. They chose a single species of mold and chose a detection method for that species which was well known to under-represent that species and even miss the airborne spores of that species ~85% of the time when they were found in the same room,[39] at the same time, by other detection methods. This under-represented the effect of this single species' toxin by many thousands to millions. They ignored the contribution of fragments,[40,41] which are much more numerous than spores in a given indoor airspace by 320–514 times.

A "half-life" is a measure used to estimate how long the effect of a single dose of a substance would persist in an organism. It literally refers to the amount of time needed for the organism to metabolize and/or excrete one-half of the original concentration. If the half-life for a substance was 1 month, at the end of 1 month, half the original concentration would still remain. At the end of 2 months, one-fourth would still be present in the organism, and one-eighth at 3 months, etc. This calculation assumes only a single dose was given. The authors of ACOEM 2002 used metabolic half-lives of mold toxins in the human body at hours to days, when other evidence now shows other mycotoxins to have half-lives in mouse tissues[42] lasting decades. The latter underestimated the half-life of toxins by 10,000 in just the first half-life and is an exponential error in subsequent half-lives. Complicating calculations, humans in WDB have repeated and chronic dosing.

When combining these errors of constants, they are multiplied by each other (a conservative calculation is $10,000 \times 320 \times 10,000 = 32,000,000,000$ or 32 billion times), easily making the underestimation at least a billion times or more. That is nine or more orders of magnitude! That degree of error alone makes the paper unreliable. Factoring in the assumptions also makes the entire proof invalid, as well as its conclusions. The ACOEM 2002 hypothesis has been shown to be unreliable and, *even more damning*, no successful testing of that hypothesis has ever graced the pages of peer-reviewed publications, to this author's knowledge. The article and its hypothesis should have been publicly rejected, not just quietly sunsetted.

Virtually every naysayer article cited in courts that this author has seen uses the ACOEM 2002 article as its backbone. The ACOEM 2002 paper is the very chassis that these other articles are built upon, making it clear that those naysayer articles are unreliable too. Since the naysayer articles are typically not the result of new human or animal data gleaned from actual studies the authors performed, these reports are merely opinion pieces and poorly valued as evidence-based medicine (because they provide little or no "evidence" or data). What is left for the defense expert to stand upon? Not much.

Since there is little or no reliable published data for the defense expert, and rarely any case-specific data to help, defense attorneys should conceivably lose every case where mold exposure is documented, peer-reviewed published mold-based illnesses such as chronic inflammatory response syndrome (CIRS) are established, and some degree of negligence, such as faulty remediation, construction defects or failure to attempt to abate the mold, is also shown. All the more so considering that the vast majority of scientific publications support indoor mold causing serious human illness, and since there is always data on the side of the plaintiff, such as mold testing in the alleged WDB and blood or other objective tests showing abnormalities from the plaintiff. Here again, the difference between justice and truth, the nuances of the law and the relative lack of scientific concepts within the education of most jurors gives the defense, and astute lawyers, an advantage.

An extension of this is the understanding that an expert can say almost anything, be it truth, opinion or mistruth. Judges act as gatekeepers and determine the credibility of such witnesses. But, a witness's expertise, by definition, typically falls outside of the common knowledge of judges, juries and even the trying attorneys, who often extensively research these fields. Hence, only an opposing expert witness might know the extent of the other expert's "errors."

As an example, a recently published report[27] evaluated all the epidemiologic papers published in an 8-year period. The major finding was that 98.2% of the published human studies were supportive of chronic exposure to inhaled indoor mold leading to single and multisystem illness in humans. However, defense expert witnesses almost always insist that ingestion is the primary cause of toxicity, not inhalation, even though that concept was decided in the literature, in the other direction, by 2008.

Further, several defense experts are on the record in their reports stating that in the medical literature, there is little or no support for the idea that indoor mold from WDB leads to human illness other than mostly nuisance respiratory issues. The 98.2% is data published in a peer-reviewed journal. These defense experts were giving an opinion (or possibly bias) that is contrary to the published data. But, how is a gatekeeping judge, a trying plaintiff's attorney or a deciding juror supposed to know that the defense expert's statement is contrary to the sum of the published literature? These deciders do not know the literature. If the witness sounds credible, appears believable and is likeable, what they say will often be believed. As such, there is little accountability for expert witnesses (potentially from both sides of the case), and data is the only thing that separates truth from opinions based in ignorance (failure to have read the literature) or bias (failure to accept the literature when it is contrary to one's opinions).

12.8   MOLD IN THE COURTROOM TODAY: DEPOSITION AND COURTROOM TACTICS

The system assumes that experts from both sides will offer honest and well-read, well-reasoned testimony that is in accordance with the literature in question. As long as witnesses are honest, and truly expert in the field in question, the lack of apparent accountability is trivial. For instance, it is possible that experts could disagree on the meaning of some findings in the literature. Differing interpretations could be a legitimate source of differing testimonies. It is also possible that one expert is not well-read in the literature of the subject area, and disagreement could occur. However, one would have to question whether the less literate expert was truly an expert. It could also be possible that an expert possesses an undeclared bias and offers testimony that is counter to the subject matter's literature. The judge could disqualify the witness or consider the testimony unreliable; the opposing attorney could impeach the witness; or the jurors could discount the testimony in their own minds. The question remains, however: If the expert witness seems credible while discussing highly technical information, and the bias is hidden, how would any of these persons discern a bias was being presented? The answer is that they likely would not detect the bias and would accept the corrupted testimony as believable. Only data can be used to overcome.

As stated earlier, in mold cases, plaintiffs typically have significant data to support their case, and the defense rarely does. After all, the defendant's attorney is arguing that the mold, if they cede it was present, did not harm the plaintiff. How does one develop data for an event that supposedly did not occur? One possible scenario is that mold testers are sometimes hired by the defense. Testers hired by the plaintiffs often present a differing story than mold testers hired by the defense. Mold testing often requires consent of the defendant, particularly if a landlord is involved. Mold testing can be expensive. The defendant may not give permission for expensive but more comprehensive testing but will allow methods that are less expensive and less sensitive. Defendants may also disallow invasive, destructive means of testing that leave ¼-inch holes in walls or removal of areas of sheetrock. Of course, there are also testing companies that are aware that chronic exposure can cause more health damage than respiratory issues and other companies that are ignorant of this.

Additionally, the defendant in many cases can limit access to certain areas of the structure involved. For example, the attic above, or crawl space below, may be deemed off limits. Testing and visual inspection of these areas is then blocked. In the end, if the defendant owns the property in question, they control the scope of testing any mold tester is allowed to perform, and this can limit the efficacy of detection. Landlords have also been known to remove moldy materials and dispose of them so that contact testing cannot be performed on the most relevant items. In these manners, the defendant can manipulate even objective testing results to their favor.

Further, the defense need not prove its case or even that exposure to mold did not cause the plaintiff's injury. All the defense needs to do is successfully sow seeds of doubt in one or more of the jurors' minds that the data being presented by the plaintiff's witnesses is inaccurate or somehow tainted. There are a number of mechanisms by which this is attempted and frequently accomplished. For instance, the defense's expert will insist that mold may be dangerous by ingestion but not by inhalation. Eating mold is bad; breathing it is not a matter for concern. This line of thinking is straight from the ACOEM 2002 dictum that sufficient inhaled mycotoxin cannot be amassed to make humans seriously ill. Exposure studies nearly always show that when comparing ingestion with inhalation with skin contact, the route of choice for poisoning is inhalation. Inhaled toxins are absorbed directly into the bloodstream from the lungs. Skin contact usually comes in second place, as toxins are more slowly absorbed through the skin layers and then into the blood. Ingestion often comes in a distant third place, as high-pH saliva in the mouth interacts with and detoxifies some toxins, low-pH stomach acids may affect others, digestive enzymes mess with still others, and toxins not detoxified through those mechanisms can be absorbed and sent directly to the liver for first-pass detoxification before the poison in question ever sees the whole body. The GAO 2008 report[43] (United States Government Accountability Office) on indoor mold should have closed this door, as it reported that inhalational exposure is the more concerning.

If that were not enough, a systematic review of every epidemiological article published between 2011 and 2018 referencing indoor microbial growth or dampness and adverse human health effects[27] was published in early 2020. Of the 114 studies reviewed, 98.2% supported the idea of single and multisystem illness as a result of exposure to indoor mold. All 114 studies looked at inhalational mold – not one even bothered to study ingested molds or mycotoxins, likely because the researchers knew inhalation was the problem, not ingestion. The scientific community has spoken. Yet, mold expert defense witnesses still insist that ingestion exposure is the worst route. Again, the defense do not have to prove their point; they merely have to plant seeds so that one or more jurors doubt the published data.

Another technique used to spread doubt is that there is no demonstrated toxin dose–response. Toxicologists use linear dose–response as a pillar of toxin exposure medicine. The more of the toxin, the greater the direct effect on the human. The primary mechanism of injury in inhalational mold exposure is through the immune system, not direct toxicity, however. The defense is speaking oranges, while the plaintiff's expert discusses apples. Discussing oranges, instead of apples, is irrelevant, and may possibly be intended to mislead or confuse the jurors.

The immune system is not a linear system; it functions through a series of cascades that amplify geometrically. A small exposure can yield a huge immune response in a person appropriately primed. Think anaphylaxis after a bee sting or sniffing a peanut odor by one who is allergic. These persons are primed, usually from previous exposure, and their responses are super-exaggerated – geometric – not linear. Another way to understand this is that the dose of bee venom injected is roughly the same every time a person receives a sting. Why does one sting lead to minor swelling in a person and another cause death by anaphylaxis? Was it a linear dose–response? Of course not. It was the primed, geometric, non-linear response of the immune system reacting far more furiously to a similar amount of toxin, leading to anaphylaxis.

However, for the doubters out there, there *is* an increased dose in a WDB. Molds, bacteria and *Actinomycetes* feeding on indoor paper-containing building materials, given exposure to water for just 24–48 hours, explosively reproduce by a factor of thousands. This reproductive mayhem is called amplification and leads to a serious dose acceleration of antigenic material, which can trigger innate immune responses, and toxin production in toxigenic species. Both reproduction and toxin production occur because mold spores are metabolically inactive, requiring both food and water to reverse their intentional inactivity. The food is the paper of the building materials. The water is never supposed to be present, and building systems, such as roofs and water vapor barriers (WVB), are put in place to prevent moisture from reaching the paper-containing building materials. However, nail (or larger) holes in the roof, high inside humidity, poorly installed windows, broken pipes, nail holes piercing pipes, condensation in the heating, ventilation and air conditioning (HVAC) or windows, construction shortcuts like not installing WVB, and numerous other routes of water intrusion can cause water to become available to microbes in buildings. When water is present, the spores become metabolically active, both reproducing and making toxins in less than 48 hours. Do not forget that microbially produced toxins are also considered foreign antigens by the human immune system and trigger the innate immune system to activity. Chronic exposure in the predisposed causes chronic innate immune system activation. That is the pathway to CIRS.

Other techniques used to spread seeds of doubt are bringing up trivial points, criticizing the strength of the journal some articles are published in (or insinuating that the journal in question does not use peer review) and outright obfuscation. One example of the last is a common defense expert witness ploy, citing that some of the laboratory tests used in diagnosing CIRS are not Food and Drug Administration (FDA) approved. That sounds like it is really a big deal. Touché. Yet if one understands how laboratories in medicine really work, one understands this is a trivial, even meaningless, molehill of a point, made out to be a mountain.

The FDA does approve test kits created for sale into physicians' office laboratories. But, the laboratory tests that confirm or disprove CIRS are not performed in physicians' offices. They are performed at national laboratories like Quest, LabCorp and National Jewish. These laboratories are regulated and monitored by CLIA (Clinical Laboratory Improvement Amendments), not the FDA. Laboratories of this scale are allowed to develop their own laboratory tests, which do not need FDA approval unless they are going to sell these as kits to physicians' office laboratories. They do require CLIA oversight, however. CLIA audits every clinical laboratory in the United States at least every 2 years, evaluating their quality assurance and ensuring precision and accuracy for every test.

CLIA is overseen by three agencies – the Centers for Disease Control (CDC), FDA and CMS (the Centers for Medicare and Medicaid). The oversight of the FDA, according to its own website,[44] falls in the areas of categorizing tests based on complexity, reviewing requests for waivers and developing the rules for CLIA complexity. Nowhere in there is the FDA required to approve these national laboratory–developed laboratory tests. Some of these tests have been run for 30+ years and used for diagnostic purposes – like antidiuretic hormone (ADH) being used to diagnose SIADH (syndrome of inappropriate ADH). HLA haplotypes are used to determine whether a patient and a potential donor are appropriate for transplanting an organ.

Defense expert witnesses who have never ordered or used some of the tests diagnostic of CIRS offhandedly state that these objective laboratory tests are not clinically relevant. However, these tests have been run on thousands of CIRS patients and hundreds of controls. These tests faithfully separate healthy controls from ill cases, and these results have been published repeatedly. Normal ranges developed by laboratories are created from statistical analysis of healthy patients. Elevations from normal and depressions from normal are both seen in ~2.5% of healthy persons, by definition. When the published CIRS literature routinely shows that 60%, 70%, 80% or even 90+% of the CIRS cases demonstrate elevations, or depressions, of a particular test, this *defines* clinical significance. However, apparently, this is not sufficient in the minds of some defense experts.

Additionally, almost all of the tests performed for diagnosis of CIRS are paid for by Medicare, and they are all paid for by most Medicaid providers. These fall under CMS. If CMS is OK with the tests, how could lack of FDA approval mean anything? It does not. Bringing up lack of FDA approval is merely a smoke screen attempting to discredit a test that is in full compliance with CLIA in an attempt to discredit the CIRS diagnosis.

In addition, many experts write rebuttals of another physician's expert witness report. A defense expert's rebuttal often will not include any human data but will attack the opposing expert personally, using pejorative adjectives, calling mold-based illness medicine "fringe medicine" and using other insults. Many of these experts will call the founder of CIRS medicine "discredited" and state that his medical license was taken, suspended or surrendered, when no such action ever took place. One unnamed expert has written in his expert witness reports, on three separate occasions that this author has witnessed, that this founding doctor's license was taken in one report, in another that it was suspended, and in the third report, that the license was surrendered. These are easily verifiable facts, and yet this so-called "expert" refused to take the 5 minutes needed to fact-check before impugning another doctor's reputation, inferring that the science the attacked physician had discovered was also bogus. Not only did this defense expert witness do it once, he did it at least three separate times, in three separate cases, and changed his story each time! That is the definition of unreliable! While not all defense expert witnesses sink to these levels, most of the experts used over and over again revert to most or all of these strategies over and over again – and without any accountability.

Another tactic used by attorneys is to try pinning a testifying medical or environmental expert into using a specific word in a certain way when the legal vernacular will have a different definition for that word. The medical expert, unaware of the legal meaning because of lack of legal training, might fall for this. Then, the attorney will attempt to split hairs to impeach the expert or make them look inept. Yet another strategy is the use of a compound question. A portion of the question is true; a portion is not. If the expert answers yes to the whole question, the attorney will presume it is a yes to the untrue section. If the answer is no, the no will be applied to the true section too. Additionally, defense medical experts typically prepare their reports from medical records and never see the plaintiff, never interview the allegedly injured person and never perform a physical exam. A record review is sufficient. But, Heaven forbid if the plaintiff's expert merely reviewed the same record, or even interviewed the plaintiff but did not perform a physical exam. According to the defense, such behavior would be worthy of throwing out that expert's opinions completely.

If this does not seem too much already, large legal firms (and other sites) maintain webpages devoted as a source of go-to information on how to defeat a mold-based illness claim. Included on some of these pages are the very tactics referred to earlier as well as defamatory information on some of the more active treating physicians who are also willing to testify.

While the legal system attempts to ensure justice, medicine is still based on the pursuit of truth and helping one's patients get better. Doctors diagnose and treat by pursuing truth – what actually happened to the patient. Many treating physicians are offended, or intimidated, by the adversarial process of the legal system. Doctors are not used to the truth they espouse being challenged by persons who do not have their training, and particularly by persons employing obfuscatory methods that may serve justice but do not serve truth. Many physicians, after their first taste of the legal system, are unwilling to subject themselves to it again. Who then will stand up for the allegedly injured plaintiff? It is like fighting Goliath and his four brothers. Perhaps that is why David gathered five smooth stones.

A moment to consider mycotoxins is in order. Within the world of providers treating mold-based illnesses, there appear to be two camps. The members of one camp emphasize the toxic effects of mold and elucidate their proof of CIRS or mycotoxin-based illness by measuring urinary mycotoxin levels. They also acknowledge immune system alterations. The other camp considers mold illness as primarily caused by normal innate immune system regulation becoming disrupted; toxin effects are a distant and irrelevant-for-diagnosis secondary issue. They demonstrate illness by showing multiple innate immune system abnormalities and downstream effects like the presence of autoantibodies and multiple hypothalamic–pituitary–end organ axis problems. The two schools of thought are not mutually exclusive; rather, they are like looking at the same coin from different sides. Both groups accept immune problems and toxic effects, just in differing degrees of priority. Treatment strategies may also differ.

However, in the courtroom, these two views play out differently. This is primarily due to the concept of "specific causation." Mold cases are generally tried under the law of toxic torts. Specific causation refers to determining the exact causative entity. Where the innate immune system is concerned, the causative entity is the increased microbial biomass in the WDB. Literature, such as the GAO 2008 report, states it is probably impossible to ferret out a single harmful microbe or chemical from all the chemical stew of potentially harmful microbes and chemicals found in a WDB. That document also discusses potential synergies between multiple species of microbes and their components. As such, there is not a single organism or chemical responsible for illness; rather, the WDB and all the amplified microbes and their products are causative.

However, in assuming direct toxicity of mycotoxins as the primary health detractor, one might be required to demonstrate a particular toxin in the patient and the same toxin in the air of the alleged offending building, as well as amplified growth of a species that is capable of making that mycotoxin in the indoor space alleged to be at fault. Detection of these substances in air and body fluids is relatively new and will no doubt become more sensitive in time. Failure to detect said substances may be a function of these detection limits as opposed to an actual absence of the substance. Additionally, there are fundamental questions raised about the detection of mycotoxins in the urine[45] of patients. Specifically, how does one determine whether an elevated level of mycotoxin in one's urine is not because of eating peanuts, drinking coffee or ingesting other food and beverages known to contain mycotoxins? Certainly, remarkably high levels of multiple urinary mycotoxins are more suspicious of chronic environmental exposure, but urinary possession of a single slightly elevated mycotoxin could be just due to normal metabolism of a mycotoxin-containing foodstuff.

12.9   WHERE IS THE CDC IN ALL OF THIS?

One might wonder, "Where is the CDC in all of this?" Since there is so much published data, why hasn't the government, or some other governmental body, stepped in? Help was on the way, then COVID. In 2019, furor over military housing conditions, and subsequent environmental illness in soldiers and their families, reached the hallowed halls of Congress. The GAO was charged with investigating. Two CIRS-knowledgeable physicians were invited to speak to the GAO. The Navy was completing a document for guidance to Navy physicians regarding mold-based illnesses. One of the references for that guidance document was a naysayer article mentioned in this text. That was brought to the Navy's attention, and within 24 hours, that reference was removed, just prior to final printing. In December 2019, one of those CIRS-knowledgeable physicians was invited to speak, with Bill Hayward (developer of the Hayward Score) and David Bloom (Chief Science Officer of Green Home Solutions), to a combined grouping of the House and Senate Armed Services Committees' aides regarding GI housing. The Congressional staffers knew the problems, had visited base and off-base housing at several sites and were very aware of the abysmal housing conditions and the political hurdles. Issues such as troop readiness, troop health and GI suicide were addressed. The GAO gave its report on military housing to both Houses the next day. Fifteen days later, Congress, in an overwhelmingly bipartisan effort (a major accomplishment nowadays, and especially considering the House was also voting on the impeachment of President Trump concurrently), approved $300 million for 2020 to investigate and begin changing the conditions of GI housing. The Housing Bill of Rights for GIs was established. Things were moving forward, then COVID-19 came, and Washington D.C. shut down for well over a year.

Where is the CDC in all of this? Good question. Guidance documents created by the CDC state that if mold[46] is seen or smelled, commercial testing is usually not necessary. The owner(s) should implement remediation as a next step. Environmental Protection Agency (EPA) guidance information[47] states that the remediators should wear personal protective equipment similar to a Hazmat suit. Apparently, inhaled mold is not safe.

While there is much published epidemiologic information out there, the single best epidemiologic study validating the claims of CIRS (multisystem illness with visual contrast sensitivity, or VCS, deficits as a result of exposure to WDB) comes from the National Institute for Occupational Safety and Health (NIOSH), a branch of the CDC. Published in 2012, this study evaluated the health of the staffs of two high schools. One was severely water damaged as demonstrated by visual inspection, spore trap testing, contact samples and Environmental Relative Moldiness Index (ERMI). The other was minimally water damaged as evidenced by the same. A VCS test and a 22-symptom health survey covering 4 body systems were administered to each participating staff member. Employees working in the WDB had statistically significantly lower VCS testing in all five columns of the test. They also had statistically significantly increased levels of symptoms in 18 of the 22 surveyed symptoms and all 4 body systems tested. This is CIRS. This study was published in 2012; curiously, the CDC has not had any further scientific articles on indoor mold published since then to this author's knowledge. The reader may draw their own conclusions as to the reasons for this silence.

The last time the Institutes of Medicine (IOM) looked at indoor mold was 2004, at the request of the CDC. At that time, the IOM found that some symptoms or illnesses, such as asthma, had clear associations with chronic exposure to indoor mold. Per the IOM, other symptoms and illnesses needed more data to confirm similar links. It has been 18 years since the IOM report was released, and there are hundreds of other studies, since published, showing associations with cognitive deficits, neurological issues, dermatological lesions, gastrointestinal symptoms, chronic fatigue, headaches, chronic myalgias and more. There are rumors that the IOM may be asked to look into indoor mold again. Should that happen, and their report extend the associations to some or all of these multisystem symptoms, the atmosphere in the courtroom would change dramatically.

As stated earlier, the ACOEM no longer have a position statement on mold, having sunsetted theirs in late 2014. The American Academy of Allergy, Asthma and Immunology (AAAAI), another well-respected medical organization, also had a position statement[48] regarding indoor mold published in 2006. This statement cited the ACOEM 2002 paper as authoritative (the untested hypothesis) and went on to suggest that persons with supposed inhaled mold illness likely had psychiatric disease. It was archived in 2011. The archive page[49] states that positions older than 5 years "are not to be considered to reflect current AAAAI standards or policy." As such, this organization no longer carries a mold position. The ACMT (American College of Medical Toxicologists) also published a position statement[50] in 2006 regarding mold. It cited the IOM paper and the ACOEM 2002 and AAAAI 2006 papers. The ACMT paper stated:

> With respect to mycotoxins in indoor air, exposure modeling studies have concluded that even in moldy environments, the maximum inhalation dose of mycotoxins is generally orders of magnitude lower than demonstrated thresholds for adverse health effects.

> The ACMT would also like to emphasize the importance of acknowledging that the diet is the most important source of human exposure to mycotoxins.

The first quote is a direct reference to the ACOEM 2002 paper "proving" there is insufficient mycotoxin amassed in a WDB to cause serious human illness. The preceding discussion showed that the calculations in ACOEM 2002 were off by at least nine orders of magnitude, and the modeling referred to has never been tested. The second quote has also been shown earlier to be incorrect. The ACMT have not sunsetted or reviewed this position statement, and it appears to be the oldest position statement on their site. By report, the CDC funds the ACMT to provide toxicological training materials to medical schools. One last bit of trivia: Most of the authors of the ACOEM 2002, AAAAI 2006 and ACMT 2006 papers were, and still are at the time of this writing, expert mold witnesses who testify primarily for the defense.

12.10 CONCLUSIONS

This chapter was written based on the observations of a non–legally trained medical professional. The legal system in the United States is an amalgamation of numerous doctrines from several legal traditions dating back thousands of years. The earliest of these traditions focused on discerning the truth, the actual events that occurred. While medical practitioners still pursue truth, the American justice system now focuses more on meting out justice – ensuring that the rights of all parties are upheld. Many procedures have been created to aid in this process, and millions of trained and untrained participants are involved, providing unprecedented protections to the parties.

Several large mold litigation cases were decided or settled in the late 1990s and early 2000s. In the pursuit of fairness, experts for plaintiffs and for the defendants state their opinions. The plaintiff's experts typically have considerable data showing the state of the WDB and the state of health of the plaintiff before the exposure, during the exposure and after appropriate treatment of a mold-based illness. Additionally, the plaintiff's expert has the vast majority of the medical literature supporting their opinions. There is little medical literature and typically little case-specific data with which the defense's attorney and medical expert witness may work. Some of these experts resort to criticizing the plaintiff's treating physician's and/or expert's methods; state the patient has some other illness that explains a fraction of the patient's new symptoms; claim that the plaintiff has a psychiatric illness; plant seeds of doubt about the objective testing; and offer in reference only naysayer articles built upon the failed hypothesis of the ACOEM 2002 former position statement and a negative view of other cited literature.

Plaintiff's and defense experts in mold-based cases typically offer diametrically opposed opinions. This is a dilemma putting the decision making in the hands of judges and juries, the latter of which may not have any of the scientific training needed to ferret out the pertinent issues. Because the nature of the law is to provide justice, i.e., ensuring each parties' rights is of paramount importance, the system also allows a relative lack of accountability for medical experts. While this is likely not an issue in the testimony of most experts, the potential for unintentional or even intentional bias in expert testimony does exist. In complex medical cases, the system of law may be insufficiently equipped to discern when this happens, in which case truth may be disbelieved, and the verdict, while just by legal standards, might not reflect the truth of what actually happened.

REFERENCES

1. The Hebrews and the foundation of western law. Constitutional Rights Foundation. Available at: https://www.crf-usa.org/bill-of-rights-in-action/bria-16-4-a-the-hebrews-and-the-foundation-of-western-law
2. Code of Hammurabi. *History.com.* Available at: https://www.history.com/topics/ancient-history/hammurabi
3. Stockton R. Who wrote the Bible? This is what the actual historical evidence says. 2/22/2018. Available at: https://allthatsinteresting.com/who-wrote-the-bible
4. The Law anterior to Moses. Bible Hub. Available at: https://biblehub.com/library/tertullian/an_answer_to_the_jews/chapter_ii_the_law_anterior_to.htm
5. Spitzer J. The Noahide Laws. Seven commandments which, according to Jewish tradition, are incumbent upon all humankind. My Jewish Learning. Available at: https://www.myjewishlearning.com/article/the-noahide-laws/
6. Green JP Sr. *Modern King James Version.* 1962. Numbers 35:30. Retrieved from Myers R.e-Sword Bible software. Version 11.0.6. 2000.
7. Green JP Sr. Modern King James Version. 1962. Deuteronomy 19:15. Retrieved from Myers R. e-Sword Bible software. Version 11.0.6. 2000.
8. Exodus 20:16 (NKJV). Blue Letter Bible. Web. 10 Oct. 2020. Available at: https://www.blueletterbible.org.nkjv/exo/20/16/t_conc_70016.
9. Plebeian. Ancient Rome. Encyclopaedia Britannica. Available at: https://www.britannica.com/topic/plebeian
10. Satterfield S. The "Viri Sacris Faciundis" and the consulship. *The Classical World.* 2014;107(2):217–235.
11. Lex Aquilia law and legal definition. *USLegal.com.* Available at: https://definitions.uslegal.com/l/lex-aquilia/
12. Quintus Mucius Scaevola – Roman law scholar. Encyclopaedia Britannica. Available at: https://www.britannica.com/biography/Quintus-Mucius-Scaevola-Roman-law-scholar
13. The mathematics of jury size. Inside Science. Available at: https://insidescience.org/news/mathematics-jury-size
14. Green JP Sr. Modern King James Version. 1962. Acts 1:18–26. Retrieved from Meyers R. e-Sword Bible software. Version 11.0.6. 2000.
15. Why did Jesus choose 12 Disciples? 10 minute apologetics. Available at: https://www.historicalbiblesociety.org/jesus-choose-12-disciples/
16. The free dictionary by Farlex. Available at: https://legal-dictionary.thefreedictionary.com/Truth#:~:text=TRUTH.,generally%20avoid%20the%20contract%3B%20Newl.
17. Law.com legal dictionary. Available at: https://dictionary.law.com/Default.aspx?selected=1086#:~:text=justice,rights%2C%20both%20natural%20and%20legal.
18. Deuteronomy 28:1–68 (NIV). Blue Letter Bible. Web. 10 Oct. 2020. Available at: https://www.blueletterbible.org.niv/deu/28/22/s_181022.
19. Merhoff CG, Porter JM. Ergot Intoxication: Historical Review and Description of Unusual Clinical Manifestations. *Ann Surg.* 1974 Nov; 180(5): 773–779.
20. Meyer CF. Epidemic panmyelotoxicosis in the Russian grain belt. II. The botany, phytopathology, and toxicology of Russian cereal food. *Mil Surg.* 1953 Oct;113(4):295–315.
21. Klepeis NE, Nelson WC, Ott WR, Robinson JP, Tsang AM, Switzer P. Behar JV, Hera SC, Engelmann WH. The national human activity pattern survey (NHAPS). 1994. Available at: https://indoor.lbl.gov/sites/all/files/lbnl-47713.pdf
22. Rae H. An exciting history of Drywall. *The Atlantic.* 7/29/2016. Available at: https://www.theatlantic.com/technology/archive/2016/07/an-exciting-history-of-drywall/493502/
23. Shoemaker RC. *Surviving Mold: Life in the Era of Dangerous Buildings.* Otter Bay Books. Baltimore, MD. 2010. Pages 253–291.
24. Available at: https://en.wikipedia.org/wiki/Tobacco_Master_Settlement_Agreement
25. Williams A. Spore war. *New York Magazine.* 2/27/2004. Available at: http://nymag.com/nymetro/real-estate/features/realestate2004/n_9985/
26. Guccione J. Ed McMahon settles suit over mold for $7.2 million. *Los Angeles Times.* 5/9/2003. Available at: https://www.latimes.com/archives/la-xpm-2003-may-09-me-mold9-story.html
27. Brandys RC, Brandys GM. *Worldwide Exposure Standards for Mold and Bacteria with Assessment Guidelines for Air, Water, Dust, Ductwork, Carpet, Insulation and Bulk Materials.* 10th Ed. OEHCS, Inc., Publications Division. Hinsdale. 2017. Pages 23–84.

28. Dooley M, McMahon SW. A comprehensive review of mold research literature from 2011–2018. *Intern Med Rev.* 2020;3(1):1–39.

29. Personal communication. Email string between OSHA and ACOEM officials from 4/6/2016, available upon request.

30. Craner J. A critique of the ACOEM statement on mold: undisclosed conflicts of interest in the creation of an "evidence-based" statement. *Int J Occup Environ Health.* 2008 Oct–Dec;14(4):283–98.

31. Armstrong D. Amid suits over mold, experts wear two hats. *Wall Street Journal.* 1/9/2007. Available at: https://www.survivingmold.com/docs/Resources/ACOEM/WSJ_1_9_07.pdf

32. McGarity TO, Wagner WE. *Bending Science: How Special Interests Corrupt Public Health Research.* Harvard University Press. Cambridge, MA. 2008. Pages 191–192.

33. LaDou J, Teitelbaum DT, Egilman DS, Frank AL, Kramer SN, Huff J. American College of Occupational and Environmental Medicine (ACOEM): a professional association in service to industry. *Int J Occup Environ Health.* 2007;13(4):4040–426.

34. Penttinen P, Pelkonen J, Huttunen K, Hirvonen MR. Co-cultivation of Streptomyces with Streptomyces californicus and Stachybotrys chartarum stimulates the production of cytostatic compound(s) with immunotoxic properties. *Toxicol Appl Pharmacol.* 2006;217:342–351.

35. Huttunen K, Pelkonen J, Nielsen KF, Nuutinen U, Jussila J, Hirvonen MR. Synergistic interaction in simultaneous exposure to Streptomyces californicus and Stachybotrys chartarum. *Environ Health Perspect.* 2004;112(4):659–665.

36. Murtoniemi T, Penttinen P, Nevalainen A, Hirvonen MR. Effects of microbial cocultivation on inflammatory and cytotoxic potential of spores. *Inhal Toxicol.* 2005;17(12):681–693.

37. Zughaier SM, Zimmer SM, Datta A, Carlson RW, Stephens DS. Differential induction of the Toll-like receptor 4-MyD88-dependent and independent signaling pathways by endotoxins. *Infect Immun.* 2006;74(5):3077.

38. Medvedev AE, Lentschat A, Wahl LM, Golenbock DT, Vogel SN. Dysregulation of LPS-induced Toll-like receptor 4-MyD88 complex formation and IL-1 receptor associated kinase 1 activation in endotoxin-tolerant cells. *J Immunol.* 2002;169(9):5209–5216.

39. Kuhn RC, Trimble MW, Hofer V, Lee M, Nassof RS. Prevalence and airborne spore levels of Stachybotrys spp. In 200 houses with water-incursions in Houston, Texas. *Can J Microbiol.* 2005;51(1):25–28.

40. Górny RL, Reponen T, Willeke K, Schmechel D, Robine E, Boissier M, Grinshpun SA. Fungal fragments as indoor air biocontaminants. *Appl Environ Microbiol.* 2002 Jul;68(7):3522–31.

41. Cho S-H, Seo S-C, Schemechel D, Grinshpun SA, Reponen T. Aerodynamic characteristics and respiratory deposition of fungal fragments. *Atmos Environ.* 2005;39:5454–5465.

42. Sanchez-Ramos J. *Brain's DNA Repair Response to Neurotoxicants.* Tampa University, Florida. Annual report. 1 Jul 2004–30 Jun 2005. Available at: http://www.dtic.mil/dtic/tr/fulltext/u2/a452374.pdf

43. GAO Report to the Chairman, Committee on Health, Education, Labor and Pensions, U.S. Senate, Indoor Mold. In: 2008.

44. Clinical Laboratory Improvements Amendments (CLIA). U.S. Food and Drug Administration. Available at: https://www.fda.gov/medical-devices/ivd-regulatory-assistance/clinical-laboratory-improvement-amendments-clia

45. Shoemaker RC, Lark D. Urinary mycotoxins: A review of contaminated buildings and food in search of a biomarker separating sick patients from controls. *Intern Med Rev.* 2019;5(6):1–35.

46. How common is mold in buildings? Available at: https://www.cdc.gov/mold/faqs.htm#:~:text=Mold%20growth%20can%20be%20removed,ammonia%20or%20other%20household%20cleaners.

47. Mold course chapter 6: Containment and personal protective equipment (PPE). Available at: https://www.epa.gov/mold/mold-course-chapter-6#:~:text=Use%20minimum%20PPE%20when%20cleaning, available%20in%20most%20hardware%20stores.

48. Bush RK, Portnoy JM, Saxon A, Terr AI, Wood RA. The medical effects of mold exposure. *J Allergy Clin Immunol.* 2006;117:326–333.

49. Archived AAAAI statements and work group reports. Available at: https://www.aaaai.org/practice-resources/statements-and-practice-parameters/archived-aaaai-statements

50. ACMT positions, guidelines and recommendations. Available at: https://www.acmt.net/resources_position.html

13 Dying for Representation
My Own Story: Founding Just Well

Kristina Baehr

CONTENTS

13.1 KRISTINA 2.0

I felt like I had been hit by a truck. I felt drunk in the middle of the day. My hair was falling out. I had insomnia. Hormone surges. Migraines. I woke up drenched in sweat. Extreme fatigue. Dizzy. Couldn't see straight. There was a wet blanket over me. I couldn't wake up in the morning. Rashes. Candida. Sugar cravings. I couldn't remember things. Or names. I felt fuzzy and lost. I have degrees from Princeton and Yale Law, but for the first time in my life, I felt dumb.

I went to a doctor, and then another, and then another. Determined to get well and find answers. Convinced that it was the stress of my high-stakes litigation career, I left my private firm and moved to the public sector. At the US Attorneys' office, I told my new colleagues that they were looking at "Kristina 2.0." I was going to be happier, healthier, stress free. I exercised more. Went to bed earlier. Eliminated gluten and dairy – and sugar.

But then we were sent home to work during the shutdown of the spring of 2020. My headaches came in a vengeance. I was working at home, while my kids were downstairs with a babysitter. I heard screaming all day almost every day. My almost 3-year-old son started running into walls. He had bruises all over his head. He was regressing in his developmental milestones. Meanwhile, my 8-year-old daughter became aggressive. She became withdrawn, anxious, moody. She complained of stomach aches, sinus issues and headaches. She yelled often. This was sudden and different and new. My other two kids, 11-year-old son and 3-year-old daughter (the other twin), were moody and lethargic.

Kristina 2.0 was determined to get everyone well. During the summer of 2020, we got our daughter into occupational therapy. We started going to a family therapist to learn to better address behavior. We increased therapy for our 3-year-old to daily intervention to address speech and developmental delays.

And I continued my quest to find the answers for my own health. A new concierge practice ran a battery of tests. And the most abnormal result was a mycotoxin test that showed I had elevated levels of "Zearalenone" and "Ochratoxin A." I had never heard of "mycotoxins." The doctor told me to test my house.

13.2 DYING FOR REPRESENTATION

The rest is history. A mold inspector found a wall of *Stachybotrys* behind my daughter's bed, which revealed that the entire house had not been flashed properly. Upon rebuilding, we found more and more mold, including a 10-ft. swath of thick *Chaetomium* in the kitchen, mold beneath the kids' bathtub, and 26 sq. ft. of mold in the HVAC, with elevated levels of every type of mycotoxin – all caused by construction defects.

We eventually learned that the roofer knowingly omitted a critical piece of the roof (causing the wall of mold in my daughter's room) and failed to flash the vast majority of the house, the builder attached particle board to tile in the bathroom without a vapor barrier (causing the bathtub of mold), the heating, ventilation and air conditioning (HVAC) company incorrectly installed the unit without dehumidification (creating a toxic humid bubble for mold to grow), and the framer installed every window incorrectly (causing the mold growth in the kitchen). And more.

These failures caused enormous damage. We ultimately had to rebuild the house from the outside in, costing hundreds of thousands of dollars. Given the levels and types of mold, every item in the home was contaminated and discarded. Meanwhile, all six of us suffered from elevated inflammation levels, immune dysfunction and other maladies, including neurological harm and developmental delays. Systemic inflammation exacerbates whatever health issues one already has. We were, in essence, a toxic mess.

At the time, I was a personal injury defense lawyer for the United States. I knew how to evaluate a case. And if ever there was a "good" legal case, this was it: clear negligence, direct causation, enormous property damage, real personal injuries, six plaintiffs. But when I reached out to personal injury lawyers in Texas, no one would return my call. Upon some searches, I found a lawyer in my area who notes on his website that he now only handles "wrongful death" mold cases. *You have to die to get representation?!*

As my mind began to clear, I got to work defending my family and building my own case. I studied the science, called the experts, read the law. I enlisted a friend and incredibly intelligent lawyer, Kevin Terrazas, to work with me. And I ultimately found the few lawyers in the country who do these cases (to great success), including Karen Ferris and Robert McKee, who each shared great counsel for free with a fellow lawyer warrior. McKee ultimately joined my legal team.

And soon thereafter, I left the Department of Justice to build the law firm I couldn't find. We called it Just Well, a firm focused on health and financial recovery. Wellness first. Every time.

In the last 5 months alone, we have received over 1,000 calls from families who are suffering from toxic exposure all over the country. They have often lost all of their personal belongings, their home and their health to boot. They are muddling through the suffering one day at a time. Not all of them will have a case, but we will provide resources to every one of them, starting with the information that I wish I had had when I was in their shoes.

13.2.1 ELEMENTS OF A VIABLE MOLD CASE

Thankfully, the steps to building a viable mold case coincide with the steps to recover health and wellness:

1. **A third-party certified mold inspection**. First, the potential client must secure an independent assessment by a certified mold inspector. Note that a tenant should never rely on the landlord to conduct mold testing because that testing will almost always be inexpensive, biased and inaccurate. After all, an inspector hired by a landlord is incentivized to find little or no mold exposure.

   Our potential clients must hire an experienced mold inspector who understands the health implications of toxic exposure. I recommend finding an inspector through International Society for Environmentally Acquired Illness, The Mold Medic, the American Council for Accredited Certification (ACAC) (look for CIEC (council-certified indoor environmental consultant), CMI (council-certified microbial inspector) or CMC (Council-Certified Microbial Consultant), and the Institute of Inspection, Cleaning and Restoration Certification (IICRC).

The inspector should conduct a full visual inspection and then take air samples (compared with outdoor control), dust samples and mycotoxin samples. If the belongings are contaminated (and they likely are), then I recommend that they also test the belongings. And, they should run at least a test or two directly on or in the HVAC. It is the HVAC that is circulating contaminated air.

2. **A medical provider who attributes their symptoms to their exposure**. To prove personal injury, we will need a doctor to reliably attribute the patient's symptoms to their exposure. Our clients and potential clients need a health professional to walk them through the detox process. The goal is generally to Remove, Detox, Restore. We recommend finding a mold-literate doctor through the International Society for Environmentally Acquired Illness. Environmental Brain Health Clinics of America is also beginning a national practice that works well with counsel and can treat patients remotely.

3. **Client willing to leave the environment**. In a mold case, we argue that the home is so contaminated that it is uninhabitable. But, we cannot make that argument if the client still lives there. And importantly, mold-literate doctors will tell you that the single most important thing a patient can do to get better is to leave the toxic environment. Unfortunately, many of our potential clients are unable or unwilling to leave their home, even while it is remediated. Those potential clients will not have a viable legal claim – and will also have a hard time recovering physically.

4. **A solvent wrongdoer**. Trial work is storytelling, and every good story needs a villain. Who caused the mold growth? Who was responsible for maintaining the property (i.e., detecting and preventing microbial growth)? Did they paint over the mold or make some other esthetic change to conceal the toxic substance? That last action is not only an Occupational Safety and Health Administration (OSHA) violation, but it is assault: the intentional or reckless infliction of bodily harm.

   And yet, the wrongdoer must also be solvent. It is not worth spending the time and mental anguish on a lawsuit if there is no recovery to be gained. For this reason, an individual landlord is not typically a viable defendant. An institutional landlord or homebuilder, however, will be.

5. **Discovery within the statute of limitations**. Finally, the case will only be viable if the mold was discovered within the statute of limitations of the given state. In some states, the statute of limitations will begin to run upon discovery of mold illness. In others, the statute of limitations will begin to run when the plaintiff knew or should have known of the mold itself. Many of our potential clients have been battling mold illness for a long time, or have known of the mold in their homes or apartments for a long time, and may not have a viable claim.

13.2.2 UNDERSTANDING THE CAUSATION STANDARD AND THE MEDICAL LITERATURE

Many trial lawyers do not take mold cases because the legal standards seem unreasonably high or impossible to meet. Industry, insurance and defense counsel have taken scorched-earth defenses and – for a time – successfully attacked experts and medical providers who testified that mold causes very real and lasting injury.

As a general rule, one must show general causation and specific causation: That mold generally causes the types of symptoms that the plaintiff experienced, and that mold specifically caused the plaintiff's symptoms. In *Allison v. Fire Insurance Exchange*, 98 S.W.3d 227 (2002) (the "Ballard" case), the Texas Supreme Court upheld the trial court's summary judgment ruling that the plaintiff failed to show that toxic mold could cause toxic encephalopathy (general causation). The court reasoned that there were no epidemiological studies showing that mold doubles the risk of brain inflammation. Importantly, however, the court *upheld* the trial court's decision to allow testimony of the plaintiff's illness and injuries as relevant to mental anguish. (The jury had awarded $5,000,000 in mental anguish and $12,000,000 in punitive damages.)

In our view and recent research, the science has caught up to the law. Whatever the standard in any given state, the most current literature and experts can likely meet it. As to general causation, the most recent research shows – with biological and medical certainty – that mold causes respiratory damage, neurological damage, systemic inflammation, immune dysfunction and more. Another contributor to this book, Dr. Scott McMahon, has conducted a review of the literature and found 112 peer-reviewed epidemiological articles linking chronic exposure to the interior of a water damaged building and adverse health effects, including brain damage, from 2011 to 2018.[1]

For a recent case, I commissioned a literature review that found – according to the most recent peer-reviewed literature – that mold doubles the risk of chronic inflammation, immune dysfunction, developmental delays, and neurological damage and neurotoxicity.[2–6] The mechanism of injury is a cytokine storm that can affect multiple systems of the body at once.[7, 8] Mold inhalation causes innate immune activation, neural, cognitive and emotional dysfunction, altered memory, pain sensitivity and anxiety-like behavior.[9]

Meanwhile, as more and more medical providers learn about toxic mold exposure and treatment, more clients have the diagnoses that they need to prove specific causation. Once general causation has been established, a good treating provider need only conduct a differential diagnosis to determine that mold did in fact cause this patient's symptoms. Communities like CIRSx, International Society for Environmentally Acquired Illness and others equip medical providers to treat mold illness.

Indeed, in many states, a retained expert may not be required at all. A treating provider can prove the elements of both general and specific causation. Dr. Alfred Johnson, in Texas, treats hundreds of mold-injured patients every year and testifies often as the sole medical expert in the case.

13.2.3 JURIES CARE

The following cases show the potential value of mold cases when litigated well. Perhaps now, more than ever, at the tail end of Covid fear and shutdowns, juries are familiar with the notion that the encounter with a pathogen can change your life. It can determine what you can and cannot do, where you can and cannot go. The pathogen can affect one person differently than another. And, even the smallest amount can be sufficient to kill when encountered by a patient with the right pre-conditions. It is no surprise, then, that the highest verdict occurred in the very first trial in the courtroom after the Covid shutdowns.

And although the defendants are as determined as ever, plaintiffs in recent years have successfully brought scientific evidence to prove real and serious injury. In *Federico v. Lincoln Military Hous. LLC*, (E.D. Va.), Shelley and Joe Federico, through their expert Dr. David Ross, introduced the NeuroQuant to prove brain injury (brain inflammation) in federal court – the very same injury that the Texas Supreme Court rejected in *Allison* in 2002. Ross's testimony survived *Daubert* expert challenges, and the case ultimately settled in 2018.

Most recently, in *Lynette R. Jividen v. EDS*, No. CACE18011479 (Fl. State Ct. Apr. 30, 2021), a jury awarded $48 million to a single plaintiff after a leaky roof led to mold contamination in her apartment. Jividen was diagnosed with chronic inflammatory response. That inflammatory response affects the nervous system, the digestive system, muscles, joints and the immune system. Dr. Scott McMahon testified for Ms. Jividen. The damage award included $10 million for expected future medical costs, more than $1.2 million for past and future lost earnings and $35 million for loss of capacity to enjoy life. The defendant's insurer denied the claim altogether earlier in the suit rather than paying out the policy limits. As a result, the insurer will now likely face liability for the entire judgment.

13.2.3 CONCLUSION: A UNITED FRONT

Now, if only more lawyers would take these cases and collaborate. Many of the best rulings are in unpublished opinions. Lawyers can and should work together across state lines to develop the best practices to litigate these cases. At Just Well, we are actively looking for referral partners in every state, not only so that we can refer cases but also so that we can create a community of litigators committed to working together to address the problem of toxic homes in America.

This is not just personal injury litigation but impact litigation. When we hold landlords, builders and other contractors to account, we deter them from the bad behavior, and we entice them to take protective action to ensure safer homes for the next generation.

Appendix: Additional Verdicts

Gorman v. Kormick & Bourgeois, 1000 WL 81549 (Cal. State Ct.) – A 45-year-old man, his 42-year-old wife and their three minor children suffered multiple injuries, including chronic respiratory and sinus infections, fatigue and organic brain damage, due to their exposure to mold in their custom-built home. The mold exposure resulted in developmental delays for their infant son. The plaintiffs contended that one defendant was negligent when it supplied lumber that was contaminated with toxic mold. The plaintiffs further alleged that the general contractor and others involved in the construction of the home were responsible for construction defects that allowed water intrusion, which led to additional mold growth. The defendant who provided the lumber denied liability and contended that the mold found on the lumber was not the kind that would cause injuries to humans. **Before trial, the plaintiffs settled with the general contractor, construction supervisor, framer, engineer, roofing company, plumber and window installer for $9.6 million. It appears that the plaintiffs settled with the defendant who supplied the lumber for an additional $13,000,000.**

Minium v. Piller (Ariz. Supreme Court 2009) – Robin Minium had lived in and worked from her apartment for 2 years when she got sick. She was no longer able to work, and she was forced to take medical leave. Because her illness left her weak, she rarely left her apartment. She claimed to have immediately informed her apartment manager when she learned her apartment might be infected with mold. Minium also informed her physicians of the potential mold contamination. Her physician immediately confirmed that her symptoms were the result of toxic mold exposure and instructed her to vacate the premises. Minium claimed she sustained severe physical and psychological complications as a result of the mold exposure and additionally, has not had her personal belongings returned or replaced. She filed a lawsuit asserting claims of breach of contract, breach of warranty of habitability, negligence, intentional infliction of emotional distress, and replevin. And, she alleged that several defendants' failure to provide such a safe environment caused her emotional and physical distress, significant doctor bills, loss of wages, loss of continued employment and permanent physical impairment. **The jury found for Minium and awarded her $3,300,000.**

CMN v. State of Cal. Dep't of Transp. (Cal. Superior Ct. 2015) – The State of California Department of Transportation owned and managed a rental property that was rented to a family with an infant. The family noticed chipped and peeling paint throughout the exterior and interior of the property, which was readily visible. The family also reported the deteriorating paint. Despite the obvious deteriorating conditions at this older home, the Department of Transportation treated the matter as cosmetic and didn't promptly make necessary repairs. Even after the family tested for lead and the test came back positive, the Department of Transportation didn't promptly take action. A blood test later revealed that the plaintiff boy, now 4 years old, was lead poisoned. By the time he was 16 months old, he could no longer form words due to permanent neurological damage; he will require extensive care for the rest of his life, costing millions of dollars. **The parties settled for $10,000,000.**

T.D. v. Rockford Memorial Hospital (Ill. Cir. Ct. 2012) – Minor T.D. reportedly suffered neurological damage, including severe intellectual and cognitive deficits, when physicians of Rockford Memorial Hospital, as well as other hospital employees and agents, failed to properly diagnose and treat her sepsis and meningitis. **The parties settled for $5,000,000.**

Baker-Goines v. First Baptist Sch. of Charleston, 2018 WL 4611097 (S.C. Ct. Common Pleas 2018) – Brett Baker-Goines, a 15-year-old male, recovering from a sports-related concussion, suffered a second concussion while playing basketball with the First Baptist School of Charleston.

Baker-Goines suffered a traumatic brain injury and social and developmental delays as a result of the second concussion. Goines sued the First Baptist School, alleging they were negligent in deviating from the standard of care and/or in training or supervising the coach, who allegedly rushed him through the South Carolina Independent School Association's return-to-play-protocol. **A jury concluded the school was negligent and awarded Goines $5,872,583.**

REFERENCES

1. Dooley, M., McMahon, S. W. (Jan. 2020). A comprehensive review of mold research literature from 2011–2018, *Internal Med. Rev.*
2. *See, e.g.,* Jedrychowski, W., Maugeri, U., Perera, F., Stigter, L., Jankowski, J., Butscher, M., ... & Sowa, A. (2011). Cognitive function of 6-year old children exposed to mold-contaminated homes in early post-natal period. Prospective birth cohort study in Poland. *Physiology & Behavior, 104*(5), 989–995.
3. Ratnaseelan, A. M., Tsilioni, I., & Theoharides, T. C. (2018). Effects of mycotoxins on neuropsychiatric symptoms and immune processes. *Clinical Therapeutics, 40*(6), 903–917.
4. Hyvönen, S., Lohi, J., & Tuuminen, T. (2020). Moist and mold exposure is associated with high prevalence of neurological symptoms and MCS in a Finnish hospital workers cohort. *Safety and Health at Work, 11*(2), 173–177.
5. Hyvönen, S., Lohi, J., & Tuuminen, T. (2020). Moist and mold exposure is associated with high prevalence of neurological symptoms and MCS in a Finnish hospital workers cohort. *Safety and Health at Work, 11*(2), 173–177.
6. Islam, Z., Harkema, J. R., & Pestka, J. J. (2006). Satratoxin G from the black mold Stachybotrys chartarum evokes olfactory sensory neuron loss and inflammation in the murine nose and brain. *Environmental Health Perspectives, 114*(7), 1099–1107.
7. Rosenblum Lichtenstein, J. H. R., Hsu, Y. H., Gavin, I. M., Donaghey, T. C., Molina, R. M., Thompson, K. J., ... & Brain, J. D. (2015). Environmental mold and mycotoxin exposures elicit specific cytokine and chemokine responses. *PloS One, 10*(5), e0126926
8. Brain, J. D., Sieber, N. L., & Rosenblum Lichtenstein, J. H. (2020). Killing two birds with one stone: Mold-induced pulmonary immune responses and arterial remodeling. *Am J Respir Cell Mol Biol., 62*(5), 537–538.
9. Harding, C. F., Pytte, C. L., Page, K. G., Ryberg, K. J., Normand, E., Remigio, G. J., ... & Abreu, N. (2020). Mold inhalation causes innate immune activation, neural, cognitive and emotional dysfunction. *Brain, Behavior, and Immunity, 87*, 218–228.

14 The Intersection between Soil, Nutrients, Toxins and Human Health

Arden Andersen

The United States spends more money per capita on healthcare than any other country in the world: Per US government figures, $11,582 per person in 2019, the most of any country in the world. This is 17.7% of gross domestic product (GDP).[1]

Considering 2018 per capita of $10,623 (16.8% of GDP) for the United States, second would be Switzerland at $9870 (11.88% GDP), Norway at $8239 (10.05% GDP), Iceland at $6530 (8.47%) and so on to #10 Australia at $5472 (9.28%) and #13 Canada at $4994 (10.79%), #17 the United Kingdom at $4315 (10.00%) GDP and #18 Japan at $4266 (10.95%), Cuba at $986 (11.19%).[2]

According to the World Health Organization, global health spending continues to rise rapidly: $7.8 trillion in 2017 or $1080 per capita, 10% of GDP and growing faster than GDP. Of this, 60% was public and 40% was private spending.[3]

Ranking expenditures of the listed countries along with their corresponding life expectancies paints a picture of serious waste or mismanagement of healthcare in the United States: Life expectancy rankings are: United States 47th, Switzerland 4th, Norway 18th, Iceland 10th, Australia 8th, Canada 17th, United Kingdom 29th, Japan 2nd. Cuba ranks 48th at 78.69 years compared with the United States at 78.81 years of life expectancy, and we send medical missionaries to Cuba to help this "deprived" country. Cuba spends $986 per capita for 11.19% GDP per year on healthcare.[4, 5]

Though we spend thousands of dollars more per person on healthcare than the developed countries listed here, it does not translate to better health, longer life expectancy, better quality of life or lower chronic disease rates. So, what is the problem? Why do we have so much disease and ill-health when we unequivocally have the best emergency medicine system in the world and spend the most per capita, by thousands of dollars, on healthcare compared with any other country? We have the most disease-causing diet and lifestyle in the world.

A Harvard professor of genetics and metabolism at the Harvard T.H. Chan School of Public health said it well: "Chronic inflammation is uniformly damaging and is absolutely causal to the process (disease), because if you interfere with it, you can reverse the pathology."[6]

Inflammation is the underlying cause of chronic disease from cardiovascular disease to diabetes, from obesity to hypertension, from multiple sclerosis (MS) to Parkinson's and Alzheimer's. Inflammation, or the modulator of inflammation – cause or reversal – is THE link to agriculture. Food is the key. Food supplies the vital nutrients for us to live, for our mitochondria ultimately to produce ATP and our Krebs cycle to produce amino acids, fatty acids, organic acids and ultimately, all the nutrient components we need to maintain and repair cells, tissues, organs and our entire organism.

Food, the food we consume daily, determines the underlying level and type of inflammation present and often raging in our body. It is the underlying cause of all disease. Even for the 5% of diseases that are genetic in origin, systemic inflammation, determined by our diet and environment, is the primary determinant in genetic expression. It matters not whether one has the genes for breast cancer, prostate cancer, lung cancer, Alzheimer's, diabetes, MS, cystic fibrosis, myasthenia gravis or autism; environment determines genetic expression. The Standard American Diet is the most

DOI: 10.1201/b23304-15

disease-inducing diet in the world. Americans are the most obese, inherently inflamed and least healthy in all developed countries. Unfortunately, as American diet and agricultural and medical technology are exported to other countries, these people develop the same ill-health, disease-ridden, declining life expectancy as is observed in America.

It has been said that everything is connected to everything. So it is with human health and agriculture. If one draws a "mind map" with human health in the center, we see more clearly how, in fact, all things are connected. One branch off human health is inflammation. It is the underlying driver of disease or successful tissue regeneration. Off it we see drugs, electromagnetic radiation, radioactive radiation and chemicals, including agricultural pesticides, industrial and domestic chemicals. Another branch off human health and off inflammation is diet/lifestyle, off which we see food choices and exercise. Another branch off human health is climate, as it is a huge factor in our environmental determination. Off it we see the water cycle, reef death, ocean/gulf dead zones, pollution and decreasing oxygen levels, local and regional weather changes leading directly and indirectly to death and destruction, crop failures and pest pressures. Another branch off human health is agriculture, off which we see economic stability and soil health, which spins off soil compaction/tilth, nutrients, pests, crop yield, water cycle and transpiration, food quality, soil erosion and sustainability.

Agriculture has a hand in every aspect of this "mind map," at least since World War II, when synthetic nitrogen was mandated by the British government for farmers to use for growing food crops for the war effort. Synthetic nitrogen did lead to increased volumetric yields, but those yields were more susceptible to insect and disease pests and poorer shelf life. These later problems were direct consequences of lowered nutrient values of the crops; however, they opened the door to a booming business in pesticide development and sales directly out of the chemical weapons stocks from the war effort itself.

Before this period, however, American farmers had abused their power of the plow and plowed up grasslands in the western United States that never should have been tilled. There was no application of common sense to prevent erosion and the Dust Bowl. Arrogance in the belief that man could conquer nature was the prod that moved farmers to create the Dust Bowl disaster of the 1930s. It was a great opportunity, however, for government to step in to gain more control over the land and collude with chemical companies to set a new course, a course of synthetic chemical agriculture, as became law in the United Kingdom at the beginning of World War II. It is much like the power grab by governments we have seen in the COVID-19 pandemic.

Volumetric yield, measured most commonly in bushels per acre, became the mantra, and government intervened to promote commodity-based large-scale agriculture, subsidizing commodity prices and paying some farmers not to farm – if they were tied to standard commodity crops of corn, soybeans, wheat, cattle and dairy. By the early 1950s, the US Department of Agriculture (USDA) embarked upon a new policy of seeking commercially funded agricultural research for all the Land Grant Universities to replace the public-funded research in a further effort to promote the chemical industry, garner more funds for research and perpetuate a more collective, monopolistic agricultural industry. DDT and atrazine (ATZ) were two of the early "miracle" chemical weapons peddled as farm pesticides to save farmers from the devastation of insects and weeds. Rachel Carson brought to the public eye the devastation and lunacy of DDT in her book *Silent Spring* in the 1960s.

Nutrient density of crops suffered directly under this industrialized anti-organic, anti-nature model. Charles Northern MD read into the Congressional Record in 1936[7] that the nutrient value of commercially produced food in the United States had declined so significantly that he could directly correlate it with the increase in digestive diseases seen in his specialized medical practice. Trace mineral analysis of over 4000 cereal grain samples, taken from 11 Midwest states, in the early 1960s, published in the *National Hog Farmer* Swine Information Service, No. E25, 1968, revealed significant decline (as much as 70% over 4 years) in these trace minerals.[8] British research showed a similar pattern in nutrient value decline in edible foods in the United Kingdom from 1941 to 1991 (Analysis of UK Composition of Foods 1940–1991. *Nutrition and Health* 2003, Vol. 17, pp. 85–115 from The Composition of Foods, Ministry of Agriculture, Fisheries and Foods and the Royal Society of Chemistry.) This analysis showed a 16–76% reduction in vital minerals. Donald Davis PhD published a study in 2004, the December issue of the *Journal of the American College of Nutrition*, finding "six out of 13 nutrients showed apparently reliable declines between 1950 and 1999."

These nutrients included protein, calcium, phosphorus, iron, riboflavin and ascorbic acid. The declines […] ranged from 6 percent for protein to 38 percent for riboflavin.[9]

Nutrients are the reason for food consumption. These studies show that eating an 8-ounce salad with cucumber, tomato, onion, pepper, celery, mixed greens, kale, cauliflower, broccoli, carrot, pumpkin seeds and mint today will deliver to our body a significantly reduced quantity of trace minerals and vitamins than that same salad grown in 1990, which is less than if it were grown in 1950, which is less than if it were grown in 1930. That's completely on agriculture. It's not genetics, though hybrids potentially are harder to get fully mineralized than are open-pollinated varieties. It is the nutritional management of the farmer that determines the nutrient value of the crops grown.

Consequently, the level of inflammation, good or bad, associated with nutrients is determined by the farmer, and with fewer vital nutrients, we have fewer antioxidants and anti-inflammatory trace elements such as selenium, zinc, copper, manganese and so forth.

Further, the nutrient density of the crop indirectly correlates with pest attraction and pressure. Keep in mind that insect digestive systems are different than ours. Insects are not capable of digesting the same sophisticated foods we were meant to consume to keep us healthy. As nutrient levels of crops decline, they become more attractive to insects because these crops produce more free nitrogen molecules, fewer complete and complex carbohydrates, more reducing sugars, and more simple and less sophisticated amino acids because the plant doesn't have the full spectrum of nutrients needed for the production of complete proteins, complex carbohydrates, etc.

For example, when the percentage of nitrate nitrogen reaches 55% of the total nitrogen content in the plant sap, aphids attack the plant. Dr. Carey Reams was the first to suggest the use of a refractometer in the field of all crops to measure the sap brix levels. The sap brix levels roughly correlate with nutrient density and can be used to predict insect susceptibility. A brix reading of 14 or above at the weakest point of the plant will essentially ward off all pressure from insect pests in that crop WITHOUT any use of pesticides.

The point of this is that if no pesticides are needed, then no pesticide residues will be found in the food people eat. Pesticides are toxic and exhaust valuable antioxidants to detoxify via the liver Phase I and II pathways. Many pesticides, such as Roundup, ATZ and DDT, are endocrine disruptors, which means they disrupt the normal endocrine development of human fetuses, infants and children; they interfere with the normal function of adult hormone systems, leading to multiple problems, including endocrine cancers.

Thus far, we have recognized that the United States is spending much more money than any other country on healthcare, yet we have the worst citizen health of all the developed countries of the world; the agricultural model we have put in place has perpetuated and continues to perpetuate declining nutrient – especially mineral – levels while we spray millions of tons of chemical weapons – called "plant protection products" for political correctness – that we know cause their own individual and collective human and animal health problems, from endocrine disruption and gender dysphoria to cancer, birth defects and a litany of ill-health. It's Business! Many of the chemical weapons manufacturers have pharmaceutical branches that produce the drugs used to treat the diseases their chemical weapons, used in agriculture, cause in consumers.

Why do plants need "protection?" Or, do they? The answer is both yes and no; it depends upon the model in which you live. You may be in the standard, Land Grant University model – Ohio State, Perdue, University of Nebraska, University of Missouri, Iowa State and so forth, as every state has a Land Grant University where the state's official agricultural school resides, and the Cooperative Extension Service sits. As we know, over 75% of university research in the United States is now industry funded. Much of that funding comes with strings attached to the data whereby it can only be released to the public if the data supports the desires of the funding corporation. That is, until the professor retires, gaining "Emeritus" status, and can then "go public," as have several, including Drs. Don Huber and Robert Kremer, or may have simply been able to get the public data out in public forums, as has Dr. Tyrone Hayes.

"Plant protection" is predicated on the belief that insects, diseases and weeds are present in nature to randomly compete with modern agricultural foods. As such, pesticides "must" be applied to get the crop to harvest before nature gets to it first. It seems logical and is fully embraced by most consumers. Even the typical organic farmer believes in this concept. He/she merely uses "organically approved" pesticides and weed control methods, but his/her mentality and logic in solving insect, disease and weed challenges is the same as that of the chemical farmer. Herein lies the problem. The belief that nature is somehow flawed and in competition with humans for their food production is purely a business model sold to the general public and more so, the farmers.

What needs to be understood is that nature is not in competition but rather, in partnership with our wellness survival. As farming "technology" has progressed to further and further deplete the nutrient values of our foods, the food plants in the field, greenhouse, garden, lake, bog or patty become weaker and weaker and more susceptible to insect, disease and weed pressure. It is illogical that nature would evolve or God would create a nature that was self-destructive.

Let's start with insects. As the French biologist Francis Chaboussou demonstrated, insects have different digestive systems than ours and therefore seek simpler, less complex nutrients for nitrogen and carbon. If one studies the Krebs cycle or citric acid cycle, which is the foundation of the biochemistry of energy production in all of nature, from plant to human, we find it requires a full complement of nutrients, trace minerals, macro minerals, vitamins, amino acids, organic acids and so forth. If any of these nutrients is not present in sufficient balanced quantities, the Krebs cycle bogs down, and incomplete amino acids, funny proteins, simple reducing sugars and basic organic acids prevail, which are exactly what the insect digestive systems are designed to utilize. As we approach balanced sufficiency, fewer and fewer of these "insect foods" are available in the plant, and thus, there is less and less insect pressure to devour the crop. A simple instrument used to assess plant health in the field is the refractometer, measuring sap sugar levels. It is calibrated for 0–32 brix, and once the farmer or gardener achieves 14 brix, 24–7 (24 hours per day, 7 days per week) in his/her crop, *no insect will attack*. If no insects attack, we don't need any insecticide. The same goes for bacterial, viral and fungal plant diseases; once the nutrient values expressed as brix levels are up to 14 or above, no disease appears, so NO pesticides are needed to get the crop to harvest.[10]

The weed challenge is explained well by the research done by the Scandinavians on geological succession of soils from fresh volcanic rock to mature forests and everything in between. The fresh rock first becomes inhabited by bacteria that etch away at the mineral base, then algae and primitive fungi. As the process continues, lichens are soon able to occupy the rock and finally, primitive upright plants. As the sophistication of biodiversity progresses, the soil is formed, and the ratio between bacterial biomass and fungal biomass changes, favoring fungi. Once we reach a 1:1 ratio, we see our sweet prairie grasses, such as fescue. Once here, the more primitive plants we call weeds, which have a more bacterially dominated ideal soil environment, fade out, and eventually, we have forests developing that have fungal to bacterial ratios of 1000 or more to 1. Again, no herbicides are needed to control the primitive plants we call weeds, because they don't thrive in the fungal-dominated soils. What about fungal diseases such as verticillium, phytophthora, etc.? These are primitive fungi dominating primitive soils. Once we approach 1:1 bacterial and fungal biomass, we have beneficial fungi like mycorrhizae as the dominate and very protective species. Only when our agricultural/farming practice causes a reversion of soils back in the geological spectrum do we see weeds and disease organisms dominate.[11]

What the discerning reader may have grasped is that as the soil evolves with nature or farming practices, it sequesters more carbon. As pointed out in the documentary "Kiss the Soil." healthy soils sequester carbon, and agriculture has the potential to completely sequester all the excess atmospheric CO_2, ALL OF IT!

Further, as we clean up the soils and get the nutrients back into our foods, we don't have the fertilizer and pesticide runoff into our streams and into our oceans to create huge dead zones, kill carbon-sequestering and oxygen-producing cyanobacteria and algae, or kill coastline-protecting reefs and vital fisheries, leading to local and regional climatic alterations and soil erosion. It is all connected.

Now that we have the overview from soil health to crop health to human health, from soil health to environmental health to climate destruction and weather alteration, we shall delve into some of the specifics of toxins, especially pesticides and their health effects on people.

Pesticides – truly, they are chemical weapons evolving from the World War I and World War II chemical weapons industry – have become ubiquitous in our society. According to the United States Geological Survey (USGS), "About 1 billion pounds of conventional pesticides are used each year in the United States to control weeds, insects, and other pests."[12]

"A study in Texas found that mothers who lived in areas where more atrazine was used had a greater chance of giving birth to children with birth defects in their faces and skulls than mothers who did not. The more atrazine used in the county, the greater the chance of birth defects."

"Researchers collected urine from pregnant women in France. They tested the urine for atrazine or its metabolites to estimate exposure to atrazine. Babies whose mothers were exposed to atrazine while they were pregnant grew more slowly. They had a smaller head circumference than babies whose mothers were not exposed to atrazine during pregnancy."

"Women living in areas in Illinois where atrazine is heavily used had more irregular menstrual periods than women living in Vermont, where less atrazine is used. Atrazine measured in the residential water was 0.4 µg/L in Vermont but 0.7 µg/L in Illinois. The more water women in Illinois drank, the more likely they were to have delayed periods."

"Farmers have reported information on their health and use of pesticides in the Agricultural Health Study. Farmers who used atrazine were more likely to have both allergic and non-allergic wheezing. The chance of reporting wheezing increased with how often the farmers reported using atrazine."

"Researchers using Agricultural Health Study data found that people who had been exposed to more atrazine had a higher risk of end-stage renal disease (kidney failure) compared to people who had not been exposed. As atrazine use increased, risk of end-stage renal disease also increased."

"Farmers in the Agricultural Health Study who used more atrazine also had a greater increase in body-mass index (BMI) than other farmers as they got older."

"The EPA concluded that 52 out of 59 species of birds would raise fewer young if they were exposed to atrazine. Five bird species often found in cornfields might produce fewer broods of nestlings per year. The EPA's models suggested that small mammals were at long-term risk near fields sprayed with atrazine. Small mammals could be harmed at up to 250 feet away from the crop." [13]

During the most recent 5 years of available survey data (2013–2017), an annual average of 72,000,000 pounds of ATZ was applied.[12]

Results suggest that ATZ could be involved in cell homeostasis perturbation, potentially through a S100a4-dependant mechanism.[14]

Research done by Tyrone Hayes PhD at UC Berkeley has shown that concentrations of ATZ well below the Environmental Protection Agency (EPA) allowable level of 3 ppb cause complete transgenderization of male frogs. Male frogs come under the influence of ATZ at lower than 0.1 ppb.[15]

We can spend pages, no, actually, volumes of books, on various toxins to which we are exposed every day. The industry that produces these toxins pays for "scientists" to "research" the "safety" of these toxins and present to various government agencies and the public "data" and published papers to "prove" their products should be allowed unencumbered in society. After all, these toxins "enhance" our lives. I am a scientist myself, and I understand the protocol that needs to be followed to evaluate the interface between man-made products and living creatures, including humans.

It can all really be summed up by inquiring what is the biochemical and biophysical "drag" these toxins present on our metabolism, specifically our mitochondria and our organism homeostasis. Certainly, in many cases, this drag includes genetic damage/alteration/mutation, which then leads to identifiable disease processes such as cancer, cardiovascular disease, kidney disease, diabetes, asthma, Parkinson's, MS, amyotrophic lateral sclerosis (ALS), birth defects, miscarriages and allergies, to name a few. Unfortunately, each toxin is measured and evaluated independently, as if it were the one and only toxin in the mix of life's exposures. Free radical generation/damage of our metabolic engine is the determining factor at the most fundamental ion, atom and molecular level. Each and every toxin, whether or not it has been "shown" to cause cancer or some other identifiable disease, does tax the metabolism. Each toxin has a given "drag" on the nutrient/homeostatic biochemistry/biophysics. Even if not shown to cause a disease directly, these chemicals are processed through the liver via Phase I and Phase II detoxification, requiring a full complement of vitamins, minerals and antioxidants, and subsequently excreted through the bile and/or kidneys. Even if unchanged molecularly, the process of excretion by the kidneys requires energy for ionic exchange.

That energy has to come from nutrients, from antioxidants: Minerals, vitamins and enzymes. So it is in pharmacology, where every drug is cleared via the liver and/or the kidneys, each having its respective "drag" on the system, as it with every chemical in our food and environment. Few doctors take this "drag" into consideration when evaluating patients' health, diet and nutrient needs and certainly, the consequences of polypharmacy. Then again, the medical system is the third leading cause of premature death in the United States.

The discussion here is not about debating or listing chemical after chemical, study after study, for that has already been done. The literature is available for all to research and read. The focus of this chapter is on the nutrients needed to compensate for the "drag" by which all these toxins burden our bodies, specifically our biophysics and biochemistry.

Phase I detoxification in our liver converts toxins, endogenous and exogenous, into smaller molecules that are often more reactive. This is because Phase 1 uses oxygen to form a reactive site on the toxin molecule so it can be more easily neutralized in Phase II via glutathione conjugation, glucuronidation, sulphation, amino acid conjugation, acetylation and methylation. Phase II converts these metabolites to water-soluble molecules to be excreted from the body. However, the gall bladder has to be working efficiently for these Phase II metabolites to be taken from the liver and dumped into the colon for elimination. This, of course, assumes an efficiently working colon, no irritable bowel syndrome (IBS) and no constipation for effective final elimination of those toxin metabolites dumped into the bile for elimination.

Phase I particularly needs B1, B2, B3, B6, choline, vitamin C, vitamin E, magnesium and selenium. The liver's regulation of Phase I is determined by the "toxin pile" it has to convert. Since this is Phase I, it will take every available needed nutrient from the circulatory reserve to accomplish its task. Most every, not all, prescribed medication must be detoxified via the P450 Phase I enzyme pathway. Whatever the Phase I output, Phase II must keep up with the subsequent timely conjugation, glucuronidation or sulphation of these Phase I metabolites. These metabolites are highly reactive and can cause DNA damage. If not immediately detoxified, they lead to liver damage, fatty liver deposits, and spill over into the systemic circulatory system, leading to a myriad of inflammatory illnesses from cardiovascular disease to autoimmune neurological and glandular disorders, fatigue, and eventual liver and kidney failure and death.

How do we know if these metabiotic pathways are functioning as desired, and whether sufficient nutrients are being supplied for the various detoxification pathways? Standard medical blood testing looks at bilirubin – measurement of red blood cell break-down and elimination – but it is not a greatly sensitive test and often detects damage after the fact. AST (aspartate transaminase),

ALT (alanine transaminase), gamma-glutamyl transferase (GGT) and alkaline phosphatase are all found on comprehensive metabolic panels regularly drawn on blood profiles. These markers indicate whether there is a problem with the liver clearing toxins/drugs; unfortunately, often after some damage has already occurred. Even with that said, the liver is quite amenable to repair, provided it receives appropriate and sufficient nutrients for repair and the exhaustive toxins – most commonly diet, medications and environmental exposures, often work related – are reduced sufficiently for the liver to get ahead of their damaging effects.

Good physicians or clinicians determine via history and physical exam much valuable insight about liver function and detoxification by what complaints the patient expresses, what illnesses they have or have had, and how they function in the present. There are alternative liver function tests available. A common test is the caffeine clearance test. The liver detoxifies caffeine via Phase I and II and eliminates it through the kidneys and bowels. If Phase I is too slow – insufficient Phase I nutrient supply – the patient will complain of extreme sensitivity to caffeine. If, however, Phase I is too fast, the patient will express zero effect from caffeine. The problem with too fast a Phase I is that eventually, it overwhelms Phase II with reactive oxygen species of Phase I detoxification, and their damaging effects grow. These effects are expressed as inflammation.[16]

A study done in citrus between the 1959 and 1960 seasons looked at vitamin C content of citrus correlated with soil moisture (low, medium and high) and pounds of nitrogen applied per tree for the year. With 1 pound per tree per year, they found 64.7 mg/100 ml of juice in high-moisture soil conditions, 66.3 mg/100 ml in medium soil moisture and 64.4 mg/100 ml of juice in the low soil moisture conditions. Two pounds of nitrogen resulted in a little less vitamin C at each soil moisture level, 3 pounds of nitrogen lowered the vitamin C a bit more, and 4 pounds of nitrogen per tree resulted in the lowest vitamin C levels at 56.9, 57.6 and 61.3 mg/100 ml, respectively. Average fruit size was 228, 207, 213, 217 cc per 1, 2, 3, 4 pounds of N applied.[17]

Trees receiving the higher rates of nitrogen application produced fruit with higher titratable acids, lower solids to acids ratio and lower vitamin C content of the juice. Since the total soluble solids were unaffected by nitrogen application rate, the decrease in solids to acid ratio is due to the increase in acid. The solids to acid ratio is used as the index of maturity, and thus, the higher nitrogen application rates delayed the fruit maturity. Not only did the higher rates of nitrogen application delay maturity, but they also reduced the internal quality of the fruit by lowering the vitamin C content of the juice. Smith and Reuther reported that in general, a high rate of nitrogen fertilization lowers the vitamin content of fruit by an indirect method whereby the vitamin C content is diluted by the production of a greater number of fruits per tree.[17]

A Kushi Institute analysis of nutrient data from 1975 to 1997 found that average calcium levels in 12 fresh vegetables dropped 27%; iron levels 37%; vitamin A levels 21%; and vitamin C levels 30%. A similar study of British nutrient data from 1930 to 1980, published in the *British Food Journal*, found that in 20 vegetables, the average calcium content had declined 19%; iron 22%; and potassium 14%. Yet another study concluded that one would have to eat eight oranges today to derive the same amount of vitamin A as our grandparents would have gotten from one.[18]

Table 3, page 7 of *Vitamin C Intake and Mortality among a Sample of the United States Population* looked at death from all causes, all cancers and all cardiovascular diseases between 1971 and 1984 and correlated this with their categorization in a 1971 to 1974 study of intake of vitamin C. The three levels were 0–49 mg C per day, over 50 mg per day and over 50 mg plus supplementation. The healthiest group took close to 800 mg of vitamin C per day via supplementation and a diet rich in fruits and vegetables. Consequently, this group had the lowest death rate and the lowest cancer and lowest cardiovascular disease rates. After 7 years, the group consuming more than 50 mg vitamin C per day had half the death rate of those consuming less than 50 mg vitamin C per day. Further, vitamin C's inverse relation to total mortality was stronger than the relation to total fat intake and serum cholesterol.[19]

The real point of this discussion is twofold. First, disease for the most part, 95% of the time, is a direct reflection of nutritional balance/imbalance. Agronomists (Michael McNeill), plant pathologists (Don Huber), biologists (Francis Chaboussou) and entomologists (Philip Callahan and Tom Dykstra) have shown in their research and in the field that plant disease/health is dictated by nutritional management. It will be reflected in the sap refractometer reading, the sap nutrient analysis and the insect/disease presence and pressure. It will be reflected in the yield and nutrient density of the crop harvested. As the veterinarians Paul Dettloff, Dan Skow and Hugh Keraman have demonstrated in their past practices, animal health is directly related to animal diet and nutrient balance/imbalance. Neither is related to drug deficiencies/sufficiencies.

As a practicing family physician and colleague of Lisa Everett Andersen, one of the foremost recognized clinical nutritionists/clinical pharmacists, we see inflammation manifested as human disease daily and subsequently, see it resolve with appropriate dietary modification and nutritional supplementation.[20] The minimum foundation we start with is:

- Vit A (71% beta-carotene) 35,000 IU
- Vit C (ascorbic acid) 2000 mg
- Vit D3 2000 IU
- Vit E (as mixed tocopherols) 800 IU
- Vit K1 150 mg
- Thiamine (B1) 200 mg
- Riboflavin (B2 as R-5-P and Riboflavin) 100 mg
- Niacin/niacinamide 250 mg
- Vit B6 (PyridoxineP-5-P) 300 mg
- Folate (Calcium folate/5-MTHF) 800 µg
- Vit B12 (hydroxocobalamin) 1000 µg
- Biotin 500 µg
- Pantothenic acid from calcium pantothenate 500 mg
- Iodine (sea kelp and potassium iodide) 1000 µg
- Magnesium (from magnesium glycinate) 500 mg
- Zinc (from zinc picolinate) 50 mg
- Selenium (from amino acid chelate) 400 µg
- Copper (citrate) 3 mg
- Manganese (ascorbate) 20 mg
- Molybdenum (fumarate) 300 µg
- Potassium (citrate) 99 mg
- Chromium (from chromium GTF) 400 µg
- Choline (citrate) 300 mg
- Inositol 300 mg
- N-Acetyl l-cysteine 200 mg
- Betaine HCl 150 mg
- Bioflavonoids (citrus) 100 mg
- PABA 100 mg
- Natural Mixed Tocopherols 40 mg
- Glutamic acid HCl 20 mg
- L-Methionine 12.5 mg
- Co-Q10 10 mg – will add 100 mg BID separately
- Boron (citrate) 4 mg
- Vanadium (aspartate or aminomin) 300 µg
- Trace elements 100 µg

We add further supplementation depending upon the individual challenges and recommend modifying their diet to reduce inflammation to whatever degree they are motivated to achieve better health.

First is the elimination of dairy products, whether or not they are organic, A2, synthetic hormone free (all milk has endogenous estrogen from the female producing the milk) or whatever the argument. We send them to NutritionFacts.org and The Game Changers movie for further education on their diet modification.

Nutrition is the foundation of our health and disease. Figure 14.1 shows a chart I devised years ago when seeking a means to explain to farmers how/why one fertilizer helped one farmer, but not another, or helped one year, but not the next. It is the same with animals and people. Find where you reside on the chart: death – well, if you are dead, you won't be reading this anyway; disease – if you have been diagnosed with any disease, you are here; pre-disease – you are susceptible but have not contracted the disease or been diagnosed yet, you just have all the critical risk factors; and finally, health – you truly have no diagnoses, don't need and take any medications, and function to your genetic capacity.

You will see on the chart, depending on where you reside, that a product may help move you up the scale toward health but may actually be detrimental to another person healthier than you. This is why we must look for real health determinants – easier, perhaps, with plants and animals. In plants, that is no insect pressure, no diseases and brix–refractometer readings above 14. That is why we start with the preceding list for our baseline nutrient supplementation and then adjust per the need of the person according to their inflammatory levels, life stressors – causing inflammation – history of exposures, genetics and motivation – yes, mental health is very important to your success. I suggest reading Bernie Segal MD *Love, Medicine and Miracles.*

We must have sufficient nutrition to run Phase I and II detoxifications of the liver determined by what symptoms the person displays and where in their body. Much toxicity is directly generated by the Standard American Diet, which puts a lot of pressure on Phase I and doesn't provide sufficient nutrient to upregulate Phase II, so the person manifests the inflammatory degenerative symptoms of the top 16 causes of death in the United States, starting with cardiovascular disease, followed by cancer.

Health starts in the mind, with an attitude to get well. It starts in the soil, with comprehensive farming approaches to improve plant nutrition to the degree that plants were intended to have – brix

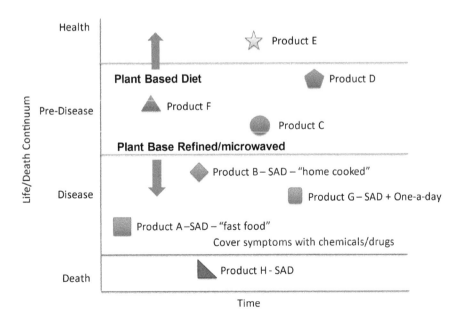

FIGURE 14.1 Life/death continuum

readings over 14 at their weakest point, 24 hours per day, 7 days per week. No gene technology, no chemical weapon or synthetic growth stimulant will ever achieve such health balance.

The chart applies equally to agriculture regarding plant and animal nutrition as well as to human health and nutrition. Specifically, as the entries state, the diet one follows correlates with one's subsequent health/disease status (Figure 14.1).

Consider this chart in regard to medicine. If you have strep throat, for example, you are in the "disease" category. For some, and in some countries, this could be life-threatening. Let's say the doctor prescribes tetracycline or doxycycline because that is all that is available or all one's insurance will cover. It is further assumed you are on the Standard American Diet, loaded with inflammation and obese; consequently, your immune system is on overload, and your liver, gall bladder, colon and kidneys are on overload. Most obese, especially morbidly obese, people have fat deposition around the vital organs, including some degree of fatty liver. Many of these people take something for reflux, as do over 50% of Americans on the Standard American Diet. Many of these people have some degree of either constipation or diarrhea, reflecting an inflamed colon. Most of them consume more soda than water, so the kidneys are further stressed. The tetracycline or doxycycline would be assigned "product A" on our chart and do little to improve the strep throat. Most doctors and mid-level practitioners are giving either amoxicillin or Augmentin, the latter because of seeing so many resistant strains of strep. Azithromycin is commonly given if the person is penicillin allergic. All these would be assigned "product C," as they will most likely successfully assist the immune system in knocking out the strep throat.

Regarding supplementation, how does the practitioner or the consumer know when enough is enough? How do we determine if the level listed earlier under the optimal daily allowance for the B vitamins is sufficient or insufficient? The answer resides in clinical practice. In other words, what is the response of the patient regarding their complaints and health? Timing and time are also factors as to how quickly the tide is turned and for how long the person has been sick. Doctors operate under this decision-making process with medication titration on every patient. There are listed ranges of dosing for every medication derived through historical experimentation, but ultimately, the medication must be, or should be, titrated per individual patient response. How does the doctor know if the patient is taking enough blood pressure medicine? Check the blood pressure over a given period.

Vitamin D has gotten a great amount of attention due to its link to immune function, and most recently, serum vitamin D was found to be deficient in a great deal of humanity. In one of my corporate clinics, where we do annual physical exams, we have been checking vitamin D levels as a matter of course and found 49% of our cooperate population from age 25 to 60 to be under the reference minimum of 30 ng/ml. Most people think that vitamin D levels are merely linked to sunshine exposure and that is it. Sunshine is certainly the primary mechanism through which humans can potentially raise their vitamin D level, but that does not guarantee anything. Even taking megadoses of vitamin D3 does not guarantee sufficiency.[21]

Vitamin D receptors have been found on over 36 areas of the body, including bones, ovaries, testes, uterus and immune cells. Vitamin D must cycle through the liver and kidneys to become fully usable by the body. Vitamin D is actually a hormone dependent upon many other nutrients to achieve its intended utilization. Vitamin K is needed to control the amount of vitamin D made, keeping it in homeostasis.[22] Other nutrients needed for vitamin D to be utilized are magnesium – an enzyme cofactor, boron – regulates blood levels of vitamin D, zinc – forms a component of the vitamin D receptor, and vitamin A – regulates the number of vitamin D receptors.[23–25]

Translating this to functional medicine/nutrition, if someone is taking 10,000 IU of vitamin D3 per day and their serum vitamin D level is still poor, it's not because of insufficient vitamin D or sunshine. It's most likely due to insufficient supporting nutrients. Clinically, we start with the dosing per the optimal daily allowance listed previously and titrate additional nutrients per patient response/need.

The same applies to agriculture, plant and animal health, and nutritional supplementation; titrate nutrients per patient response while asking how are their symptoms, how's their energy, how's their elimination? How are the complaints for which they which they originally came to the clinic?

There is a group of clinicians, Lifestyle Medicine practitioners, who promote improved lifestyle, physical and mental fitness, and a more plant-based diet while contending that one can do everything with diet, that no supplementation is needed. This is only true to the degree that the patient can get sufficient nutrition in their food to address the needs of the patient in order to reverse their health problems. It assumes that we live in a pristine world free of chemical and pesticide pollution, heavy metal toxicity, plastics and plastic leachates, electromagnetic pollution and other stressors. It makes the grand assumption that the food automatically contains fully sufficient nutrient levels.

Nice theories, and many people by just changing their diets will have great health improvements. Yet, many need more nutrition than what the food delivers to achieve health and to do so in a reasonable amount of time. Vitamin D is often a good example, as are magnesium, various B vitamins, glutathione and so forth. They must be supplemented to get the therapeutic doses needed to overcome acute degenerative/life-threatening symptoms.

An excellent case in point is that during a measles epidemic, vitamin C was used prophylactically at 1000 mg every 6 hours by vein or intramuscularly and prevented the development of measles in the test cases. Taken orally, it must be given at 1000 mg every 2 hours around the clock. If Koplik's spots and fever had already begun, the administration of these doses of vitamin C completely resolved all signs and symptoms in 48 hours.[26]

One will not get such levels of vitamin C from any diet or food concentrate.

Another example of having to titrate dosing to achieve the desired outcome is in regard to hormones, specifically bioidentical hormone replacement therapy. Most young girls today after starting their menstrual cycles have 2 good weeks out to the month and 2 weeks of misery with severe cramping, migraines, heavy bleeding and significant premenstrual syndrome (PMS) mood swings. These young girls are put on birth control pills (BCPs) to stop their symptoms. BCPs do this by significantly reducing endogenous hormone production, as they are synthetic molecules that will occupy the hormone receptors but not function as the natural hormones. This leads to the multitude of potential hazardous side-effects experienced by these young women, including anxiety, depression, malaise, infertility, blood clots, female cancers and a variety of other side-effects listed on the package inserts.

As doctors are not very well trained in functional biochemistry – I admit I was not in medical school – they merely follow the protocol of patient symptom complaint, drug prescription, have a nice day. Most of these young girls are progesterone deficient, attributed directly to being the third and fourth generation exposed to a multitude of endocrine disruptors, including ATZ, glyphosate, plastics, synthetic animal hormones and industrial chemicals. Further, their diets, as with most Americans, and especially teenagers, are deficient in the building blocks necessary to produce sufficient steroid sex hormones while also countering the multitude of environmental endocrine disruptors. For many, diet and nutrition supplementation are not sufficient to completely resolve these menstrual symptoms.

Bioidentical progesterone – meaning it is derived from plant sterols that are enzyme reacted to form the exact human molecule produced by the human body – is taken as a troche dissolved between the cheek and gum to get directly into the blood stream via the mucous membrane on days 12–26 of their cycle. The progesterone is titrated until the cramping, heavy bleeding, depression and PMS are resolved. The same applies to most miscarriages, pregnancy morning sickness symptoms, pre-eclampsia/eclampsia and post-partum depression.

The intersection between soil, nutrients, toxins and human health is intimate. Soil health/illhealth is reflected directly in the human population, in the tons of chemical weapons applied to our food in the name of "plant protection" and in the amount of pharmaceuticals consumed by people daily throughout their lives. As much as people would like to believe that human illness is out of their own control, and more importantly, responsibility, the truth is that it is fully in their control and responsibility. Consumers vote daily at the grocery store and vending machines with their dollars.

The mere fact that nearly every grocery store in urban and suburban American now has an organic section is purely driven by consumer buying habits, voting with their dollars. As consumers become more educated on the nutrient quality of food and what they can expect, they continue to vote in favor of more nutritious, more flavorful, higher-brix foods. Consumers are the drivers of agricultural change, of soil management change, of plant nutritional changes. Genetic engineering of crops is a bait and switch maneuver by industry to continue to avoid solving plant production problems at the soil nutrition level so that they can continue to sell patented, profitable wares, now to include "seeds" and "plants" in addition to chemical weapons.

In conclusion, nutrition is fundamentally about the Krebs cycle, also known as the citric acid cycle, and what is required to run it completely and efficiently, because out of it comes every biological molecule necessary for life to exist; necessary to feed the mitochondria for the production of ATP, the most vital molecule to sustain life. A number of factors contribute to less-than-ideal ATP output and inferior Krebs cycle functioning. Low–nutrient dense food is foundational to nutrient deficiency, coupled with ubiquitous chemical toxins that directly and indirectly generate free radicals that further deplete the Krebs cycle, in addition to poor diet choices, endocrine disruptors, societal stressors. and electrical, magnetic and microwave radiation that directly induce free radical generation. It is no wonder that people are so depleted and sick today. Supplementation is vital to any hope of recovery, but most importantly, we must regenerate agriculture, leading to regenerating nutrient density in our food. Only then will we find health or at a minimum, potential health.

REFERENCES

1. Centers for Medicare & Medicaid Services Official Website. https://www.cms.gov/files/document/highlights.pdf. Accessed May 16, 2021.
2. The World Bank. Current health expenditure per capita (current US$). https://data.worldbank.org/indicator/SH.XPD.CHEX.PC.CD?most_recent_value_desc=true. Accesses online May 16, 2021.
3. Global Spending on Health: A World in Transition 2019. https://www.who.int/health_financing/documents/health-expenditure-report-2019.pdf?ua=1. Accessed online May 16, 2021.
4. https://data.worldbank.org/indicator/SH.XPD.CHEX.GD.ZS
5. The World Bank. "Current health expenditure per capita (current US$)" and "Current health expenditure (% of GDP). https://data.worldbank.org/indicator/SH.XPD.CHEX.PC.CD
6. Shaw, J. Raw and red-hot: Could inflammation be the cause of myriad chronic conditions? *Harvard Magazine* May–June 2019. https://www.harvardmagazine.com/2019/05/inflammation-disease-diet
7. (U.S. Senate Document #264) United States Senate Document No.264 (sare.org)
8. National Hog Farmer, Swine Information Service, No. E25, 1968
9. Study suggests nutrient decline in garden crops over past 50 years. *UT News*. The University of Texas at Austin. https://news.utexas.edu/2004/12/01/study-suggests-nutrient-decline-in-garden-crops-over-past-50-years/
10. Chaboussou, F. *Healthy Crops: A New Agricultural Revolution*. Carpenter Publishing. 2005.
11. Pennanen, T, Strommer, R, Markkola, A, Fritze, H. Microbial and plant community structure across a primary succession gradient. *Scand J For Res* January 2001;16(1):37–43.
12. https://www.usgs.gov/centers/oki-water/science/pesticides?qt-science_center_objects=0#qt-science_center_objects. Accessed online July 11, 2021.
13. National Pesticide Information Center, Atrazine Fact Sheet. http://npic.orst.edu/factsheets/atrazine.html. Accessed online July 11, 2021.
14. Peyre, L et al. Atrazine. *Toxicol In Vitro* 2014;28(2):156–63. PMID:24211529https://pubchem.ncbi.nlm.nih.gov/compound/atrazine#section=Mechanism-of-Action accessed online July 11, 2021.
15. Hayes, T, Haston, K, Tsui, M, Hoang, A, Haeffele, C, Vonk, A. Atrazine-induced hermaphroditism at 0.1 ppb in American leopard frogs (Rana pipiens): Laboratory and field evidence. https://ehp.niehs.nih.gov/doi/10.1289/ehp.5932. Published:1 April 2003. https://doi.org/10.1289/ehp.5932. Accessed online July 11, 2021.

16. Shyu, JK, Wang, YJ, Lee, SD, Lu, RH, Lo, KJ. Caffeine clearance test: A quantitative liver function assessment in patients with liver cirrhosis. *Zhonghua Yi Xue Za Zhi.* 1996 May;57(5):329–34. PMID: 8768380.

17. Hales, TA. Valencia orange fruit growth and quality as affected by moisture tension and level of nitrogen nutrition. A Thesis Submitted to the Faculty of the Department Of Horticulture in Partial FuJ.fillment of the Requirements For the Degree of Master of Science. In the Graduate College: University of Arizona' I960. https://repository.arizona.edu/bitstream/handle/10150/551442/AZU_TD_BOX191_E9791_1960 _136.pdf;jsessionid=CBAC0C76943292DDE1DDF6E14228D7FA?sequence=1. Accessed online July 25, 2021.

18. Dirt poor: Have fruits and vegetables become less nutritious? Because of soil depletion, crops grown decades ago were much richer in vitamins and minerals than the varieties most of us get today. April 27, 2011. https://www.scientificamerican.com/article/soil-depletion-aND-NUTRITION-LOSS/

19. Enstrom, JE, Kanim, LE, Klein, MA. Vitamin C intake and mortality among a sample of the United States population. *Epidemiology* May 1992;3(3):194–202. http://www.scientificintegrityinstitute.org/ EPID1992.pdf. Accessed online July 25, 2021.

20. Everett Andersen, L. *Learning How to Thrive in a Toxic World and the Impact of Clinical Endocrinology and BHRT.* Mission Point Press. Traverse City. 2020.

21. Norman, AW. From vitamin D to hormone D: Fundamentals of the vitamin D endocrine system essential for good health. *Am J Clin Nutr* 2008;88(2):491S–499S.

22. Vitamin K2. *Altern med Rev* 2009;14(3):284–293.

23. Matsuzaki, H, et al. Magnesium deficiency regulates vitamin D metabolizing enzymes and type II sodium-phosphate cotransporter mRNA expression in rats. *Magnes Res* 2013;26(2):8–86.

24. Pizzorno, L. Nothing boring about boron. *Integr Med* 2015;14(4):35–48.

25. Ng, KY, et al. "Vitamin D and vitamin A receptor expression and the proliferative effects of ligan activation of these receptors on the development of pancreatic progenitor cells derived from human fetal pancreas. *Stem Cell Rev Rep* 2011;7(1):53–63.

26. Klenner, FR. The treatment of poliomyelitis and other virus disease with vitamin C. *South Med Surg* July 1949; 111(7):209–214.

15 Current Clinical and Research Considerations for ME/CFS

Maria A. Vera-Nunez and Kenneth J. Friedman

CONTENTS

15.1 INTRODUCTION

Myalgic encephalomyelitis/chronic fatigue syndrome (ME/CFS) is a complex, multifactorial condition characterized by unexplained, persistent and disabling fatigue, which must be present in adults for at least 6 months. The diagnosis may be made in children after 3 months.[80] Post-exertional malaise is now considered a cardinal symptom of ME/CFS and requires other symptoms to be present, depending upon case definition, which include cognitive issues, non-restorative sleep, orthostatic intolerance, chronic pain and gastrointestinal problems.[33, 34, 47] This challenging, chronic disease impacts the patient's ability to function, study or work. Up to 75% of patients with ME/CFS cannot work, and an estimated 25% are consistently housebound or bedbound.[5] These patients are at increased risk of death by suicide.[20] All these factors have a negative economic and social impact on the patients, their families and society.

Although the etiology of ME/CFS is uncertain, there is ample evidence that multiple body systems are affected (immune, nervous, gastrointestinal, cardiovascular and endocrine/metabolic systems)[9, 97] and that there are contributing environmental and lifestyle factors.[13, 80]

15.2 NUTRITIONAL AND ENVIRONMENTAL ASPECTS IN THE EVALUATION AND TREATMENT OF ME/CFS

A specific nutrient deficiency has not been identified as a cause of ME/CFS. However, several studies demonstrate the presence of metabolic abnormalities,[68, 69] which can be worsened by the deficit of nutrients that act as cofactors in metabolic pathways.

In addition, several factors may increase the risk of nutrient deficiency in ME/CFS patients. Some of them can be suspected after completing a detailed medical history and/or a thorough physical exam. Still, due to this population's heterogeneity, we recommend objectively evaluating the patient's nutritional status, using laboratory tests to identify nutrient deficiencies and possible etiologies.

15.2.1 RISK FACTORS FOR NUTRITIONAL DEFICIENCIES IN PATIENTS WITH ME/CFS

Socio-economic: A recent study sponsored by the Centers for Disease Control and Prevention (CDC)[94] reported that 74.9% of patients with ME/CFS were unemployed, and 69.9% were disabled. Another study found that only 13% of patients maintained full-time employment, and 25% were house- or bedbound.[73] Food insecurity[35] (due to work-related impairment, job loss, or unemployment) and decreased energy for grocery shopping and meal preparation[90] may affect these patients' food intake and access to nutrient-dense foods.

Long-term use of medication: Patients with ME/CFS usually take medications chronically to manage their symptoms. Certain medications may impact the patient's metabolic status, increasing the need for particular nutrients, resulting in subclinical and clinically relevant nutrient deficiencies.[64, 104]

Inflammation: The acute and chronic inflammation present in ME/CFS may cause nutrient deficiencies due to abnormal absorption or metabolism[76] and increased nutrient allocation to the activated immune system.[36] Reciprocally, abnormal nutrient levels can contribute to immune dysfunction.[3, 8, 37, 44, 81]

Gastrointestinal dysfunction: The digestion and absorption of nutrients may be affected by the following disorders observed in ME/CFS:

Dysbiosis is the change of the commensal microbiota relative to the community found in healthy individuals and has been associated with an abnormal immune response towards environmental and self-antigens.[74, 99] Dysbiosis has been described in patients with ME/CFS, including reduction or loss of beneficial bacteria, small intestinal bacterial overgrowth (SIBO), increase of potentially pathogenic bacteria [55] and loss of microbiota diversity.[39]

Impaired gastrointestinal mucosal integrity[66] and *microbial translocation* may cause an increased antigenic exposure (food particles or bacteria) to the gastrointestinal immune tissue, which could result in loss of oral tolerance and immune activation,[39] developing food allergies and sensitivities. Ghali et al. reported that the frequency of food sensitivities increased with the severity of post-exertional malaise (PEM) in patients with ME/CFS, present in up to 11% of patients with very severe PEM,[38] possibly due to worsening immune dysfunction in severe disease.

Dysautonomia affecting the enteric nervous system causes motility issues (nausea, dysphagia, gastroesophageal reflux, gastroparesis, constipation, diarrhea) and abnormal secretion of digestive enzymes.[11, 14] These result in malabsorption, abdominal discomfort, bloating and pain. Patients with ME/CFS may reduce their food intake to avoid these symptoms.

Dental and orofacial problems. Patients with ME/CFS report xerostomia, dental caries, periodontal disease, bruxism, temporomandibular joint disorder and impacted third molar teeth.[80] These issues may affect food intake, mastication and digestion.

Tube feeding: Severely affected patients may need tube feeding due to severe nausea or dysphagia.[80]

Eating disorders: Pendergrast compared characteristics of housebound and non-housebound ME/CFS patients and found a prevalence of eating disorders in 4.8% and 4.4%, respectively.[73]

15.2.2 ENVIRONMENTAL EXPOSURE

Some cases of ME/CFS are precipitated by or occur after toxic exposure.[80] Glutathione deficiency is observed in patients exposed to water-damaged buildings, mold and mycotoxins and is associated with mitochondrial damage. Also, these patients are frequently deficient in nutrients necessary to support detoxification pathways. Deficiencies in vitamin D, magnesium, zinc, coenzyme Q10 and B vitamins have been reported.[45]

15.2.3 GENETIC PREDISPOSITION

Several studies have reported the association of single nucleotide polymorphisms (SNPs) with the metabolism and bioavailability of nutrients,[4, 64, 89] in some cases affecting their absorption or increasing the needed concentration. This may result in nutrient deficiency, especially during increased metabolic states, like the chronic inflammation present in ME/CFS. However, our literature search did not identify recent studies that evaluate the prevalence of SNPs associated with nutrient metabolism in patients with ME/CFS.

15.2.4 NUTRITIONAL EVALUATION OF PATIENTS WITH ME/CFS

ME/CFS is a condition known to be precipitated by various triggers and involves the malfunction of several interconnected body systems. A methodical evaluation of these patients should identify the clinical cause of a nutrient deficiency and help create a customized therapeutic intervention. Once a nutrient deficiency is identified, we should correct it and address its cause to break the dysfunction cycle. The factors detailed earlier illustrate that patients with ME/CFS are at higher risk for malnutrition and nutrient deficiencies. Jones and Probst (2017) found that 95% of patients with ME/CFS had low fiber intake, and 70% consumed unhealthy levels of fat, vegetables and fruit.[49]

The clinical evaluation of these patients should include obtaining information from their medical histories to identify factors that predisposed them to nutrient deficiencies and factors that precipitated or maintain dysfunction. The clinician may use patient recall, food journals, surveys or other instruments to assess these risk factors. This information can be obtained during the intake visit or more passively retrieved using electronic medical record tools, online instruments, or mobile apps like PhenX, Living matrix and My Fitness Pal.[42, 62, 72]

The physical exam may also provide clues to malnutrition or dietary deficits. Calculating the patient's body mass index (BMI) and measuring body composition to determine the fat and lean mass percentage will give objective measurements to assess risk and need for intervention.[46, 75] Also, nutrient deficiencies can cause changes in the skin, nails and hair, and other organ abnormalities. However, due to this population's heterogeneity, we recommend that the clinical evaluation of a patient with ME/CFS include an objective nutritional status evaluation, with the measurement of biomarkers to identify the presence of malnutrition and nutrient deficiencies. These biomarkers will allow the intervention to be personalized according to the patient's clinical phenotype. Also, these test results can help identify other conditions that may develop after the ME/CFS diagnosis. Providing documentation of abnormal laboratory results will help communicate the need for further testing to other clinicians. For example, a referral to a gastroenterologist for an upper and lower endoscopy is appropriate for a ME/CFS patient with a newly diagnosed iron-deficiency anemia refractory to iron replacement and without objective blood loss.

15.2.5 NUTRITIONAL DEFICIENCIES FOUND IN PATIENTS WITH ME/CFS

Studies that evaluated the frequency of nutrient deficiency in patients with ME/CFS found the following deficiencies.

Joustra et al. completed a meta-analysis of studies evaluating nutritional deficiencies in patients with ME/CFS. They identified studies showing a significantly lower level of vitamin B1, manganese and vitamin A in patients with ME/CFS versus controls. No significant difference was identified in the levels of vitamin B12, folic acid, iron, magnesium, molybdenum, phosphorus, sodium, iodine, potassium or selenium in patients with ME/CFS[53] However, the authors acknowledge issues with the quality and heterogeneity of the studies included. The evaluation did not include genomic variations that may affect the patients' nutrient requirements, where tissue deficiencies are not reflected by serum level concentrations.

> **Essential fatty acids:** Higher omega 6 polyunsaturated fatty acids (PUFAs) (linoleic and arachidonic acid) and mono-unsaturated fatty acids (MUFAs) (oleic acid), as well as a lower omega 3/omega 6 ratio, have been reported in ME/CFS compared with controls. The severity of illness was found to positively correlate with linoleic, arachidonic and oleic acid levels.[49] Castro-Marrero et al. found a low omega-3 index in 92.6% of the ME/CFS patients studied, suggesting a pro-inflammatory state and a possible increased risk to cardiovascular health.[18]
>
> **Vitamin D** has an immunomodulatory action, decreasing autoimmunity and chronic inflammation (promoting dendritic cell and regulatory T-cell differentiation, and reducing T helper (Th) 17 cell response and inflammatory cytokines secretion).[81]. Patients with chronic pain and fibromyalgia are at higher risk for vitamin D deficiency than healthy controls.[53] Jones and Prost reported a suboptimal level of vitamin D in 60% of patients with ME/CFS compared with controls,[49] and Witham et al.'s RCT (randomized control trial) study in patients with ME/CFS found a (deficient) baseline 25-hydroxy vitamin D level of 18 ng/mL.[102] Two studies found a significantly higher visual analog score for pain in patients with ME/CFS and vitamin D deficiency.[53]
>
> **Coenzyme Q10 (Ubiquinol)** is an essential factor for cellular energy production and antioxidant activity. Decreased levels have been reported in patients with ME/CFS compared with healthy controls.[15]

Based on our clinical experience, we recommend a comprehensive initial laboratory evaluation to measure vitamins (Thiamine-B1, Riboflavin-B2, Niacin-B3, Pyridoxine-B6, folic acid, Cobalamin-B12, Biotin (Vitamin B7)IBO, A, C, D, E, K), minerals (magnesium, manganese, molybdenum, iron, zinc, copper, iodine, selenium), antioxidants/cofactors (alpha-lipoic acid, coQ10), essential fatty acids and amino acids. We also recommend the measurement of toxic elements (lead, arsenic, mercury, cadmium and aluminum) and mycotoxins. Follow-up laboratory tests should be ordered and tailored to monitor the resolution of previously identified deficiencies or toxic exposures.

A patient's medical history may support the use of tests to evaluate the gastrointestinal function (celiac disease, food intolerance, allergy and non-IgE mediated sensitivity, markers for intestinal malabsorption, inflammatory bowel disease, SIBO and tests to evaluate gastrointestinal dysmotility). Also, some patients may have been exposed to non-metal toxins, some of which can be tested for by commercial laboratories (atmospheric pollutants, food preservatives, hormonal disruptors, agricultural pesticides and pharmaceutical excipients).[10]

In patients who have refractory nutrient deficiencies, a strong family history of ME/CFS or autoimmunity, or severe impairment, consider genomic testing to evaluate SNPs that may affect nutrient bioavailability. For example, the level of vitamin D in the serum varies after supplementation, dependent upon the presence of CYP2R1, CYP24A1 or VDR SNP variations.[4] Other studies identified 59 vitamin B-12-related gene polymorphisms associated with vitamin B12 status[89] and serum magnesium levels.[63] There are commercially available clinical decision support systems that help the clinician identify SNPs relevant to the patient's case.[48]

15.2.6 Nutritional Therapeutic Approach

Joustra et al. report that 35–68% of patients with ME/CFS and fibromyalgia take nutritional supplements. There is no evidence of a nutrient deficiency as a sole etiology of ME/CFS.[53] There is some evidence of nutritional interventions improving fatigue and other symptoms, but not sustained recovery[15]. However, the available studies have limitations in the sample size, study duration, diversity of instruments used, and quality. In our ME/CFS clinical practice, we frequently identify nutrient deficiencies, and the targeted replenishment of a nutrient deficiency, identified by testing, may result in significant fatigue improvement. There is a need for large, higher-quality studies that evaluate the prevalence of nutrient deficiencies in ME/CFS. Some efforts are underway to standardize the data collection of ME/CFS studies (NINDS Common Data elements)[88] and create an ME/CFS registry.[61] Some studies have reported the effect of nutritional interventions in ME/CFS. Patients who received hydroxocobalamin, an active form of vitamin B12, had significant improvement of fatigue and well-being, not observed with cyanocobalamin.[16] Another study found a benefit in the use of parenteral vitamin B12 (hydroxo- or methylcobalamin) and oral folic acid, with the most favorable response in a subgroup according to methylenetetrahydrofolate reductase status (C677T and A1298C).[78] Therapy with vitamin D for 6 months increased the serum vitamin D levels in patients with ME/CFS, but there were no changes in fatigue or depression. [53] Treatment with amitriptyline and magnesium citrate improved fatigue and pain more effectively than amitriptyline alone.[53] Oral nicotinamide adenine dinucleotide hydride (NADH) supplementation improved fatigue symptoms and reduced anxiety at 3 months.[16] A combination of NADH and coenzyme Q10 improved perception of fatigue and resulted in a significant reduction in the maximum heart rate during the exercise test.[17] Also, there was a therapeutic benefit on fatigue levels with the supplementation of high cocoa polyphenol–rich chocolate[15], d-ribose and omega-3 fatty acids.[49]

Patients with ME/CFS are a heterogeneous population at risk for nutrient deficiencies. Stratifying these patients by subgroups, based on history, physical exam and the objective biomarkers obtained during testing, is helpful to personalize the intervention according to the patient's metabolic, genomic and environmental phenotype. We encourage the patient to incorporate unprocessed foods that contain the needed nutrients as much as possible. However, the patient may have intolerance or sensitivity to these foods or other digestive issues that affect motility and absorption. In these situations, using a supplement in the form of a capsule or tablet may provide the needed nutrient without incurring the negative consequences of digesting a food in which this nutrient is found.

In some cases, there is no change in the laboratory results after nutrient supplementation, which may indicate an issue with nutrient absorption. In our experience, some patients may benefit from adding digestive enzymes, especially with lipid-soluble nutrients like vitamin D and essential fatty acids. Some patients absorb or tolerate other formulations better (liquid, powder, chewable, parenteral, nebulized or intranasal). If the patient reports an adverse reaction to a nutritional supplement, consider that the patient may be sensitive to excipients present in that product and may need to try a different brand or route of administration.

The correction of nutrient deficiencies should not be isolated. The clinician should manage the patient's expectations. There is no magic supplement that will resolve all the patient's symptoms. Other interventions are necessary to create an infrastructure for a healthy lifestyle (nutrient-rich diet, adequate sleep, effective stress management and some degree of physical activity – as tolerated). Correcting only one dysfunction while others still exist will not result in a steady or consistent improvement. In addition to advocating for foundational lifestyle factors, the clinician should also progressively identify and treat other body systems' dysfunctions, such as toxic exposure, chronic infection, dysautonomia, autoimmunity and others that have been associated with ME/CFS. The persistence of any of these other factors will perpetuate a vicious cycle that affects nutrient bioavailability.

There are few studies evaluating the effect of dietary modifications on the symptoms of patients with ME/CFS.[15] Food sensitivity is frequent in the ME/CFS population. Eliminating the foods that trigger symptoms may decrease the gastrointestinal immune activation and improve digestive and immune symptoms. The foods most frequently associated with reactivity are gluten/grains, dairy,[49] eggs, soy, sugar and nightshades/high-histamine foods. To test for a suspected food sensitivity, ideally, the patient avoids the chosen food entirely for 3 weeks and then completes a reintroduction challenge. If the patient notices improvement of symptoms, and the symptoms recur after reintroducing the food, it is recommended to avoid this food for 3 to 6 months. We do not want to restrict the patient's diet for a prolonged time and may re-challenge when symptoms have improved. Sometimes, the patient reacts to several foods. In this case, commercial laboratory tests are helpful to recognize severe sensitivity and start with the avoidance of those foods.

ME/CFS patients with autoimmune features may benefit from avoiding lectin-containing foods,[98] especially during symptom relapse episodes. Also, calorie restriction, intermittent fasting and ketogenic diets may protect mitochondrial function.[23] It is, therefore, worth considering a trial of these dietary interventions.

In managing chronic diseases like ME/CFS, it is paramount that the healthcare provider recognizes the importance of evaluating the patient's nutritional status and has the training and skills to provide nutritional education that empowers patients and enhances their self-management skills.[25] Education is an essential tool to create a structure in the patients' lives that will empower them to choose foods that meet their dietary requirements, identify/avoid foods that they do not tolerate, and conserve sufficient energy for meal preparation. The use of teaching kitchens has proven useful in preparing patients for self-management.[25] Group educational activities help with engagement and accountability.[7] Members of the patient's support network should be included in these educational activities. It is also crucial to create a healthcare provider network to support the patient's efforts. Referring the patient to providers who use a whole person health approach, with integrative and functional medicine training, including a nutritionist, health coach, nurse, psychologist, and physical and occupational therapist, will create a sustainable healthcare structure that will support the patient in between clinical visits.

15.3   AUTOIMMUNITY

Autoimmune disease may manifest with multiple unspecific symptoms in different body systems. These symptoms can overlap with the ME/CFS diagnostic criteria. It is recommended to look for markers for chronic inflammation and autoantibodies during the initial evaluation of a patient complaining of chronic fatigue and pain. Once the ME/CFS diagnosis has been established, we recommend testing autoantibodies for known autoimmune conditions periodically (at least yearly), as the patient may have been diagnosed with ME/CFS in an early stage of an autoimmune disease. We have observed cases that presented positive autoantibodies and symptoms compatible with conditions like systemic lupus erythematosus (SLE) and rheumatoid arthritis (RA) years after an ME/CFS diagnosis with negative titers.

Some patients with ME/CFS may have positive autoantibody titers but do not meet the criteria for the diagnosis of an established autoimmune pathology; therefore, they do not qualify for the standard of care therapeutics. Antibodies against nuclear and membrane structures and neurotransmitter receptors have been reported in ME/CFS.[87] The presence of autoantibodies indicates immune dysfunction, and there is a need for clinical trials that evaluate the correlation of the antibody presence and dysfunction before permanent end-organ damage occurs. Integrative and functional medicine approaches are fundamental to the treatment of these patients, who are on a continuum. One end is a frank, autoimmune disease, and the other end is being symptom free. The closer they are to the disease end, the easier it is for unanticipated factors (like infections or stress) to trigger a relapse or crisis period. Lifestyle changes can contribute to decreased immune reactivity and chronic inflammation and keep the patients closer to the symptom-free end of the spectrum. Clinicians should provide guidance and implement interventions to achieve restorative sleep, exercise, physical activity as tolerated, a low-inflammatory diet and avoidance of foods that cause immune reactivity. Clinicians should provide stress and trauma management, and support efforts to create a social network which provides the patients with a sense of connection and purpose.

There is evidence to suggest a clinically phenotypic subgroup of ME/CFS patients in whom autoimmunity is the main pathophysiological mechanism.[87] Fluge et al. used Rituximab to achieve B-cell depletion and decrease autoantibody production in ME/CFS patients. In earlier studies (a single-arm and an RCT with a small sample), approximately 60% of patients experienced a variable degree of clinical remission.[28, 30] However, in a recent RCT with a larger sample (n = 151), there was not a significant difference between the Rituximab treatment and control groups for levels of fatigue and function.[29] However, these results could have been due to the heterogeneity of ME/CFS patients enrolled in the trial. A clinical trial that uses Rituximab on ME/CFS patients with an autoimmune clinical phenotype could provide more information about the disease etiology.

Loebel et al.'s observations [60] may support this hypothesis and explain the dysautonomia symptoms in some patients. They identified anti-G protein-coupled receptor autoantibodies to the autonomic nervous system in patients with ME/CFS.[101] Moreover, ME/CFS patients reported symptom improvement after immunoadsorption to remove autoantibodies against $\beta2$-adrenergic receptors.[82, 93] Other immunosuppressants have been used for therapy. Rekeland et al. completed an open-label phase II trial giving intravenous cyclophosphamide to patients with ME/CFS.[79] They reported significant fatigue improvement, increased physical activity and up to 68% of remission after 4 years of treatment. Patients with positive HLA-DQB1*03:03 and/or HLA-C*07:04 had a significantly higher response rate.

Identifying an ME/CFS subgroup with a predominant autoimmune etiology could help clinicians start targeted therapies earlier. Low-dose naltrexone (LDN) has an immunomodulatory effect, decreasing chronic inflammation, increasing immune tolerance and modulating microglial activation.[92, 103] In our clinical practice, we have observed the benefit of LDN in pain and fatigue; however, not all patients respond to it. LDN could be eliciting a favorable response in patients of the autoimmune subgroup. Larger studies are needed to measure autonomic autoantibodies in healthy controls and patients with other autoimmune conditions, including testing for genetic variants associated with autoimmunity. Further clinical trials that evaluate targeted immunotherapy in the subgroup of ME/CFS patients with autoimmune antibodies are needed.

15.4   DYSAUTONOMIA

Dysautonomia is frequently found in ME/CFS patients and is a cause of multiple symptoms. An objective evaluation to document the presence of autonomic dysfunction is recommended. Consider including the NASA 10-minute lean test or a tilt-table test and taking a skin biopsy for small fiber neuropathy. Symptoms associated with orthostatic intolerance, gastrointestinal motility issues and temperature dysregulation should all be documented.

15.4.1   ANTIBODIES AGAINST THE AUTONOMIC NERVOUS SYSTEM

As mentioned in the autoimmunity section, there is evidence of autoimmune neurosensory dysautonomia: Autoantibodies against the $\beta2$-adrenergic receptors and M1, M3 and M4 muscarinic acetylcholine receptors are found in patients with ME/CFS.[101] The removal of these antibodies by immunoadsorption seems to be a promising therapy.[52, 57] Testing for these antibodies is available commercially.[19, 58]

15.4.2 SMALL FIBER NEUROPATHY (SFN)

Recent observations by Dr. Oaklander and Dr. Systrom's research group reported a 30% (definite) and 13% probable frequency of SFN in patients with ME/CFS and low biventricular cardiac filling pressures during exercise.[52, 86] The depressed cardiac output from impaired venous return and impaired peripheral oxygen extraction could explain the presence of post-exertional intolerance in ME/CFS. Also, 31% of these patients had biopsies consistent with SFN, which could contribute to oxygenated blood shunting from capillary beds due to neuropathic dysregulation.[52] Intravenous immunoglobulin therapy has been used in the therapy of SFN with response rates of 77% to 83%.[86] There is an ongoing study to evaluate the exercise response to pyridostigmine in ME/CFS patients diagnosed with cardiac preload cardiac.[21] Dr. Oaklander's work outlines the specific standards for the evaluation and biopsy for SFN to avoid false-negative results.[22, 71]

15.4.3 CRANIOCERVICAL INSTABILITY (CCI) AND MAST CELL ACTIVATION

Clinicians who specialize in the management of ME/CFS have observed that craniocervical instability can be a comorbidity in patients with dysautonomia. Bragee et al. evaluated ME/CFS patients and found 50% of the patients exhibited hypermotility, 73% exhibited positive signs of possible intracranial hypertension by brain magnetic resonance imaging (MRI) and 80% exhibited craniocervical obstruction of the cervical spine as detected by MRI.[12]

Craniocervical instability (CCI) may be associated with cervical medullary syndrome symptoms such as headache, vertigo, difficulties with speech, hearing, swallowing and balance, and dysautonomia.[26] All of these symptoms have been reported by ME/CFS patients as well. It is possible that chronic immune dysfunction caused by autoimmunity,[57] chronic inflammation,[1] toxic exposure[2, 100] and other factors could increase the laxity of cervical ligaments over time in patients with or without Ehlers–Danlos Syndrome (EDS). We also have observed in our practice that mast cell activation is a frequent comorbidity in patients with CCI. Mast cells release vasoactive, angiogenic and profibrotic chemicals in response to hypoxia, mechanical stimulation, or neurological and inflammatory mediators.[84] An increase in the number of mast cells in tendinopathy biopsies has been described.[6, 84] Also, mast cell–derived prostaglandin E2 (PGE2) has been found to reduce collagen synthesis and enhance the expression and activity of metalloproteinases in human tendon fibroblasts.[6, 24] Future studies are needed to evaluate the effects of these factors on the progression of CCI in patients with ME/CFS and therapeutic interventions to prevent it.

Based on current evidence, we recommend neurological imaging evaluation to evaluate for CCI and neurosurgery referral if needed[43] in ME/CFS patients suspected of having hypermobility/EDS or whose dysautonomia symptoms do not respond to standard therapeutic interventions.

15.4.4 REDUCED CEREBRAL BLOOD FLOW

Van Campen et al.[96] measured cerebral blood flow of ME/CFS patients with orthostatic intolerance symptoms during a 30-minute head-up tilt test measured by Doppler flow imaging of the carotid and vertebral arteries. They found a reduction of cerebral blood flow of 90% in ME/CFS patients during orthostatic testing (some had a delayed response). There was a significant linear correlation between orthostatic intolerance symptoms and reduced cerebral blood flow.

15.5 INFECTIONS

ME/CFS symptoms may start after an infection (viral or bacterial) with a subgroup of patients presenting chronic flu-like symptoms. Some hypotheses about ME/CFS etiology postulate that chronic infection may perpetuate the symptoms associated with chronic inflammation and immune dysfunction.[51] A recent study found that subjective sickness behavior in ME/CFS patients was similar to patients injected experimentally with bacterial endotoxin at peak inflammation.[50] The initial evaluation of ME/CFS patients should include testing for pathogens including Epstein–Barr virus (EBV),[85] human herpesvirus 6 (HHV-6), cytomegalovirus (CMV), human parvovirus B19 and intracellular bacteria. Other infections like Lyme disease should be ruled out. Some patients present with persistent viral-like symptoms and serology indicating chronic viral reactivation.[77] [87] Schreiner et al. observed that human herpesvirus 6 reactivation induced mitochondrial fragmentation and dysfunction in vitro,[83] which may be the link between chronic viral reactivation and mitochondrial cell-danger response that causes ME/CFS symptoms.

An ongoing study at the National Institutes of Health (NIH) is focused on ME/CFS subsequent to known infection compared with post-Lyme disease and healthy control groups.[41] This study will provide valuable information about ME/CFS occurring after an initial infection. The Open Medicine Foundation (OMF) is sponsoring a study to evaluate herpes simplex encephalopathy and the development of ME/CFS.[31]

More recently, there have been reports of patients who have persistent illness after SARS-CoV-2 infection (mild/moderate and severe)[5] without an obvious organ injury.[56] They are called "Long-Haulers" in the community or post-acute sequelae of SARS-CoV-2 infection (PASC) by the NIH. Some of these patients present symptoms similar to ME/CFS, indicating a possible pathophysiology overlap,[56] and may benefit from treatment approaches used for this condition.[59] The NIH and other funding agencies are sponsoring studies to evaluate these patients with post-viral fatigue, which will hopefully provide valuable information about the pathophysiology, diagnosis and treatment of PASC and ME/CFS.

15.6   SLEEP/PAIN/NEUROINFLAMMATION

Unrefreshing sleep is a criterion in the diagnosis of ME/CFS. Gotts et al. evaluated 343 ME/CFS patients and found that 30% met diagnostic criteria for obstructive sleep apnea (OSA) and periodic limb movement (PLM) disorder. Moreover, they found that 89.1% of patients without OSA or PLM had quantitative evidence of insomnia or hypersomnia, with four specific sleep phenotypes by polysomnography.[40] We recommend a referral to sleep medicine for polysomnography during the initial evaluation of a patient with ME/CFS.

Patients with ME/CFS report musculoskeletal pain frequently. An ongoing study sponsored by the Open Medicine Foundation (OMF) is evaluating skeletal muscle dysfunction in ME/CFS[32] To evaluate PEM, muscle biopsy samples are being taken at rest and during recovery from exercise. Morikawa et al. found that compression at myofascial neck trigger points significantly reduced subjective musculoskeletal pain relief via prefrontal cortex activity and reduction of sympathetic activity (which exacerbates chronic pain).[65] Van Campen et al. found that the pressure pain threshold (the degree of pressure required before the individual experiences pain) in patients with ME/CFS (with or without fibromyalgia) decreased after head-up tilt testing.[95]

Recent studies have provided imaging evidence of central nervous system changes in ME/CFS. Thapaliya et al. found increased T1weighted/T2weighted ratio values (to assess tissue microstructure integrity) in ME/CFS patients' brain MRIs. These results indicate increased myelin and/or iron levels in both white and subcortical gray matter and basal ganglia.[91] Similar findings have been described in neurodegenerative diseases. Mueller et al. used whole-brain magnetic resonance spectroscopy to look for metabolite and temperature markers for neuroinflammation in ME/CFS patients. They identified abnormal metabolic ratios (choline/creatine in the left anterior cingulate) that correlated with fatigue levels and a significant increase in the temperature of several brain regions (right insula, putamen, frontal cortex, thalamus and cerebellum) in ME/CFS patients.[67] There is also evidence of abnormalities of the functional connectivity within the brainstem and with other brain regions.[70] Further clinical trials are needed to identify specific neuroimaging changes in ME/CFS and their underlying causes.

15.7 HORMONES

Gender differences have been observed in ME/CFS, with women being predominantly affected.[27] However, no specific hormonal pattern has yet been identified. We recommend a comprehensive hormone profile evaluation during the initial visit. It should include cortisol levels, a thyroid hormone profile, insulin resistance markers and sex hormones to rule out endocrine/exocrine insufficiency or dysfunction. Patients with frank hormonal abnormalities should be referred to a specialist for evaluation. If a patient has borderline hormonal abnormalities, the clinician should address lifestyle factors and environmental exposures that may affect these results before considering hormonal replacement therapy.

15.8 INTEGRATIVE TREATMENT MODALITIES

Mind-body interventions have been shown to improve fatigue severity, depression and anxiety symptoms, and quality of life in patients with ME/CFS. These include mindfulness-based stress reduction, mindfulness-based cognitive therapy, relaxation, Qigong, cognitive-behavioral stress management, acceptance and commitment therapy, and isometric yoga.[54]

15.9 CONCLUSION

ME/CFS is a complex multi-symptom condition that affects several body systems. Current clinical and research observations point to possible clinical phenotypes or subgroups with different main physiopathologic mechanisms.[10] Clinicians evaluating ME/CFS patients should complete a comprehensive clinical evaluation of all the body systems, identify which system is more likely to be driving the mechanism of disease, and start therapies to address it. Then, they can incorporate other interventions gradually, starting with low doses (nutrients, supplements or medications) and increasing them slowly, as tolerated by the patient. ME/CFS patients frequently have chemical sensitivities and may report side effects to medications, supplements and/or alternative therapies.

ME/CFS is a chronic condition that is challenging to manage for both the patient and the treating clinician. The clinician should support these patients, teach them self-management skills to identify triggers and symptoms of dysfunction, and intervene early to avoid relapse. There has been a recent increase in research funding for ME/CFS, and there are several promising clinical trials that could help elucidate the etiology and management of this disease.

REFERENCES

1. Abate, M., et al., 2009, Pathogenesis of tendinopathies: inflammation or degeneration? *Arthritis Res Ther*, **11**(3): p. 235.
2. Akpinar, H.A., H. Kahraman, and I. Yaman, 2019, Ochratoxin A sequentially activates autophagy and the ubiquitin-proteasome system. *Toxins*, **11**(11).
3. Avery, J.C. and P.R. Hoffmann, 2018, Selenium, selenoproteins, and immunity. *Nutrients*, **10**(9).
4. Barry, E.L., et al., 2014, Genetic variants in CYP2R1, CYP24A1, and VDR modify the efficacy of vitamin D3 supplementation for increasing serum 25-hydroxyvitamin D levels in a randomized controlled trial. *J Clin Endocrinol Metab*, **99**(10): p. E2133–7.
5. Bateman, L., et al., 2021, Myalgic encephalomyelitis/chronic fatigue syndrome: essentials of diagnosis and management. *Mayo Clin Proc*, **96**(11): p. 2861–2878.
6. Behzad, H., et al., 2013, Mast cells exert pro-inflammatory effects of relevance to the pathophyisology of tendinopathy. *Arthritis Res Ther*, **15**(6): p. R184.
7. Beidelschies, M., Association of a shared medical appointment program focused on nutrition and lifestyle interventions with patient-reported health-related quality of life and biometric outcomes, in Institute for Functional Medicine 2020 Annual International Conference. 2020.
8. Bird, R.P., 2018, The emerging role of vitamin B6 in inflammation and carcinogenesis. *Adv Food Nutr Res*, **83**: p. 151–194.

9. Bjorklund, G., et al., 2019, Chronic fatigue syndrome (CFS): suggestions for a nutritional treatment in the therapeutic approach. *Biomed Pharmacother*, **109**: p. 1000–1007.

10. Blitshteyn, S. and P. Chopra, 2018, Chronic fatigue syndrome: from chronic fatigue to more specific syndromes. *Eur Neurol*, **80**(1–2): p. 73–77.

11. Bonaz, B., T. Bazin, and S. Pellissier, 2018, The vagus nerve at the interface of the microbiota-gut-brain axis. *Front Neurosci*, **12**: p. 49.

12. Bragee, B., et al., 2020, Signs of intracranial hypertension, hypermobility, and craniocervical obstructions in patients with myalgic encephalomyelitis/chronic fatigue syndrome. *Front Neurol*, **11**: p. 828.

13. Brown, B.I., 2014, Chronic fatigue syndrome: a personalized integrative medicine approach. *Altern Ther Health Med*, **20**(1): p. 29–40.

14. Camilleri, M., Gastrointestinal function, in *Primer on the Autonomic Nervous System*, D.R.I. Biaggioni, Editor. 2012, Elsevier: London, UK.

15. Campagnolo, N., et al., 2017, Dietary and nutrition interventions for the therapeutic treatment of chronic fatigue syndrome/myalgic encephalomyelitis: a systematic review. *J Hum Nutr Diet*, **30**(3): p. 247–259.

16. Castro-Marrero, J., et al., 2017, Treatment and management of chronic fatigue syndrome/myalgic encephalomyelitis: all roads lead to Rome. *Br J Pharmacol*, **174**(5): p. 345–369.

17. Castro-Marrero, J., et al., 2016, Effect of coenzyme Q10 plus nicotinamide adenine dinucleotide supplementation on maximum heart rate after exercise testing in chronic fatigue syndrome - A randomized, controlled, double-blind trial. *Clin Nutr*, **35**(4): p. 826–34.

18. Castro-Marrero, J., et al., 2018, Low omega-3 index and polyunsaturated fatty acid status in patients with chronic fatigue syndrome/myalgic encephalomyelitis. *Prostaglandins Leukot Essent Fatty Acids*, **139**: p. 20–24.

19. Celltrend, *POTS-CFS/ME-CRPS-SFN Diagnostics*. Available from: https://www.celltrend.de/en/pots -cfs-me-crps/.

20. Chu, L., et al., 2021, Identifying and managing suicidality in myalgic encephalomyelitis/chronic fatigue syndrome. *Healthcare*, **9**(6).

21. ClinicalTrials.gov, *The Exercise Response to Pharmacologic Cholinergic Stimulation in Myalgic Encephalomyelitis/Chronic Fatigue Syndrome*. 2020; Available from: https://clinicaltrials.gov/ct2/show /NCT03674541.

22. Commons, N., *Getting a Diagnostic Skin Biopsy*. Available from: https://neuropathycommons.org/get -tested/skin-biopsy.

23. Craig, C., 2015, Mitoprotective dietary approaches for myalgic encephalomyelitis/chronic fatigue syndrome: Caloric restriction, fasting, and ketogenic diets. *Med Hypotheses*, **85**(5): p. 690–3.

24. Del Buono, A., et al., 2013, Metalloproteases and tendinopathy. *Muscles Ligaments Tendons J*, **3**(1): p. 51–7.

25. Eisenberg, D.M. and J.D. Burgess, 2015, Nutrition education in an era of global obesity and diabetes: Thinking outside the box. *Acad Med*, **90**(7): p. 854–60.

26. F.C., H., 2016, Cranio-cervical instability in patients with hypermobility connective disorders. *Journal of Spine*, **5**(2).

27. Faro, M., et al., 2016, Gender differences in chronic fatigue syndrome. *Reumatol Clin*, **12**(2): p. 72–7.

28. Fluge, O., et al., 2011, Benefit from B-lymphocyte depletion using the anti-CD20 antibody rituximab in chronic fatigue syndrome. A double-blind and placebo-controlled study. *PLoS One*, **6**(10): p. e26358.

29. Fluge, O., et al., 2019, B-lymphocyte depletion in patients with myalgic encephalomyelitis/chronic fatigue syndrome: A randomized, double-blind, placebo-controlled trial. *Ann Intern Med*, **170**(9): p. 585–593.

30. Fluge, O., et al., 2015, B-lymphocyte depletion in myalgic encephalopathy/ chronic fatigue syndrome. An open-label phase II study with rituximab maintenance treatment. *PLoS One*, **10**(7): p. e0129898.

31. Foundation, O.M., *Herpes Simplex Encephalopathy and the Development of ME/CFS*. Available from: https://www.omf.ngo/herpes-simplex-encephalopathy-and-the-development-of-me-cfs/.

32. Foundation, O.M., *Skeletal Muscle Dysfunction Research*. Available from: https://www.omf.ngo/skel-etal-muscle-dysfunction-research/.

33. Friedman, K.J., 2019, Advances in ME/CFS: Past, present, and future. *Front Pediatr*, **7**(131).

34. Fukuda, K., Straus, S.E., Hickie, I., Sharpe, M.C., Dobbins, J.G., and Komaroff, A. T 1994, The chronic fatigue syndrome: a comprehensive approach to its definition and study. International Chronic Fatigue Syndrome Study Group. *Ann Intern Med*, **12**: p. 953–959.

35. Fuller-Thomson, E., R. Mehta, and J. Sulman, 2013, Long-term parental unemployment in childhood and subsequent chronic fatigue syndrome. *ISRN Family Med*, **2013**: p. 978250.

36. Furman, D., et al., 2019, Chronic inflammation in the etiology of disease across the life span. *Nat Med*, **25**(12): p. 1822–1832.

37. Gammoh, N.Z. and L. Rink, 2017, Zinc in Infection and Inflammation. *Nutrients*, **9**(6).

38. Ghali, A., et al., 2020, Epidemiological and clinical factors associated with post-exertional malaise severity in patients with myalgic encephalomyelitis/chronic fatigue syndrome. *J Transl Med*, **18**(1): p. 246.

39. Giloteaux, L., et al., 2016, Reduced diversity and altered composition of the gut microbiome in individuals with myalgic encephalomyelitis/chronic fatigue syndrome. *Microbiome*, **4**(1): p. 30.

40. Gotts, Z.M., et al., 2013, Are there sleep-specific phenotypes in patients with chronic fatigue syndrome? A cross-sectional polysomnography analysis. *BMJ Open*, **3**(6).

41. Health, N.I.o., *NIH Intramural Study on Myalgic Encephalomyelitis/Chronic Fatigue Syndrome.* Available from: https://mecfs.ctss.nih.gov/.

42. Health, N.I.o., n.d., *PhenX Toolkit – Nutrition and Dietary Supplements*; Available from: https://www.phenxtoolkit.org/domains/view/50000.

43. Henderson Sr., F.C., et al., 2019, Cervical medullary syndrome secondary to craniocervical instability and ventral brainstem compression in hereditary hypermobility connective tissue disorders: 5-year follow-up after craniocervical reduction, fusion, and stabilization. *Neurosurg Rev*, **42**(4): p. 915–936.

44. Hewison, M., 2012, Vitamin D and immune function: an overview. *Proc Nutr Soc*, **71**(1): p. 50–61.

45. Hope, J., 2013, A review of the mechanism of injury and treatment approaches for illness resulting from exposure to water-damaged buildings, mold, and mycotoxins. *ScientificWorldJournal*, **2013**: p. 767482.

46. Hoskin, L., et al., 2000, Bone density and body composition in young women with chronic fatigue syndrome. *Ann N Y Acad Sci*, **904**: p. 625–7.

47. Institute-of-Medicine, *Beyond Myalgic Encephalomyelitis/Chronic Fatigue Syndrome: Redefining an illness.* 2015, National Academies Press, Washington, DC.

48. IntellxxDNA, n.d., *IntellxxDNA – Clinicians*; Available from: https://www.intellxxdna.com/clinicians/.

49. Jones, K. and Y. Probst, 2017, Role of dietary modification in alleviating chronic fatigue syndrome symptoms: a systematic review. *Aust N Z J Public Health*, **41**(4): p. 338–344.

50. Jonsjo, M.A., et al., 2020, Patients with ME/CFS (Myalgic Encephalomyelitis/Chronic Fatigue Syndrome) and chronic pain report similar level of sickness behavior as individuals injected with bacterial endotoxin at peak inflammation. *Brain Behav Immun*, **2**: p. 100028.

51. Jonsjo, M.A., et al., 2020, The role of low-grade inflammation in ME/CFS (myalgic encephalomyelitis/chronic fatigue syndrome) - associations with symptoms. *Psychoneuroendocrinology*, **113**: p. 104578.

52. Joseph, P., et al., 2021, Insights from invasive cardiopulmonary exercise testing of patients with myalgic encephalomyelitis/chronic fatigue syndrome. *Chest*, **160**(2): p. 642–651.

53. Joustra, M.L., et al., 2017, Vitamin and mineral status in chronic fatigue syndrome and fibromyalgia syndrome: A systematic review and meta-analysis. *PLoS One*, **12**(4): p. e0176631.

54. Khanpour Ardestani, S., et al., 2021, Systematic Review of Mind-Body Interventions to Treat Myalgic Encephalomyelitis/Chronic Fatigue Syndrome. *Medicina*, **57**(7): p. 652.

55. Kirchgessner, A., The role of the microbiota and potential for dietary intervention in chronic fatigue syndrome, in *The Gut-Brain Axis: Dietary, Probiotic and Prebiotic Interventions on the Microbiota*, H. Stanton, Editor. 2016, Elsevier: London, UK.

56. Komaroff, A.L. and W.I. Lipkin, 2021, Insights from myalgic encephalomyelitis/chronic fatigue syndrome may help unravel the pathogenesis of postacute COVID-19 syndrome. *Trends Mol Med*, **27**(9): p. 895–906.

57. Konttinen, Y.T., et al., 1989, Atlantoaxial laxity in rheumatoid arthritis. *Acta Orthop Scand*, **60**(4): p. 379–82.

58. Laboratories, M., *Autoimmune Dysautonomia Evaluation.* Available from: https://www.mayocliniclabs.com/test-catalog/Overview/92121.

59. Lapp, C.W. and J.F. John, 2021, Managing COVID-19 post viral Fatigue Syndrome. *Fatigue: Biomedicine, Health & Behavior.*

60. Loebel, M., et al., 2016, Antibodies to beta adrenergic and muscarinic cholinergic receptors in patients with Chronic Fatigue Syndrome. *Brain Behav Immun*, **52**: p. 32–39.

61. M.E, S. You + ME, n.d.; Available from: https://solvecfs.org/you-me-registry/

62. Matrix, L. *Empowering Personalized, Therapeutic Partnerships to Effectively Address Chronic Conditions.* n.d.; Available from: https://livingmatrix.com/practitioners/.

63. Meyer, T.E., et al., 2010, Genome-wide association studies of serum magnesium, potassium, and sodium concentrations identify six Loci influencing serum magnesium levels. *PLoS Genet*, **6**(8).

64. Mohn, E.S., Kern, H.J., Saltzman, E., Mitmesser, S.H., & McKay, D.L., 2018, Evidence of drug-nutrient interactions with chronic use of commonly prescribed medications: an update. *Pharmaceutics*, **10**(1).

65. Morikawa, Y., et al., 2017, Compression at myofascial trigger point on chronic neck pain provides pain relief through the prefrontal cortex and autonomic nervous system: A pilot study. *Front Neurosci*, **11**: p. 186.

66. Morris, G., et al., 2019, Myalgic encephalomyelitis/chronic fatigue syndrome: From pathophysiological insights to novel therapeutic opportunities. *Pharmacol Res*, **148**: p. 104450.

67. Mueller, C., et al., 2020, Evidence of widespread metabolite abnormalities in Myalgic encephalomyelitis/chronic fatigue syndrome: assessment with whole-brain magnetic resonance spectroscopy. *Brain Imaging Behav*, **14**(2): p. 562–572.

68. Nagy-Szakal, D., et al., 2018, Insights into myalgic encephalomyelitis/chronic fatigue syndrome phenotypes through comprehensive metabolomics. *Sci Rep*, **8**(1): p. 10056.

69. Naviaux, R.K., et al., 2016, Metabolic features of chronic fatigue syndrome. *Proc Natl Acad Sci U S A*, **113**(37): p. E5472–80.

70. Nelson, T., et al., 2021, Brainstem abnormalities in myalgic encephalomyelitis/chronic fatigue syndrome: A scoping review and evaluation of magnetic resonance imaging findings. *Front Neurol*, **12**: p. 769511.

71. Oaklander, A.L. and M. Nolano, 2019, Scientific advances in and clinical approaches to small-fiber polyneuropathy: A review. *JAMA Neurol*.

72. MyFitnessPal, Inc. (2022). MyFitnessPal (Version 22.23.1) [Mobile app] Google Play App Store https://play.google.com/store/apps/details?id=com.myfitnesspal.android.

73. Pendergrast, T., et al., 2016, Housebound versus nonhousebound patients with myalgic encephalomyelitis and chronic fatigue syndrome. *Chronic Illn*, **12**(4): p. 292–307.

74. Petersen, C. and J.L. Round, 2014, Defining dysbiosis and its influence on host immunity and disease. *Cell Microbiol*, **16**(7): p. 1024–33.

75. Pietrangelo, T., et al., 2018, Old muscle in young body: an aphorism describing the Chronic Fatigue Syndrome. *Eur J Transl Myol*, **28**(3): p. 7688.

76. Raiten, D.J., et al., 2015, Inflammation and Nutritional Science for Programs/Policies and Interpretation of Research Evidence (INSPIRE). *J Nutr*, **145**(5): p. 1039S–1108S.

77. Rasa, S., et al., 2018, Chronic viral infections in myalgic encephalomyelitis/chronic fatigue syndrome (ME/CFS). *J Transl Med*, **16**(1): p. 268.

78. Regland, B., et al., 2015, Response to vitamin B12 and folic acid in myalgic encephalomyelitis and fibromyalgia. *PLoS One*, **10**(4): p. e0124648.

79. Rekeland, I.G., et al., 2020, Intravenous cyclophosphamide in myalgic encephalomyelitis/chronic fatigue syndrome. An open-label phase II study. *Front Med*, **7**: p. 162.

80. Rowe, P.C., et al., 2017, Myalgic encephalomyelitis/chronic fatigue syndrome diagnosis and management in young people: a primer. *Front Pediatr*, **5**: p. 121.

81. Sassi, F., C. Tamone, and P. D'Amelio, 2018, Vitamin D: Nutrient, hormone, and immunomodulator. *Nutrients*, **10**(11).

82. Scheibenbogen, C., et al., 2018, Immunoadsorption to remove ss2 adrenergic receptor antibodies in chronic fatigue syndrome CFS/ME. *PLoS One*, **13**(3): p. e0193672.

83. Schreiner, P., et al., 2020, Human herpesvirus-6 reactivation, mitochondrial fragmentation, and the coordination of antiviral and metabolic phenotypes in myalgic encephalomyelitis/chronic fatigue syndrome. *Immunohorizons*, **4**(4): p. 201–215.

84. Scott, A., et al., 2008, Increased mast cell numbers in human patellar tendinosis: correlation with symptom duration and vascular hyperplasia. *Br J Sports Med*, **42**(9): p. 753–7.

85. Shikova, E., et al., 2020, Cytomegalovirus, Epstein-Barr virus, and human herpesvirus-6 infections in patients with myalgic small ie, Cyrillicncephalomyelitis/chronic fatigue syndrome. *J Med Virol*.

86. Shoenfeld, Y., et al., 2020, Complex syndromes of chronic pain, fatigue and cognitive impairment linked to autoimmune dysautonomia and small fiber neuropathy. *Clin Immunol*, **214**: article number 108384.

87. Sotzny, F., et al., 2018, Myalgic encephalomyelitis/chronic fatigue syndrome - evidence for an autoimmune disease. *Autoimmun Rev*, **17**(6): p. 601–609.

88. Stroke, N.I.F.N.D.A., *Common Data Elements: Myalgic Encephalomyelitis/Chronic Fatigue Syndrome*. n.d.; Available from: https://www.commondataelements.ninds.nih.gov/Myalgic%20Encephalomyelitis/Chronic%20Fatigue%20Syndrome.

89. Surendran, S., et al., 2018, An update on vitamin B12-related gene polymorphisms and B12 status. *Genes Nutr*, **13**: p. 2.

90. Taylor, R.R., & Kielhofner, G.W., 2005, Work-related impairment and employment-focused rehabilitation options for individuals with chronic fatigue syndrome: a review. *Journal of Mental Health*, **14**(3): p. 253–267.

91. Thapaliya, K., et al., 2020, Mapping of pathological change in chronic fatigue syndrome using the ratio of T1- and T2-weighted MRI scans. *Neuroimage Clin*, **28**: p. 102366.

92. Toljan, K. and B. Vrooman, 2018, Low-dose naltrexone (LDN)-review of therapeutic utilization. *Med Sci*, **6**(4).

93. Tolle, M., et al., 2020, Myalgic encephalomyelitis/chronic fatigue syndrome: efficacy of repeat immuno-adsorption. *J Clin Med*, **9**(8).

94. Unger, E.R., et al., 2017, Multi-site clinical assessment of myalgic encephalomyelitis/chronic fatigue syndrome (MCAM): design and implementation of a prospective/retrospective rolling cohort study. *Am J Epidemiol*, **185**(8): p. 617–626.

95. van Campen, C., et al., 2021, Orthostatic stress testing in myalgic encephalomyelitis/chronic fatigue syndrome patients with or without concomitant fibromyalgia: effects on pressure pain thresholds and temporal summation. *Clin Exp Rheumatol*, **39**(Suppl 130(3)): p. 39–47.

96. van Campen, C., et al., 2020, Cerebral blood flow is reduced in ME/CFS during head-up tilt testing even in the absence of hypotension or tachycardia: A quantitative, controlled study using Doppler echography. *Clin Neurophysiol Pract*, **5**: p. 50–58.

97. VanElzakker, M.B., S.A. Brumfield, and P.S. Lara Mejia, 2018, Neuroinflammation and cytokines in myalgic encephalomyelitis/chronic fatigue syndrome (ME/CFS): a critical review of research methods. *Front Neurol*, **9**: p. 1033.

98. Vojdani, A., D. Afar, and E. Vojdani, 2020, Reaction of lectin-specific antibody with human tissue: possible contributions to autoimmunity. *J Immunol Res*, **2020**: p. 1438957.

99. Vojdani, A.V.E., Oral tolerance failure, food immune reactions and the autoimmune connection, in *Food-associated Autoimmunities: When Food Breaks Your Immune System*. 2019, A&G Press, Los Angeles.

100. Wang, X., et al., 2016, Elevation of IGFBP2 contributes to mycotoxin T-2-induced chondrocyte injury and metabolism. *Biochem Biophys Res Commun*, **478**(1): p. 385–391.

101. Wirth, K. and C. Scheibenbogen, 2020, A unifying hypothesis of the pathophysiology of myalgic encephalomyelitis/chronic fatigue syndrome (ME/CFS): recognitions from the finding of autoantibodies against ss2-adrenergic receptors. *Autoimmun Rev*, **19**(6): p. 102527.

102. Witham, M.D., et al., 2015, Effect of intermittent vitamin D3 on vascular function and symptoms in chronic fatigue syndrome: a randomised controlled trial. *Nutr Metab Cardiovasc Dis*, **25**(3): p. 287–94.

103. Younger, J., L. Parkitny, and D. McLain, 2014, The use of low-dose naltrexone (LDN) as a novel anti-inflammatory treatment for chronic pain. *Clin Rheumatol*, **33**(4): p. 451–9.

104. Zielinski, D.C., et al., 2015, Pharmacogenomic and clinical data link non-pharmacokinetic metabolic dysregulation to drug side effect pathogenesis. *Nat Commun*, **6**: p. 7101.

16 Allostatic Load/Overload and Myalgic Encephalitis/Chronic Fatigue Syndrome (ME/CFS)

Jeffrey Moss

CONTENTS

16.1 INTRODUCTION

16.1.1 LACK OF CONSENSUS ON VIRTUALLY ALL ASPECTS OF ME/CFS

One of the most current papers on the subject of myalgic encephalitis/chronic fatigue syndrome (ME/CFS) published in a major medical journal was "Advances in understanding the pathophysiology of chronic fatigue syndrome" by Komaroff.[1] This paper begins with an interesting question and answer that perfectly summarizes why, for several decades now, both the patients suffering from the fatigue and other symptoms that have now been broadly classified as ME/CFS and the health care professionals who have been trying to assist them have been, more often than not, frustrated in the goal of obtaining significant, long-term symptomatic improvements:

> When does an illness become a disease? When the underlying biological abnormalities that cause the symptoms and signs of the illness are clarified.

As will be demonstrated in this introductory section, there is far from a consensus on "the underlying biological abnormalities" that create what is currently known as ME/CFS. Therefore, as noted by McManimen et al. in their paper "Dismissing chronic illness: A qualitative analysis of negative health care experiences,"[2] all too many health care practitioners seem to be either confused or unwilling to address patients who maintain they have ME/CFS as if they have a legitimate disease. As noted by the authors, 77% of patients experiencing symptoms consistent with ME/CFS reported a negative interaction with a health care professional. In addition, 57% reported poor treatment by doctors, and 66% believed that treatment by a doctor worsened the condition. McManimen et al.[2] continue by pointing out that many ME/CFS patients perceive that health care professionals believe that ME/CFS is primarily a psychological illness because very often, symptoms cannot be objectively measured. In contrast, ME/CFS patients tend to strongly believe that their illness is not psychosomatic.

In discussing papers summarizing physicians' perception of ME/CFS, the authors point out that because physicians often could not objectively measure symptoms, they would often report that ME/CFS patients were exaggerating their symptoms and malingering for some other purpose. This would lead to characterizations of ME/CFS patients as "lacking fortitude" and "low symptom threshold." Why the dismissive attitudes? One reason, as noted by several studies reported by McManimen et al.,[2] is lack of knowledge about the condition due to poor training in medical schools and minimal inclusion in medical textbooks.

What is known and is generally not disputed by both patients and practitioners is the following, as noted in the paper "Onset patterns and course of myalgic encephalomyelitis/chronic fatigue syndrome" by Chu et al.[3]

16.1.2 Basic Epidemiologic Data

ME/CFS affects 0.76 to 3.28% of the worldwide population and up to 2.5 million residents of the United States. The average age of onset is during the fourth decade of life, with women being affected two to three times more often than men. However, CFS has been reported in children. In addition, despite the moniker "yuppie flu," ethnic minorities and individuals in lower socioeconomic classes are affected.

16.1.3 Typical Patient Presentation

Chu et al.[3] point out that severe fatigue is accompanied by musculoskeletal pain, headaches, sore throat, tender lymph nodes, concentration/memory difficulties and unrefreshing sleep. In addition, these symptoms are exacerbated by minimal physical and/or cognitive exertion (termed post-exertional malaise [PEM]). As might be expected, these symptoms affect quality of life, with unemployment statistics as high as 81% in ME/CFS patients. Furthermore, ~25% of patients may be confined to their homes and beds. To put the loss of quality of life into perspective, quality of life scores in ME/CFS patients have been reported to be lower than those of patients suffering from multiple sclerosis, rheumatoid arthritis, congestive heart failure and myocardial infarction. Finally, according to Chu et al.,[3] long-term prognosis for this patient population is poor, with the median rate of full recovery reported to be 5%. In turn, this decades-long illness costs the United States ~$18–$54 billion annually in terms of direct medical costs, lost productivity and taxes.

16.2 CURRENTLY ACCEPTED GUIDELINES FOR DIAGNOSIS

Interestingly, the title of this section is misleading because, as frustratingly noted by Friedman in his paper "Advances in ME/CFS: Past, present, and future,"[4] there are no universally accepted guidelines for diagnosis. Instead, several sets of diagnostic criteria have been proposed. However, simplified diagnostic criteria proposed by the Institute of Medicine have not been widely accepted. Therefore, according to the author, diagnosis is most often purely based on symptoms, some of which are considered mandatory for diagnosis and others are considered adjunctive. In addition, there appears to be a consensus that patients must experience symptoms for at least 6 months despite treatment for co-morbidities in order to be classified as ME/CFS patients.

16.3 TRADITIONAL APPROACHES TO ASSESSMENT AND TREATMENT OF ME/CFS

As noted by Friedman,[4] ME/CFS in the United States was first reported in the medical literature in 1934. Early thinking on causation revolved around infection with the Epstein–Barr virus (EBV), Ross River Virus and Q fever; it was reported that 6% of patients suffering from these conditions developed ME/CFS. In addition, the severity of these infections was the best predictor of developing the condition. As time progressed, attitudes about causation degraded when according to Friedman,[4] some authors labeled an outbreak of ME/CFS as "mass hysteria." Then, as mentioned earlier, thanks to a report in the *New York Times*, ME/CFS became known as "Yuppie Flu," despite the fact that all socioeconomic groups of the American population are affected, most especially those in socioeconomically disadvantaged populations.

These hostile attitudes towards ME/CFS, though, were not limited to the public and popular mass media. Friedman [4] goes on to point out that scientists, clinicians and educators who pursued ME/CFS often jeopardized careers and livelihood. For example, clinicians in medical schools have been advised to discontinue seeing ME/CFS patients, because of the time involved in addressing their needs, or find employment elsewhere. Researchers have been told that research on ME/CFS will not qualify for promotion consideration, and without promotion, the researchers will need to leave the institution. Finally, medical educators have been told that educational activities involving ME/CFS are not "professional" and therefore, will be banned from the workplace.

These mischaracterizations and dismissive attitudes predictably led to poor and sometimes harmful treatment. As was noted earlier, the misrepresentations just discussed have led many to conclude that ME/CFS is a psychosomatic illness that can be cured with cognitive behavioral therapy (CBT) and exercise therapy. Friedman[4] points out that more current published research is disputing this assumption. Of even more concern is potentially harmful treatment, such as the situation where parents of children diagnosed with ME/CFS have been accused of Munchausen's Syndrome by Proxy, leading to removal of the children from the home, resulting in increased illness severity.[4].

While it is virtually impossible to conceive of a circumstance where removal from the home of children suffering from ME/CFS would be justified, what about CBT? In disputing and discarding the use of CBT with ME/CFS patients, could we be "throwing out the baby with the bathwater?" As will be hypothesized later in this chapter, we must avoid the common thinking that because a therapeutic intervention is not a universal cure for everyone, it cannot be a portion of the cure for some. Papers on the allostatic load model of illness that will be discussed in following sections of this chapter present a compelling argument that illnesses such as ME/CFS occur as the result of metabolic responses to cumulative environmental stress, where patient perceptions and thought processes, even though they are not the total cause, as suggested by the psychosomatic theories on ME/CFS, may be an important contributor to the total causational picture. In turn, when therapies such as CBT and exercise therapy are combined with therapies that address environmental stressors such as chronic infection, exposure to chemical and heavy metal toxins, poor nutrition, etc. and therapies that address responses to these environmental stressors such as chronic inflammation, gastrointestinal (GI) dysfunction, and imbalances of hormones such as cortisol and insulin, the data on CBT and exercise therapy is more likely to be positive.

16.4   WHY A NEW MODEL OF ASSESSMENT AND PATIENT MANAGEMENT IS NEEDED

As was suggested earlier, prevailing medical views about ME/CFS are often incorrect, leading to treatments that demonstrate poor efficacy. These errors in judgement by the medical community were explored in detail in the paper "Rethinking the standard of care for myalgic encephalomyelitis/chronic fatigue syndrome" by Friedberg et al.[5] The first error in judgement noted by the authors is the generally accepted definition of the illness. An often reported and accepted definition is known as the Oxford criteria, which define ME/CFS as solely an issue of chronic fatigue. In contrast, the reality of ME/CFS is a multisystem presentation consisting of issues such as non-restorative sleep, cognitive difficulties and very importantly, as will be described later, PEM (sustained post-exertion worsening of symptoms). This limited definition has led to the assumption, as noted by Friedberg et al.,[5] that ME/CFS is primarily a psychological disease that results from deconditioning related to fear of activity and false assumptions that the illness has a physical basis. This false belief about the nature of ME/CFS has led to a standard of care revolving around CBT and graded exercise therapy (GET). Why? The authors point out mistaken thinking that since ME/CFS is a behavioral disease related to false assumptions, changing beliefs about the illness will lead to increased activity. In contrast, Friedberg et al. point out the true nature of ME/CFS:

> This model stands in stark contrast to the harsh reality of this disabling condition and the significant evidence of neurological, immunological, autonomic, and energy metabolism impairment, as reviewed in an influential 2015 Institute of Medicine Report.

Does this mean that CBT is of no use to the ME/CFS patient? Not really. CBT can actually have great value for ME/CFS patients when it is used as it was originally intended, which is not as a stand-alone cure for disease. It was, in reality, devised as a tool to promote, for people with chronic diseases, the ability to cope with illness, along with other therapeutic interventions, in order to improve quality of life. As noted by Friedberg et al.,[5] it was never designed to convince ME/CFS patients that they are either psychologically ill or not really ill at all. Friedberg et al.[5] conclude their paper with an affirmation of the main premise of this book chapter that ME/CFS is a complex, multifactorial illness, which requires a multi-disciplinary treatment team that has expertise in key areas such as immunology, infectious disease, cardiology, neurology, psychology, occupational therapy and social work.

16.5   THE REALITY OF THE ME/CFS PATIENT EXPERIENCE

As was suggested earlier, according to "Assessment of post-exertional malaise (PEM) in patients with myalgic encephalomyelitis (ME) and chronic fatigue syndrome (CFS): A patient driven survey" by Holtzman et al.,[6] the most important symptom experienced by ME/CFS patients is not fatigue per se. Rather, it is what is known as post-exertional malaise (PEM), which is considered to be a hallmark symptom of ME/CFS. The authors go on to point out that the PEM experienced by the ME/CFS patient is not just a simple matter of excessive fatigue after routine exercise activities such as walking or jogging. Rather, typical daily activities most people take for granted can trigger PEM. These include toileting, bathing, dressing, communicating and even reading. What can trigger PEM? Again, it not just negative thinking, as is too often assumed. These triggers include infections and exposure to certain chemicals, foods and metals. Furthermore, ME/CFS patients are unique in that PEM can often have a delayed onset after these triggers are encountered and a longer recovery time than might be expected in a non-ME/CFS population.

To get more detail on the true nature of PEM, a hallmark symptom of ME/CFS, Holtzman et al.[6] conducted a study via questionnaire on 1,534 adults with a mean age of 51 years who identified as having ME and/or CFS. The respondents were from over 35 countries, with 41.1 currently living in the United States. Of these, 84.6% were females and 97.5% were white/Caucasian; 2% identified as being of Latino or Hispanic origin; 56.6% were married or living with a partner; 39.3% had a college degree and 45.7% were receiving disability payments. Concerning the specifics of diagnosis, 50.7% had a diagnosis of CFS, 22% had a diagnosis of ME and 27.2% had a diagnosis of both; 94.4% were diagnosed by a medical doctor. Concerning the specifics of PEM, 72.3% reported symptom exacerbation immediately after exertion, with others having varying degrees of delayed onset.

What were the triggers of symptom exacerbation? The answer to this question is particularly important given traditional medical thinking that ME/CFS is largely a psychological illness. Interestingly, in support of this explanation of ME/CFS, 93.2% of respondents indicated good or bad emotional stress as a trigger. However, in line with the hypothesis being presented in this book chapter, there were many other triggers besides exertion:

- 78.2% reported "basic activities of daily living" as a trigger.
- 64.5% reported "positional changes" as a trigger.
- 85.5% reported noise being a trigger.

Furthermore, in support of the hypothesis that ME/CFS is a complex, multisystem metabolic disorder that includes, but is not limited to, psychological stress, Holtzman et al.[6] point out that a large percentage of the study population indicated heat, light, cold, foods, chemicals, vibration, mold, medications and dietary supplements as PEM triggers. Which symptoms were most often worsened by physical or cognitive exertion? The most common were reduced stamina and/or functional capacity (99.4%), physical fatigue (98.9%), cognitive exhaustion (97.4%), problems with thinking (97.4%), unrefreshing sleep (95.0%), muscle pain (87.9%), insomnia (87.3%), muscle weakness/instability (87.3%), temperature dysregulation (86.9%) and flu-like symptoms (86.6%).

What is the duration of PEM after onset? Holtzman et al.[6] report that 58% of respondents indicated an average of 3–6 days. Other durations reported by respondents were 1–2 days and 1 week to 1 month.

Of most concern, 30.3% reported 1–6 months. How long had the disease of ME/CFS been present with the respondents? The majority reported over 10 years with illness being present over 50% of the time.

Finally, one of the most important and interesting questions on the survey was how the respondents felt concerning the accuracy of the survey in terms of reflecting their true PEM experiences. Of all respondents, 29.8% indicated that the survey was very accurate, 57.7% indicated it was accurate, 10.7% were neutral, 1.2% felt it was not accurate, and 0.1% reported it was not at all accurate. Thus, as can be seen, the Holtzman et al.[6] study appears to be a reliable "in the trenches" barometer of the reality of ME/CFS and highly supports the hypothesis that ME/CFS is a complex metabolic disorder with many possible primary causes and pathophysiological mechanisms that will vary greatly in priority from patient to patient, even though clinical presentations will often be similar from patient to patient.

16.6 HOW EFFICACIOUS HAVE PHARMACEUTICAL THERAPIES BEEN WITH ME/CFS?

Still another indication that the traditional medical approach to ME/CFS does not optimally address the needs of the ME/CFS patient population is the poor results seen with pharmaceutical interventions, as reported by Richman et al. in their paper "Pharmaceutical interventions in chronic fatigue syndrome: A literature-based commentary."[7] What were the authors' findings? First, they note that most drugs are directed not at causation but at symptom management. The drugs most often employed, according to the authors, are antivirals, pain relievers, antidepressants and oncologic agents, all used as single-intervention treatments. All were suggested to demonstrate little efficacy. What do Richman et al.[7] suggest as a solution? In further support of the hypothesis put forth in this book chapter, they suggest that there is no single solution that can be addressed by a single drug. Rather, they suggest that ME/CFS may be more effectively treated with combination therapies tailored to specific causes and symptoms unique to each individual patient. To do so will require a better understanding of the systems biology underlying the biological drivers behind ME/CFS.

16.7 RESEARCH SUPPORTING THE HYPOTHESIS THAT ME/CFS HAS MANY POSSIBLE PATHOPHYSIOLOGIC MECHANISMS THAT VARY FROM PATIENT TO PATIENT

16.7.1 OVERVIEW

The paper "Pathological mechanisms underlying myalgic encephalomyelitis/chronic fatigue syndrome" by Missailidis et al.[8] provides excellent support for the hypothesis that ME/CFS has multiple pathophysiologic mechanisms that vary from patient to patient. The paper begins by pointing out that ME/CFS has far from the often-assumed clinical presentation of systemic uniformity from patient to patient. Rather, it can affect multiple body systems and organs at different times with varying levels of intensity. In turn, this leads to different patterns of symptoms that can vary greatly from person to person. Therefore, while on the surface, there is a general perception of similar case presentations from patient to patient, the reality is that the ME/CFS population is highly heterogeneous. Why does the symptomatic presentation vary so greatly from patient to patient? One reason, as noted by Missailidis et al.,[8] is that the common assumption that causation is generally infective in nature is inaccurate. In fact, there is no known single, uniform causative cause. In contrast, the initial insult may have nothing to do with infective pathogens but instead, could be any number of alternative stresses of large enough intensity to disrupt homeostatic regulation loops that lead to disturbed muscle function, mitochondrial function, immune function, neurological function, adrenal function and gut function in a way that will be unique from patient to patient.

Missailidis et al.[8] go on to describe some of these disruptions in homeostatic regulation loops in greater detail, as seen in the following subsections.

16.7.2 Dysregulated Amino Acid Metabolism and Krebs Cycle Substrates

Blood samples of some ME/CFS patients have demonstrated low glutamine and ornithine concentrations, suggesting urea cycle dysregulation. A similar study has demonstrated elevations in ornithine and decreases in citrulline in some patients.

Other researchers have found impaired glycolytic formation of pyruvate, which in turn, leads to lower levels of pyruvate derivatives for utilization for energy production in the Krebs cycle. It has also been suggested that lower levels of pyruvate derivatives may be due to poor pyruvate dehydrogenase function.

16.7.3 Dysregulated Krebs Cycle Function

When provision of pyruvate metabolites is impaired, it has been suggested that in some ME/CFS patients, there is compensatory elevation of fatty acid metabolism in the Krebs cycle via beta oxidation, which is fairly slow in nature in terms of the provision of ATP. Therefore, when exertion calls for a switch to glycolytic processes that can meet the sometimes immediate need for increased energy production, this switch is unable to occur in the ME/CFS patient. This would explain the common complaint of extreme fatigue with exertion. The authors go on to note that this switch to increased reliance on lipid oxidation may be mediated by increased and pathologic inflammation.

16.7.4 Dysregulation of Inflammatory Mediators

Missailidis et al.[8] make it clear that chronic, system-wide inflammation is central to the clinical presentation of ME/CFS and is clearly linked with symptom severity. The chronic inflammatory pattern, though, does not result in uniform elevation of all inflammatory cytokines. In fact, interleukin-8 and transforming growth factor-beta1 have been found to be suppressed. Other research has demonstrated that immune globulins such as IgM and IgA may be elevated, and when this is addressed with anti-inflammatory and antioxidant medications, patients who demonstrate increased gut permeability may experience significant symptom improvement. These findings have been used to support the connection between increased gut permeability and inflammation in ME/CFS patients.

16.7.5 Dysregulation of Gut Microflora

Missailidis et al.[8] point out that disturbances of gut microbiota can play a role in ME/CFS. This can lead to gut abnormalities such as impaired motility, increased gut permeability and irritable bowel syndrome (IBS)-type symptoms. The authors go on to point out that disturbances in gut microflora, increased gut permeability and mitochondrial dysfunction may be linked.

Disturbances in gut microflora can also have an impact on brain function. This can happen when physiological stresses cause a reduction in numbers of *Bifidobacterium* and *Lactobacillus* microflora species. Since these species reduce commensal microflora that produce endotoxin, increased levels of endotoxin caused by a reduction in *Bifidobacterium* and *Lactobacillus* organisms can translocate into the bloodstream, leading to increased systemic inflammation and increased production of stress hormones such as cortisol in the brain.

16.7.6 Interactions of All of the Above

It is often assumed that when multiple metabolic imbalances exist, they function in a relatively isolated, "parallel universe" manner. Unfortunately, the reality of ME/CFS suggests that this is not the case, adding even more complexity to the ME/CFS dysmetabolism presentation. Missailidis et al.[8] elegantly point out ways these metabolic interactions can occur:

> For example, the elevated oxidative stress reported in the disorder may be entangled with perturbed immune-inflammatory pathways, gut inflammation, and dysfunctional mitochondria. This may be exacerbated by other disturbances, such as the reported reduction in creatine kinase (CK) levels, which can lead to the absence of CK-mediated reactive oxygen species suppression. This raises the possibility of a vicious cycle of immunodysregulation and gut dysbiosis accompanied by poor physiological gut function that contribute to the perpetuation of a chronic bowel disease state. Such an altered state could interact with the previously suggested HPA dysregulation and contribute to the perpetuation of an alternative resting homeostasis.

With this in mind, the authors close their paper by stating the following:

> It is likely that the inflammation and immune dysfunction classically studied in ME/CFS are entangled with dysfunctional energetics, gut health, or autonomic and adrenal dysregulation. The evidence for metabolic and mitochondrial dysfunction indicates inefficient respiration, impaired provision of TCA cycle substrate, and metabolic shifts towards the utilization of alternative metabolites. Immune effector cell dysfunction, chronic inflammation, defective signaling, and elevated oxidative stress may interact with not only the dysfunctional energetics but also with abnormal gut physiology and microbiota composition. These effects on the gut may also tie back to mitochondrial function and vice versa. The reciprocal interactions between these affected systems and the varied clinical presentation of relevant symptoms between individuals make it difficult to postulate cause-effect relationships with confidence.

16.7.7 AN IN-DEPTH EXAMINATION OF THE KEY METABOLIC IMBALANCES OFTEN ENCOUNTERED IN ME/CFS PATIENTS

As was eloquently conveyed by Missailidis et al.,[8] the reality of ME/CFS is far from the general allopathic model of disease, which operates on the assumption that similar clinical presentations are one-dimensional entities that involve uniform causation and metabolic imbalances. Rather, the authors make it clear that even though ME/CFS patients often experience similar symptomatic presentations, the underlying causes, metabolic imbalances and interactions between different metabolic imbalances result in a level of patient uniqueness that necessitates virtually complete elimination of practitioner assumptions and agendas about causation and metabolic imbalances/interactions seen with other patients and the adoption of an assessment and treatment protocol that is completely and totally based on each individual patient presentation. In agreement, Rivera et al.[9] suggest that the pathophysiology of ME/CFS involves "three pillars" that continuously interact with each other. These three pillars are the immune system, the nervous system and the neuroendocrine network. Finally, Jeffrey et al.[10] suggest another version of a three-pillar pathophysiology involving oxidative stress, immune dysregulation and potassium inequity.

Fortunately, as noted by Missailidis et al.,[8] the metabolic imbalances seen with different ME/CFS patients are not entirely random and unpredictable. Some do occur more often than others.

16.8 ADDITIONAL RESEARCH ON THE PATHOPHYSIOLOGY OF ME/CFS

16.8.1 DYSREGULATION OF INFLAMMATORY MEDIATORS

Several studies beyond that performed by Missailidis et al.[8] have made it clear that ME/CFS patients often demonstrate increased levels of pro-inflammatory cytokines and acute phase reactants, typically associated with an infectious pathogen, especially a viral infection.[9, 11, 12] The elevation of pro-inflammatory cytokines greatly explains the common findings of fatigue and flu-like symptoms.[9-11] In addition, the presence of unregulated inflammatory mediators is often accompanied by dysfunctional mitochondria, increased translocation of Gram-negative bacteria, and alteration of intracellular signal transduction and apoptosis pathways.[9] Other evidence of upregulation/dysregulation of immunoinflammatory pathways is the following:[9–13]

- Increases in tumor necrosis factor (TNF)-α, interleukin (IL)-1α, IL-1β, IL-4, IL-5, IL-6 and IL-12.
- Decreases in IL-8, IL-13 and IL-15.
- Activation of cell-mediated immunity as evidenced by increased neopterin levels.
- A Th1 to Th2 shift and alteration of Th17 pathways.
- Increased translocation of bacteria through the leaky gut, which is accompanied by increased levels of IgA and IgM.
- Increased levels of NF-κB, which can be induced by viral infections. This increase can greatly propel the inflammatory cascade in ME/CFS patients.
- Decreased levels of total IgG and IgG subclasses such as IgG1 and IgG3.
- Increased high sensitivity C-reactive protein (hsCRP).
- Dysfunctional natural killer (NK) cells.

Inflammatory mediators that instigate neuroinflammation are also dysregulated in ME/CFS patients,[14] which would help explain the neuropathic pain and the common occurrence of neuropsychologic symptoms such as cognitive impairment, decreased alertness, impaired memory, concentration and depressive symptoms seen in this patient population.[9, 10] Upregulation of neuroinflammation often involves activation of central nervous system (CNS) glial cells, specifically microglia and astrocytes.[9] This neuroinflammatory upregulation is suggested to result in a phenomenon known as "sickness behavior," which consists of clinical findings such as malaise, lassitude, fatigue, numbness, reduced appetite, reduced social interactions, fatigue and weight loss.[9] This neuroinflammatory upregulation leading to "sickness behavior" has been suggested to be associated with a shift towards an allergic T-helper type-2 (TH2) pattern.[9] Similarly to systemic inflammation, upregulation of neuroinflammation in ME/CFS patients can be triggered by an immunologic response to an infectious process.[9] Finally, the inflammatory mediators that trigger upregulated glial cell activity can also link with neuronal glutamate receptors, leading to enhanced neuroexcitation.[9]

16.8.2 OXIDATIVE/NITROSATIVE STRESS INDUCED BY INFLAMMATION

Systemic inflammation in ME/CFS patients can result in increased oxidative and nitrosative stress (O&NS), which in itself, has been considered to be a critical pathophysiologic feature in this disease.[12] Specifically, O&NS can lead to decreased levels of antioxidants.[9] These diminished antioxidants include zinc, coenzyme Q10 and antioxidant enzymes.[9] In addition, oxidative stress in ME/CFS patients has been linked with damage to fatty acids, proteins and DNA.[9] A lowered omega-3:omega-9 polyunsaturated fatty acid ratio has also been reported.[9]

Markers of O&NS that are often elevated are blood isoprostane, oxidized LDL, 4-hydroxynonenal (HNE), malondialdehyde (MDA), oxidatively modified proteins and iso-prostaglandin.[9,12] Low levels of glutathione have also been reported.[9]

Further evidence of a link between fatigue and oxidative stress has been provided by studies which have demonstrated that antioxidant supplementation can be helpful in fatigue patients.[15] Specifically, supplementing CFS patients with coenzyme Q10 and nicotinamide adenine dinucleotide (NADH) reduced fatigue, whereas a placebo did not.[15]

16.8.3 NEUROTRANSMITTER DISTURBANCES

Rivera et al.[9] point out that the central fatigue seen with ME/CFS patients is highly correlated with increased serotonin (5-HT) and its metabolites in the CNS, largely as a consequence of inflammatory activity. Inflammatory cytokines can alter the metabolism and release of neurotransmitters, including serotonin.[9] More specifically, TNF-α and IL-1β have been demonstrated to acutely activate the serotoninergic transporter (SERT).[9]

How does increased 5-HT lead to fatigue? Rivera et al.[9] suggest that 5-HT spills over to reach the extra-synaptic receptor sites in the initial axon segment. This inhibits the generation of action potentials. This appears to be a protective mechanism against excessive 5-HT activity, as this inhibition of action potentials also prevents hyperactivity of motor neurons and reduces detrimental muscle activity. Unfortunately, as with so many of the other metabolic adjustments to long-term, chronic inflammation, this excessive 5-HT activity and consequent inhibition of action potentials that prevent 5-HT-induced hyperactivity of motor neurons also can contribute to central fatigue.[9]

Finally, it has been suggested that in certain ME/CFS patients, particularly adolescents, there may be a significant prevalence of methylation issues in the form of catechol-O-methyltransferase (COMT) polymorphisms. Given that optimal COMT activity is necessary for optimal catecholamine metabolism, elevated levels of norepinephrine and epinephrine have been noted in adolescent ME/CFS patients with low COMT activity.[9]

Inflammation can also alter dopamine neurotransmission by creating oxidative stress and mitochondrial damage in dopaminergic neurons, thus leading to an impairment in dopaminergic neurotransmission.[15]

16.8.4 Neuroendocrine Imbalances

As was mentioned earlier, neuroendocrine imbalances are one of the pathophysiologic "three pillars" that underly ME/CFS.[9] While studies have been conflicting, it appears most likely that ME/CFS patients demonstrate hypofunction of the hypothalamic/pituitary/adrenal (HPA) axis, which is manifested by a low salivary cortisol-awakening response.[9] In addition, ME/CFS patients often demonstrate aberrant diurnal hormone variation, reduced HPA response to both physical and psychological stressors, and enhanced sensitivity to glucocorticoids.[9] However, while these are important pathophysiologic findings, Rivera et al. make it clear that HPA axis disturbances are not a primary causational factor but rather, a consequence or comorbidity of ME/CFS.[9]

Why is the HPA axis hypofunctioning in ME/CFS patients? It has been suggested that this is the result of a "stressed crash" or "exhaustion" phenomenon whereby the hyperfunctioning HPA axis that is the result of acute stress switches to an exhaustion phase when the stress becomes prolonged.[9]. This results in an HPA axis that loses its ability to cope with environmental stress, with attendant low cortisol output.[9]

What came first – chronic inflammation that leads to HPA axis disturbances, or HPA axis hypofunction that leads to activation of immune/inflammatory pathways? In actuality, either scenario could be present, and as has been repeatedly suggested earlier, ME/CFS patients, despite similar clinical presentations, can be unique from a pathophysiologic perspective. Therefore, it certainly possible in some cases that HPA axis hypofunction will contribute to an activation of immune-inflammatory pathways as well as attenuation of Th1 cell-mediated immune responses and promotion of Th2-mediated responses.[9] However, it is equally possible that because of bidirectional communication between immune-inflammatory pathways and the HPA axis, pro-inflammatory cytokines can induce the HPA axis to produce more HPA axis–related hormones.[9] Evidence of neuroendocrine dysfunction caused by increased systemic inflammation is elevated levels of IL-6 and CRP.

Disturbances in adrenal hormone receptors have also been reported in ME/CFS patients.[16] Specifically, the impaired HPA response seen in ME/CFS patients may be overactivity of glucocorticoid receptors (GR) and mineralocorticoid receptors (MR), which leads to increased suppression of the hypothalamus and anterior pituitary.[16] This receptor dysfunction, along with the other HPA imbalances discussed earlier, can reduce the ability of HPA hormones to reduce inflammatory activity, leading to a scenario where even slight stressors can trigger an inflammatory response.[16]

Other neuroendocrine imbalances reported in 90% of ME/CFS patients are elevated sympathetic activity, reduced parasympathetic activity and hypoactivity of the vagus nerve.[12] Morris et al.[12] go on to point out that the most frequently reported manifestation of disturbances in neuroendocrine function among ME/CFS patients is chronically blunted heart rate variability (HRV).

16.8.5 SUBOPTIMAL MITOCHONDRIAL FUNCTION AND ENERGY PRODUCTION

Another downstream effect of inflammation reported in ME/CFS patients, as suggested earlier, is reduction in mitochondrial function and energy production.[15] Specifically, it has been proposed that chronic low-grade inflammation creates and maintains a state of persistent fatigue by inducing a metabolic switch away from energy-efficient oxidative phosphorylation to fast-acting but less efficient aerobic glycolytic energy production, with attendant increases in reactive oxygen species (ROS) and decreased cellular energy.[15] The reason for this is that inflammation upregulates the need of immune cells for rapid creation of cellular energy.[15] To do this, immune cells shift to aerobic glycolysis, which is a less efficient but fast-acting pathway for energy production.[15] This prolonged reliance on aerobic glycolysis also leads to lower energy availability due to reduced nutrient availability, which in turn, leads to lower energy availability for other key organ systems.[15] Also, the increase in inflammation-induced energy needs of immune cells decreases the availability of "behavioral" energy, which is the energy spent on daily activities.[15]

Interestingly, prolonged inflammation, over time, will eventually lead to a decrease in aerobic glycolysis even in immune cells, because eventually, inflammation will lead to insulin resistance, reducing the uptake of glucose by immune cells. This in turn will lead to reduced ATP production in immune cells even by the inflammation-induced aerobic glycolysis pathway.[15]

Are there compensatory energy production pathways that non-immune organ systems can rely upon when chronic inflammation is leading to increased aerobic glycolysis in immune cells at the expense of other organ systems? Lipid and protein metabolism is one way the body compensates.[15] Unfortunately, lipid metabolism is slow and cannot respond to rapid energy requirements.[15] Compounding the problem is the fact that increased reliance on protein metabolism for the production of energy reduces protein availability for promotion of growth and repair.[15]

What happens to the cells and cellular components involved in energy production in the presence of chronic inflammation? First, inflammation-induced ROS can harm both mitochondria and mitochondrial DNA.[15] Also, neurons that are heavily dependent on mitochondrial oxidative phosphorylation for ATP needs are harmed. Chronic inflammation also harms neurons by an indirect mechanism, because neurons also rely on lactate for energy production, and that is provided by astrocytes. Chronic inflammation leads to insulin resistance, which in turn, decreases astrocyte glucose and protein metabolism, leading to decreased lactate production for use by neurons.[15]

What about behavioral energy availability? Chronic low-grade inflammation can increase systemic energy expenditure by 10%, leading to a reduction of energy available for daily activities.[15] Several studies have shown that this inflammation-induced reprioritization of energy can have a direct impact on motivation to exert effort.[15]

McGregor et al.[17] noted similar findings to those of Lacourt et al.,[15] in that females suffering from ME/CFS demonstrate deregulated glycolysis activity, with increases in fasted first morning serum glucose and decreases in lactate and acetate. Furthermore, these researchers also noted deregulation of urea cycle activity, as evidenced by reductions in the purine metabolite hypoxanthine. Still more evidence of disturbed glycolysis and urea cycle activity noted by McGregor et al.[17] was increased urine excretion of mannitol, methylhistidine, acetate and glucose. These findings led the author to conclude that PEM in ME/CFS patients is associated with changes in glycolysis and acetylation that are consistent with a hypoacetylation state.

Other findings in ME/CFS patients that are indicative of mitochondrial dysfunction are denuded ATP production, lower levels of coenzyme Q10 and intracellular acidosis.[12]

16.8.6 GI Microbiome Imbalances, Increased Intestinal Permeability, and Bacterial Translocation

As was suggested earlier, many researchers have reported that disturbances in GI function are common in ME/CFS patients. Several papers[12, 18] point out that many ME/CFS patients demonstrate increased permeability of the intestinal mucosa and translocation of lipopolysaccharide (LPS) and peptidoglycan into the bloodstream. Furthermore, Morris et al.[12] note that translocation of commensal antigens correlates directly with increased markers of inflammation. Morris et al. [12] go on to point out that O&NS disrupt the tight junctions that maintain the integrity of the intestinal mucosal barrier. Under these conditions, translocation of commensal antigens can occur as well as intact Gram-negative bacteria, including *Pseudomonas aeruginosa, Hafnia alvei, Morganella morganii* and *Citrobacter koseri*.[12] This antigen and bacterial translocation can, in turn, cause translocation of bacterial LPS into the systemic circulation.[12]

Finally, it is important to note that the translocated LPS is an important cause of the depressed and unresponsive HRV reported earlier.[12]

Clinical evidence of the link between ME/CFS and GI dysfunction includes the fact that the risk of CFS is significantly higher in patients with inflammatory bowel disease compared with the general population.[18] There is clinical evidence of microbiome disturbances as a major contributing factor to ME/CFS in the form of data suggesting that irritable bowel syndrome related to previous exposure to *Giardia lamblia* can often be accompanied by chronic fatigue.[19, 20]

16.8.7 Cardiovascular Disturbances

As noted by Bozzini et al.,[21] patients with CFS often demonstrate orthostatic intolerance and abnormal sympathetic predominance in the autonomic cardiovascular response to gravitational stimuli. Furthermore, small left ventricular size with low cardiac output has been observed.[21] Adolescents with CFS have demonstrated reduced systolic blood pressure variability and sympathetic predominance of baroreflex heart rate control during orthostatic stress.[21] Finally, CFS patients tend to present with low blood pressure.[21]

16.8.8 Thyroid Dysfunction

In a study of 98 CFS patients aged 21–69 years and 99 age- and sex-matched controls, Ruiz-Nunez et al.[22] noted that CFS patients tend to exhibit lower free T3, total T4, total T3, T3/T4 ratios, protein binding of thyroid hormones, and 24-h urinary iodine excretion compared with controls. In contrast, percentage reverse T3 tends to be higher in CFS patients than in controls.[22] These results led the authors to conclude that many CFS patients demonstrate a mild form of "non-thyroidal illness syndrome" and "low T3 syndrome." Furthermore, in contrast to the trend of increased inflammation and increased immune function that has, as suggested earlier, been reported in many studies of CFS patients, Ruiz-Nunez[22] noted in the CFS patients an association between low T3 and low hsCRP. These findings led the authors to hypothesize that CFS patients are less responsive to inflammatory stimuli. In addition, the CFS patients demonstrating a "low T3 syndrome" again, in contrast to what is reported in so many ME/CFS patients, do not appear to present convincing evidence of chronic low-grade inflammation.[22]

16.8.9 Genetic Polymorphisms

As with so many other chronic illnesses, the presence of genetic polymorphisms can quite possibly create a predisposition to many of the metabolic imbalances and clinical findings reported in ME/CFS patients, as noted by Perez et al.[23] Specifically, in their pilot study, Perez et al.[23] found that 5693 single nucleotide polymorphisms (SNPs) had at least a 10% frequency in at least one ME/CFS cohort. The most clinically relevant of the SNPs reported in the Perez et al.[23] study may be that relating to cytochrome P450 2D6 (CYP2D6), which is an important enzyme involved in the metabolism of xenobiotics. Furthermore, CYP2D6 plays a vital role in androgen and estrogen biosynthesis and metabolism, tyrosine metabolism, and metabolism of codeine and morphine.[23] From a clinical standpoint, SNPs of CYP2D6 were found more often in ME/CFS patients who also exhibited fibromyalgia.[23] Given that studies have suggested a relationship between exposure to chemical toxins and incidence of ME/CFS (see later), it may be that detoxification enzyme SNPs are a significant part of the pathophysiologic picture in ME/CFS patients.

16.9 ALLOSTATIC OVERLOAD – A MORE ACCURATE MODEL THAT REFLECTS THE TRUE NATURE OF ME/CFS

It is clear, based on the research outlined earlier, that ME/CFS, with its lack of a standard, across-the-board, well-defined cause and many pathophysiologic manifestations that can vary from patient to patient, does not fit the traditional model of illness that suggests diseases are well-defined entities with similar clinical presentations that always have a singular cause, pathophysiology and treatment protocol. Does another model of disease exist that is more consistent with the true nature of ME/CFS? This question was answered by Arroll[24] in her paper "Allostatic overload in myalgic encephalomyelitis/chronic fatigue syndrome (ME/CFS)." In this hypothesis paper, the allostatic overload model of illness is presented with an explanation of why it is uniquely appropriate to reflect the true nature of ME/CFS, which can result in both a more accurate clinical assessment of any individual patient and more efficacious, cost-effective and practical treatment modalities.

16.9.1 ALLOSTASIS AND ALLOSTATIC OVERLOAD – A DEFINITION

As noted by Arroll,[24] to understand the concept of allostasis and allostatic overload, it is first important to understand how the body responds to any stressor, which may be physical or psychological in nature. She goes on to point out that the classic work by Hans Selye on the human stress response provides an explanation. Briefly, Selye proposed a three-phase theory called the "general adaptation syndrome." In the first "alarm" phase, the stressor is accompanied by physiologic changes but no permanent damage. If the stressor persists, the second "resistance" phase occurs, in which physiological adaptation takes place to cope with the stressor. However, even in this second phase, there is no significant damage to the organism that would yield perceptible signs and/or symptoms. In contrast, with a persistent, long-term stressor, the third "exhaustion" phase can occur, which often does lead to clinical illness and sometimes, mortality. Arroll[24] goes on to suggest that the signs and symptoms that define an illness are not caused by the stressor per se but by overactive and prolonged activity of the physiologic changes that compose the general adaptation syndrome proposed by Selye. This suggestion leads Arroll[24] to a discussion of the work by Bruce McEwen and colleagues on what is known as allostasis and allostatic load/overload.

In defining allostasis, McEwen and colleagues[25] first point out that allostasis basically defines how the body responds to environmental stressors to maintain a constant internal environment, or homeostasis, which it does by continually adjusting the "internal physiologic milieu." Furthermore, depending on the demands of the environment, "different physiological systems will interact with different levels of activity." More precisely, according to "What's in a name? Integrating homeostasis, allostasis and stress" by McEwen and Wingfield,[26] allostatic mechanisms act in response to environmental stressors to maintain homeostasis. Thus, allostasis is needed to maintain homeostasis. An example would be jumping into a 65°F pool on a summer day with an air temperature of approximately 90°F. Upon entering the pool, there is an instantaneous decrease of 25°F in the external milieu. Why is it that thermogenic shock does not immediately occur in a healthy individual? The answer is that hundreds and possibly thousands of allostatic mechanisms just as quickly become activated to adjust the internal milieu to maintain homeostatic constants such as body temperature, blood pressure and pulse, so that the net cognitive effect is a pleasurable, refreshing experience. Thus, with this in mind, allostatic responses to stressors are not inherently negative in nature. In contrast, with short-term stresses, allostatic responses promote health. An example of this would be increases in muscle mass and strength in response to physiologic amounts of exercise. The body's allostatic responses increase muscle mass and strength in order to "cope" with the stress of exercise. However, if the exercise is excessive, these initial allostatic coping mechanisms will start to become overwhelmed, leading to a secondary allostatic response of muscle pain and inflammation. What is one of the purposes of this secondary allostatic response? This secondary allostatic response is designed to send a cognitive message to stop the excessive exercise. What if this cognitive message is not heeded? The allostatic response of inflammation and pain are very metabolically expensive, in that energy reserves will be taken from other parts of the body to maintain inflammation and pain, leading to potential suboptimal function of these other body parts. This situation, where the body needs to compromise health in response to ongoing stress, is called "allostatic load/overload," where the response to prolonged stressors leads to suboptimal metabolic activity and signs and symptoms that are consistent with illness. The following two quotes by McEwen and Wingfield[26] provide excellent definitions of allostasis and allostatic load/overload:

> [A]llostasis refers to the ability of the body to produce hormones (such as cortisol, adrenalin) and other mediators (e.g., cytokines, parasympathetic activity) that help an animal adapt to a new situation/challenge. This includes the predictable and unpredictable.

> Allostatic load is defined as the cumulative result of an allostatic state. It can be considered the result of the daily and seasonal routines organisms have to obtain food and survive, and extra energy needed to migrate, molt, breed, etc. as well as deal with unpredictable perturbations.

At what point does allostasis become allostatic load? As noted by Fava et al.,[25] this transition from tolerable stress that leads to a tolerable allostatic response to a toxic stress that leads to allostatic load/overload is highly variable from person to person. However, the authors point out that allostatic load/overload is defined as "the transition to this extreme state."

Before leaving this introductory section on allostasis and allostatic load/overload, it should be emphasized that the allostatic response and resultant load/overload can occur with any stressor or combination of stressors, not just psychological stress, as mistakenly assumed by many. As noted by Fava et al.,[25] allostatic load can result from stressors as varied as poor sleep, social isolation, lack of exercise, poor diet and income equality.

16.9.2 Allostatic Load and ME/CFS

As pointed out by Arroll,[24] ME/CFS patients tend to demonstrate metabolic indicators consistent with allostatic load that are due to the cumulative effects of years of excessive and/or prolonged environmental stressors. Then, a significant stressor occurs, such as a viral or bacterial infection that acts as a "straw that breaks the camel's back" of sorts, leading to symptoms consistent with ME/CFS. Arroll[24] points out that the following, which are often seen in ME/CFS patients, strongly suggest that allostatic load is present:

- Low levels of urinary cortisol that is not linked with the usual causes such as psychiatric comorbidity, sleep problems, medication use and disability.
- Elevated dehydroepiandrosterone (DHEA).
- Increased parameters of inflammation such as IL-1, IL-6 and TNF.
- Decreased NK cell cytotoxic activity.
- Elevations in IL-1B, IL-12, IL-6, IL-8, IL-10 and IL-13 in those ME/CFS patients reporting high post-exertional fatigue.

Can stressful life events other than infection act as "the straw that breaks the camel's back" in ME/CFS patients, leading to the transition from a physiologic, benign allostatic response to a symptom producing allostatic load/overload scenario? Arroll[24] points out that research has noted that the following have been reported to initiate symptoms in ME/CFS patients:

- Change of residence.
- Marriage.
- Divorce.
- Change of jobs.
- Death of a loved one.
- Job-related conflict.

Arroll [24] goes on to point to another important aspect of environmental stress-induced allostatic load that is rarely considered. Basically, being stressed is stressful. More precisely, ME/CFS patients often experience a vicious circle effect whereby environmental stressors lead to an allostatic response that eventually becomes allostatic load/overload, leading to symptoms. However, it does not end there. The symptoms themselves, such as fatigue, pain, sleep disturbance, etc., act as another stress "increasing allostatic load and eventually maintaining allostatic overload," completing the vicious circle. Another aspect of this vicious circle, according to Arroll,[24] is fear of experiencing symptoms. This would explain, according to the author, why even after the "straw that breaks the camel's back" stressor has ceased, ill health can persist.

Arroll[24] concludes her paper by discussing the value of the allostasis/allostatic load/allostatic overload model in terms of more accurately assessing and more efficaciously treating the ME/CFS patient. This model allows for the fact that there is no single environmental stressor that leads to ME/CFS in all patients. Rather, a whole host of environmental stressors can be inducing agents, the combination of which will vary from patient to patient. What virtually all the ME/CFS patients do share in common is the allostatic responses to any particular patient-specific stressor or set of stressors plus the eventual excessive allostatic responses that lead to allostatic load/overload and accompanying symptomatology. With this concept in mind, Arroll[24] concludes with the following insightful statement:

> This paradigm shift will lead us away from the search for the holy grail of the sole pathogen and in doing so, may allow the development of effective symptom-alleviating treatments.

Do other publications support the idea that ME/CFS is an allostatic load phenomenon? In "Allostatic load is associated with symptoms in chronic fatigue syndrome patients" by Goertzel et al.,[27] the authors devised an allostatic load index. Using this index, it was concluded that high levels of allostatic load were significantly associated with bodily pain, physical functioning, and generally, symptom frequency/intensity. In an accompanying publication by the same group of researchers entitled "Chronic fatigue syndrome and high allostatic load" by Maloney et al.,[28] the authors again discussed the use of their allostatic load index. This index is comprised of the following measurements plus the levels that are indicative of the presence of CFS:

- Diastolic blood pressure (recumbent 30 min) greater than 90.
- Systolic blood pressure (recumbent 30 min) greater than 140.
- Aldosterone less than or equal to 4.5 ng/dl.
- Waist to hip ratio (males) greater than 0.95.
- Waist to hip ratio (females) greater than 0.87.
- Albumin lower than 3.6 g/dL.
- C-reactive protein greater than or equal to 5.0 mg/L.
- Interleukin-6 greater than or equal to 82.2.

- Urinary cortisol in males lower than 26.5 μg/24 h.
- Urinary cortisol in females lower than 13.0 μg/24 h.
- DHEA sulfate in males lower than or equal to 79.5 mg/dL.
- DHEA sulfate in females lower than or equal to 15.5 mg/dL.
- Epinephrine greater than 24.0 pg/mL.
- Norepinephrine greater than or equal to 433.0 pg/mL.

Based on this index, it was concluded that CFS is associated with a high level of allostatic load. The authors also reported that the three components of the index that best discriminated CFS cases from controls are waist to hip ratio, aldosterone and urinary cortisol.

16.10   KEY ENVIRONMENTAL STRESSORS THAT LEAD TO ALLOSTATIC LOAD IN ME/CFS PATIENTS

As was mentioned earlier, allostasis and the excessive allostatic responses that are the basis for allostatic load are responses to one or more significant environmental stressors. Which stressors, based on published research, appear to be most significant for ME/CFS patients? Consider the following.

16.10.1   Infectious Disease

As was noted earlier, it has been long suggested that ME/CFS may be caused by EBV or cytomegalovirus. However, as pointed out by Underhill,[29] infectious diseases such as influenza and mononucleosis can be followed by symptoms resembling ME/CFS. In addition, Melenotte et al.[30] point out research that suggests the presence of post-infectious CFS that can be induced, in addition to EBV, by Chikungunya virus infection, hepatitis A and B infections, brucellosis, Q fever caused by *Coxiella burnetii*, and Lyme disease caused by the *Borrelia burgdorferi* group.

16.10.2   Chemical and Metal Toxins

Underhill[29] points out the following chemical and metal toxins that have been linked with ME/CFS:

- Organophosphate pesticides.
- Solvents.
- Ciguatera fish poisoning.
- Cadmium.
- Mycotoxins from water damaged buildings.

Interestingly, research has also demonstrated that ME/CFS can also be linked with environmental chemicals whose toxicology is either controversial and/or seldom recognized. An example of this is the paper by Khoo et al.[31] that suggests CFS is more common in patients with silicone breast implants compared with systemic sclerosis controls. Even more interesting and controversial are two papers that suggest a relationship between ME/CFS and aluminum adjuvants used in hepatitis B vaccines.[32, 33] Gherardi et al. [32] propose the following:

> Instead of being rapidly solubilized in the extracellular space, injected aluminum particles are quickly captured by immune cells and transported to distant organs and the brain where they elicit an inflammatory response and exert selective low dose long-term neurotoxicity. Clinical observations and experiments in sheep, a large animal like humans, confirmed both systemic diffusion and neurotoxic effects of aluminum adjuvants. Post-immunization ME/CFS represents the core manifestation of "autoimmune/inflammatory syndrome induced by adjuvants" (ASIA).

16.10.3 Disturbances in Gut Microflora

As was mentioned earlier, ME/CFS has been found to be associated with disturbances in gut micro-flora. Nagy-Szakal et al. explored this relationship in detail in their paper "Fecal metagenomic profiles in subgroups of patients with myalgic encephalomyelitis/chronic fatigue syndrome."[34] The authors begin their paper by pointing out that disturbances in GI function are very common in ME/CFS patients, in that 35% to 90% report abdominal discomfort consistent with IBS. Furthermore, previous research has reported that post-infective fatigue states have been linked with acute giardiasis. To ascertain the impact of disturbances of gut microflora as a contributor to this relationship, the authors evaluated 50 ME/CFS patients and 50 healthy controls using DNA-based stool analysis. The ME/CFS patients were subdivided into those patients with IBS (ME/CFS + IBS) and those without IBS. Among all the ME/CFS cases, increases in the following microflora were associated with better vitality, health change and motivation scores: *Ruminococcus gnavus*, *Coprobacillus bacterium*, *Clostridium bolteae* and *Clostridium asparagiforme*. Among all ME/CFS cases, a decrease in relative abundance of the following was associated with worse emotional wellbeing scores: *Fecalibacterium prausnitzii* and *Coprococcus catus*. Finally, in all ME/CFS cases, decreases in the following were associated with improved motivation scores: *Rosburia inulinivorans* and *Dorea formicigenerans*.

In the ME/CFS + IBS cases, the decreases in the following were associated with improved vitality, health change and fatigue scores: *Alistipes*, *Dorea longicatena* and *Rosburia inulinivorans*. In these patients, decreases in *Coprococcus comes* were associated with worse fatigue scores, and decreases in *Faecalibacterium* species were associated with worse pain scores.

In ME/CFS without IBS cases, increases in *Pseudoflavorifractor capillosus* were associated with worse vitality, emotional wellbeing, health changes and motivation scores. Finally, in this group, relative abundances of *Dorea formicigenerans* and *Clostridium scindens* were associated with improved motivation scores.

16.11 PUTTING IT ALL TOGETHER: A PATIENT-SPECIFIC APPROACH THAT ADDRESSES BOTH THE ENVIRONMENTAL STRESSORS THAT INCREASE ALLOSTATIC LOAD AND THE SPECIFIC METABOLIC IMBALANCES THAT COMPRISE ALLOSTATIC LOAD

While allostatic load is not mentioned specifically, the paper "Chronic fatigue syndrome: A personalized integrative medicine approach" by Brown presents an excellent review of the literature not only on the identification and treatment of the various environmental stressors that create allostatic load in ME/CFS patients but also on the identification and treatment of the various metabolic imbalances that comprise allostatic load.[35] First, consider the literature on major environmental stressors that create allostatic load in ME/CFS patients.

16.12 ENVIRONMENTAL STRESSORS THAT CREATE ALLOSTATIC LOAD IN ME/CFS PATIENTS

16.12.1 Nutrient Deficiency

Vitamin D – Brown[35] points out that several studies have documented that vitamin D deficiency is prevalent in ME/CFS patients compared with the general population. He goes on to note that the suggested association is that vitamin D deficiency may contribute to ME/CFS oxidative stress and inflammation with generation of subsequent fatigue symptoms. In fact, symptoms of severe vitamin D deficiency are so similar to those seen with ME/CFS that people with vitamin D deficiency are often misdiagnosed as having ME/CFS. In terms of treatment of ME/CFS patients who are deficient in vitamin D with vitamin D supplements, modest clinical improvement in some individuals has been reported.

Impaired long-chain fatty acid metabolism – Brown[35] reports literature suggesting that functional impairment of fatty acid metabolism may explain, in part, functional changes in the CNS as well as clinical symptoms in ME/CFS patients. A suggested mechanism is that viral infection associated with ME/CFS "may impair the biosynthetic pathway for long-chain fatty acids." In support of this hypothesis, case reports have demonstrated improvement of ME/CFS symptoms with gamma linolenic acid (GLA), eicosapentaenoic acid (EPA) and/or docosahexaenoic acid (DHA) supplementation.

Functional B vitamin deficiency – Functional deficiencies in ME/CFS patients of folate, pyridoxine (vitamin B6), riboflavin (vitamin B2) and thiamine (vitamin B1) have been reported. Unfortunately, intervention trials of B vitamins with ME/CFS patients have been mixed in terms of clinical improvement.

Magnesium deficiency – Several studies have reported low magnesium status in ME/CFS patients. A suggested mechanism for the contribution of magnesium deficiency to ME/CFS symptoms is contribution to a pro-oxidant, low-grade inflammatory state. Evidence supporting the use of magnesium supplementation to improve ME/CFS symptoms is limited, with two case reports suggesting that intravenous magnesium supplementation resulted in significant clinical improvement.

Functional amino acid deficiency – Brown[35] points out hypotheses suggesting that amino acids required for neurotransmitter synthesis and production of ATP might be deficient in ME/CFS patients. Based on this hypothesis, a study was conducted in which fasting levels of plasma amino acids were measured in ME/CFS patients, and based on the findings of this assessment on each patient, a unique, 15-gram mixture of free-form amino acids was given for 3 months. Twenty participants completed the study. Of those individuals, 90% experienced at least a 25% improvement in symptoms, and 75% reported a 50% to 100% improvement.

Carnitine deficiency – Brown[35] points out one study noting that plasma carnitine status of ME/CFS patients was 30% to 40% lower in certain forms of carnitine compared with controls, with carnitine concentrations highly correlating with clinical symptoms. Brown[35] goes on to report two studies using carnitine supplementation in ME/CFS patients. One study employing 3 g per day of carnitine demonstrated significant improvement in symptoms, especially between the fourth and eighth weeks of treatment. A second study compared supplementation of 2 g per day of acetyl-L-carnitine, 2 g per day of propionyl-L-carnitine, and a combined treatment of 2 g of each per day. All treatments yielded beneficial effects on fatigue, pain and cognitive function.

Zinc deficiency – Brown[35] notes that serum zinc has been reported to be significantly lower in ME/CFS patients compared with healthy controls. In addition, low levels of zinc have been correlated with symptom severity and immunological dysfunction. Concerning intervention, even though no controlled clinical trials have been conducted using zinc supplementation with ME/CFS patients, clinical evidence, according to Brown,[35] has suggested that zinc supplementation may have a positive impact on fatigue, immune function, mood, inflammation and oxidative stress.

16.12.2 Psychological Stress

Brown[35] notes that adverse life events and related neuroendocrine dysfunction have preceded development of ME/CFS symptoms in some cases, leading to the allostatic response of HPA axis dysfunction. This HPA axis dysfunction is often demonstrated by low cortisol levels. However, Brown[35] also notes that most typically, HPA axis dysfunction develops after the onset of ME/CFS symptoms. Interventions reported to be effective are the following:

Cognitive behavioral therapy (CBT) – Brown[35] points out that some patients have reported improvements in symptoms and cortisol levels with CBT. However, some ME/CFS patients have also reported worsening of symptoms with CBT.

Mind-body medicine – Brown[35] reports evidence that mind-body therapies can improve HPA axis dysfunction and bring about a reduction in symptoms and/or improvements in physical functioning. Specifically, a randomized, controlled study on qigong exercise demonstrated improvements in fatigue and mental functioning compared with controls.

16.12.3 Environmental Pollutants

Brown[35] suggests, as noted earlier, that a number of studies have demonstrated that environmental toxins can be a major environmental stressor that contributes to the development of ME/CFS. These toxins include pesticides, insecticides, mercury, lead, nickel, cadmium, tobacco smoke and ciguatera poisoning. One study provided evidence of this relationship by showing that serum organophosphates were higher in ME/CFS patients compared with controls. Brown[35] goes on to note that interventions to reduce toxic load include nutritional detoxification, which employs dietary changes and supplemental nutrients that support endogenous detoxification pathways. Studies on this approach have reported enhancement of hepatic metabolism and reduction in subjective symptoms of fatigue. Another study using a detoxification program consisting of ascorbic acid and choline supplementation reported that ME/CFS symptoms improved as blood levels of pesticides decreased. Finally, it has been suggested, according to Brown,[35] that infrared sauna therapy may benefit ME/CFS patients by "diaphoretic elimination of persistent organic pollutants."

16.12.4 Disturbances of Gut Microflora

As has been mentioned earlier, disturbances in gut microflora can be a major environmental stressor that can dramatically increase allostatic load. Brown[35] points out that in ME/CFS patients, low levels of *Bifidobacterium* and high levels of *Enterococcus* and *Streptococcus* have been reported, as well as small intestinal bacterial overgrowth (SIBO). A related finding in ME/CFS patients, according to Brown,[35] is that compared with healthy controls, higher levels of serum antibodies against lipopolysaccharide (endotoxin) correlated closely with symptom severity. Brown[35] goes on to point out that high levels of circulating endotoxin can be significantly reduced with healthy dietary patterns. In fact, according to the author, one study demonstrated a reduction in circulating endotoxin by 31% within 1 month. Furthermore, dietary changes plus treatment with anti-inflammatory and antioxidative nutrients such as glutamine, N-acetylcysteine and zinc over 10 to 14 months significantly reduced antibodies to endotoxin, "with over 50% of participants showing significant clinical improvement or remission."

Several studies, according to Brown,[35] have also demonstrated that probiotic supplementation can have a significant impact. Specifically, supplementation with *Lactobacillus* and *Bifidobacterium* significantly decreased anxiety symptoms in ME/CFS patients to a greater degree than in controls. Another trial, according to Brown,[35] demonstrated that supplementation of *Lactobacillus paracasei* sp. Paracasei F19, *Lactobacillus acidophilus* NCFB 1748 and *Bifidobacterium lactis* Bb12 in ME/CFS patients resulted in significant improvement in neurocognitive function and a trend towards "improvement in general symptoms and quality of life in some individuals."

16.12.5 Chronic Infection

As has been repeatedly demonstrated, chronic infection can be a significant environmental stressor leading to the creation of ME/CFS symptoms. Brown[35] points out that certain infectious pathogens can produce a significant, often lifelong, infection, stimulating continued immune responses. Furthermore, some of these long-term pathogens can act as neuropathogens that directly or indirectly affect the CNS, leading to ME/CFS symptoms.

As has also been repeatedly mentioned, EBV can be one of those instigators of lifelong infection in ME/CFS patients. Brown[35] points out that long-term treatment with the antiviral drug valacyclovir "led to decreased serum antibodies to EBV and a significant improvement in a subgroup of individuals with CFS/ME with persistent EBV infection."

16.13 KEY METABOLIC RESPONSES TO ENVIRONMENTAL STRESSORS THAT COMPRISE ALLOSTATIC LOAD IN ME/CFS PATIENTS

16.13.1 INFLAMMATION

As was noted earlier, a key aspect of the allostatic response is inflammation and free radical production. When in excess, they can be powerful contributors to allostatic load/overload. In ME/CFS patients, according to Brown,[35] higher levels of the inflammatory mediators CRP and 8-isoprostaglandin F_{2a} isoprostanes have been reported compared with healthy controls. Brown[35] goes on to suggest that a traditional Mediterranean diet has been shown to reduce chronic, low-grade inflammation and may be beneficial to ME/CFS patients.

16.13.2 MITOCHONDRIAL DYSFUNCTION

A key aspect of allostatic load/overload is mitochondrial dysfunction.[36] With this in mind, Brown[35] points out that mitochondrial dysfunction may be central to the pathology of ME/CFS. The author goes on to point out research demonstrating that measurements of availability of ATP and efficiency of mitochondrial oxidative phosphorylation are reduced in ME/CFS patients compared with controls. Furthermore, these reductions are correlated with severity of illness. Further support for the suggestion of mitochondrial dysfunction in ME/CFS patients, according to Brown,[35] is evidence of a deficiency of coenzyme Q10, a key factor in mitochondrial energy metabolism and membrane potential.

According to Brown,[35] several studies have suggested that nutritional supplementation can improve mitochondrial function. In relation to ME/CFS, one study employing supplementation of D-ribose, "a structural component of intermediate metabolites required for mitochondrial energy metabolism," for 3 weeks reported improvements in energy, wellbeing, sleep and mental clarity, and decreased pain. Another study on ME/CFS patients using a nutritional formula to support mitochondrial function containing vitamins, minerals, amino acids, plant extracts, phospholipids and fatty acids "reported a 43% reduction in fatigue in individuals with CFS/ME and fibromyalgia after 8 weeks of treatment." Finally, according to Brown,[35] a paper that audited ME/CFS patients who had evidence of mitochondrial dysfunction found that improvements in symptoms and mitochondrial function often occurred with the use of an integrative treatment plan that frequently included the mitochondrial nutrients D-ribose, magnesium, acetyl-L-carnitine and coenzyme Q10.

Brown[35] concludes his paper with some final thoughts about ME/CFS patients that strongly support an individualized, allostatic load approach to their assessment and treatment:

> Currently accepted treatments for CFS/ME have modest clinical benefits and for most patients the disease prognosis remains poor. Because CFS/ME is a heterogeneous disorder with diverse etiological factors and pathological features, a patient-centered integrative framework based on modifiable physiological and environmental factors may offer hope for more effective management and better clinical outcomes. An individualized approach to patient management may also help identify patient subgroups that are more likely to respond favorably to specific treatments. A personalized integrative approach to CFS/ME deserves further consideration as a template for patient management and future research.

16.14 SOME FINAL THOUGHTS

According to an August 18, 2020 posting on the Mayo Clinic website:

> The cause of chronic fatigue syndrome is unknown, although there are many theories – ranging from viral infections to psychological stress. Some experts believe chronic fatigue syndrome might be triggered by a combination of factors.

Can the research-based allostatic load hypothesis that ME/CFS is a "combination of factors," as suggested by Brown[35] and so many other clinicians and researchers whose publications are reviewed in this book chapter, be dismissed as a mere belief, as suggested by the Mayo Clinic website? Clearly, the research presented in this book chapter on the allostatic load model of ME/CFS makes it clear that it is more than a belief system.

While Brown[35] and many of the other authors whose work was highlighted earlier did not use the specific terms "allostasis" and "allostatic load," they make a strong case that the essence of the allostatic load/overload model of ME/CFS best explains ME/CFS pathophysiology. What is the essence of the allostatic load/overload model? Very simply, even though patients share similar symptomatic patterns, the underlying basis for these symptoms, which are environmental stressors and the metabolic imbalances that result from these stressors, is unique to each patient. Furthermore, with this apparent reality of pathophysiologic uniqueness despite similar symptomatic patterns in mind, it is clear that the path to the most efficacious and cost-effective assessment and treatment will not be the all too common, preconceived, "one size fits all" agendas about causes, mechanisms and cures. In contrast, the published literature reviewed earlier makes it clear that the best path to efficacious and practical assessment and treatment of the ME/CFS patient will be patient centered. What does "patient centered" mean? Very succinctly, it means that rather than using the traditional "this is the way we've always done it" approach, patient diagnostic data and patient needs will be individually considered using the lens of the width and breadth of pathophysiologic research on ME/CFS, of which this book chapter is but a brief overview.

REFERENCES

1. Komaroff AL. Advances in understanding the pathophysiology of chronic fatigue syndrome. *JAMA* 2019;Published online July 5, 2019.
2. McManimen S et al. Dismissing chronic illness: A qualitative analysis of negative experiences. *Health Care Women Int* 2019;40:241–58.
3. Chu L et al. Onset patterns and course of myalgic encephalomyelitis/chronic fatigue syndrome. *Front Pediatr* 2019;7.
4. Friedman KJ. Advances in ME/CFS: Past, present, and future. *Front Pediatr* 2019;7.
5. Friedberg F, Sunnquist M, Nacul L. Rethinking the Standard of Care for Myalgic Encephalomyelitis/ Chronic Fatigue Syndrome. *J Gen Intern Med* 2019.
6. Holtzman CS et al. Assessment of post-exertional malaise (PEM) in patients with myalgic encephalomyelitis (ME) and chronic fatigue syndrome (CFS): A patient driven survey. *Diagnostics* 2019;9.
7. Richman S et al. Pharmaceutical interventions in chronic fatigue syndrome: A literature-based commentary. *Clin Ther* 2019;41:798–805.
8. Missailidis D et al. Pathological mechanisms underlying myalgic encephalomyelitis/chronic fatigue syndrome. *Diagnostics* 2019;9.
9. Rivera M et al. Myalgic encephalomyelitis/chronic fatigue syndrome: A comprehensive review. *Diagnostics* 2019;9.
10. Jeffrey MG et al. Treatment avenues in myalgic encephalomyelitis/chronic fatigue syndrome: A split gender pharmacogenomic study of gene-expression modules. *Clin Ther* 2019;41:815–35.
11. Sotzny F et al. Myalgic encephalomyelitis/chronic fatigue syndrome - evidence for an autoimmune disease. *Autoimmun Rev* 2018;17:601–9.
12. Morris G et al. Myalgic encephalomyelitis/chronic fatigue syndrome: From pathophysiological insights to novel therapeutic options. *Pharmacol Res* 2019;148.
13. Groven N et al. Patients with fibromyalgia and chronic fatigue syndrome show increased hsCRP compared to healthy controls. *Brain Behav Immun* 2019;Published online ahead of print.
14. Mueller C et al. Evidence of widespread metabolite abnormalities in myalgic encephalomyelitis/chronic fatigue syndrome: Assessment with whole-brain magnetic resonance spectroscopy. *Brain Imaging Behav* 2019;Published online ahead of print January 7, 2019.
15. Lacourt TE et al. The high costs of low-grade inflammation: Persistent fatigue as a consequence of reduced cellular-energy availability and non-adaptive energy expenditure. *Front Behav Neurosci* 2018;12.

16. Tsai S et al. Increased risk of chronic fatigue syndrome following psoriasis: A nationwide population-based cohort study. *J Translational Med* 2019;17.

17. McGregor NR et al. Post-exertional malaise is associated with hypermetabolism, hypoacetylation and purine metabolism deregulation in ME/CFS cases. *Diagnostics* 2019;9.

18. Tsai S et al. Increased risk of chronic fatigue syndrome in patients with inflammatory bowel disease: A population-based retrospective study. *J Translational Med* 2019;17.

19. Litleskare S et al. Quality of life and its association with irritable bowel syndrome and fatigue ten years after giardiasis. *Neurogastroenterol Motil* 2019;31.

20. Litleskare S et al. Prevalence of irritable bowel syndrome and chronic fatigue 10 years after Giardia infection. *Clin Gastroenterol Hepatol* 2018;16:1064–72.

21. Bozzini S et al. Cardiovascular characteristics of chronic fatigue syndrome. *Biomed Rep* 2018;8:26–30.

22. Ruiz-Nunez B et al. Higher prevalence of "Low T3 Syndrome" in patients with chronic fatigue syndrome: A case-control study. *Front Endocrinol* 2018;9.

23. Perez M et al. Genetic predispositoin for immune system, hormone, and metabolic dysfunction in myalgic encephalomyelitis/chronic fatigue syndrome: A pilot study. *Front Pediatr* 2019;7.

24. Arroll MA. Allostatic overload in myalgic encephalomyelitis/chronic fatigue syndrome (ME/CFS). *Med Hypotheses* 2013;81:506–8.

25. Fava GA, McEwen BS, Guidi J, Gostoli S, Offidani E, Sonino N. Clinical characterization of allostatic overload. *Psychoneuroendocrinology* 2019;108:94–101.

26. McEwen BS, Wingfield JC. What is in a name? Integrating homeostasis, allostasis and stress. *Horm Behav* 2010;57:105–11.

27. Goetzel BN et al. Allostatic load is associated with symptoms in chronic fatigue syndrome patients. *Pharmacogenomics* 2006;7:485–594.

28. Maloney EM et al. Chronic fatigue syndrome and high allostatic load. *Pharmacogenomics* 2006;7:467–73.

29. Underhill RA. Myalgic encephalomyelitis, chronic fatigue syndrome: An infectious disease. *Med Hypotheses* 2015;85:765–73.

30. Melenotte C et al. Post-bacterial infection chronic fatigue syndrome is not a latent infection. *Med Mal Infect* 2019;49:140–9.

31. Khoo T et al. Silicone breast implants and depression, fibromyalgia and chronic fatigue syndrome in a rheumatology clinic population. *Clin Rheumatol* 2019;38:1271–6.

32. Gherardi RK et al. Myalgia and chronic fatigue syndrome following immunization: Macrophagic myofasciitis and animal studies support linkage to aluminum adjuvant persistency and diffusion in the immune system. *Autoimmun Rev* 2019;18:691–705.

33. Agmon-Levin N et al. Chronic fatigue syndrome and fibromyalgia following immunization with the hepatitis B vaccine: Another angle of the 'autoimmune (auto-inflammatory) syndrome induced by adjuvants' (ASIA). *Immunol Res* 2014;60:376–83.

34. Nagy-Szakal D et al. Fecal metagenomic profiles in subgroups of patients with myalgic encephalomyelitis/chronic fatigue syndrome. *Microbiome* 2017;5.

35. Brown BI. Chronic fatigue syndrome: A personalized integrative medicine approach. *Altern Ther* 2014;20:29–40.

36. Picard M, Juster RP, McEwen BS. Mitochondrial allostatic load puts the 'gluc' back in glucocorticoids. *Nat Rev Endocrinol* 2014;10:303–10.

Section II

Functional and Integrative Medicine: Perspectives in Deep Healing

17 Soil Health Impacts on Water and Nutrient Use Efficiency

Jerry L. Hatfield, Peter L. O'Brien and Kenneth M. Wacha

CONTENTS

17.1 INTRODUCTION

Soil health, the continued capacity of soil to function as a vital living ecosystem that sustains plants, animals and humans,[1] is of increasing importance to researchers and land managers worldwide, as forces of global change are leading to land degradation.[2] Maintaining soil health is especially important in agricultural areas, as increasing human populations continue to demand more food, fuel and fiber from agricultural land.[3, 4] This increased demand has led to extensive land conversion to agricultural production and the continuation of disruptive management practices,[5, 6] both of which have the potential to diminish soil health and reduce sustainable, long-term success in agronomic systems.[2, 7]

The act of converting land to agricultural production affects the soil in numerous ways, including altering soil structure and hydrology,[8, 9] degrading biological communities[10] and decreasing soil C stocks.[11] Further, many common practices that increase the productivity potential of agricultural systems, including tillage, fertilizer application and agrochemical applications, also threaten environmental quality by increasing erosion,[12] greenhouse gas emissions[13] and nutrients in surface runoff.[14] Thus, these practices that are implemented to meeting rising demand, when used incorrectly, actually contribute to land degradation and pose a threat to long-term food security and environmental quality. These negative consequences associated with agronomic systems have spurred a resurgence in understanding how to manage soils to maintain high productivity and reduce environmental impact.

One important way to quantify how successful management practices are at reducing impacts to environmental quality may be to assess metrics of efficiency. Two critical resources in agricultural systems that dictate productivity are nutrients and water, and they may be understood in the context of water use efficiency (WUE) and nutrient use efficiency (NUE). Broadly, increasing resource use efficiency will be associated with reduced losses to other sources, such as greenhouse gas emissions, evaporation, runoff, leaching and erosion. Thus, maintaining or increasing crop production while increasing WUE and NUE will necessarily result in fewer resources lost and more efficient systems.

The potential of agronomic systems to increase WUE and NUE is directly related to many soil parameters that are also indicative of soil health. Notably, the relationship between soil health and

DOI: 10.1201/b23304-19

both WUE and NUE has not been comprehensively investigated. In this chapter, we 1) provide a brief overview of soil health, including discussions of terminology, methods of quantification and frameworks of soil health assessment; 2) describe how soil health indicators relate to metrics of agroecosystem efficiency, including WUE and NUE; and 3) highlight research directions that connect soil health with both WUE and NUE to show how this connection may improve our understanding of agroecosystem resilience and sustainability.

17.2   SOIL HEALTH

The Natural Resources Conservation Service (NRCS) definition of soil health, the continued capacity of soil to function as a vital living ecosystem that sustains plants, animals and humans, naturally begs the question: What functions does the soil perform? Many of the functions that soils perform are so ubiquitous and reliable that they often go unnoticed. Nonetheless, these functions are critical in delivering ecosystem services and regulating environmental quality. In agricultural systems specifically, soils (1) serve as suitable habitat capable of sustaining biodiversity, (2) provide structure and a resource medium for biomass production, (3) store and filter water resources, and (4) degrade, detoxify and manage wastes through both nutrient cycling and long-term resource storage.[15–17]

The manner in which soils function is closely regulated by their composition. Soils comprise a series of different materials, including minerals, solid organic matter, biota, air and water, so they serve as an interface between the lithosphere, biosphere, atmosphere and hydrosphere.[18] The largest pool, mineral matter, is typically defined by classifying the sizes of each abiotic particle into sand-, silt- or clay-sized particles. The distribution of these size fractions, as well as the amount of pore space (i.e., the volume of air and water), governs the transfer of air, water, nutrients and root growth that are associated with the various soil functions. Notably, the composition of these different soil materials varies widely in space and time due to the influence of soil forming factors, including climate, topography, parent material, time and interactions with living organisms.[19]

Assessment of soil health typically begins with quantifying parameters that describe physical, chemical and biological properties Table 17.1.

TABLE 17.1

Commonly Measured Soil Physical, Chemical and Biological Parameters to Serve as Soil Health Indicators and Inform Soil Health Assessments[21,22,23]

Physical	Chemical	Biological
• Aggregate stability	• Base saturation	• Enzyme analysis
• Available water capacity	• Soil C	• (e.g., Arylsulfatase, beta-
• Bulk density	• Total, organic, inorganic,	glucosidase, phosphatase)
• Soil depth	• permanganate-oxidizable	• C mineralization rate
• Erosion rating	• Cation exchange capacity	• N mineralization rate
• Infiltration	• Electrical conductivity	• Earthworms
• Hydraulic conductivity	• Extractable P, K, Ca, Mg, Na	• Fatty acid methyl esters
• Saturated, unsaturated	• Heavy metals	• Faunal community indices (e.g.,
• Penetration resistance	• Extractable micronutrients	nematode maturity index)
• Porosity	• pH	• Genomics
• Reflectance	• Reflectance	• Microbial biomass carbon
• Soil stability index	• Sodium absorption ratio	• Phospholipid fatty acids
• Texture	• Soil N	• Quantitative polymerase chain
	• Total, inorganic, organic,	reaction (qPCR)
	• potentially mineralizable	• Soil respiration
		• Soil protein index

Identifying what parameters specifically should be included as soil health indicators has been the subject of extensive research. Generally, these indicators should meet several criteria: 1) they must be related to a soil ecosystem service, a soil function or a soil threat; 2) they must be measurable by reliable, reproducible procedures; 3) they must be sensitive enough to indicate changes; and 4) they must be interpretable across space and time to provide meaningful information.[20-22] Some disagreement over how (or if) to apply these criteria still exists, precisely because the variability of soils is such that the same parameter will not be meaningful in every instance. Nonetheless, the body of literature attempting to identify a minimum dataset for soil health assessment continues to grow. The incomplete understanding of bio-physicochemical parameters, however, makes it critical to understand that a static minimum dataset may be unrealistic; rather, the minimum dataset must remain adaptable in the face of evolving knowledge and methodological advances.[21]

The final two steps of soil health assessment involve 1) a qualitative analysis of each soil health indicator (e.g., low, medium, high or poor, good, very good) when compared with similar soils; and 2) consolidation of the assessment of all indicators into a comprehensive soil health score. Two leading soil health frameworks used in the United States are the Soil Management Assessment Framework[23] and the Cornell Soil Health Assessment,[18] although many other frameworks have been developed worldwide.[22, 24]

17.3 RESOURCE USE EFFICIENCY

Many of the soil parameters included as soil health indicators are critical in determining the resource use efficiency of the agroecosystem, including both WUE and NUE. In fact, while soil health is a valuable framework for understanding soil water and nutrient cycling, it does not provide any context for vegetation growth or resource uptake. Thus, if the goal is to understand how management practice influences systemwide sustainability and resource balances, relating soil health to WUE and NUE is especially informative.

17.3.1 WATER USE EFFICIENCY

WUE is a concept introduced over 100 years ago by Briggs and Shantz[25] to demonstrate the relationship between plant productivity and water use. They coined the term "water use efficiency" as a metric to quantify the amount of biomass produced per unit of water used by a plant. WUE can be mathematically described as:

$$WUE = \frac{total\ biomass\ or\ grain\ yield}{water\ transpired\ by\ the\ plant}$$

This is a simple relationship that relates plant production in proportion to the amount of water transpired by the crop canopy. Thus, WUE increases as plant productivity increases per unit of water transpired by the plant.

In the last century of research, the primary focus has been on the variation in WUE across different systems, with the assumption that WUE was increased as a combination of increased water use and increased plant growth. This assumption was challenged by Basso and Ritchie[26] after they found that maize (*Zea mays* L.) productivity could be increased with no change in water use rate and result in increased WUE. This finding occurred because transpiration rate reaches a limit when the crop canopy completely covers the surface; this limit is imposed by the canopy reaching the maximum amount of intercepted net radiation, which typically occurs when the leaf area index of the canopy exceeds 4. This observation provides support for the argument that enhancing soil health to supply more water to the plant would increase WUE, as increased biomass production could occur after transpiration rate reaches its limit.

Shifting the focus onto the ability of the soil to supply water for plant production necessarily involves a shift away from the traditional understanding of WUE, as the original equation requires that soil water extracted by the roots and transpired by the plant be separated from all other processes at the soil surface, especially evaporation. A closely related concept that may be useful in understanding WUE moving forward is precipitation use efficiency (PUE), given by:

$$PUE = \frac{total\ biomass\ or\ grain\ yield}{seasonal\ precipitation}$$

The use of PUE is especially important in rain-fed agriculture, as precipitation supplements stored soil water as the only sources for biomass production. Therefore, PUE may be a useful link between WUE and soil health, which plays an important role in the infiltration and storage of precipitation.

17.3.2 Nutrient Use Efficiency

NUE is similar to WUE but is often more complex because of the processes linked with nutrient cycling in the soil. The water balance in the soil is relatively simple because the amount of water available is directly input from either precipitation or irrigation. This is not the case for nutrients, because the amount of a nutrient in the soil could be from application of the nutrient, released from the soil or recycled from organic material in the root zone.[27] Hawkesford et al.[28] provided a comprehensive analysis of NUE in plants, which was an extension of the overview provided by Cassman et al.[29] These summaries identified improving NUE as a goal of agronomic management practices, which requires definition of a variety of NUE metrics. Dobermann[30] provided a synopsis of the different NUE metrics that offer an idea of how we can link nutrient use efficiency to soil health. These metrics are:

$$Recovery\ Efficiency\ (RE) = (U - U_o)/F$$

$$Physiological\ Efficiency\ (PE) = (Y - Y_o)/(U - U_o)$$

$$Internal\ Utilization\ Efficiency\ (IE) = Y/U$$

$$Agronomic\ Efficiency\ (AE) = (Y - Y_o)/F\ or\ RE\ x\ PE$$

$$Partial\ Factor\ Productivity\ (PFP) = Y/F\ or\ Y_o/F + AE$$

where F is the fertilizer applied, Y the crop yield with nutrients applied, Y_o the crop yield without nutrients applied, U the total nutrient uptake in the above-ground biomass with nutrients applied, and U_o the total nutrient uptake in the above-ground biomass with no nutrients applied.

One limitation to the approaches suggested by Dobermann[30] is the focus on applied nutrients; the definitions provided here pertain only to fertilizer applied and do not account for nutrient cycling or availability within the soil matrix. However, for many nutrients, the availability within the soil can be regulated by decomposition and mineralization of crop residues and soil organic matter, or they can be supplied by primary and secondary minerals. In the case of nitrogen, which has been the focus of most research on NUE because it is one of the most limiting nutrients in crop production,[29, 31] numerous sources and sinks of nitrogen in the soil make estimating nitrogen use efficiency more difficult. Berendse and Aerts[32] proposed that nitrogen use efficiency in perennial crops was complex because of the turnover of root systems along with the dynamics of processes affecting nitrogen availability in the soil profile. Similarly, legumes have the capacity to contribute to soil nitrogen pools via atmospheric N_2 fixation, and these contributions may be overlooked if the focus remains only on applied nutrients.

17.4   RELATIONSHIP OF SOIL HEALTH WITH RESOURCE USE EFFICIENCY

The primary effect of soil health on either WUE or NUE can be simply related to the effect of soil health on plant growth. Generally, improvements in soil health to supply either water or nutrients to the plant will benefit plant growth and alleviate stresses that would limit productivity; these improvements would then increase plant biomass or harvestable yield. Thus, if we assume that management to improve soil health results in increased soil water or nutrient availability without increased inputs, then any increases in plant productivity reflect improved resource use efficiency. A review by Hatfield et al.[33] summarized the potential role of soil management in WUE. Soil management practices that impact WUE can be divided into two large categories; 1) practices that alter the water balance to decrease soil water evaporation and increase the amount available for transpiration through the plant, which results in a reduction in water stress, and 2) practices that improve soil conditions and result in enhanced plant growth. This latter aspect would be expected to influence not only WUE but NUE as well and should be the focus of how we manage agricultural systems.

Improving soil health can greatly alter soil hydraulic properties, including infiltration and water retention, especially in rain-fed agricultural systems.[34] This can be especially important in the upper surface layers of the soil, which serves as either a regulator or a restrictor of water entry based on the ability of soil aggregates to retain pore spacing under imposed water stress.[35] Management practices influence the soil aggregate characteristics (i.e., size distribution and stability) in surface layers through varying levels of tillage intensity and amount of surface cover.[36] Tillage events can break apart soil aggregates and reduce aggregate stability, causing soil consolidation.[37] When soil aggregates rupture, encapsulated material is released, which can clog pore spaces, impede infiltration and prompt runoff conditions to develop rapidly.[38] These interactions can become more pronounced when considering extreme weather events, including water overabundance through increased rainfall intensity or lack of plant-available water during extended dry periods. Management practices that promote surface cover through residue or cover crops can help dissipate the energy of falling raindrops and decrease splash effects and erosion events. Improving soil health promotes stable aggregates and infiltration, thereby maximizing the amount of water going into the soil for crops. Similarly, water retention and storage can be improved by management practices that increase soil porosity and soil organic matter. As soil health improves, more water infiltrates into the soil, and more water is retained within the profile for plants to access throughout the growing season.

The linkage of NUE to soil health is evidenced by studies that show the positive impacts of plant growth–promoting rhizobacteria and arbuscular mycorrhiza fungi on plant growth and yield.[39] These effects were found across tillage systems in the study by Adesemoye et al. but show the value of examining the soil systems more completely than by simply measuring the amount of fertilizer added to the soil. Mandal et al.[40] showed that adding biochar as a soil amendment increased nitrogen use efficiency because of changes in the chemical and physical conditions of the soil that would be associated with soil health.

Further, many researchers have linked soil health with increased plant biomass and grain production. For example, Meena et al.[41] showed that maize and chickpea (*Cicer arietinum* L.) productivity was increased by practices that increased soil health to supply more nutrients to these crops. In a previous study, Novak et al.[42] observed that adding biochar to the soil to enhance soil health had a direct impact on crop productivity. In a review of the literature, Dias et al.[43] summarized that practices oriented toward soil health had a positive impact on crop productivity. This increase in plant production represents a possible synergistic effect between soil health and resource use efficiency. More plant production increases soil organic matter via residue and root inputs, improves soil pore networks via root growth and aggregate formation, and increases soil nutrient transformations due to increased biological activity; these improvements in soil quality indicators create a positive feedback loop with resource use efficiency by promoting plant production without requiring additional external inputs.

17.5   LINKAGE OF SOIL HEALTH, WUE, AND NUE TO NUTRITION

The linkage among soil health, WUE and NUE has not been investigated and offers the potential to understand the dynamics of future crop production systems that could enhance food security. For example, Lal[44] evaluated the potential use of pulses in cropping systems to provide a stable food source of nutritious food while also impacting soil health and having an effect on the efficiency of growth of other crops in the rotation. Kerr et al.[45] observed that adoption of legumes into cropping systems was of benefit to the overall productivity of the system because of the increased soil fertility and the diversity of the foods grown in supplying protein. Upadhyay et al.[46] compared different commercial fertilizer with organic manures and in combination on a diverse crop rotation of a rice (*Oryza sativa* L.) system that included durum wheat (*Triticum durum* Desb.), sunhemp (*Crotolaria juncea* L.), potato (*Solanum tuberosum* L.), berseem (*Trifolium alexandrium* L.), vegetable pea (*Pisum sativum* L.) and sorghum (*Sorghum bicolor* L. Moench) as part of the cropping system. They found productivity was increased with commercial fertilizers compared with the organic manures; however, after five cropping cycles, the manure treatments had higher soil organic carbon and more available N, P, and K compared with the commercial fertilizer plots. There was an increase in soil microorganisms under the organic manure treatments after five cropping cycles. These changes in the soil increased the water productivity of the cropping systems because of the enhanced soil health. These results are similar to those reported by Patel et al.[47] when they observed that continual use of organic amendments improved soil health and the overall crop productivity of vegetable-based systems. These studies didn't measure WUE or NUE; however, we could estimate that enhancing productivity would increase both of these parameters.

Management of cropping systems to enhance soil health does provide benefits to the crop and the nutritional quality of the produce. The results from research studies are limited and do not permit the development of firm guidelines for these relationships to be assessed. It will remain a challenge for the next generation of research studies to develop these relationships.

17.6   CHALLENGES

Water use and NUE are metrics to compare among cropping systems for their ability to efficiently utilize natural resources. However, the linkage to soil health can only be surmised based on the observation that enhanced soil health increases crop productivity, water availability and nutrient availability. If we increase either water or nutrient availability, we can increase the efficiency of water or nutrient use because we will have increased plant productivity. The challenge remains to develop a series of more integrated studies that define and quantify these relationships. The benefit would be to more efficiently and effectively utilize our natural resources to sustain plant productivity to meet the world's food and nutritional needs for the expanding population.

REFERENCES

1. USDA-NRCS. 2020. United States Department of Agriculture: Natural Resources Conservation Services: Soil. *Health.* http://www.nrcs.usda.gov/wps/portal/nrcs/main/soils/health/. Accessed 23 May 2020.
2. Karlen, D.L., and C.W. Rice. 2015. Soil degradation: Will humankind ever learn? *Sustainability.* 7:12490–12501. https://doi.org/10.3390/su70912490
3. Hatfield, J.L., and C.L. Walthall. 2015. Meeting global food needs: Realizing the potential via genetics x environment x management interactions. *Agron. J.* 107:1251–1226.

4. Hatfield, J.L., T.J. Sauer, and R.M. Cruse. 2017. Soil: The forgotten piece of the water, food, energy nexus. In: Donald L. Sparks, editor, *Advances in Agronomy, Vol. 143*, Burlington: Academic Press, 2017, pp. 1–46. ISBN: 978-0-12-812421-5

5. O'Brien, P.L., J.L. Hatfield, C. Dold, E. Kistner-Thomas, and K. Wacha. 2020. Cropping pattern changes diminish agroecosystem services in North and South Dakota, USA. *Agron. J.* 1–24. https://doi.org/10.1002/agj2.20001

6. Alexander P., M.D.A. Rounsevell, C. Dislich, J.R. Dodson, K. Engstrom, and D. Moran. 2015. Drivers for global agricultural land use change: The nexus of diet, population, yield and bioenergy. *Glob. Environ. Chang.* 35:138–147. https://doi.org/10.1016/j.gloenvcha.2015.08.011

7. Lal, R. 2015. Restoring soil quality to mitigate soil degradation. *Sustainability.* 7: 5875–5895. https://doi.org/10.3390/su7055875

8. Schilling, K.E., K.S. Chan, H. Liu, and Y.K. Zhang. 2010. Quantifying the effect of land use land cover change on increasing discharge in the Upper Mississippi River. *J. Hydrol.* 387: 343–345. https://doi.org/10.1016/j.jhydrol.2010.04.019

9. Cambardella, C.A., and E.T. Elliott. 1993. Carbon and nitrogen distribution in aggregates from cultivated and native grassland soils. *Soil Sci. Soc. Am. J.* 57:1071–1076.

10. Postma-Blaauw, M.P., R.G.M. de Goede, J. Bloem, J.H. Faber, and L. Brussard. 2010. Soil biota community structure and abundance under agricultural intensification and extensification. *Ecology* 9:460–473.

11. Tang, S., J. Guo, S. Li, J. Li, S. Xie, X. Zhai, C. Wang, Y. Zhang, and K. Wang. 2019. Synthesis of soil carbon losses in response to conversion of grassland to agriculture land. *Soil Till. Res.* 185:29–35. https://doi.org/10.1016/j.still.2018.08.011

12. Mhazo, N., P. Chivenge, and V. Chaplot. 2016. Tillage impact on soil erosion by water: Discrepancies due to climate and soil characteristics. *Agric. Ecosyst. Environ.* 230:231–241. https://doi.org/10.1016/j.agee.2016.04.033

13. Snyder, C.S., T.W. Bruulsema, T.L. Jensen, and P.E. Fixen. 2009. Review of greenhouse gas emissions from crop production systems and fertilizer management effects. *Agric. Ecosyst. Environ.* 133:247–266. https://doi.org/10.1016/j.agee.2009.04.021

14. Hatfield, J.L., L.D. McMullen, and C.S. Jones. 2009. Nitrate nitrogen patterns in the Raccoon River Basin related to agricultural patterns. *J. Soil Wat. Conserv.* 64: 19–199. https://doi.org/10.2489/jswc.64.3.190

15. Bone, J., M. Head, D. Barraclough, M. Archer, C. Scheib, D. Flight, and N. Voulvoulis. 2010. Soil quality assessment under emerging regulatory requirements. *Environ Int.* 36, 609–622.

16. Kibbelwhite, M.G., K. Ritz, and M.J. Swift. 2008. Soil health in agricultural systems. *Phil. Trans. R. Soc. B.* 363:685–701. https://doi.org/10.1098/rstb.2007.2178

17. Blum, W.E.H. 2005. Functions of soil for society and the environment. *Rev. Environ. Sci. Bio/Tech.* 4:75–79. https://doi.org/10.1007/s11157-005-2236-x

18. Moebius-Clune, B.N., D.J. Moebius-Clune, B.K. Gugino, O.J. Idowu, et al., 2016. *Comprehensive Assessment of Soil Health. The Cornell Framework Manual.* 3rd ed. Cornell University, Geneva.

19. Schaetzl, R.J., and M.L. Thompson. 2015. *Soils: Genesis and Geomorphology.* 2nd ed. Cambridge University Press, Cambridge, UK.

20. Rinot, O., G.J. Levy, Y. Steinberger, T. Svoray, and G. Eshel. 2019. Soil health assessment: A critical review of current methodologies and a proposed new approach. *Sci. Tot. Environ.* 648:1484–1491. https://doi.org/10.1016/j.scitotenv.2018.08.259

21. Wander, M.W., L.J. Cihacek, M.Coyne, R.A. Drijber, et al., 2019. Developments in agricultural soil quality and health: Reflections by the research committee on soil organic matter management. *Fron. Environ. Sci.* 7:109. https://doi.org/10.3389/fenvs.2019.00109

22. Bunemann, E.K., G. Bongiorno, Z. Bai, R.E. Creamer, et al., 2018. Soil quality: A critical review. *Soil Biol. Biochem.* 120:105–125. https://doi.org/10.1016/j.soilbio.2018.01.030

23. Andrews, S.S., D.L. Karlen, and C.A. Cambardella. 2004. The soil management assessment framework: A quantitative soil quality evaluation method. *Soil Sci. Soc. Am. J.* 68:1945–1962. https://doi.org/10.2136/sssaj2004.1945

24. Karlen, D.L., K.S. Veum, K.A. Sudduth, J.F. Obryki, and M.R. Nunes. 2019. Soil health assessment: Past accomplishments, current activities, and future opportunities. *Soil Till. Res.* 195:104365. https://doi.org/10.1016/j.still.2019.104365

25. Briggs, L.J., and H.L. Shantz. 1913. *The Water Requirement of Plants.* Bureau of Plant Industry Bulletin. US Department of Agriculture, Washington, DC, pp. 282–285.

26. Basso, B., and J.T. Ritchie. 2018. Evapotranspiration in high-yielding maize and under increased vapor pressure deficit in the US Midwest. *A&EL* 3. https://doi.org/10.2134/ael2017.11.0039.

27. Baligar, V.C., N.K. Fageria, and Z.L. He. 2001. Nutrient use efficiency in plants. *Comm. Soil Sci. and Plant Anal.* 32:921–950. https://doi.org/10.1081/CSS-100104098

28. Hawkesford, M., S. Kopriva, and L. De Kok. 2014. Nutrient use efficiency in plants: Concepts and approaches. *Plant Ecophysiology Series.* Springer ISBN: 978-3-319-10634. https://doi.org/10.1007/978-3-319-10635-9

29. Cassman, K.G., A. Dobermann, and D.T. Walters. 2002. Agroecosystems, nitrogen-use efficiency, and nitrogen management. *AMBIO: J Hum Environ.* 31:132–140. https://doi.org/10.1579/0044-7447-31.2.132

30. Dobermann, A. 2007. Nutrient use efficiency, measurement and management. In *Fertilizer Best Management Practices General Principles, Strategy for their Adoption and Voluntary Initiatives vs Regulations.* International Fertilizer Industry Association, Paris, France, 2007, pp. 1–28, ISBN 2-9523139-2-X

31. Fageria, N.K., and V.C. Baligar. 2005. Enhancing nitrogen use efficiency in crop plants. *Adv. Agrono.* 88:97–185. https://doi.org/10.1016/S0065-2113(05)88004-6

32. Berendse, F., and R. Aerts. 1987. Nitrogen-use-efficiency: A biologically meaningful definition? *Funct Ecol.* 1:293–296. https://www.jstor.org/stable/2389434

33. Hatfield, J.L., T.J. Sauer, and J.H. Prueger. 2001. Managing soils to achieve greater water use efficiency: A review. *Agron. J.* 93:271–280

34. Blanco-Canqui, H., B.J. Wienhold, V.L. Jin, M.R. Schmer, and L.C. Kibet (2017). Long-term tillage impact on soil hydraulic properties. *Soil Till. Res.* 170:38–42.

35. Amezketa, E. 1999. Soil aggregate stability: A review. *J Sustain. Agric.* 14(2–3):83–151.

36. Kasper, M., G.D. Buchan, A. Mentler, and W.E.H. Blum (2009). Influence of soil tillage systems on aggregate stability and the distribution of C and N in different aggregate fractions. *Soil Till. Res.* 105:192–199.

37. Unger, P.W. (1992). Infiltration of simulated rainfall: Tillage system and crop residue effects. *Soil Scie. Soc. Am. J.* 56:283–289.

38. Wacha, K.M., A.N. Papanicolaou, C.P. Giannopoulos, B.K. Abban, C.G. Wilson, S. Zhou, ... and T. Hou (2018). The role of hydraulic connectivity and management on soil aggregate size and stability in the Clear Creek Watershed, Iowa. *Geosciences.* 8:470.

39. Adesemoye, A.O., H.A. Torbert, and J.W. Kloepper. 2008. Enhanced plant nutrient use efficiency with PGPR and AMF in an integrated nutrient management system. *Canadian J Microbiol.* 54:876–886. https://doi.org/10.1139/W08-081

40. Mandal, S., R. Thangarajan, N.S. Bolan, B. Sarkar, N. Khan, Y.S. Ok, and R. Naidu. 2016. Biochar-induced concomitant decrease in ammonia volatilization and increase in nitrogen use efficiency by wheat, *Chemosphere.* 142:120–127. https://doi.org/10.1016/j.chemosphere.2015.04.086

41. Meena, B.P., A.K. Biswas, M. Singh, R.S. Chaudhary, A.B. Singh, H. Das, and A.K. Patra. 2019. Long-term sustaining crop productivity and soil health in maize–chickpea system through integrated nutrient management practices in Vertisols of central India. *Field Crops Res.* 232:62–76. https://doi.org/10.1016/j.fcr.2018.12.012

42. Novak, J.M., J.A. Ippolito, R.D. Lentz, K.A. Spokas, C.H. Bolster, K. Sistani, K.M. Trippe, C.L. Phillips, and M.G. Johnson. 2016. Soil health, crop productivity, microbial transport, and mine spoil response to biochars. *Bioenergy Res.* 9: 454–464. https://doi.org/10.1007/s12155-016-9720-8

43. Dias, T., A. Dukes, and P.M. Antunes. 2014. Accounting for soil biotic effects on soil health and crop productivity in the design of crop rotations. *J Sci. Food and Agric.* 95:3 https://doi.org/10.1002/jsfa.6565

44. Lal, R. 2017. Improving soil health and human protein nutrition by pulses-based cropping systems. *Adv. Agron.* 145:167–204. https://doi.org/10.1016/bs.agron.2017.05.003

45. Kerr, R.B., S. Snappe, M. Chirwas, L. Shumba, and R. Msachi. 2007. Participatory research on legume diversification with Malawian smalholder farmers for improved human nutrition and soil fertility. *Expt. Agric.* 43:437–453. https://doi.org/10.1017/S0014479707005339

46. Upadhyay, V.B., V. Jain, S.K. Vishwakarma, and A.K. Kumhar. 2011. Production potential, soil health, water productivity and economics of rice (*Oryza sativa*)-based cropping systems ujnder different nutrient sources. *Indian J. Agron.* 56:311–316.

47. Patel, D.P., A. Das, M. Kumar, G.C. Munda, S.V. Ngachan, G.I. Ramkrushna, J. Layek, N. Pongla, J. Buragihain, and U. Somireddy. 2014. Continuous application of organic amendments enhances soil health, produce quality and system productivity of vegetable-based cropping systems in subtropical Eastern Himalayas. *Expt. Agric.* https://doi.org/10.1017/S0014479714000167

18 Mitochondrial Correction as a Cancer Therapy

Michael J. Gonzalez and Jorge R. Miranda-Massari

CONTENTS

DOI: 10.1201/b23304-20

18.1 INTRODUCTION

Cancer and degenerative diseases in general are increasing to epidemic proportions in all industrialized countries. Cancer has been widely considered a genetic disease involving nuclear mutations in oncogenes and tumor suppressor genes; this view persists despite the numerous inconsistencies associated with the somatic mutation theory. In contrast to the somatic mutation theory, emerging evidence suggests that cancer is a metabolic disease of mitochondrial origin (1–4). According to Warburg's theory, respiratory insufficiency seems to be the main originator of cancer. We are proposing cancer as a mitochondrial disease where diseased or damaged mitochondria become more dependent on glucose and glutamine for energy. A shift from oxidative phosphorylation (OXPHOS) to fermentation can cause cellular de-differentiation, the most relevant characteristic of malignancy.

As described already in the 1920s by Otto Warburg, cancer cells often show a shift in energy production from mitochondrial oxidative phosphorylation to cytosolic glycolysis (3). This so-called aerobic glycolysis, in which glucose is converted to pyruvate and lactate in spite of the presence of oxygen, is a major characteristic of most tumor cells. Importantly, this increase in glycolytic activity similar to that observed in early embryonic cells. Thus, cancer cells seem to resume a more primitive metabolic pattern (4). Albert Szent Gyorgi interpreted malignancy as a reversion to the primordial state (Alpha State) from the oxidative (Beta State) of normal cell function. We support this change of paradigm by providing information about the nature, etiology and function of mitochondria in normal and cancer cells.

Not only does aerobic glycolysis provide the cell with adenosine triphosphate (ATP) from the readily available substrate glucose, but the rapid glycolytic flux can also provide the cells with the necessary substrates and metabolic intermediates for lipid, amino acid, and DNA synthesis that are needed for rapid growth. For example, NADPH, ribose, acetyl-CoA and glucose-derived non-essential amino acids can be provided by aerobic glycolysis. In addition to an altered use of glucose, cancer cells make energetically inefficient use of glutamine to supply the nitrogen for the synthesis of nucleotides and non-essential amino acids and to facilitate import of essential amino acids and support NADPH production. Glycolytic metabolism and the associated metabolic reprogramming not only support rapid growth, even at the expense of other cells, but also make the cancer cell less dependent on oxygen availability while generating an acidic microenvironment that enhances cell division and thus, malignancy. It has been long appreciated that under hypoxic conditions, glycolytic rates are markedly enhanced, with a resulting increase in lactate production.

Cancer cells produce far less ATP per molecule of glucose by simple aerobic glycolysis (i.e., reduced efficiency); nevertheless, they can produce a substantial amount of ATP at a much faster rate due to rapid consumption of substrates. Cancer cells produce ATP almost 100 times faster than normal cells (5). Cancer cells actively have more glucose transporters on their cell surface membranes, so that more glucose is brought inside the cell. This increase in glucose metabolism through glycolysis allows the generation of glycolytic intermediates that funnel into biosynthetic pathways that support the production of NADPH, lipids, proteins and nucleotides.

Respiration cannot operate smoothly unless all of the delicate interior structures inside mitochondria are intact and functional. Mitochondria have evolved with a process called retrograde response (RTG), which helps them deal with temporary stress or damage. The retrograde response was designed for temporary emergency use, not for long-term use; nevertheless, cancer cells appear to stay in this mode. Whereas the RTG response evolved to protect cells from sudden energy failure, a persistent RTG response with inadequate respiration can cause genomic instability, and eventually, this can result in tumorigenesis (6). Genome instability is linked to mitochondrial dysfunctions through retrograde signaling and to the perpetuation of the malignant state. Thus, this emerging evidence supports an important role for metabolic aberrancies and mitochondrial dysfunction in cancer; in general, suggesting that cancer is primarily a mitochondrial metabolic disease (4, 7).

18.2   MITOCHONDRIA AND CANCER

The mitochondria are considered ancient bacterial symbionts with their own mitochondrial DNA (mtDNA), RNA and protein synthesizing systems. Each human cell contains hundreds of mitochondria. Margulis theorized that mitochondria are probably descended from free-living bacteria that survived endocytosis by a eukaryotic host cell. Such mutualistic symbiosis is a potent and largely unappreciated and unrecognized force in evolution.

Mitochondria play a much greater physiological role than has been previously thought. Some important mitochondrial functions are: (a) energy production by manufacturing ATP, (b) regulation of membrane potential, (c) signaling and messaging through reactive oxygen species, (d) calcium signaling, (e) apoptosis and autophagy, (f) cellular metabolism, (g) iron metabolism and heme synthesis, and (h) steroid synthesis (7).

Mitochondria synthesize the universal energy molecule ATP. They accomplish this through glycolysis, oxidative phosphorylation and electron transport in conjunction with the oxidation of metabolites by the Krebs cycle and the breakdown of fatty acids by beta-oxidation. Because of their capacity to generate ATP, mitochondria are known exclusively for their ability to produce this important energy molecule, the main fuel for all energy demands of the cell. We inherit our mitochondrial DNA from our mothers. Although mitochondria are present in sperm, they are not transferred to the ova during the process of fertilization, since most of them are concentrated in the tail, which is lost in the process.

Mitochondria are so efficient at producing energy that their arrival on the evolutionary scene is thought to be responsible for the increase in complexity of living things. Building and supporting elaborate new creatures with specialized organs and capabilities requires a superabundance of usable energy (for organization, compartmentalization, order and communication). If large quantities of energy are not constantly produced to maintain form, function, order and organization; then complex organisms will gradually succumb to entropy or chaos. For cells, this will mean a regression, with their DNA becoming unstable; they will lose their shape and become disorganized, intercellular communication will be impaired, and they start reproducing uncontrollably as a survival mechanism (4).

Mitochondria are active, mobile intracellular organelles that undergo constant fission and fusion. They form an interconnected network with other cellular organelles, and their functions extend beyond the cell membranes so as to influence the organism's entire physiology. Mitochondria can achieve this by affecting communication between cells, tissues and organs. Predictably, any small defect in any of these functions could elicit mitochondrial dysfunction and promote a combination of diseases including cancer, metabolic disorders and neurodegenerative diseases (8).

Mitochondria are continually confronted with factors and environmental variables that can jeopardize their function. These factors include chronic stress, sleep disturbances, hyperglycemia, xenobiotics such as drugs, antibiotics, organic pollutants and environmental toxins. These factors and/or variables can cause mitochondrial dysfunction. This can be characterized in four ways: (a) an insufficient number of mitochondria, (b) insufficient substrate or nutrient cofactors needed for oxidative phosphorylation (e.g., nutrient deficiency due to poor diet or drug-induced nutrient depletion), (c) acquired dysfunction in the ATP synthesis machinery or (d) damage to the mitochondrial membranes. Mitochondrial dysfunction will result in a number of cellular consequences, including:

(i) decreased ATP production; (ii) increased reliance on alternative anaerobic energy sources; and (iii) increased production of reactive oxygen species (ROS) and reactive nitrogen species (RNS). Of interest is that ROS/RNS can also have a variety of normal roles, which include regulation of gene expression (9, 10). At physiological concentrations, ROS/RNS can function as "redox messengers" in intracellular signaling and regulation. ROS/RNS molecular recognition occurs at both the atomic and the macromolecular level, which expands the potential number of ROS/RNS-specific receptors and interaction sites. Nevertheless, an unbalanced production of ROS/RNS can be detrimental to mitochondrial function and viability.

At the molecular level, a reduction in mitochondrial function occurs as a result of the following changes: (a) loss of maintenance of the electrical and chemical transmembrane potential of the inner mitochondrial membrane, (b) alterations in the function of the electron transport chain, including those due to insufficiencies of nutrients and cofactors/coenzymes essential for mitochondrial function, such as magnesium, thiamine, ubiquinone and lipoic acid, or (c) a reduction in the transport of critical metabolites into mitochondria. In turn, these changes result in reduced efficiency of oxidative phosphorylation and a reduction in the production of ATP (11). Many of the organic cofactors/coenzymes and structural fatty acids and phospholipids essential for mitochondrial function are damaged or destroyed. Several components of this system require routine replacement, and this need may be facilitated with specific dietary/substrate supplements.

The importance of metabolic and mitochondrial dysfunction in the cellular etiology of cancer is evidenced by the observations that damaged mitochondria can turn healthy cells into transformed cells and that healthy mitochondria can reverse cancerous behavior in tumor cells. These observations provide an insight that cancer is not simply or exclusively a genetic disease but more a mitochondrial-originated disease (4, 7). Mitochondrial dysfunction may play a central role in a wide range of diseases in addition to cancer. These diseases include neurodegenerative diseases, such as Alzheimer's disease, Parkinson's disease, Huntington's disease, amyotrophic lateral sclerosis and Friedreich's ataxia; cardiovascular diseases, such as atherosclerosis and other heart and vascular conditions; diabetes and metabolic syndrome; autoimmune diseases, such as multiple sclerosis, systemic lupus erythematosus and type 1 diabetes; neurobehavioral and psychiatric diseases, such as autism spectrum disorders, schizophrenia, and bipolar and mood disorders; gastrointestinal (GI) disorders; fatiguing illnesses, such as chronic fatigue syndrome and Gulf War illnesses; musculoskeletal diseases, such as fibromyalgia and skeletal muscle atrophy; and chronic infections (12).

Many pharmaceuticals have been identified as mitochondrial toxicants (13–15). The high lipid content of mitochondrial membranes facilitates the accumulation of lipophilic compounds and also of organic chemicals, particularly amphiphilic xenobiotics such as pharmacologic agents, including anti-bacterials, anti-psychotics, anti-depressants, anti-arrhythmics, anorexic agents, cholesterol-lowering agents and others. Cationic metal ions, such as lead, cadmium, mercury and manganese, have also been shown to accumulate in mitochondria. Another factor contributing to mitochondrial susceptibility is the presence of cytochrome P450s in mitochondria, which can activate chemicals that are relatively non-reactive prior to metabolism. At the same time, mitochondria can also be protected in several ways, including greater redundancy of their contents and ability to replace defective components via mitophagy, biogenesis, complementation and apoptosis.

An important property in mitochondria is their controlled leak of matrix protons. Leaky mitochondria cause uncoordinated electron transport, which causes energy to be wasted as heat instead of being converted into ATP. This mitochondrial uncoupling has been shown in faster-growing tumors that are actually warmer because of this effect. Increased proton leak will increase oxygen consumption (uncoupled respiration, UCR), and the energy will be dissipated as heat instead of being trapped as useful energy.

Metabolic normalization of cancer cells and concomitant inhibition of carcinogenesis may potentially also be attained by induction of mitochondrial biogenesis and mitochondrial correction. Moreover, studying the role of mitochondria in cancer cell de-differentiation/differentiation processes may allow further insight into the pathophysiology of transformation and could lead to the development of new cancer therapies. Increases in mitochondrial respiration, restoration of mitochondrial membrane potential, increases in population doubling times, and reduction of cell proliferation may be important steps in overcoming the cancer state. By restoring failing mitochondrial energetics, cancer morphogenesis may be reversed.

An example of the process of cancer re-differentiation via mitochondrial correction is the repair of aconitase dysfunction using frataxin, which reverses cell transformation (16, 17). Aconitase is an enzyme that catalyzes the stereo-specific isomerization of citrate to isocitrate via cis-aconitate in the tricarboxylic acid cycle within the mitochondria. Frataxin, a highly conserved protein found in prokaryotes and eukaryotes, is required for efficient regulation of cellular iron homeostasis and functions to activate mitochondrial energy conversion and oxidative phosphorylation. Frataxin functions as an activator of oxidative phosphorylation, leading to increased mitochondrial membrane potential and an elevated cellular ATP content.

Additional evidence shows that normalizing mitochondrial function is capable of suppressing tumorigenesis. The strongest evidence that cancer may be a mitochondrial-originated disease has been demonstrated by nuclear-cytoplasm transfer studies. Many of these studies, even those done in cell cybrids, have shown that a nucleus from a malignant cell when placed in a cell with normal cytoplasm will not produce malignant daughter cells (i.e., mutations in nuclear DNA are insufficient to cause cancer when placed within a normally functioning cellular context with normal mitochondria). It was also demonstrated that normal cell nuclei could not suppress tumorigenicity when placed in the tumor cell cytoplasm (i.e., in the context of dysfunctional metabolism and mitochondria, cancer can be induced despite normal nuclear DNA). Therefore, in these studies, normal nuclear gene expression was unable to suppress malignancy. These studies establish that it was the cytoplasm and not the nucleus that dictated the malignant state of the cell (18–23). If this is the case, and tumor cells have defective or dysfunctional mitochondria, as Warburg suggested, then malignant suppression should result from the introduction of normal mitochondria from normal cells to the malignant cell. Indeed, these nuclear-cytoplasmic transfer studies in various cell types confirm that the integrity of mitochondrial respiration prevents carcinogenesis. In other words, cancer arises from respiratory insufficiency, just as Warburg postulated many decades ago (24). In summary, the origin of tumorigenesis requires damaged or ineffective mitochondria. Normal isolated mitochondria co-cultured with cancer cells could be taken into the cancer cells, where they can then reverse aerobic glycolysis and inhibit cell growth (25–30). This can in theory be done in conjunction with exosomes carrying pro-differentiation information in a complementary biological synergistic action.

18.3   MITOCHONDRIAL CORRECTION

The first step in correcting damaged mitochondria involves addressing lifestyle factors. Studies show that increasing physical activity improves mitochondrial function, so encouraging regular, moderate exercise is essential (25, 29, 31). Combining exercise with a diet rich in organic vegetables, moderate in organic, grass-fed meats, free-range poultry and wild-caught fish, and very low in refined carbohydrates and sugar may be essential part of the equation. In addition, implementing practices that reduce stress, such as meditation or yoga, as well as ensuring good sleeping habits is also important. Finally, detoxifying the body by removing xenobiotics that inhibit mitochondrial function while replacing necessary essential components should substantially help improve mitochondrial function.

When the mitochondria become unable to adequately perform their functions, cells will either die, become dormant or undergo malignant transformation. The possibility exists to cause such cells to revert back (re-differentiate) to normal aerobic cells, capable of normal function via metabolic and mitochondrial correction, which may be accomplished in a number of ways. The current genocentric pharmacologic approach has been to kill cancer cells with toxic therapies – chemotherapy and radiation – rather than attempt to reconvert them back to normal. This cytotoxic approach has been largely unsuccessful; therefore, considering other paradigms that may yield unconventional but more effective approaches may prove to be useful and less damaging.

18.4 DIET

Nutrition is an important part of cancer treatment, because the components of the diet are determinants of cell functionality. For cancer patients, eating the right kinds of foods can help them feel better, stay stronger and most importantly, overcome and survive the disease. All tumors depend heavily on glucose for survival. Research shows a strong connection between high blood sugar (hyperglycemia), diabetes and cancer. High blood glucose raises insulin levels. High blood glucose also raises levels of Insulin-like Growth Factor 1 (IGF-1). Cancer cells with receptors on their surfaces for IGF-1 grow more rapidly, because IGF-1 activates metabolic pathways that drive tumor cell growth (26–28).

Studies have consistently estimated that 30% or more of all cancers may be due to dietary factors (25). Bioactive food components that affect various aspects of metabolism may be important tools to reverse glycolytic to oxidative metabolism and enhance sensitivity to apoptosis. The success of such a strategy may depend on several factors acting in concert. Glycolytic metabolism and the associated metabolic reprogramming not only support rapid growth of cancer cells, but they also make the cancer cells less dependent on oxygen availability and generate a favorable (acidic) microenvironment for growth. Inhibition of glycolysis may have therapeutic implications in cancer treatment as a strategy to suppress or even eliminate cancer cells. Such a strategy may also make use of bioactive food components.

One class of bioactive food components that affect energy metabolism and may have anti-cancer effects are polyphenols. Quercetin, a polyphenol present in apples, onions, tea and wine, affects energy metabolism. Another polyphenol with anti-cancer potential is resveratrol. Resveratrol is well known as a compound that is present in red wine. Bioactive food molecules that affect energy metabolism may also function as anti-cancer agents using mechanisms distinct from their effect on energy metabolism. Despite being categorized as antioxidants, most dietary antioxidant compounds exhibit their functional effects through specific cellular mechanisms rather than though general, direct antioxidant effects. Mechanisms such as cancer cell growth limitation, anti-angiogenesis and normalization of the glycolytic metabolism are possible.

Carbohydrates provide rapidly usable cellular energy but unlike proteins and fat, also stimulate potent insulin signals that can be powerful mitogens. A carbohydrate-restricted diet will slow cancer growth in patients by decreasing the secretion and circulating levels of insulin. Tumor glucose uptake can be stabilized and decreased with a carbohydrate-restricted diet. Hyperglycemia activates monocytes and macrophages to produce inflammatory cytokines that play an important role in the progression of cancer (26–32). High plasma glucose concentrations elevate the levels of circulating insulin and free IGF1, two potent anti-apoptotic and growth factors for most cancer cells (30).

Paleolithic-type diets, which by definition exclude grain products, have been shown to improve glycemic control and therefore, are expected to help against cancer. A low-carbohydrate, high-fat diet to increase the blood levels of ketones, along with supplements or foods rich in citric acid, can impair glycolysis and may prove a beneficial adjunct in the treatment of many cancers (29).

A ketogenic diet characterized by minimal carbohydrate intake, a moderate amount of protein and higher amounts of fat seems to limit cancer cell growth. This shift in macronutrients causes the body to switch to utilizing ketones (produced by burning fats) instead of glucose as its primary source of fuel. Ketones (e.g., acetoacetate, β-hydroxybutyric acid and acetone) are produced in the liver when lipids are burned instead of glucose. Low-carbohydrate diets reduce the extreme glucose peaks and help patients avoid both hyperglycemia and rebound hypoglycemia, providing more sustained energy throughout the day. Ketones are efficiently used for the generation of ATP (energy) in mitochondria. Cancer cells cannot use ketones as an energy source (33). The ketogenic diet mimics the metabolic state of starvation, forcing the body to utilize fat as its primary source of energy.

The ketogenic diet may be beneficial in optimizing mitochondrial function. The transition from glucose metabolism to ketone metabolism is also a powerful anti-inflammatory strategy. The goal of this diet is to shift the body from burning mostly glucose (sugar) to burning mostly ketones (fat). The quickest way to get into the therapeutic zone is to start by fasting (water only) for 3–5 days. During the induction phase, carbohydrate withdrawal symptoms may occur, which typically include lightheadedness, nausea and headaches (Keto Flu). An alternative to this fasting is to limit carbohydrates to less than 12 grams per day and limit protein to 0.8 to 1.2 grams per kg body weight per day (0.4 to 0.6 grams per pound body weight). With this less extreme keto plan, patients may need up to several weeks to reach the recommended therapeutic zone values (urinary ketones). Ketogenic diets may also facilitate easier surgical reduction in tumor burden, as ketosis can reduce blood vessel mass, inflammation and tumor size, thereby facilitating surgical removal of the tumor mass. The increase of ketones in the blood can also inhibit the activity of phosphofructokinase, an enzyme that plays a key role in the regulation of glycolysis. Citric acid, an intermediary product of the Krebs cycle metabolism, has also been reported to block the actions of phosphofructokinase.

To support mitochondrial function, cancer patients should be advised to eat 8–12 servings daily of a variety of whole, colorful vegetables and fruits; among different plants, color variation indicates phytochemical variety, thereby allowing the diet to provide a wide range of anti-cancer and metabolism-enhancing phytochemicals. Vegetables should be the primary focus, especially the bitter foods in the cruciferous family (such as broccoli, watercress and arugula), as these foods provide numerous anti-cancer benefits. Coconut oil, a brain-healthy saturated fat that contains medium-chain triglycerides (MCTs), also supports mitochondrial function via production of ketones.

Calorie and carbohydrate restriction, along with eating lean, clean (pesticide and toxin-free) proteins, high-quality fats and oils, and more plant foods may help to prevent or slow down all degenerative diseases. All grains are minimized or avoided on a mitochondria restoration diet in order to achieve the desired goals of mild ketosis and low glycemic impact. Most malignant cells lack key mitochondrial enzymes necessary for the conversion of ketone bodies and fatty acids to ATP (30–32).

Maintaining a lower and consistent insulin level is key to optimal mitochondrial health. A heavily processed, high–glycemic load diet of too many grains and added sugars can lead to increased insulin and inflammation with associated and accelerated mitochondrial dysfunction. Minimizing grains, especially highly processed ones, and using low-glycemic vegetables and fruits as the main source of carbohydrates helps to stabilize blood sugar and protect mitochondria.

High-quality proteins are the best choice, including grass-fed, organic, non–genetically modified organism (GMO) sources. For fish, patients should choose wild-caught salmon, as farmed salmon (fish in general) may contain hormones and toxic chemicals. We encourage the consumption of minimally refined, cold-pressed, organic, non-GMO fats and liquid oils whenever possible. When possible, we advise phytonutrient-dense, unfiltered, extra-virgin olive oil, avocado oil or coconut oil to dress salads and vegetables. MCT oil is another option that can also be used for cooking and for dressings.

Cancer patients should aim for a minimum of 4–6 servings of organic vegetables every day (ideally, 10–12 servings per day). A serving is only ½ cup of cooked vegetable or 1 cup of raw leafy greens. Patients get four servings of vegetables in one meal by filling a plate with vegetables or eating a hearty salad. All greens (including collard, dandelion, kale, mustard and turnip greens), along with chard/Swiss chard, spinach, sea vegetables, and the many green vegetables in the cruciferous family have been found to support the mitochondria via effects such as antioxidant protection, anti-inflammatory benefits and enhancement of xenobiotic clearance.

Patients are instructed to eat a rainbow of colors: Red peppers, tomatoes and radishes; orange carrots, peppers and pumpkin; yellow summer squash and peppers; green asparagus, avocado and green beans; blue/purple eggplant and cabbage; and white/tan mushrooms, jicama and onions. Patients are also counseled to purchase organic vegetables (and fruits) when possible. Foods should be "organic," grown without chemical pesticides, given that many pesticides are neurotoxins, mitochondrial toxins, carcinogens and endocrine disruptors.

Fruits with a low to moderate glycemic response can be consumed when patients are feeling the need for something sweet. All berries, along with pomegranate seeds and grapes with the skin, have been shown to increase levels of glutathione in the body. Fruit juices are not encouraged, as they are dense sources of sugar and can increase blood sugar levels, thereby promoting oxidative stress, immunosuppression and hyperinsulinemia.

Patients should drink plenty of pure, filtered water daily. It is generally recommended to drink at least six to eight glasses. (One glass = 1 cup = 8 ounces.) For variety and additional antioxidant and anti-cancer benefits, patients may consider adding at least 2 cups of green tea daily, with the general recommendation being to include herbal teas, especially those prepared from adaptogenic herbs like cordyceps, schizandra, ginseng, astragalus and licorice, which can be used as desired and tolerated. The importance of pesticide- and toxin-free food from local, free-range, grass-fed and organic sources cannot be stressed enough.

Also considered should be intermittent fasting; the benefits provided by fasting are crucial for the plasticity of mitochondrial energy networks. If the cells detect the presence of macronutrients, especially carbohydrates; autophagy is suppressed due to the elevation of growth factors such as insulin, IGF-1 and mammalian target of rapamycin (mTOR) (33). Therefore, the key is to elevate fuel sensors of energy preservation such as 5' AMP-activated protein kinase (AMPK) and to lower mTOR, which can be accomplished with strict intermittent fasting. Fasting increases AMPK, which promotes fatty acid oxidation, which produces ketone bodies. The mitochondria run more efficiently on ketone bodies, because they can get into the mitochondria faster via the electron transport chain, and they yield more ATP than glucose. Fasting increases FOXO proteins, which are transcription factors that regulate longevity through the insulin and IGF-1 pathway. FOXO1 and FOXO3 promote mitophagy. Fasting increases sirtuins, which are a family of proteins that act as metabolic sensors. SIRT1 regulates mitochondrial biogenesis and peroxisome proliferator-activated receptor-gamma coactivator (PGC)-1alpha. Sirtuins regulate fat and glucose metabolism in response to physiological changes in energy levels; thus, they are crucial determinants of energy homeostasis (34). Suppressing SIRT2 restricts fatty acid metabolism, reduces mitochondrial activity and promotes obesity. The key to keeping mitochondria healthy is to maintain clean energy homeostasis and remove dysfunctional cellular components that cause inflammation. Time-controlled fasting prevents mitochondrial aging and deterioration. It can also promote the longevity of mitochondria by eliminating the production of ROS and free radicals by dysfunctional organelles (35). Intermittent fasting protects against telomere shortening and DNA damage. Telomeres are protective caps on top of chromosomes that shorten as you age. Fasting increases sirtuins, which promote fat burning and mitochondrial functioning.

18.5   DIETARY SUPPLEMENTATION: DESCRIPTIONS AND SUGGESTIONS FOR ADULT DOSAGES

Several supplements are important in any regimen designed to boost mitochondrial health (36).

Dietary supplements can reduce the oxidative burden of ATP generation, provide additional substrate for oxidative phosphorylation and repair leaky membranes that interrupt the electron transport system. In addition, mitochondrial biogenesis, or the generation of new mitochondria, can also be stimulated (37).

18.5.1   CoQ10 (Ubiquinone)

Coenzyme Q10 (CoQ) is a small lipophilic molecule critical for the transport of electrons from complexes I and II to complex III in the mitochondrial respiratory chain. Furthermore, CoQ is essential for the stability of complex III in the mitochondrial respiratory chain, functions as an antioxidant in cell membranes and is involved in multiple aspects of cellular metabolism. CoQ10 also reduces lactic acid levels, improves muscle strength and decreases muscle fatigability. CoQ10 protects against beta-amyloid-induced mitochondrial malfunction. Statin drugs are thought to cause mitochondrial damage in part by lowering levels of CoQ10, and supplementation with CoQ10 has been shown to counteract some of the negative effects of statins. CoQ10 is an important supplement to counteract the adverse effects of cancer therapy (38). CoQ10 is probably the most widely used cofactor for treating mitochondrial-related diseases. CoQ10 is also a strong antioxidant in its reduced form, and it can affect the expression of certain genes involved in cell signaling, metabolism and transport. However, the main role of CoQ10 is its involvement in the transfer of electrons along the multiple complexes of the mitochondrial electron transport chain. In combination with lipoic acid, CoQ10 may increase ATP production by oxidative phosphorylation, resulting in decreased utilization of alternative energy sources and less efficient energy-generating pathways. CoQ10 may also diminish plasma lactate concentrations (36, 39).

Suggested amount 100 mg tid (three times a day)

18.5.2   L-CARNITINE (3-HYDROXY-4-N-TRIMETHYLAMINOBUTYRATE)

L-Carnitine is a naturally occurring fatty acid transporter. It is directly involved in the transport of fatty acids into the mitochondrial matrix for subsequent β-oxidation; but it also functions in removal of excess acyl groups from the body and in the modulation of intracellular coenzyme A (CoA) homeostasis. L-carnitine helps fatty acids cross the inner mitochondrial membrane to be used as energy. It also scavenges reactive oxygen and binds iron. L-carnitine also has been shown to prevent the damaging effects of statins on the mitochondria. L-carnitine protects against mitochondrial dysfunction associated with oxidative stress caused by a series of conditions such as aging, ischemia reperfusion, inflammation, degenerative diseases, cancer and drug toxicity (11, 39, 40). L-carnitine has been used to increase the rate of mitochondrial oxidative phosphorylation. L-carnitine also is essential for the detoxification of environmental pollutants, meaning that it can protect the mitochondria in several different scenarios.

Suggested dose 500 mg bid (twice a day)

18.5.3   ACETYL-L-CARNITINE

Acetyl-L-carnitine (ALCar) is an ester of the tri-methylated amino acid L-carnitine. It is better absorbed compared with L-carnitine and crosses the blood–brain barrier more efficiently. Dietary supplementation with acetyl-L-carnitine might reverse age-related mitochondrial changes. ALCar helps restore mitochondrial membrane potential and cardiolipin levels. Cardiolipin is an important component of the inner mitochondrial membrane, and it constitutes about 20% of the total lipid composition. ALCar facilitates fatty acid transport into mitochondria, and it increases overall cellular respiration. ALCar enhances cognitive performance, increases production of neurotransmitters, and helps restore levels of certain hormone receptors to more youthful levels. ALCar reverses many aspects of age-related cellular dysfunction, principally through maintenance of mitochondrial function (41).

Suggested dose 250 mg bid (twice a day)

18.5.4   IDEBENONE (2,3-DIMETHOXY-5-METHYL-6-(10-HYDROXYDECYL)-1,4-BENZOQUINONE)

Idebenone is a CoQ10 analog that while sharing some of CoQ10's properties, offers unique mitochondrial-protective benefits of its own. Idebenone is a powerful mitochondrial free radical quencher that reduces the ever-increasing damage to mitochondrial membranes and DNA that occurs with aging. Idebenone has also been shown to be more effective than CoQ10 in protecting the electron transport chain. When cellular oxygen levels are low, idebenone is actually superior to CoQ10 for preventing free radical damage while helping cells maintain relatively normal ATP levels (42).

Suggested dose 150 mg qd (once a day)

18.5.5 N-Acetyl Cysteine

N-Acetyl cysteine (NAC) is the acetylated precursor of both the amino acid L-cysteine and reduced glutathione (GSH). A major cause of mitochondrial dysfunction is due to oxidative changes that take place in the respiratory chain where oxidative phosphorylation occurs. NAC has a positive effect on key elements of the respiratory chain. It increases the activities of mitochondrial complexes I, IV and V. NAC also helps maintain levels of glutathione, an important antioxidant capable of preventing damage to important cellular components caused by ROS. NAC protects cells by promoting oxidative phosphorylation, improving mitochondrial membrane integrity and enhancing mitochondrial homeostasis (43).

Suggested dose 600 mg qd (once a day)

18.5.6 (R) Alpha-Lipoic Acid (1,2-Dithiolane-3-Pentanoic Acid)

Alpha-lipoic acid (ALA) is a potent antioxidant, transition metal ion chelator, redox transcription regulator and anti-inflammatory agent. It acts as a critical cofactor in mitochondrial α-keto acid dehydrogenases and is important in mitochondrial oxidative-decarboxylation reactions. ALA is an amphipathic molecule with both hydrophilic and hydrophobic properties. This makes ALA a perfect molecule to establish communication between the cytoplasm and mitochondria. ALA may also have mitochondrial-resuscitating properties. By providing ALA for 2 weeks, mitochondrial oxygen consumption has been completely restored in deficient mitochondria. It was also found that ALA, like ALCar, increased mitochondrial membrane potential by up to 50%. ALA supplementation also increased mitochondrial glutathione and vitamin C concentrations, indicating that ALA may have the ability to reverse the age-associated decline of low–molecular weight antioxidants, therefore reducing the risk for oxidative damage that occurs with aging. ALA supplementation improves mitochondrial function, alleviates some of the age-related loss of metabolic activity, increases ATP synthesis and blood flow, and increases glucose uptake. Furthermore, ALA supplementation may be a safe and effective means to improve general metabolic function (44).

Suggested dose 300 mg bid (twice a day)

18.5.7 Omega 3 Fatty Acids (Eicosapentaenoic acid [EPA] and Docosahexaenoic acid [DHA])

Omega-3 fatty acids from fish oils are cardio-protective. They minimize the increase in mitochondrial calcium content, increase levels of phosphatidylcholine and prevent the decrease in cardiolipin content. Omega-3s may also be important in mitochondrial membrane restoration. An omega-3-rich diet directly increases mitochondrial membrane cardiolipin concentrations, increases the ratio of mitochondrial membrane omega-3 to omega-6, and increases the tolerance of the heart to ischemia and reperfusion (45). The propensity for ROS/RNS emissions increases with omega-3 supplementation, although there are no changes in markers of lipid or protein oxidative damage. These results demonstrate that omega-3 supplementation improves mitochondrial ADP kinetics, suggesting post-translational modification of existing proteins (46).

Suggested dose 1 g tid (molecularly distilled)

18.5.8 Vitamin C (Ascorbic Acid)

Vitamin C may improve mitochondrial function by providing needed H (electrons) for the conversion of ascorbic acid to dehydroascorbic acid (46). Also related to vitamin C's electron transfer ability, it has the capacity to advance electrons in the electron transport system; thus functioning as an ergogenic aid (47). Vitamin C is taken up by the mitochondria and is able to preserve mitochondrial membrane potential (48–50). Even modest blood glucose elevations, as typically occur after a Western diet meal, competitively impair the transport of ascorbic acid into immune cells (49, 50) and probably into the mitochondria. Vitamin C is structurally similar to glucose, so it competes with glucose for the Glut receptors (51–54).

Suggested dose 500 mg tid; in disease state, consider bowel tolerance oral dosing or intravenous administration

18.5.9 B-Complex Vitamins

The B vitamins are water-soluble vitamins required as cofactors for enzymes essential in cell function and energy production (55).

18.5.9.1 Thiamine (Vitamin B1)

Thiamine is active in the form of thiamine pyrophosphate (TPP). As a cofactor, TPP is essential to the activity of cytosolic transketolase and pyruvate dehydrogenase as well as mitochondrial dehydrogenases – ketoglutarate dehydrogenase and branched chain keto acid dehydrogenase. Large doses of thiamine (vitamin B1) have been used to stimulate NADH, which then augments oxidative phosphorylation at complex I, a very important reaction in energy production (55, 56).

Suggested dose 100 mg qd (once a day)

18.5.9.2 Riboflavin (Vitamin B2)

Riboflavin is a precursor to flavin adenine dinucleotide (FAD) and flavin mononucleotide (FMN). As prosthetic groups, they are essential for the activity of flavoenzymes, including oxidases, reductase and dehydrogenases. Riboflavin is a water-soluble B vitamin (B2). It is a key building block in complexes I and II and a cofactor in several other key enzymatic reactions involving fatty acid oxidation and in the Krebs cycle. Riboflavin improved exercise capacity in a patient with a mitochondrial myopathy due to a complex I dysfunction (57, 58).

Suggested dose 100 mg qd (once a day)

18.5.9.3 Niacin (Vitamin B3)

Niacin is a precursor to reducing groups nicotinamide adenine dinucleotide (NAD+) and nicotinamide adenine dinucleotide phosphate (NADP+). These molecules are involved in more than 500 enzymatic reactions. For the focus of this review, it is important to note that NAD/NADP are involved in reactions pertaining to mitochondrial respiration, glycolysis and lipid beta-oxidation. Niacin ameliorated age-related changes in bioenergy (58, 59).

Suggested dose 50 mg qd (once a day)

18.5.9.4 Pantothenic acid (Vitamin B5)

Pantothenic acid is the precursor of coenzyme A (CoA), a molecule essential for 4% of known enzymatic reactions. In the interest of this review, it is important to note the role of CoA in heme synthesis, in lipid metabolism and as a prosthetic group in the TCA cycle (60).

Suggested dose 50 mg qd (once a day)

18.5.9.5 Magnesium

Magnesium ion plays an important role in a wide variety of biochemical processes, including optimizing mitochondrial function and the creation of ATP, regulation of blood sugar, and the activation of muscles and nerves. Over 300 enzymes require the presence of magnesium ions for their catalytic action, including all enzymes utilizing or synthesizing ATP. Magnesium ions are critical for the optimization of the mitochondria, which has enormous potential to influence cancer. In fact, optimizing mitochondrial metabolism may be at the core of effective cancer treatment (61).

Suggested dose magnesium citrate 500 mg tid; dose may be reduced as needed per osmotic laxative effect.

18.5.9.6 Phospholipids

Phospholipids are an important class of lipids found in all cellular membranes. Glycerolphospholipids, the type of phospholipid found in cellular and intracellular membranes, are made up of two fatty acids (long chains of hydrogen and carbon molecules), which are attached to a glycerol head. The glycerol molecule is also attached to a phosphate group, and this is the hydrophilic part of the molecule. The glycerolphospholipids help cellular membranes and act not only as diffusion barriers but also as dynamic cell organelles, contributing to the synthesis of intracellular mediators, such as arachidonic acid and inositol phosphates. Glycerolphospholipids interact and work with integral membrane proteins to modulate various cellular activities. As membrane phospholipids are known to be essential to cellular membrane function and cell viability, their modification and restoration by exogenous dietary phospholipids remains a useful approach for maintaining and restoring cellular membrane function.

Cell membranes control a variety of cellular processes as well as the maintenance of structural and ionic barriers and intercellular communication networks (as mentioned earlier). They are also involved in cell transport, secretion, recognition, adhesion and other important cell functions. Membrane lipids provide at least four major requirements for cellular health. They are used as: (1) an important energy storage reservoir; (2) the matrix for all cellular membranes, enabling separation of enzymatic and chemical reactions into discrete cellular compartments; (3) bioactive molecules in certain signal transduction and molecular recognition pathways; and (4) important functional molecules that undergo interactions with other cellular constituents, such as proteins and glycoproteins. This latter characteristic is an absolute requirement for the formation, structure and activities of biological membranes (40, 62–65). Phospholipids contribute to the physicochemical properties of the membrane and thus influence the conformation and function of membrane-bound proteins, such as receptors, ion channels, enzymes and transporters, and they also influence cell function by serving as precursors for prostaglandins and other signaling molecules. Finally, they can modulate gene expression through the activation of transcription.

One of the fundamental biochemical differences between tumor cells and normal cells is the composition of the membrane lipid matrix, including glycophospholipids and other lipids, and their oxidation state. Membrane peroxidation can modify phospholipid structure, affecting lipid fluidity, permeability and membrane function (62–65). In addition, the intracellular trafficking of phospholipids, which plays a crucial role in phospholipid homeostasis, can also be modified by peroxidation events. In the mitochondria, the activities of the enzymes involved in cellular respiration are markedly influenced by the composition and oxidation state of the phospholipids of the inner mitochondrial membrane. Oxidation of inner mitochondrial membrane phospholipids can result in increased leakiness of the inner mitochondrial membrane. Leaky mitochondrial membranes cause mitochondrial impairment and loss in the production of ATP. When there is progressive functional loss of mitochondrial function, such as in the excessive oxidative modification of the mitochondrial membrane phospholipids, this can cause changes in health that could progress to disease.

The outer mitochondrial membrane encloses the entire organelle and has a protein-to-phospholipid ratio similar to that of eukaryotic plasma membranes. The outer mitochondrial membrane contains transport proteins called porins (66). The inner mitochondrial membrane is rich in the phospholipid cardiolipin, which is characteristic of the bacterial plasma membrane and is important in electron transport function and provides yet more evidence suggesting the mitochondrion's bacterial origin.

Maintenance of the appropriate phospholipid composition in the mitochondrial membranes is essential for mitochondrial structure and function. Thus, mitochondria depend on phospholipid metabolism, the transport of phospholipids into mitochondria and supply of appropriate lipids from the diet. Regulation of the synthesis, trafficking and degradation of phospholipids is essential to maintain phospholipid homeostasis in the mitochondria. An important element of phospholipid homeostasis is that the phospholipids in the mitochondria can be modified by dietary glycerolphospholipids and fatty acids.

Membrane lipid replacement (MLR), the use of functional oral supplements containing cell membrane glycerolphospholipids and antioxidants, can safely replace damaged membrane phospholipids. Most, if not all, clinical conditions are characterized by membrane phospholipid oxidative damage, resulting in loss of membrane and cellular function (62–65). Orally ingested phospholipids can be degraded into their constituent parts and absorbed; they can be taken in as intact molecules without degradation, or they can be absorbed as small phospholipid droplets and micelles (62–65). Eventually, they are delivered to tissues and cells, where they are transferred by membrane contact and carrier or transport proteins to various cellular and organelle membranes.

MLR plus antioxidants has been used to reverse ROS/RNS damage and increase mitochondrial function in certain clinical disorders, such as chronic fatigue syndrome (CFS) and fibromyalgia (62–65). In these disorders, MLR has been found to be effective in preventing ROS/RNS-associated changes and reversing mitochondrial damage and loss of function (62). MLR is possible because cellular lipids are in dynamic equilibrium in the body. Thus, functional oral MLR supplements containing cell membrane glycerolphospholipids and antioxidants have been used to replace damaged, usually oxidized, membrane glycerophospholipids that accumulate during aging and in various clinical conditions. Once delivered to membrane sites, they naturally replace and stimulate the removal of damaged membrane lipids. Various chronic clinical conditions are characterized by membrane damage, mainly oxidative but also enzymatic, resulting in loss of cellular function. This is readily apparent in mitochondrial inner membranes, where oxidative damage to phospholipids like cardiolipin and other molecules results in loss of transmembrane potential and electron transport function and generation of high-energy molecules.

Suggested dose mixed phospholipids 1 g tid (three times a day) for anti-aging and 2 g tid for chronic illnesses

18.5.9.7 *Ginkgo biloba* (*Salisburia adiantifolia*)

Ginkgo biloba is one of the oldest living tree species. It is also one of the best-selling herbal supplements in the United States and Europe. Ginkgo leaves contain flavonoids and terpenoids. A growing volume of data confirms that *Ginkgo biloba* extract (GBE) reduces oxidative stress and improves mitochondrial respiration (67). GBE has been found to protect mtDNA against oxidative damage and oxidation of mitochondrial glutathione (68).

Suggested dose 40 mg bid (twice a day)

18.5.9.8 Succinate (Succinic Acid)

Succinate is a tricarboxylic acid (Krebs) cycle intermediate that donates electrons directly to complex II. Succinates have been widely used for their alleged ability to enhance athletic performance (69, 70). Succinate ameliorates energy deficits (70). It seems that the use of succinates is even more effective when a balance of several salts is used, especially combinations with magnesium and potassium.

Suggested dose 125 mg qd (once a day)

18.5.9.9 Pyrroloquinoline Quinone (PQQ)

PQQ is a small molecule that acts as a redox agent in cells. It can modify cell signaling and support mitochondrial function. PQQ is reported to participate in a range of biological functions. PQQ protects mitochondria from oxidative stress. It also promotes the spontaneous generation of new mitochondria, a process known as mitochondrial biogenesis or mitochondriogenesis (71–73). This effect is an improvement in mitochondrial function.

Suggested dose 20 mg qd (once a day)

18.5.9.10 Sodium Bicarbonate

Sodium bicarbonate ($NaHCO_3$) is a salt composed of sodium ions and bicarbonate ions. The glycolytic nature of malignant tumors contributes to high levels of extracellular acidity in the tumor microenvironment. The extracellular pH of malignant tumors is acidic (pH 6.5–6.9) compared with normal tissue (pH 7.2–7.4). Tumor acidity is a driving force for cellular division, invasion and metastasis (74–78). Recently, it has been shown that buffering of extracellular acidity through systemic administration of oral bicarbonate may inhibit the spread of metastases.

Dose to individualized effect to achieve urine pH of 7.5–8 while not consuming excess sodium

18.5.9.11 Nicotinamide Adenine Dinucleotide (NADH)

NADH functions as a cellular redox cofactor in over 200 cellular redox reactions and as a substrate for certain enzymes. NADH delivers electrons from metabolite hydrolysis to the electron transport chain, but in its reduced form, it can also act as a strong antioxidant. Pyruvate is converted to lactate, which requires all the glycolytic NADH output to be converted to NAD+, and this lactate is then excreted from the cell. Thus, aerobic glycolysis does not produce any net output of NADH. NADH can be successfully administered orally or by intravenous/intraperitoneal infusion (78). NAD precursors such as nicotinamide riboside (NR) or nicotinamide mononucleotide (NMN) should be considered.

Suggested dose 20 mg qd (once a day)

18.5.9.12 D-Ribose

Ribose is a naturally occurring five-carbon sugar produced in the body from glucose. In addition to serving as the carbohydrate backbone for ribonucleic acid (RNA) and deoxyribonucleic acid (DNA), ribose is also an essential ingredient in the manufacture of ATP. Thus, ribose provides the key building block of ATP. The mitochondria of high–energy output organs such as the heart, liver, adrenals, GI tract, brain, muscles and endocrine glands utilize two methods for building or conserving cyclic nucleotides like ATP, ADP and AMP. The first process by which these nucleotides are synthesized is the de novo pathway, in which nucleotides are made using ribose. This is the slower of the two pathways. The second or faster pathway is the salvage pathway, in which the mitochondria pick up ATP metabolites to form new ATP. In this manner, ribose enables the cells to more quickly and efficiently recycle (i.e., salvage) the end products formed by the breakdown of ATP to form new ATP molecules. Thus, the ribose salvage pathway is known as the salvage pathway of ATP formation. Ribose is essential for both the salvage and de novo reactions to work, and it is formed in the body from glucose through the pentose phosphate pathway. Aside from this relatively time-consuming pathway, there are no foods that are able to provide enough ribose to rapidly restore ribose levels should the need arise, as when exercising or working, and especially during a heart attack or stroke.

D-ribose is another excellent addition to the mitochondrial resuscitation regimen. D-ribose reduces markers of oxidative stress that can form after high-intensity exercise (79). It also boosts post-exercise ATP levels (80) and has been shown to have beneficial effects in heart disease patients (81). D-ribose replenishes low myocardial energy levels, improving cardiac dysfunction following ischemia. Studies also have shown that it can improve ventilation efficiency in patients with heart failure (79). The presence of ribose in the cell stimulates the metabolic pathway to actually produce ATP. If the cell does not have enough ribose, it cannot make ATP.

Oral or intravenous ribose has been found to rapidly restore ribose levels in nerves and muscles. Ribose supplementation can dramatically improve recovery of failing ATP levels during and following acute or chronic anoxia or ischemia. Research has shown that taking ribose has a positive effect on ATP production in all muscle fiber types, especially the heart. Ribose supplementation increases the de novo production of ATP through oxidative phosphorylation by more than 300%. Ribose also activates the salvage pathway, causing nucleotides to be revitalized into the manufacture of ATP by over 500% (82).

Ribose has also been shown to increase athletic performance. Supplementation (10 grams per day) in young male recreational bodybuilders resulted in significant increases in muscular strength and total work performance after 4 weeks compared with pre-treatment levels. No changes were noted in those using a placebo (83).

Suggested dose 5 g qd (once a day)

18.5.9.13   Citrate

A citrate is a derivative of citric acid. Citric acid is a weak organic tricarboxylic acid. It occurs naturally in citrus fruits. It is an intermediate in the citric acid cycle, which occurs in the metabolism of all aerobic organisms. Citrate inhibits the phosphofructokinase enzyme, blocking glycolysis at the start; citrate also inhibits the pyruvate dehydrogenase enzyme complex and the succinate dehydrogenase enzyme. These citrate or citric acid properties have the capacity to inhibit glycolysis and a step in the Krebs cycle; the citrate inhibits three base enzymes in the mitochondrial metabolism of the Krebs cycle (84–88).

No suggested dose

18.5.9.14   Creatine

Creatine is an essential, natural substance that is synthesized in the body from three amino acids: Glycine, arginine and methionine. Creatine plays a very powerful role in energy metabolism as a muscle fuel in its role in regenerating ATP. Creatine combines with phosphate in the mitochondria to form phosphocreatine. It serves as a source of high-energy phosphate, released during anaerobic metabolism. It also acts as an intracellular buffer for ATP and as an energy shuttle for the movement of high-energy phosphates from mitochondrial sites of production to cytoplasmic sites of utilization (89–99). Operating through the ATP/ADP cycle, creatine phosphate maintains ATP levels by serving as a reservoir of high-energy phosphate bonds in muscle and nerve tissues. The energy required to rephosphorylate ADP into ATP depends on the amount of phosphocreatine (PCr) stored in muscle tissues. As phosphocreatine is depleted during exercise, energy availability declines due to a loss of ability to resynthesize ATP at the rate required.

In 1943, it was shown that creatine supplementation extended the cycling times of athletes (89). Creatine enhances both strength and endurance in athletes (89–99). Some researchers have shown strength gains with as little as 5 to 7 days of supplementation (99). In a double-blind study that examined the effects of creatine in a weight training program in men over 70, it was shown that creatine had a significant advantage over placebo in terms of increased lean body mass, reduction in body fat, increased muscular strength and endurance (95, 97). In Italy, physicians administered 6 grams of creatine each day to 13 patients hospitalized with congestive heart failure. After 4 days, they noted a reduction in heart size, reduced vascular resistance and increased ejection fraction, all indicators of improved heart function (96).

In a review article, Tarnopolsky concluded that creatine monohydrate supplementation results in an increase in skeletal muscle total and phosphocreatine concentrations, increased fat-free mass and enhanced high-intensity exercise performance in young healthy men and women (97). He also noted neuroprotective effects, which have been proposed to be of benefit in Parkinson's disease, Alzheimer's disease and amyotrophic lateral sclerosis and after ischemia. He concluded that creatine appeared to have potential to attenuate age-related muscle atrophy and strength loss as well as to protect against neurodegenerative disorders. The U.S. Food and Drug Administration (FDA) has granted orphan drug status to creatine as a treatment for patients with amyotrophic lateral sclerosis (Lou Gehrig's disease) based on creatine's demonstrated ability to enhance cellular energy production. In addition, a European patent has also recently been issued for the use of creatine compounds to prevent aging effects and to treat muscle atrophy (98).

Suggested dose 5 g qd (once a day)

18.5.9.15   Shilajit

Shilajit is a thick, sticky, tar-like substance with a color ranging from white to dark brown (the latter is more common) found predominantly in Himalaya and Tibetan mountains. It is an ancient Indian adaptogen. Shilajit enhances CoQ10's mitochondrial benefits and supports levels of the active ubiquinol form. Components of shilajit can serve as electron reservoirs, replenishing electrons lost by CoQ10 and allowing this vital coenzyme to remain active longer (100).

Suggested dose 200 mg qd (once a day)

18.5.9.16 Mushrooms

Coriolus versicolor (Turkey tail) is a mushroom of the Basidiomycetes class, from which the extracts Polysaccharide-K and Polysaccharide-Peptide (PSK, PSP, respectively) have been demonstrated to inhibit various carcinomas in animals and humans. This is achieved by inducing apoptosis and activating a cascade of pathways involving the activation of p38 MAPK signaling cascades and over-expression of pro-apoptotic protein Bax (101). PSK was approved for clinical use in various cancers in Japan in the 1980s. Other mushrooms that seem to have analogous effects on mitochondria are Reishi (*Ganoderma lucidum*; 102–104) Maitake (*Grifola frondosa*; 105, 106) Shiitake (*Lentinula edodes*; 107), Cordyceps (*Ophiocordyceps sinensis*; 108), Chaga (*Inonotus obliquus*; 109) and Lion's Mane (*Hericium erinaceus*; 110).

No suggested dose

18.5.9.17 Herbs

Certain herbs, such as *Rhodiola rosea* (111), *Leuzea carthamoides* (112), *Eleutherococcus senticosus* (113) and *Schisandra chinensis* (114), have shown some capacity to activate the synthesis and resynthesis of ATP.

Suggested dose: Rhodiola has been taken as 200 mg qd of an extract standardized to contain rosavins and salidrosides in a 3:1 ratio; for the rest of the herbs, there is no suggested dose

18.5.9.18 Melatonin

Melatonin (N-acetyl-5-methoxytryptamine) is a methoxyindole, which is synthesized in the pineal gland of vertebrates through a multistep process starting from hydroxylation of tryptophan and culminating with transformation of serotonin to N-acetyl serotonin, followed by methylation to the final substance, melatonin. Melatonin is a ubiquitous molecule with a variety of functions, including potent reductive properties. Due to its lipophilic character, it easily crosses cellular and intracellular membranes and reaches all subcellular organelles. Melatonin has been shown to protect the bioenergetic function of mitochondria (115–118).

Suggested dose 10 mg qd before sleep

18.5.9.19 Arginine

Arginine is a basic amino acid and is classified as a conditionally essential amino acid. One of the main functions of arginine is its participation in protein synthesis. Arginine is utilized by a number of metabolic pathways that produce a variety of biologically active compounds, such as nitric oxide, creatine, agmatine, glutamate, polyamines, ornithine and citrulline. Also, arginine is involved in a number of roles in the body, such as the detoxification of ammonia formed during the nitrogen catabolism of amino acids via the formation of urea; its potential to be converted to glucose (hence, its classification as a glycogenic amino acid); and its ability to be catabolized to produce energy (119, 120). Many of the benefits of arginine stem from its ability to generate nitric oxide (NO), aided by an enzyme called nitric oxide synthase. NO acts as a signaling molecule that induces smooth muscle cells to relax, expanding the blood vessels (vasodilation); blood pressure drops, and blood flow is improved. More blood is delivered to the tissues, which are then better nourished with oxygen.

Suggested dose 500 mg tid (three times a day)

18.5.9.20 Resveratrol

Resveratrol (3,5,4′-trihydroxy-trans-stilbene) is a plant-derived polyphenol that exerts diverse physiological activities, mimicking some of the molecular and functional effects of dietary restriction.

Resveratrol has been shown to increase cellular mitochondrial content and induce apoptosis (121–123).

Suggested dose 20 mg qd (once a day)

18.5.9.21 Quercetin

Quercetin is a naturally occurring flavonoid that has a broad spectrum of bioactive effects. Among these, quercetin can impact mitochondrial biogenesis by modulating enzymes and transcription factors. Quercetin is now recognized as a phytochemical that can modulate pathways associated with mitochondrial biogenesis, mitochondrial membrane potential, oxidative respiration and ATP anabolism, intra-mitochondrial redox status and subsequently, mitochondria-induced apoptosis (124).

Suggested dose 500 mg bid (twice a day)

18.5.9.22 Glutathione

Glutathione (GSH), the major intracellular thiol compound, is a ubiquitous tripeptide produced by most mammalian cells, and it is the main mechanism of antioxidant defense against ROS and electrophiles. GSH's versatility permits it to counteract hydrogen peroxide, lipid hydroperoxides or xenobiotics, mainly as a cofactor of enzymes such as glutathione peroxidase or glutathione-S-transferase (GST). GSH (γ-glutamyl-cysteinyl-glycine) serves as a cofactor for a number of antioxidant and detoxifying enzymes. GSH in the mitochondrial matrix plays a key role in defense against respiration-induced ROS and in the detoxification of lipid hydroperoxides and electrophiles. Moreover, as mitochondria play a central strategic role in the activation and mode of cell death, mitochondrial GSH has been shown to critically regulate the level of sensitization to secondary hits that induce mitochondrial membrane permeabilization and release of proteins confined in the intermembrane space necessary to induce cell death (apoptosis) (125).

Oral glutathione supplementation does not efficiently increase intracellular glutathione levels; it can be absorbed intact into the blood stream. Since increased glutathione levels in the blood have been shown to slow the breakdown of nitric oxide, glutathione supplementation may be useful to augment nitric oxide boosters such as L-citrulline or L-arginine. NAC is a prodrug for L-cysteine, which is used with the intention of allowing more glutathione to be produced when it would normally be depleted. Through glutathione buffering, NAC provides antioxidative effects and other benefits, so it is both more efficient and cheaper than glutathione. Liposome-encapsulated glutathione (Lypo-GSH) seems to be a more effective way to supplement this nutrient.

Suggested dose 250 mg qd in liposomal form

18.5.9.23 Dichloroacetate (DCA)

DCA is a potent lactate-lowering drug. It activates the pyruvate dehydrogenase complex by inhibiting the activity of pyruvate dehydrogenase kinase, which normally phosphorylates and inhibits the enzyme. The ability of DCA to keep the pyruvate dehydrogenase complex in an active state reduces the accumulation of lactate in body tissues (23, 126, 127). DCA can switch a cell from aerobic glycolysis to oxidative respiration. This drug induced apoptosis of cancer cells (128) by reducing mitochondrial membrane potential, blocking aerobic glycolysis (Warburg effect), and activating mitochondrial potassium-ion channels (129). Other mechanisms of DCA action against cancer cells have also been proposed. These include: (a) inhibition of angiogenesis; (b) alteration of expression of hypoxia-inducible factor 1-α (HIF1-α) (21); and (c) alteration of the pH regulators vacuolar-type H+-ATPase (V-ATPase) and monocarboxylate transporter 1 (MCT1) and other regulators of cell survival, such as p53-upregulated modulator of apoptosis (PUMA), glucose transporter 1 (GLUT1), B-cell lymphoma 2 (BCL2) protein and cellular tumor antigen p53 (130).

An oral DCA regimen that included the natural neuroprotective medications acetyl-L-carnitine, R-α-lipoic acid and benfotiamine (DD) has been used clinically. Intravenous DCA up to 100 mg/kg/dose has been confirmed as safe. Shifts in ATP production from glycolysis to oxidative phosphorylation by inhibition of PDK1 with dichloroacetate (DCA) was shown to shift metabolism from glycolysis to glucose oxidation. Treatment with DCA increased mitochondrial production of ROS/RNS in all tested cancer cells, but not in normal cells (130). It is important to mention that DCA in high doses can damage mitochondria and produce peripheral neuropathy. Peripheral neuropathy is not uncommon with prolonged DCA treatment.

No suggested dose

18.5.9.24   3-Bromopyruvate

Bromopyruvic acid and its alkaline form, bromopyruvate, are synthetic brominated derivatives of pyruvic acid. They are lactic acid and pyruvate analogs. 3-Bromopyruvate (BP) has been shown by others to inhibit hexokinase (131). Being a lactate analogue, it is likely taken up by cells via lactate transporters, which are over-expressed in tumor cells (131). This drug may have significant side effects.

No suggested dose

18.5.9.25   2-Deoxyglucose

2-Deoxyglucose (DG) is a non-metabolizable glucose analog. DG is easily taken up by tumor cells via glucose transporters and is then phosphorylated by hexokinase, but it is not further metabolized in the glycolytic process (132). DG will thus titrate endogenous glucose and thereby, block glycolysis (133, 134).

No suggested dose

18.5.9.26   EPI-743

EPI-743 is a new drug that is based on vitamin E. EPI-743 is a para-benzoquinone analog. Tests have shown that it can help improve the function of cells with mitochondrial problems. It works by improving the regulation of cellular energy metabolism through targeting the enzyme NADPH quinone oxidoreductase (135).

No suggested dose

18.6   LIFESTYLE AND MITOCHONDRIA

18.6.1   EXERCISE

Dietary interventions are just one part of the overall picture of optimizing mitochondrial function. Other lifestyle considerations like exercise, movement, stress and sleep also play a role in mitochondrial health. Exercise and movement have been shown to improve cellular energy production (136). Both aerobic and anaerobic exercise should be performed on a regular basis. Exercise also has an important role in mitochondrial disease therapy, as it has been shown to reduce the burden of unhealthy mitochondria; increase the percentage of healthy, non-mutated mtDNA; and improve endurance and muscle function.

Suggested exercise: combine aerobic exercises (such as cycling, walking, running, hiking and playing tennis and basketball, which focus on increasing cardiovascular endurance) and anaerobic exercises (such as weight training to increase muscle strength) for 45 min 3× a week.

18.7   HYPERBARIC (HIGH PRESSURE, 100%) OXYGEN THERAPY (HBOT)

Hyperbaric oxygen treatment (HBOT) involves inhaling up to 100% oxygen at a pressure greater than 1 atm in a pressurized chamber. Excess oxygen reduces the activity of an enzyme called hexokinase II, which grabs onto glucose after it enters cells and traps it inside so it can be burned for energy. Also, HBOT significantly ameliorates mitochondrial dysfunction (137–142). When cells are proliferating, DNA is unwound, unprotected and being replicated; if high ROS levels are sensed at this time, the process is aborted, and the cell can be driven into apoptosis.

Suggested treatment 45 min 1.5–2.5 atm twice a week

18.8 INTRAVENOUS LASER THERAPY (IVLT)

Laser therapy works on the principle of inducing a biological response through energy transfer, in that the photonic energy delivered into the tissue by the laser modulates the biological processes within the tissue. Light energy is transmitted through space as waves that contain tiny "energy packets" called photons (duality). Each photon contains a definite amount of energy depending on its wavelength (color).

Intravenous or intravascular laser blood irradiation involves the in-vivo illumination of the blood by feeding low-level laser light. It is a minimally invasive laser procedure in which a small needle is placed into the vein in the forearm, under the assumption that any therapeutic effect will be circulated through the circulatory system.

It works similarly to photosynthesis; the correct wavelengths and power of light at certain intensities for an appropriate period of time can increase ATP production, and cell membrane alterations could lead to permeability changes and second messenger activity, resulting in functional changes (143–146).

Acupuncture treatment (needles in cardinal points) increases the patient's energy but only by mobilizing reserve energy (meridians); in contrast, laser therapy introduces additional energy into the system.

Mitochondria are the key to photobiomodulation. Cytochrome c oxidase can absorb red light, converting the photonic energy into biological energy (ATP). Cytochrome c oxidase is commonly accepted as a photo acceptor that catalyzes cellular-level activity when exposed to red to near-infrared light.

The absorption of different colors within the mitochondrial respiratory chain is as follows:

Complex 1 (NADH dehydrogenase) absorbs blue and ultraviolet light.
Complex 3 (cytochrome c reductase) absorbs green and yellow light.
Complex 4 (cytochrome c oxidase) absorbs red and infrared light.

Mitochondria changed to "giant mitochondria" after laser irradiation with activation of various metabolic pathways and increased production of ATP due to activation of the respiratory chain and increased ATP synthesis. ATP is also used as a signaling molecule in communications between nerve cells and other tissues.

There is a normalization of the tissue metabolism due to increased O_2. There is also an increase of enzymes. An increase of ATP synthesis occurs with a normalization of cell membrane potential. Irradiation in the red range is effective to increase the absorption spectrum of cytochrome C oxidase in the respiratory chain with a concomitant stimulation of ATP synthesis.

There is an increased change of the redox potential in mitochondria and cytoplasm by oxidation at the NADH. Thereby, the proton motor force is increased, which drives the backflow of the protons into the matrix and by doing so, increases the ATP turnover. In addition, the electron transfer is accelerated; both effects cause an increase of ATP synthesis.

IVLT has pleiotropic action that produces a cascade of events due to increased energy.

Suggested Tx IVLT 10 min of each color twice a week. We recommend that this therapy is accompanied by mitochondria-supporting supplements.

18.9 CONCLUSIONS

Mitochondrial dysfunction has been identified as one of the principal causes of bio-energetic decline. Although there is no single silver bullet or exact combination of substances or supplements that will unfailingly resuscitate all aspects of failing mitochondria, it has been reported that a number of nutrients, supplements and prescription substances may alleviate or restore many aspects of mitochondrial dysfunction. Combinations of these, acting on multiple targets, may normalize and/or improve mitochondrial function, increase cellular and systemic energy production, alleviate mitochondrial-related disease and delay age-related decline in many organs and systems of the body.

The rise in the incidence of cancer and deaths from cancer parallels the rise not only of the development and use of toxic chemicals and materials in the environment, but also of toxins in our food and water supplies and pharmaceuticals. The rise in cancer incidence and deaths is thought to be directly caused by such toxic ingestion and the body's increasing inability to cope with the toxic overload of xenobiotics, which profoundly damages the mitochondria. It is conceivable that combinations of various mitochondrial enhancers/resuscitators, acting on various segments of the mitochondrial energy production pathway, will have complementary/additive effects and decrease the cancer incidence and death rates.

Here, we have proposed a combination of diet, exercise and supplements containing a mixture of nutrients mentioned herein to significantly enhance mitochondrial function in order to help restore oxidative respiration to a level of favoring malignant cell re-differentiation, or at least restore apoptotic mechanisms, since the intrinsic apoptotic pathway in cells is regulated largely by functional mitochondria. In restoring mitochondrial function, we may reverse aerobic glycolysis, inhibit cancer cell growth and possibly, reverse malignancy.

Scientific support for the use of vitamin-based and cofactor-based mitochondrial therapies is accumulating. This mitochondrial correction (mitochondrial rescue, mitochondrial repair) approach is intended to promote critical enzymatic reactions, reduce putative sequelae of excess free radicals and scavenge toxic metabolic molecules, which tend to accumulate in mitochondrial diseases. Some supplements also may act as alternative energy fuels or may bypass biochemical blocks within the respiratory chain. We believe this concept can have an important repercussion in the treatment of degenerative diseases that present the common characteristic of mitochondrial dysfunction.

REFERENCES

1. Wallace DC. A mitochondrial paradigm of metabolic and degenerative diseases, aging, and cancer: a dawn for evolutionary medicine. *Ann Rev Genet* 2005;39:359–407.
2. Warburg O. On the origin of cancer cells. *Science* 1956;123 (3191):309–314.
3. Warburg O, Posener K, Negelein E. *Ueber den Stoffwechsel der Tumoren; Biochemische Zeitschrift*, Vol. 152, pp. 319–344, 1924. (German). Reprinted in *English in the Book: On Metabolism of Tumors by O. Warburg, Publisher*: Constable, London, 1930.
4. Gonzalez MJ, Massari JRM, Duconge J, Riordan NH, Ichim T, Quintero-Del-Rio AI, Ortiz N. The bioenergetic theory of carcinogenesis. *Med Hypotheses* 2012;79:433–439.
5. Demetrius LA, Coy JF, Tuszynski JA. Cancer proliferation and therapy: the Warburg effect and quantum metabolism. *Theor Biol Med Model* 2010;7:2.
6. Butow RA, Avadhani NG. Mitochondrial signaling: the retrograde response. *Mol Cell* 2004;14:1–15.
7. Seyfried TN, Shelton LM. Cancer as a metabolic disease. *Nutr Metab* 2010;7:7.
8. Elliott RL, Jiang XP, Head JF. Mitochondria organelle transplantation: a potential cellular biotherapy for cancer. *J Surg* 2015; S(2):9.
9. Turpaev KT. Reactive oxygen species and regulation of gene expression. *Biochemistry* 2002;67(3):281–292.
10. Dalton TP, Shertzer HG, Puga A. Regulation of gene expression by reactive oxygen. *Ann Rev Pharmacol Toxicol* 1999;39:67–101.
11. Nicolson GL. Mitochondrial dysfunction and natural supplements. *Integr Med* 2014;13 (4):36–43.
12. Pagano G, Talamanca AA, Castello G, Cordero MD, d'Ischia M, Gadaleta MN, Pallardó FV, Petrović S, Tiano L, Zatterale A. Oxidative stress and mitochondrial dysfunction across broad-ranging pathologies: toward mitochondria-targeted clinical strategies. *Oxid Med Cell Longev* 2014;541230.
13. Meyer JN, Leung MCK, Rooney JP, Sendoel A, Hengartner MO, Kisby GE, Bess AS. Mitochondria as a target of environmental toxicants. *Toxicol Sci* 2013;134(1):1–17.
14. Goodson WH III, Lowe L, Carpenter DO, et al. Assessing the carcinogenic potential of low-dose exposures to chemical mixtures in the environment: the challenge ahead. *Carcinogenesis* 2015;36(suppl 1):S254–S296.

15. Narayanan KB, Ali M, Barclay BJ, et al. Disruptive environmental chemicals and cellular mechanisms that confer resistance to cell death. *Carcinogenesis* 2015;36(Suppl 1):S89–S110.

16. Schulz TJ, Thierbach R, Voigt A, Drewes G, Mietzner B, Steinberg P, Pfeiffer AF, Ristow M. Induction of oxidative metabolism by mitochondrial frataxin inhibits cancer growth: Otto Warburg revisited. *J Biol Chem* 2006;281:977–981.

17. Ristow M, Pfister MF, Yee AJ, Schubert M, Michael L, Zhang CY, Ueki K, Michael II MD, Lowell BB, Kahn CR. Frataxin activates mitochondrial energy conversion and oxidative phosphorylation. *Proc Natl Acad Sci* 2000;97(22):12239–12243.

18. McKinnell RG, Deggins BA, Labat DD. Transplantation of pluripotential nuclei from triploid frog tumors. *Science* 1969;165:394–396.

19. Mintz B, Illmensee K. Normal genetically mosaic mice produced from malignant teratocarcinoma cells. *Proc Natl Acad Sci* 1975;72:3585–3589.

20. Li L, Connelly MC, Wetmore C, Curran T, Morgan JI. Mouse embryos cloned from brain tumors. *Cancer Res* 2003;63:2733–2736.

21. Minocherhomji S, Tollefsbol TO, Singh KK. Mitochondrial regulation of epigenetics and its role in human diseases. *Epigenetics* 2012;7:326–334.

22. Elliott RL, Jiang XP, Head JF. Mitochondrial organelle transplantation: introduction of normal epithelial mitochondria into human cancer cells inhibits proliferation and increases drug sensitivity. *Breast Cancer Res Treat* 2015;136:347–354.

23. Parikh S, Saneto R, Falk MJ, Anselm I, Cohen BH, Haas R. Medicine society TM. A modern approach to the treatment of mitochondrial disease. *Curr Treat Options Neurol* 2009;11(6):414–430.

24. John AP. Dysfunctional mitochondria, not oxygen insufficiency, cause cancer cells to produce inordinate amounts of lactic acid: the impact of this on the treatment of cancer. *Med Hypotheses* 2001;57(4):429–431.

25. Anand P, Kunnumakara AB, Sundaram C, Harikumar KB, Tharakan ST, Lai OS. Cancer is a preventable disease that requires major lifestyle changes. *Pharm Res* 2008;25:2097–2116.

26. Shanmugam N, Reddy MA, Guha M, Natarajan R. High glucose-induced expression of proinflammatory cytokine and chemokine genes in monocytic cells. *Diabetes* 2003;52:1256–1264.

27. Wen Y, Gu J, Li SL, Reddy MA, Natarajan R, Nadler JL. Elevated glucose and diabetes promote interleukin-12 cytokine gene expression in mouse macrophages. *Endocrinol* 2006;147:2518–2525.

28. Dandona P, Chaudhuri A, Ghanim H, Mohanty P. Proinflammatory effects of glucose and anti-inflammatory effect of insulin: relevance to cardiovascular disease. *Am J Cardiol* 2007;99:15B–26B.

29. Klement RJ and Kämmerer U. Is there a role for carbohydrate restriction in the treatment and prevention of cancer? *Nutr Metab* 2011;8:75.

30. Pollak M. Insulin and insulin-like growth factor signaling in neoplasia. *Nat Rev Cancer* 2008;8:915–928.

31. Seyfried TN. Cancer as a mitochondrial metabolic disease. *Front Cell Develop Biol* 2015;3:43.

32. Tisdale MJ, Brennan RA. Loss of acetoacetate coenzyme A transferase activity in tumours of peripheral tissues. *Br J Cancer* 1983;47:293–297.

33. Yang H, Yang T, Baur JA, Perez E, Matsui T, Carmona JJ, Lamming DW, Souza-Pinto NC, Bohr VA, Rosenzweig A, de Cabo R, Sauve AA, Sinclair DA. Nutrient-sensitive mitochondrial NAD+ levels dictate cell survival. *Cell* 2007;130(6):1095–1107.

34. Houtkooper RH, Pirinen E, Auwerx J. Sirtuins as regulators of metabolism and healthspan. *Nat Rev Mol Cell Biol* 2012;13(4):225–238.

35. Lettieri-Barbato D, Cannata SM, Casagrande V, Ciriolo MR, Aquilano K. Time-controlled fasting prevents aging-like mitochondrial changes induced by persistent dietary fat overload in skeletal muscle. *PLoS One* 2018;13(5):e0195912.

36. Zhou W, Mukherjee P, Kiebish MA, Markis WT, Mantis JG, Seyfried TN. The calorically restricted ketogenic diet, an effective alternative therapy for malignant brain cancer. *Nutri & Metabol* 2007;4:5.

37. Tarnopolsky MA. The mitochondrial cocktail: rationale for combined nutraceutical therapy in mitochondrial cytopathies. *Adv Drug Delivery Rev* 2008;60:1561–1567.

38. Conklin KA, Nicolson GL. Molecular replacement in cancer therapy: reversing cancer metabolic and mitochondrial dysfunction, fatigue and the adverse effects of therapy. *Curr Cancer Therapy Rev* 2008;4:66–76.

39. Rodriguez MC, MacDonald JR, Mahoney DJ, Parise G, Beal MF, Tarnopolsky MA. Beneficial effects of creatine, CoQ10, and lipoic acid in mitochondrial disorders. *Muscle Nerve* 2007;35(2):235–242.

40. Nicolson GL. Mitochondrial dysfunction and chronic disease: treatment with natural supplements. *Altern Ther Health Med* 2013:at5027.

41. Ames BN, Liu J. Delaying the mitochondrial decay of aging with acetyl L-Carnitine. *Ann NY Acad Sci* 2004;1033:108–116.

42. Giorgio V, Petronilli V, Ghelli A, Carelli V, Rugolo M, Lenaz G, Bernardia P. The effects of idebenone on mitochondrial bioenergetics. *Biochimica et Biophysica Acta.* 2012;1817(2):363–369.

43. Banaclocha M. Therapeutic potential of N-acetylcysteine in age-related mitochondrial neurodegenerative diseases. *Med Hypotheses* 2001;56(4):472–477.

44. Hagen TM, Ingersoll RT, Lykkesfeldt J, Liu J, Wehr CM, Vinarsky V, Bartholomew JC, Ames AB. (R)-alpha-lipoic acid-supplemented old rats have improved mitochondrial function, decreased oxidative damage, and increased metabolic rate. *FASEB J* 1999;13(2):411–418.

45. Hansford R, Naotaka T, Pepe S. Mitochondria in heart ischemia and aging. *Biochem Soc Symp,* 1999;66:141–147.

46. Herbst EA, Paglialunga S, Gerling C, Whitfield J, Mukai K, Chabowski A, Heigenhauser GJ, Spriet LL, Holloway GP. Omega-3 supplementation alters mitochondrial membrane composition and respiration kinetics in human skeletal muscle. *J Physiol* 2014;592 Pt 6:1341–1352.

47. González MJ, Miranda JR, Riordan HD. Vitamin C as an ergogenic aid. J Orthomolec *Med* 2005;20(2):100–102.

48. González MJ, Rosario-Pérez G, Guzmán AM, Miranda-Massari JR, Duconge J, Lavergne J, Fernandez N, Ortiz N, Quintero A, Mikirova N, Riordan NH, Ricart CM. Mitochondria, energy and cancer: the relationship with ascorbic acid. *J Orthomol Med* 2010;25(1):29–38.

49. Ohta S. Molecular hydrogen is a novel antioxidant to efficiently reduce oxidative stress with potential for the improvement of mitochondrial diseases. *Biochim Biophys Acta* 2012;1820:586–594.

50. Heaney ML, GardnerJR, Karasavvas N, Golde,DW, Scheinberg DA, Smith E A, O'Connor OA. Vitamin C antagonizes the cytotoxic effects of antineoplastic drugs. *Cancer Res* 2008;68(19):8031–8038.

51. Krone CA, Ely JT. Controlling hyperglycemia as an adjunct to cancer therapy. *Integr Cancer Ther* 2005;4:25–31.

52. Ely JT, Krone CA. Glucose and cancer. *N Z Med J* 2002;115:U123.

53. Kc S, Cárcamo JM, Golde DW. Vitamin C enters mitochondria via facilitative glucose transporter 1 (Glut1) and confers mitochondrial protection against oxidative injury. *FASEB J* 2005;19:1657–1667.

54. González MJ, Miranda-Massari JR, Mora EM, Guzmán A, Riordan NH, Riordan HD, Casciari JJ, Jackson JA, Román-Franco A. Orthomolecular oncology review: ascorbic acid and cancer 25 years later. *Integr Cancer Ther* 2005;4:32–44.

55. Depeint F, Bruce WR, Shangari N, Mehta R, O'brien PJ. Mitochondrial function and toxicity: role of the B vitamin family on mitochondrial energy metabolism. *Chem Biol Interact* 2006;163:94–112.

56. Lou HC. Correction of increased plasma pyruvate and lactate levels using large doses of thiamine in patients with Kearns-Sayre Syndrome. *Arch Neurol* 1981;38:469.

57. Arts WFM, Scholte HR, Bogaard JM, Kerrebijn KF, Luyt-Houwen IEM. NADH-CoQ reductase deficient myopathy: successful treatment with riboflavin. *Lancet* 1983;2:581–582.

58. Driver C, Georgiou A. How to re-energize old mitochondria without shooting yourself in the foot. *Biogerontology* 2002;3:103–106.

59. HUSKISSON E, MAGGINI S, RUF M. The Role of Vitamins and Minerals in Energy Metabolism and Well-Being. *J Intern Med Res* 2007;35:277 –289.

60. Bratman S, Kroll D, eds. *Panthothenic Acid and Pantethine. Natural Health Bible.* Roseville, CA: Prima Publishing;2000:275–276.

61. Gröber U, Schmidt J, Kisters K. Magnesium in prevention and therapy. *Nutrients* 2015;7(9):8199–8226.

62. Nicolson GL, Ash ME. Lipid replacement therapy: a natural medicine approach to replacing damaged lipids in cellular membranes and organelles and restoring function. *Biochim Biophys Acta* 2014;1838:1657–1679.

63. Nicolson GL, Rosenblatt S, Ferreira de Mattos G, Settineri R, Breeding PC, Ellithorpe RR, Ash ME. Clinical uses of membrane lipid replacement supplements in restoring membrane function and reducing fatigue in chronic diseases and cancer. *Discoveries* 2016, January–March;4(1):e54.

64. Nicolson GL. Mitochondrial dysfunction and chronic disease: treatment with natural supplements. *Integr Med: A Clini J* 2014;13(4):35–43.

65. Nicolson GL, Ash ME. Lipid replacement therapy: a natural medicine approach to replacing damaged lipids in cellular membranes and organelles and restoring function. *Biochim Biophys Acta* 2014;1838(6):1657–1679.

66. Kühlbrandt W. Structure and function of mitochondrial membrane protein complexes. *BMC Biol* 2015;13:89.

67. Eckert A. Mitochondrial effects of Ginkgo biloba extract. *Int Psychogeriatr* 2012;24(Suppl 1):S18–S20.

68. Eckert A, Keil U, Kressmann S, Schindowski K, Leutner S, Leutz S, Müller WE. Effects of EGb 761 Ginkgo biloba extract on mitochondrial function and oxidative stress. *Pharmacopsychiatry* 2003;36(1) Supplement 1:S15–S23.

69. Sastre J, Pallardo F, De la Asuncion J, Vina J. Mitochondria, oxidative stress and aging. *Free Radical Res* 2000, 32: (3), 189–198.

70. Nowak G, Clifton GL, Bakajsova D. Succinate Ameliorates energy deficits and prevents dysfunction of complex I in injured renal proximal tubular cells. *J Pharmacol Exp therapeut* 2008;324(3):1155–1162.

71. Rucker R, Chowanadisai W, Nakano M. Potential physiological importance of pyrroloquinoline quinone. *Altern Med Rev* 2009 Sep;14(3):268–277.

72. Stites TE, Mitchell AE, Rucker RB. Physiological importance of quinoenzymes and the O-quinone family of cofactors. *J Nutr* 2000;130:719–727.

73. Chowanadisai W, Bauerly K, Tchaparian E, Rucker RB. Pyrroloquinoline quinone (PQQ) stimulates mitochondrial biogenesis. *FASEB J* 2007;21:854.

74. Griffiths JR. Are cancer cells acidic? *Br J Cancer* 1991;64(3):425–427.

75. Vaupel P, Kallinowski F, Okunieff P. Blood flow, oxygen and nutrient supply, and metabolic microenvironment of human tumors: a review. *Cancer Res* 1989;49(23):6449–6465.

76. Wike-Hooley JL, Haveman J, Reinhold HS. The relevance of tumour pH to the treatment of malignant disease. *Radiother Oncol* 1984;2(4):343–366.

77. Robey IF and Martin NK. Bicarbonate and dichloroacetate: evaluating pH altering therapies in a mouse model for metastatic breast cancer. *BMC Cancer* 2011;11:235.

78. Rex A, Hentschke MP, Fink H. Bioavailability of reduced nicotinamide-adenin-dinucleotide (NADH) in the central nervous system of the anaesthetized rat measured by laser-induced fluorescence spectroscopy. *Pharmacol Toxicol* 2002;90(4):220–225.

79. Seifert JG, Subudi AW, Fu MX, Riska KL, John JC, Shecterle LM, St Cyr JA. The role of ribose on oxidative stress during hypoxic exercise: a pilot study. *J Med Food* 2009;12:690–693.

80. Dhanoa TS and Housner JA. Ribose: more than a simple sugar? *Curr Sports Med Rep* 2007 Jul;6(4):254–257.

81. MacCarter D, Vijay N, Washam M, Shecterle L, Sierminski H, St Cyr JA. D-ribose aids advanced ischemic heart failure patients. *Int J Cardiol* 2009;137:79–80.

82. Berg JM, Tymoczko JL, Stryer L. *Biochemistry.* 5th edition. New York: W H Freeman; 2002.

83. Van Gammeren D, Falk D, Antonio J. The effects of four weeks of ribose supplementation on body composition and exercise performance in healthy, young, male recreational bodybuilders: a double-blind, placebo-controlled trial. *Curr Therapeut Res* 2002; 63(8):486–495.

84. Tornheim K, Lowenstein JM. Control of phosphofructokinase from rat skeletal muscle. Effects of fructose diphosphate, AMP, ATP and citrate. *J Biol Chem* 1976;251(23):7322–7328.

85. Taylor WM, Halperin ML. Regulation of pyruvate dehydrogenase in muscle. Inhibition by citrate. *J Biol Chem* 1973;248(17):6080–6083.

86. Hillar M, Lott V, Lennox B. Correlation of the effects of citric acid cycle metabolites on succinate oxidation by rat liver mitochondria and submitochondrial particles. *J Bioenerg* 1975;7(1):1–16.

87. Velichko MG, Trebukhina RV, Ostrovskii IuM. Features of pyruvate and lactate metabolism in tumorbearing rats following citrate administration. *Vopr Med Khim* 1981;27(1):68–72.

88. Bucay AH. The biological significance of cancer: mitochondria as a cause of cancer and the inhibition of glycolysis with citrate as a cancer treatment. *Med Hypotheses* 2007;69:826–828.

89. Keys A. Physical performance in relation to diet. *Fed Proc* 1943;2:164.

90. Kreider RB, Ferreira M, Wilsoln M, Grindstaff P, Plisk S, Reinardy J, Cantler E, Almada AL. Effects of creatine supplementation on body composition, strength, and sprint performance. *Med Sci Sports Ex* 1998;30:73–82.

91. Vandenberghe K, Goris M, Van Hecke P, Van Leemputte M, Vangerven L, Hespel P. Long-term creatine intake is beneficial to muscle performance during resistance training. *J Appl Physiol* 1997;83:2055–2063.

92. Stone MH, Sanborn K, Smith LL, O'Bryant HS, Hoke T, Utter AC, Johnson RL, Boros R, Hruby J, Pierce KC, Stone ME, Garner B. Effects of in-season (5 weeks) creatine and pyruvate supplementation on anaerobic performance and body composition in American football players. *Int J Sport Nutr* 1999;9:146–165.

93. Urbanski RL, Vincent WJ, Yuaspelkis BB. Creatine supplementation differentially affects maximal isometric strength and time to fatigue in large and small muscle groups. *Int J Sport Nut* 1999;9:136–145.

94. Volek JS, Kraemer WJ, Bush JA, Boetes M, Incledon T, Clark KL, Lynch JM. Creatine supplementation enhances muscular performance during high intensity resistance exercise. *J Am Diet Assoc* 1997;97:765–770.

95. Cooke MB, Brabham B, Buford TW, Shelmadine BD, McPheeters M,. Hudson GM, Stathis C, Greenwood M, Kreider R, Willoughby DS. Creatine supplementation post-exercise does not enhance training-induced adaptations in middle to older aged males. *Eur J Appl Physiol* 2014;114(6):1321–1332.

96. Ferraro S, Codella C, Palumbo F, Desiderio A, Trimigliozzi P, Maddalena G, Chiariello M. Hemodynamic effects of creatine phosphate in patients with congestive heart failure: a double-blind comparison trial versus placebo. *Clin Cardio* 1996;19(9):699–703.

97. Tarnopolsky MA. Potential benefits of creatine monohydrate supplementation in the elderly. *Curr Opin Clin Nutr Metab Care* 2000;3(6):495–502.

98. Hespel PJL, KU Leuven Research & Development, Belgium. Creatine compounds for prevention of aging effects and treatment of muscle atrophy. *Eur Pat Appl. EP* 2000;1(002):532, 24 May.

99. Cooper R, Naclerio F, Allgrove J, Jimenez A. Creatine supplementation with specific view to exercise/ sports performance: an update. *J Intl Soc Sports Nutr* 2012;9:33.

100. Surapaneni DK, Adapa SR, Preeti K, Teja GR, Veeraragavan M, Krishnamurthy S. Shilajit attenuates behavioral symptoms of chronic fatigue syndrome by modulating the hypothalamic-pituitary-adrenal axis and mitochondrial bioenergetics in rats. *J Ethnopharmacol* 2012;143:91–99.

101. Kobayashi H, Matsunaga K, Oguchi Y. Antimetastatic effects of PSK (Krestin), a protein-bound polysaccharide obtained from basidiomycetes: an overview. *Cancer Epidemiol Biomarkers Prev* 1995;4(3):275–281.

102. Ko KM, Leung HY. Enhancement of ATP generation capacity, antioxidant activity and immunomodulatory activities by Chinese Yang and Yin tonifying herbs. *Chin Med* 2007;2:3.

103. Cherian E, Sudheesh NP, Janardhanan KK, Patani G. Free-radical scavenging and mitochondrial antioxidant activities of Reishi-Ganoderma lucidum (Curt: Fr) P. Karst and Arogyapacha-Trichopus zeylanicus Gaertn extracts. *J Basic Clin Physiol Pharmacol* 2009;20(4):289–307.

104. Sudheesh NP, Ajith TA, Mathew J, Nima N, Janardhanan KK. Ganoderma lucidum protects liver mitochondrial oxidative stress and improves the activity of electron transport chain in carbon tetrachloride intoxicated rats. *Hepatol Res* 2012;42(2):181–191.

105. Soares R, Meireles M, Rocha A, Pirraco A, Obiol D, Alonso E, Joos G, Balogh G. Maitake (D fraction) mushroom extract induces apoptosis in breast cancer cells by BAK-1 gene activation. *J Med Food.* 2011;14(6):563–572.

106. Zhang Y, Sun D, Meng, Guo W, Chen Q, Zhang Y. Grifola frondosa polysaccharides induce breast cancer cell apoptosis via the mitochondrial-dependent apoptotic pathway. *Int J Mol Med* 2017;40(4):1089–1095.

107. Fang N, Li Q, Yu S, Zhang J, He L, Ronis MJ, Badger TM. Inhibition of growth and induction of apoptosis in human cancer cell lines by an ethyl acetate fraction from Shiitake mushrooms. *J Altern Complement Med* 2006;12(2):125–132.

108. Lee HH, Lee S, Lee K, Shin YS, Kang H, Cho H. Anti-cancer effect of Cordyceps militaris in human colorectal carcinoma RKO cells via cell cycle arrest and mitochondrial apoptosis. *DARU J Pharmaceut Sci* 2015;23(1):35.

109. Sun Y, Yin T, Chen XH, Zhang G, Curtis RB, Lu ZH, Jiang JH. In vitro antitumor activity and structure characterization of ethanol extracts from wild and cultivated chaga medicinal mushroom, Inonotus obliquus (Pers:Fr.) Pilát (Aphyllophoromycetideae). *Int J Med Mushrooms* 2011;13(2):121–130.

110. Kim SP, Nam SH, Friedman M. Hericium erinaceus (Lion's Mane) mushroom extracts inhibit metastasis of cancer cells to the lung in CT-26 colon cancer-tansplanted mice. *J Agric Food Chem* 2013;61(20):4898–4904.

111. Abidov M, Crendal F, Grachev S, Seifulla R, Ziegenfuss T. Effect of extracts from Rhodiola rosea and Rhodiola crenulata (Crassulaceae) roots on ATP content in mitochondria of skeletal muscles. *Bull Exp Biol Med* 2003;136(6):585–587.

112. Azizov AP, Seifulla RD, Chubarova AV. Effects of leuzea tincture and leveton on humoral immunity of athletes. *Eksp Klin Farmakol* 1997;60(6):47–48.

113. Eschbach LF, Webster MJ, Boyd JC, McArthur PD, Evetovich TK. The effects of Siberian ginseng (Eleutherococcus senticosus) on substrate utilization and performance. *Int J Sport Nutr Exerc Metab* 2000;444–451.

114. Panossian A, Wikman G. Pharmacology of Schisandra chinensis Bail: an overview of Russian research and uses in medicine. *J Ethnopharmacol* 2008;118(2):183–212.

115. Acuña-Castroviejo D, Martín M, Macías M, Escames G, León J, Khaldy H, Reiter RJ. Melatonin, mitochondria, and cellular bioenergetics. *J Pineal Res* 2001;30(2):65–74.

116. León J, Acuña-Castroviejo D, Escames G, Tan DX, Reiter RJ. Melatonin mitigates mitochondrial malfunction. *J Pineal Res* 2005;38(1):1–9.

117. Petrosillo G, Di Venosa N, Pistolese M, Casanova G, Tiravanti E, Colantuono G, Federici A, Paradies G, Ruggiero FM. Protective effect of melatonin against mitochondrial dysfunction associated with cardiac ischemia- reperfusion: role of cardiolipin. *FASEB J* 2006;20(2):269–276.

118. Kleszczyński K, Zillikens D, Fischer TW. Melatonin enhances mitochondrial ATP synthesis, reduces reactive oxygen species formation, and mediates translocation of the nuclear erythroid 2-related factor 2 resulting in activation of phase-2 antioxidant enzymes (γ-GCS, HO-1, NQO1) in ultraviolet radiation-treated normal human epidermal keratinocytes (NHEK). *J Pineal Res* 2016;61(2):187–197.

119. Nagaya N, Uematsu M, Oya H, Sato N, Sakamaki F, Kyotani S, Ueno K, Nakanishi N, Yamagishi M, Miyatake K. Short-term oral administration of L-arginine improves hemodynamics and exercise capacity in patients with precapillary pulmonary hypertension. *Am J Resp Crit Care Med* 2001;163:887–891.

120. Xu W, Ghosh S, Comhair SAA, Asosingh K, Janocha AJ, Mavrakis DA, Bennett CD, Gruca LL, Graham BB, Queisser KA, Kao CC, Wedes SH, Petrich JM, Tuder RM, Kalhan SC, Erzurum SC. Increased mitochondrial arginine metabolism supports bioenergetics in asthma. *J Clin Invest* 2016;126(7):2465–2481.

121. Lagouge M, Argmann C, Gerhart-Hines Z, et al. Resveratrol improves mitochondrial function and protects against metabolic disease by activating SIRT1 and PGC-1alpha. *Cell* 2006;127(6):1109–1122.

122. de Oliveira MR, Nabavi SF, Manayi A, Daglia M, Hajheydari Z, Nabavi SM. Resveratrol and the mitochondria: from triggering the intrinsic apoptotic pathway to inducing mitochondrial biogenesis, a mechanistic view. *Biochim Biophys Acta* 2016;1860(4):727–745.

123. Ungvari Z, Sonntag WE, de Cabo R, Baur JA, Csiszar A. Mitochondrial protection by resveratrol. *Exercise Sport Sci Rev* 2011;39(3):128–132.

124. de Oliveira MR, Nabavi SM, Braidy N, Setzer WN, Ahmed T, Nabavi SF. Quercetin and the mitochondria: a mechanistic view. *Biotechnol Adv* 2016;34(5):532–549.

125. Ribas V, García-Ruiz C, Fernández-Checa JC. Glutathione and mitochondria. *Front Pharmacol* 2014;5:151.

126. Khan NA, Govindaraj P, Meena AK, Thangaraj K. Mitochondrial disorders: challenges in diagnosis & treatment. *Indian J Med Res* 2015;141(1):13–26.

127. Avula S, Parikh S, Demarest S, Kurz J, Gropman A. Treatment of mitochondrial disorders. *Curr Treat Options Neurol.* 2014;16(6):292.

128. Bonnet S, Archer SL, Allalunis-Turner J, Haromy A, Beaulieu C, Haromy A, Beaulieu C, Thompson R, Lee CT, Lopaschuk GD, Puttagunta L, Bonnet S, Harry G, Hashimoto K, Porter CJ, Andrade MA, Thebaud B, Michelakis ED. A mitochondria-K+ channel axis is suppressed in cancer and its normalization promotes apoptosis and inhibits cancer growth. *Cancer Cell* 2007;11(1):37–51.

129. Khan A, Marier D, Marsden E, Andrews D, Eliaz I. A novel form of dichloroacetate therapy for patients with advanced cancer: a report of 3 cases. *Altern Ther Health Med* 2014;20(suppl 2):21–28.

130. Michelakis ED, Webster L, Mackey JR. Dichloroacetate (DCA) as a potential metabolic-targeting therapy for cancer. *Br J Cancer* 2008;99:989–994.

131. Ihrlund LS, Hernlund E, Khan O, Shoshan MC. 3-Bromopyruvate as inhibitor of tumour cell energy metabolism and chemopotentiator of platinum drugs. *Mol Oncol* 2008;2:94–101.

132. Pedersen PL. The cancer cell's "power plants" as promising therapeutic targets: an overview. *J Bioenerg Biomembr* 2007;39:1–12.

133. Zhao Y, Wieman HL, Jacobs SR, Rathmell JC. Mechanisms and methods in glucose metabolism and cell death. *Methods Enzymol* 2008;442:439–457.

134. Cantor JR, Sabatini DM. Cancer cell metabolism: one hallmark, many faces. *Cancer Discov* 2012;2(10):881–898.

135. Enns GM, Cohen BH. Clinical trials in mitochondrial disease: an update on EPI-743 and RP103. *J Inborn Errors Metab Screening* 2017;5.

136. Sahlin K. Muscle energetics during explosive activities and potential effects of nutrition and training. *Sports Med* 2014;44(Suppl 2):167–173.

137. Dave KR, Prado R, Busto R, Raval AP, Bradley WG, Torbati D, Pérez-Pinzón MA. Hyperbaric oxygen therapy protects against mitochondrial dysfunction and delays onset of motor neuron disease in Wobbler mice. *Neuroscience* 2003;120(1):113–120.

138. Rossignol DA, Bradstreet JJ, Van Dyke K, Schneider C, Freedenfeld SH, O'Hara N, Cave S, Buckley JA, Mumper EA, Frye RE. Hyperbaric oxygen treatment in autism spectrum disorders. *Med Gas Res* 2012;2:16.

139. Palzur E, Zaaroor M, Vlodavsky E, Milman F, Soustiel JF. Neuroprotective effect of hyperbaric oxygen therapy in brain injury is mediated by preservation of mitochondrial membrane properties. *Brain Res* 2008;1221:126–133.

140. Moen I, Stuhr LEB. Hyperbaric oxygen therapy and cancer: a review. *Targeted Oncol* 2012;7(4):233–242.

141. Poff AM, Ari C, Seyfried TN, D'Agostino DP. The ketogenic diet and hyperbaric oxygen therapy prolong survival in mice with systemic metastatic cancer. *PLoS One* 2013;8:e65522.

142. Poff AM, Ward N, Seyfried TN, Arnold P, D'Agostino DP. Non-toxic metabolic management of metastatic cancer in VM mice: novel combination of ketogenic diet, ketone supplementation, and hyperbaric oxygen therapy. *PLoS One* 2015;10:e0127407.

143. Ferraresi C, Kaippert B, Avci P, Huang YY, de Sousa MV, Bagnato VS, Parizotto NA, Hamblin MR. Low-level laser (light) therapy increases mitochondrial membrane potential and ATP synthesis in C2C12 myotubes with a peak response at 3–6 hours. *Photochem Photobiol.* 2015;91(2):411–416.

144. Xu X, Zhao X, Liu TC, Pan H. Low-intensity laser irradiation improves the mitochondrial dysfunction of C2C12 induced by electrical stimulation. *Photomed Laser Surg* 2008;26(3):197–202.

145. Momenzadeh S, Abbasi M, Ebadifar A, Aryani M, Bayrami J, Nematollahi F. The intravenous laser blood irradiation in chronic pain and fibromyalgia. *J Lasers Med Sci* 2015;6(1):6–9.

146. Huang SF, Tsai YA, Wu SB, Wei YH, Tsai PY, Chuang TY. Effects of intravascular laser irradiation of blood in mitochondria dysfunction and oxidative stress in adults with chronic spinal cord injury. *Photomed Laser Surg* 2012;30(10):579–586.

19 The Impact of Untreated Sleep Disorders on Children's Cognition, Academics, Behaviors, Health and Safety – Screening, Identification and Treatment

Marsha L. Luginbuehl and Alyse Shockey

CONTENTS

DOI: 10.1201/b23304-21

19.1   INTRODUCTION

There are many medical and educational studies investigating the incidence rate and negative impact of major sleep problems/disorders on children and adolescents' cognition, academics, behaviors, health and safety. Pediatric sleep disturbances occur frequently and persist in 12–35% of young children and up to 60% of school-age children.[1–3] In a 1999 epidemiology study, it was found that 20–25% of children and adolescents not only had a sleep disturbance but developed a serious sleep disorder.[4] Most sleep researchers today would agree with Mindell and Owens[5] that approximately 25–33% of elementary school-aged children experience significant sleep problems or sleep disorders (many studies). The incidence rate and severity of these sleep disorders usually increase in adolescence[6] and adulthood if not treated and corrected early, thus having an increasingly negative impact on cognition, academics, behaviors, moods, health and later, work performance.[6–20] If not aggressively screened, identified and corrected by a variety of pediatric professionals, these unidentified sleep disorders will negatively impact personal relationships, work success, health and safety in adulthood.

This chapter will discuss the major sleep disorders requiring professional screening of all children and adolescents, and the possible treatment or interventions to resolve them. Also, there will be a discussion of the incidence rate of each sleep disorder, short- and long-term negative consequences of these untreated sleep disorders, and then a brief discussion of an accurate, easy-to-use screening tool that can be implemented by pediatric professionals to identify these major sleep disorders.

The ideal time for screening would be in early childhood between 3 and 8 years of age to prevent significant cognitive, academic, behavioral and health problems from arising.[6, 15] Of course, if the child is already beyond 8 years old, it is critical to screen him or her immediately, because any of these major sleep disorders will negatively impact their daytime functioning. The second most important screening time is between 12 and 18 years of age, because two of these major sleep disorders usually have onset within this time period. Unfortunately, only a small percentage of the pediatric population with a major sleep disorder are being screened, identified and treated at this time. The average time that elapses from onset of a sleep disorder until diagnosis is approximately ≥10–15 years.[21, 22] By then, a great deal of collateral damage has occurred.

19.2   MAJOR PEDIATRIC SLEEP DISORDERS, PREVALENCE RATES, NEGATIVE IMPACT ON DAYTIME FUNCTIONING AND HEALTH, AND POSSIBLE TREATMENTS OR INTERVENTIONS

There are many types of sleep disturbances and sleep disorders that can occur in children, and some of them will disappear within a short time or before the child reaches elementary school. However, there are five or six major sleep disorders in children and adolescents that will rarely disappear without identification and professional interventions. Based on extensive research and collaboration with many renowned pediatric sleep specialists, Luginbuehl[6, 15] enumerated these major pediatric sleep disorders that result in negative consequences and must be identified as early as possible. They are (1) sleep-related breathing disorders (SRBD) (such as upper airway resistance syndrome [UARS] and obstructive sleep apnea [OSA]), (2) periodic limb movement disorder (PLMD), (3) restless legs syndrome (RLS), (4) narcolepsy and (5) behavioral insomnia of childhood (BIC) or delayed sleep phase syndrome (DSPS). Any of these major sleep disorders can cause a daytime condition called excessive daytime sleepiness (EDS), but young children are more likely to exhibit signs of attention deficit hyperactivity disorder (ADHD)-like characteristics when the sleep disorder is still milder.[7, 8] All usually result in difficulties with school and work functioning, long-term health, safety and quality of life if they are not corrected early.[6, 7, 13–29]

19.3   SLEEP-RELATED BREATHING DISORDERS (SRBDS)

On a bell-shaped curve, SRBDs range from mild snoring at the lowest or mildest end of the spectrum, to UARS, to OSA at the moderate-to-severe or most harmful end of the spectrum. In English, snoring is defined as: "to breathe during sleep with harsh, snorting noises caused by vibration of the soft palate."[30] Primary snoring also includes the criteria that the snoring is without associated apneas, hypopneas, hypoxemia, hypercapnia or sleep fragmentation.[31] However, this snoring may not be harsh but barely audible, raspy breathing.

The latest criteria for OSA in children provided by the International Classification of Sleep Disorders Diagnostic and Coding Manual – Third Edition (ICSD-3; American Academy of Sleep Medicine [AASM])[32] is as follows: "Complete or nearly complete cessation of airflow in the presence of respiratory effort; obstructive hypopnea is considered ≥50% reduction in airflow with arousal or oxygen desaturation of ≥3%, with obstructive events lasting ≥1 respiratory cycle." In other words, the child stops breathing in sleep for ≥1+ times per hour or has numerous hypopnea events during sleep (partial blockage of breathing and ~50% decrease in oxygen during a hypopnea event).

UARS does not meet this criterion and is milder. In the case of UARS, the person is experiencing a narrowing of the airway that causes belabored breathing at night and sometimes even during the daytime. This can cause disruptions to sleep, resulting in a few nighttime apnea events and/or some hypopnea events, but they do not occur frequently enough for a diagnosis of OSA. Nevertheless, it may still result in daytime problems such as lowered cognitive and academic performance and more behavioral, safety and health problems if not corrected. UARS may also increase in severity and become more serious OSA if untreated.

OSA often results in more frequent and louder snoring than UARS (93% of OSA children experience snoring), restless sleep (79%), ADHD (58%), open mouth breathing (46%) and more serious sleep disruptions and apnea events causing EDS. These breathing problems can be a result of numerous factors such as enlarged tonsils, tongue or adenoids, a narrowed nasal passage, mandibular deformities causing airway crowding, a tumor growing in an airway, a recessive chin, etc. If any of these problems exist, it results in too much effort to breathe, waking the person from deep, restful sleep and/or causing a deficit of oxygen or CO_2 from reaching the arterial blood flow and brain. This reduction in oxygen to the person's arterial blood flow and brain often has serious consequences for a person's daytime functioning, health and safety.

19.3.1 PREVALENCE RATE OF SRBDs

There have been many studies trying to determine the prevalence rate of snoring, and particularly OSA due to its harmful consequences. Because these sleep problems/disorders are currently under-identified, the prevalence rates provided here may be under-estimates.

Estimations of habitual snoring in children and teens vary across many studies depending on the definition of snoring and who is rating the snoring. The estimated population prevalence is about 1.5% to 6% by parents reporting that the child "always" snores, and this could include children with OSA.[33] Some estimates range as high as 12%. Most professionals ignore snoring, especially mild snoring or raspy breathing, but snoring is a symptom that there is something wrong within the airways causing belabored breathing at night, which can result in daytime performance deficits.

The OSA prevalence rate in children is from at least 2.5%[26] to as high as 4%,[33] and it is as high as 6% in adolescence.[34] On the average, 67% of children with Down syndrome (DS) have OSA, often caused by a thicker, enlarged tongue blocking the airways or their problematic neck structure.[35]

The OSA incidence rate is two to three times higher in African American children than in Caucasians, possibly due to a different structure of their airways.[34, 36] Thus, the AASM recommends that all children with DS or who are African American be screened for OSA. Though more studies of UARS are needed, the rate may be higher than OSA.

19.3.2 NEGATIVE IMPACT OF OSA ON DAYTIME FUNCTIONING AND HEALTH

OSA is the most harmful of all the major sleep disorders.[37] Thus, sleep specialists and pediatricians focus primarily on identifying this sleep disorder while sometimes almost disregarding the other major sleep disorders that also have negative daytime performance and health consequences.[6] There are hundreds of studies measuring the harmful effects of OSA on children; too many to mention them all. Only some of the relevant studies will be discussed, but they are supported by many later studies.

Untreated OSA results in many developmental delays.[6, 37–40] It significantly decreases cognitive scores on intelligence tests by approximately 8–11 points in elementary-aged students.[11, 12] These deficits frequently occur in skills such as processing speed, listening, memory, visual-motor coordination (which impacts work completion), verbal fluency, verbal comprehension and executive functioning.[18, 23, 41] As a result, many of these students have delayed academic skills or lower grade point averages,[13, 19, 20, 23, 34, 42–44] more behavioral and emotional problems such as depression and ADHD (hyperactivity, distractibility and impulsivity), aggression, oppositional-defiant behaviors, anxiety, and lower motivation and self-esteem.[6–9, 44, 45] In a study of 11,000 children, having SRBD through 5 years of age was associated with 40% increased odds of needing special education at 8 years of age.[46]

After the OSA or other sleep disorders are corrected, especially if this correction takes place early in a student's school career, students' cognitive scores can rise 8–12 points.[11] As a result, academic scores (reading, math and writing) gradually and significantly improve.[6, 13] Also, behavior problems often decrease to normal ranges shortly after correction.[6, 16, 23]

OSA not only has a negative impact on students' daytime school functioning, but it starts to affect long-term health if not corrected early. As students' OSA becomes more severe in adolescence and adulthood, it causes EDS, which is not only detrimental to learning and work efficiency but becomes a serious safety hazard when a student begins to work or drive a vehicle.[47] Sometimes, obesity causes OSA because of too much fatty tissue in the neck narrowing the breathing airways. However, many studies have found OSA to cause significant childhood weight gains and obesity, and as a result, the beginnings of a variety of health problems such as Type II diabetes, high blood pressure and cardiovascular disease.[25, 48–51]

Children with OSA had 20–28% higher heart rates and 18–26% higher blood pressure during sleep apnea events than controls.[52] Elementary-aged students with uncorrected OSA already had the beginning symptoms of endothelial dysfunction, which is a precursor of cardiovascular disease.[25, 53]

When one considers the avalanche of neurocognitive, learning, behavioral and health problems that OSA causes children (and we have not even mentioned the severe health problems that eventually occur in adults), then it is understandable that OSA is considered the most harmful of the 84 diagnosable sleep disorders. On a positive note, many of these detrimental effects of OSA and UARS are preventable or reversible if children are screened early and treated.

19.3.3 Possible Treatment Interventions for SRBDs/OSA

There are numerous treatments that may help correct SRBDs, and various professionals who are trained in airway breathing disorders and can determine what is causing the airway breathing problems or obstruction. Because these obstructions can be caused by various problems, there are a variety of treatment options depending on the cause of the mild snoring, UARS or OSA.

Some causes of breathing problems could be enlarged tonsils or adenoids, a long uvula, tumors or a cleft palate interfering with breathing. Often in these cases, an adenotonsillectomy, surgical shortening or removal of the uvula, tumor removal or cleft palate repair is recommended and often performed by an ears, nose and throat specialist (ENT). Although these surgical procedures for tonsils and adenoids may correct the problem in the short term, they are somewhat intrusive treatment options, and surgery does not always continue to correct the problem in the long term for about 45% of people. These 45% start experiencing renewed SRBD problems later because the original cause, the incorrect breathing behaviors and habits, was never corrected with airway breathing treatment to remove the maladaptive breathing habits.

Sometimes, there could be issues with poor posture, mouth breathing or incorrect oral habits that cause craniofacial abnormalities, such as a narrow jaw, a recessive chin or a problematic mouth structure resulting in dental malocclusions, small nasal airways, etc. When there are dental malocclusions due to a narrow jaw causing overcrowding, which often causes SRBDs, there is the possibility of a specialized orthodontist widening the oral structure with teledontic treatment of pharyngorofacial disorders.[54] Once the jaw has been widened to address malocclusions or extended in the case of a recessive chin, the SRBD usually improves significantly or disappears, because this treatment has opened the airways wider for resistance-free breathing in the day and nighttime.

Other likely causes for the obstruction could be inflammation of the airways due to asthma or allergies, fatty tissue in the airways caused by obesity, or collapsing of the pharyngeal tissue in the throat. These physical problems also result in narrowing and crowding of the airways. In cases where asthma or allergies are restricting the airways, these problems need to be addressed by a pulmonologist or allergist. In cases of obesity and fatty tissue in the throat obstructing breathing, the person needs to lose weight by consulting with a dietician, physician or fitness trainer. It is sometimes difficult for the person with SRBD to lose weight without first having one of the other interventions to reduce the SRBD problem and make weight loss easier.

For the body to function in balance, it is necessary that breathing, chewing, swallowing and over-all posture perform optimally together. The jaws grow and develop as a result of balanced pressure from the lips, cheeks and tongue. Any disruption in this equilibrium can result in not only facial and skeletal changes but also changes in airway health.[5] These changes occur early in life, as the orofacial growth is particularly fast during the first 2 years of life.

Infant airways are divided into three parts: The nasopharynx (the portion of the airway associated with the nose), the oropharynx (the portion of the airway associated with the mouth and throat) and the hypopharynx (the pharyngeal airway space below the mouth). The nasopharynx develops as an infant breathes through his or her nose consistently. Therefore, mouth-breathing babies and small children will not adequately develop their nasal passages.

Long-term mouth breathing can be correlated with large tonsils and adenoids. The nose is a natural filtration system. If it is not being used, the tonsils and adenoids are being exposed to more allergens and bacteria, causing them to be inflamed. Once this tissue becomes inflamed, the child is then forced to bring the tongue forward and/or breathe with an opened mouth posture – further agitating the inflamed tonsils and/or adenoids. An anterior tongue posture can lead to flaring of the front teeth and/or a dental open bite.

Continual open mouth postures and mouth breathing will change the way a jaw will grow and develop. An open mouth posture allows supra-eruption of the posterior maxilla and downward and backward (clockwise) growth. This can lead to a long face, flaccid musculature, vertical maxillary excess and muscle strain to keep lips together. This facial pattern is often associated with airway and breathing problems. If not addressed early, the only way to correct this jaw pattern is bimaxillary surgery combined with orthodontics. Mouth breathing not only increases upper airway resistance[26] but also causes micro-trauma to the back of the throat that may induce local inflammatory reactions in the tonsils, leading to their enlargement.

The tongue is directly linked with the oropharynx. The back of the tongue makes up the front wall of the oropharynx. As the tongue moves forward and fills the oral cavity, it is moved out of the back of the throat, opening up the airway. If the tongue is tethered (tongue tied), the tongue movement is restricted. A restricted tongue, therefore, can have the following effects on skeletal growth and development as well as airway development:

- If the tongue is tethered, it cannot rise to the palate and cannot put pressure on the upper jaw. This can lead to narrow upper jaws and upper jaws that do not grow forward enough.
- Tethered tongues have been correlated with small lower jaws. If the tongue is tethered, it holds back the forward growth potential of the mandible (the lower jaw).
- If the upper jaw is narrow and small, and/or if the lower jaw is small or set back, the tongue will fill the oropharynx (the airway space in the back of the throat) and compromise the airway.

- Tethered tongues are seen to be correlated with dental and skeletal open bites. If the child is trying to open his or her airway, and the skeletal structures are blocking the airway, the child is forced to bring his or her tongue forward in order to breathe better. This will result in an open bite. Once there is space between the front teeth, the tongue will always rest there. If the underlying airway issue is not resolved, long-term correction of the open bite is unpredictable.

Early observation of the thin strip of tissue, lingual frenulum, that attaches the floor of the mouth to the ventral side of the tongue is critical since it guides the forward growth of the tongue. [55,56]

When the lingual frenulum is abnormally short or tethered, it results in ankyloglossia, commonly described as "tongue tie," which restricts tongue mobility to varying degrees Figure 19.1 [55,57]

As a child is developing, a balance needs to exist between the lingual and buccal musculature: The tongue pushes against the dentition and the jaw so it expands, and the buccal muscles counter this force to promote forward growth of the jaw. With ankyloglossia, the tongue is restricted, and therefore, the necessary force required for expansion and positioning of the jawbone[58] results in underdeveloped upper jaw bones, speech difficulty, nasal obstruction,[59] mouth breathing[60] and OSA.[61] Mouth breathing not only increases upper airway resistance [62] but also causes micro-trauma to the back of the throat that may induce local inflammatory reactions in the tonsils, leading to their enlargement. This can produce "nasal disuse," particularly during sleep, an often-missed condition[63] that will not spontaneously improve even after surgical elimination of the abnormal anatomic presentation. Daytime reeducation and retraining of nasal usage will be needed, which is the least intrusive and possibly the safest treatment option for some of these above-mentioned problems to strengthen poorly functioning or impaired muscles in the face, airways and posture. This new but promising treatment is performed by professionals trained in posture, muscles and breathing function in order to restore optimal balance. Parents and professionals may want to consider exploring this treatment option with an orofacial myofunctional therapist before turning to other treatments that require more intrusive or long-term interventions. For more information about this treatment option, please go to www.airwayhealth.org.

Another treatment option often recommended by sleep specialists is a continuous positive airway pressure apparatus (C-PAP or Bi-PAP), which is often used when surgery is not desirable, or orthodontists are gradually correcting mandibular or malocclusion issues, or less intrusive measures are not effective. This device is held over the nose by a strap and pumps a steady flow of oxygen into the person's airways at night to hold them open so that no apnea or hypopnea events occur. There are

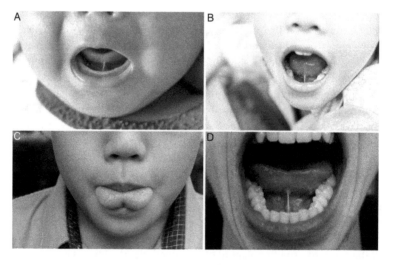

FIGURE 19.1 Tongue Tie Ankyloglossia (a) Tongue tie in an infant (b) Youth with tongue tie (c) Heart shaped tongue tip indicates the frenum is restricting function (d) Adult tongue tie can create tension on the teeth and move them

several concerns associated with this form of treatment: (1) C-PAP/Bi-PAP is a form of treatment that may cause facial or cranial deformities in children when worn for a lengthier period, which in turn may cause greater problems than SRBD; (2) some people experience panic-like attacks when using C-PAP/Bi-PAP; and (3) many teenagers and adults are not compliant when using C-PAP or Bi-PAP, especially when they go away to college or the military, or when they get married. They may fear getting ridiculed when using C-PAP.

Whatever form of treatment is necessary to correct UARS or OSA, professionals must try to identify these sleep disorders and the best possible treatment/s as early as possible. OSA is a serious sleep disorder that can disable, incapacitate or even kill if ignored.

19.4 PERIODIC LIMB MOVEMENT DISORDER (PLMD) AND RESTLESS LEGS SYNDROME (RLS)

The second and third major pediatric sleep disorders are PLMD and RLS, which tend to go together. "PLMD is characterized by the *periodic* (every 20–40 seconds) and *sustained* (0.5–4.0 seconds in duration) contractions of one or both front leg muscles in the absence of perceived arousal".[64] These contractions result in repetitive jerks of the feet, legs, arms and/or thighs during the night, disturbing the quality of sleep and often awakening or arousing the child from deep to light sleep.[65] Youth with PLMD also have difficulty falling asleep and staying asleep throughout the night.[27] PLMD is often caused by RLS.

RLS is defined as tingling, searing, crawling or irresistible urges to move the limbs, and is one of the main causes of insomnia.[65] These uncomfortable sensations begin or worsen when the student sits in class or lies down at night. They are partially relieved by leg movements (PLMD), which can disrupt sleep.

19.4.1 PREVALENCE RATES OF PLMD AND RLS

The prevalence rate of PLMD is uncertain, but it is probably about 3–6% in children and adolescents, about 9.3% in Caucasian adults and 4.3% in African American adults.[64] It is believed that PLMD may be the cause of approximately 25% of ADHD.[6, 8, 27] The prevalence of RLS has been estimated to be from about 2% in children up to 6% in older adults, with twice as many women as men having RLS.[66–68] It is sometimes difficult to diagnose RLS in young children, because they often have trouble describing their symptoms to parents and physicians.[68] Children may use an unorthodox vocabulary to describe RLS, such as "I have coke bubbles running through my legs!" or "I've got spiders crawling under my skin!" Many adults tend to ignore these unconventional descriptions because they do not realize that the child is describing RLS.

19.4.2 NEGATIVE IMPACT OF PLMD AND RLS ON DAYTIME FUNCTIONING AND HEALTH

PLMD and RLS are two of the biggest causes of insomnia and physicians prescribing lifelong insomnia medications instead of effectively treating the PLMD and RLS. The negative academic and behavioral impact of PLMD and RLS appears to be about the same as that of ADHD. This information will not be repeated here, because ADHD consequences are well known to have a negative influence on interpersonal relationships and academic and behavioral success.

19.4.3 TREATMENT OPTIONS FOR PLMD AND RLS

These sleep disorders can often be corrected or significantly improved with medication taken before bedtime that diminishes or stops the uncomfortable or painful RLS limb sensations and movements so that the student gets more restful, deep sleep. Currently, many sleep specialists are prescribing Neurontin, Mirapex, or sometimes Clonidine or L-Dopa before bedtime.[69] Neurontin, Mirapex and L-Dopa reduce or stop the periodic limb movements so that the person gets a restful night's sleep. Clonidine helps the person fall asleep more quickly so that s/he gets more hours of sleep, although

Clonidine does not stop the leg movements that can arouse the individual from his/her deep, restful levels of sleep. Both Neurontin and Clonidine have been used successfully with children and adolescents for many years, whereas Mirapex use is newer. Various sleep specialists and neurologists have reported that Neurontin has the safest and longest track record with children/teens, has few side effects and appears to be an effective treatment.

An even more benign form of treatment may be a liquid iron supplement in cases where the person may have a *serum ferritin deficiency*. In situations where a patient is complaining of RLS sensations or periodic limb movements (PLMs), the physician can check to determine whether such a deficiency exists by taking a blood sample. Liquid iron supplements for 6 to 8 weeks have been the first-line treatment solution when a serum ferritin deficiency exists, which is the case for about 25% of all people experiencing RLS or PLMD.[69] Another promising treatment may be iron given intravenously to children.[69]

When the RLS sensations and/or PLMs are decreased or stopped, the student can get a deep, restful night's sleep, usually resulting in significantly improved daytime concentration, improved work production and fewer behavior problems. The ADHD-like behaviors often decrease or disappear completely unless it is severe.

To diagnose PLMD, a sleep study using actigraphy over multiple nights may be a more accurate measure of PLMD than polysomnography (PSG) if the student is not exhibiting any symptoms of an SRBD, because PLMs can vary in frequency and intensity on different nights. Therefore, a one-night study using PSG may not provide a valid assessment if the child only exhibits PLMs a few nights per week, and the PSG is not on one of those nights. Some physicians prescribe medication for RLS or PLMD to try to stop these sleep symptoms rather than undergo the high costs of an overnight PSG study or multiple nights of actigraphy.

19.5   NARCOLEPSY

Narcolepsy sometimes exists when an individual experiences EDS resulting in frequent sleep attacks. This EDS is sometimes accompanied by episodes of cataplexy, which is sudden loss of muscle tone when experiencing emotional duress or excitement.[70] If a cataplexy attack occurs, the person often loses control of the limb muscles and may fall suddenly, risking injury. Sometimes, people's loss of muscle control is unexpectedly manifested in slurred speech or loss of neck or head control. Other symptoms that may develop in later adolescence or adulthood are sleep paralysis and hypnagogic hallucinations, which are intense, frightening, dream-like experiences that occur while falling asleep or awakening.[70] Narcolepsy often starts in adolescence, but in rare cases, it can begin in childhood with the primary symptom being EDS.[28]

19.5.1   Prevalence Rate of Narcolepsy

The exact prevalence rate of childhood or adolescent narcolepsy is uncertain, because it develops gradually and is underdiagnosed.[28] Early prevalence studies in the United States were done with adult populations and reported rates of approximately 1 in 1,500 to 1 in 2,000.[71] It is presently estimated that the number of people in the United States with narcolepsy ranges from 135,000 to 200,000 people   (www.ninds.nih.gov/Disorders/Patient-Caregiver-Education/Fact-Sheets/Narcolepsy-Fact -Sheet). However, it could be higher because of some misdiagnoses as schizophrenia due to the hypnogogic hallucinations or depression due to EDS.

19.5.2   Negative Impact of Narcolepsy on Daytime
Functioning, Health and Quality of Life

Narcolepsy is a very debilitating sleep disorder due to the EDS, frequent sleep attacks and cataplexy that makes working or driving a vehicle dangerous if untreated. There has been inadequate research focused on the effects of narcolepsy on academic performance and behaviors because it is one of the rarer sleep disorders, so the research pool is small, especially with students, who are often not diagnosed until later in high school or post high school. Due to the debilitating effects of EDS and sleep attacks on performance, many students with narcolepsy may never attend college, or if they do, they cannot take a full course load.

These students usually make normal academic progress in early childhood, elementary and middle school. However, after the onset of narcolepsy, typically in high school or young adulthood, the EDS becomes disruptive to learning and typically increases with age. These individuals usually experience a gradual deterioration in academic or job performance.[28] Teachers are often the first professionals to notice and report these problems to parents because of the EDS noted in classes.

In a retrospective study of 180 narcoleptic adult patients, 51% credited their low or falling grades to EDS resulting in poor concentration and memory difficulties; 34% indicated that they had interpersonal problems with teachers because of poor work production and EDS; 32% noted frequent embarrassment caused by social isolation in school because of ridicule from peers about their EDS, frequent sleep attacks or sudden loss of muscle control; adults with narcolepsy also had significantly higher rates of losing job promotions, getting fired from jobs, being on disability, having marriage problems or being divorced; and 25% suffered from reoccurring suicidal thoughts due to their frequent school, work and/or interpersonal relationship problems.[24] Due to these problems, these individuals struggle to maintain a rewarding career or demanding family life, especially if their narcolepsy is not successfully treated.

19.5.3 TREATMENT OF NARCOLEPSY

Due to the difficulty of diagnosing narcolepsy in the beginning stages, even by sleep specialists, this student needs to be referred to a neurologist specializing in pediatric sleep medicine who is trained to evaluate narcolepsy. Typically, these youth undergo an overnight sleep study with PSG to first rule out OSA, PLMD or other disorders that can cause EDS. If those sleep disorders are ruled out, then they may request a daytime multiple sleep latency test (MSLT).[72] This usually involves four or five daytime naps that the person is required to take, lasting 20 minutes each. During these naps, the length of time until sleep onset and REM sleep is measured. People with narcolepsy usually fall asleep much more quickly (within about 5 minutes) than those without narcolepsy ($\geq$12 minutes for sleep onset). Narcoleptic patients often achieve REM sleep within the first 20 minutes compared with those without narcolepsy, who usually require 60 to 90 minutes to achieve REM sleep.[73] In some sleep clinics, the student's hypocretin level, obtained by tapping the spinal fluid, is measured for a more accurate diagnosis.

Narcolepsy can become very debilitating if it goes untreated. When diagnosed, it is usually managed with medications designed to decrease the sleep attacks and cataplexy. In the past, Ritalin was often prescribed to help control the EDS and sleep attacks. Today, there are many other medications being used, such as Adderall and Adderall XR, Provigil, Nuvigil, Modafinil, Sodium Oxybate (Xyrem), Concerta, Dexedrine and some others. Some of these medications lessen the EDS, and others reduce the EDS and the amount or severity of cataplexy. If it appears that the student does not have narcolepsy or another sleep disorder causing these symptoms, then other causes may need to be explored, such as the student's use of good sleep hygiene, idiopathic hypersomnia (characterized by a familial history of frequent daytime sleepiness in spite of adequate nighttime sleep and good sleep hygiene, and often treated by stimulant medication), Klein–Levin Syndrome (characterized by EDS, impulsive over-eating and hyper-sexuality) or a seizure disorder. The person's sleep hygiene should be checked first because that is easy to identify and correct without expensive and time-consuming testing.

19.6 DELAYED SLEEP PHASE SYNDROME (DSPS) AND BEHAVIORAL INSOMNIA OF CHILDHOOD (BIC)

The fifth and most frequently occurring major sleep disorder in adolescence and early adulthood is DSPS. DSPS is a common form of insomnia found mainly in adolescents and young adults when their circadian rhythms are longer than the normal 24-hour sleep-wake cycle.[74] Consequently, they cannot fall asleep until midnight or later, and then they have difficulty awakening for school or staying awake in early morning classes.[74] DSPS is not only caused by biological changes in the circadian rhythm of the individual but also influenced by poor sleep hygiene, such as drinking excessive amounts of caffeine in the evening, smoking, playing computer games or watching TV late in the evening, or being awakened by cell phone communications.[74]

Children and pre-teens do not have the circadian rhythm issues causing them to fall asleep later and later each evening, but they have delayed sleep onset due to poor sleep habits that parents allow. In the case of children, this sleep disorder is more appropriately referred to as behavioral insomnia of childhood (BIC).[32] Mindell's research[75] indicates that this problem often starts early in life when parents hold their newborn baby or rock and walk with the infant on their shoulder until the baby falls asleep instead of laying the infant in bed while still awake and allowing him/her to self-soothe and fall asleep naturally. Some parents even continue to hold the baby for lengthy periods of time while s/he is asleep. These babies become programmed to believe that they cannot fall asleep or stay asleep without the parent/s being present or holding them. This sets in motion significant sleep problems with small children that often continue through elementary, such as begging to be rocked or held until asleep, demanding to sleep with the parents nightly, crying for the parents if the child wakes up in the night in his/her own bed, and demanding to stay up as late as the parents. Therefore, the child does not habituate to a set bedtime that is appropriate for children and is often irritable or tired during the daytime due to insufficient sleep at night.

19.6.1 PREVALENCE RATE OF DSPS

In 1988, it was estimated that approximately 7% of adolescents had DSPS and had developed a circadian rhythm (internal clock) longer than 24 hours, thus staying up too late on school nights, at weekends and during vacation.[76] However, the rate rose to 10.7% in 2006,[34] and it is probably even higher today with an over-abundance of modern electronic interference and poor sleep monitoring by parents. The U.S. prevalence rate of children exhibiting BIC is estimated to be at least 15% and could be higher, depending on how researchers define BIC.[77]

19.6.2 NEGATIVE IMPACT OF DSPS ON DAYTIME FUNCTIONING AND HEALTH

More studies are needed about the daytime consequences of BIC on students' daytime functioning and health. However, in one classic study comparing elementary children who received the needed 9½ hours of sleep compared with children who only received an average of 8 hours of sleep nightly, the children with 1½ hours less sleep exhibited significantly more externalizing and internalizing behavior problems ($p < 0.05$).[78] These problematic behaviors were aggressiveness, delinquent behaviors, attention problems, social problems with peers, and somatic complaints (headaches, stomachaches, etc.). Teachers also stated that these students with insufficient sleep had more memory and academic problems.[78]

There is much research on the impact of DSPS, but due to space constraints, only a few seminal studies will be mentioned. Students with DSPS are often tardy, skip morning classes due to EDS, are likely to sleep through early morning classes and receive lower grades than peers without DSPS.[29] Many students with this form of insomnia struggle with various mental health issues caused by lack of sleep.[14] Forty percent of these students reported frequent use of alcohol or drugs to help fall asleep earlier, which exacerbated this problem.[79] Many of these students dropped out of high school because of their inability to perform adequately in early morning classes resulting in poor or failing grades.[13, 29, 76, 77, 79, 80] Most attempts to move their sleep time earlier failed unless parents and professionals intervened with strategies to improve sleep habits.[80] Students' behaviors, emotional regulation, motivation, school attendance and high school graduation improved after DSPS was corrected with simple behavioral interventions or delay of high school start times to 8:30–9:00 a.m.[29]

19.6.3 TREATMENT OR INTERVENTIONS FOR DSPS AND BIC

There are many interventions parents can use to help youth correct this problem, especially if it appears that they have no other sleep disorder causing the sleep disturbance. Parents or professionals can do an online search for interventions for BIC or DSPS and find many effective interventions to do at home. Only in situations where home interventions fail is it necessary to contact a sleep psychologist.

The most important factor in correcting DSPS is for the student to develop healthy lifestyle habits and a consistent sleep/wake cycle on weeknights and weekends, and then not deviate too much from this schedule on weekends or holidays. Consistency is critical.

If online sleep hygiene tips are not successful after 2 months of consistently implementing them, then parents should consider making an appointment with a sleep specialist. This student may need the aid of daily exposure to special light therapy with a 10,000–15,000-lux lamp that can help get the student's sleep/wake cycle straightened out. Increasing the amount of direct sunlight the individual receives may also help the situation.

19.7 MISCELLANEOUS CONSEQUENCES OF ANY OF THE ABOVE-MENTIONED SLEEP DISORDERS

Approximately 33% of students in special education have one of these major sleep disorders that is causing or exacerbating many of their learning or behavioral problems.[6] Their school performance improved significantly after the sleep disorder was corrected.[6, 11, 13, 15]

Approximately 27% of college students reported significant sleep problems or possibly a major sleep disorder. They had a significantly lower grade point average (GPA) (mean < 2.0) than their classmates without sleep problems.[81]

In an extensive study conducted by the AAA Foundation for Traffic Safety from 2009 to 2013, the following statistics were gathered:

- There were 328,000 drowsy driving crashes annually (based on trained investigator reports).
- These drowsy driving accidents resulted in ~109,000 injuries and ~6,400 fatalities annually.
- The cost of these crashes was estimated at $109 billion annually in injury or death costs, which does not include additional costs of property damage to vehicles or their contents; these costs would be much higher in today's economy.
- ~50% of all sleep-related accidents involved drivers under 25 years of age.

This chapter has briefly addressed the major sleep disorders that have a negative impact on children's and adolescents' daytime performance and health. However, hundreds of studies have shown the devastating effects these sleep disorders also have on adults when they are not identified and treated in childhood. The negative impact ranges from causing or exacerbating a multitude of adulthood diseases (obesity, high blood pressure, Type II diabetes, some forms of cancer, cardiovascular problems, etc.) resulting in very costly long-term medical treatment or even causing premature death. Also, adults with untreated sleep disorders are responsible for causing employers great fiscal losses due to employees calling in sick when tired, causing a variety of on-the-job accidents, and having more illnesses and diseases, which result in higher insurance costs.

19.8 SLEEP SCREENING FOR CHILDREN AND YOUTH

Most of these academic, health and safety consequences and costs could be prevented by health professionals conducting regular screenings of all their patients, especially their pediatric patients from 2 through 18 years of age. At least one sleep screening should be conducted by a pediatrician or dentist for children by the age of about 8 years and then again when that student reaches beginning or mid-adolescence. The purpose of this second screening in adolescence is to identify narcolepsy and DSPS, which typically have onset in adolescence. Furthermore, OSA and PLMD often become more severe with increasing age and might be easier to identify in adolescence if missed in childhood. It is important that this screening includes all the major sleep disorders mentioned in this chapter, because these sleep disorders wreak havoc on daytime performance and health.

At the present time, there is only one sleep screening inventory in the world, the Sleep Disorders Inventory for Students – Revised (SDIS-R), that screens for all of these sleep disorders in children and adolescents, demonstrates high validity and reliability with coefficients in the .80s and .90s, and uses all 11 recommended steps of accurate validation[6, 15, 82, 83] (also see the website www .SleepInventory.com for published articles discussing these psychometric measures in greater detail). The SDIS-R-Children's version screens children from 2 years through 10 years of age for SRBD, PLMD, DSPS/BIC and EDS, and provides a Total Sleep Disturbance Index (SDI). The SDIS-R-Adolescent version screens youth from 11 years through 18 years of age for all the sleep disorders on the children's inventory plus narcolepsy, and some RLS symptoms have been added to the PLMD scale, making it the PLMD/RLS scale.

In addition to screening for all the major pediatric sleep disorders, the SDIS-Revised also offers parents helpful information about the following five parasomnias that worry parents, although they do not usually disrupt the child/teen's daytime functioning or health: (1) Bedwetting (nocturnal enuresis), (2) night terrors (sleep terrors), (3) sleepwalking (somnambulism), (4) sleep-talking (somniloquy) and (5) teeth grinding (bruxism).

These inventories can be quickly completed by a parent or caretaker online (it requires about 12 to 20 minutes depending on the rater's reading speed and knowledge of the child's daytime and sleep behaviors). A comprehensive written report with a visual graph of the results is computer generated immediately for both the parents and the professional, which eliminates a 2 week+ waiting period for the professional to score and supply the results to parents. These inventories are normed and available in English and Spanish, but the results are written in English. Soon, the questionnaires will also be available in French, German and possibly Russian. There is also the Sleep Disorders Inventory for Adults (SDI-A), which screens grown-ups (from 19 years through adulthood). However, this adult version has not yet been validated. It is only available online to those who would like an estimation of the adult's sleep problems.

Two of the most important features of this inventory, besides high validity and reliability coefficients and quick, accurate computer scoring, are that it was normed and validated on a broad population of 821 children and teens from 45 public schools, 2 private psychological practices and 7 leading pediatric sleep clinics in the United States (Johns Hopkins Pediatric Hospitals in MD, All Children's Hospital in St. Petersburg, FL, which is now owned and managed by Johns Hopkins Pediatric Hospitals in MD, Tampa General Hospital in FL, Stanford Sleep Disorder Clinic in Stanford, CA, Miami Children's Hospital in FL, Carle Regional Sleep Disorders Center in Urbana, IL, and University Community Hospital in Tampa, FL.[6, 15, 82, 83] The thorough 11-step validation process was guided and assisted by 16 well-known sleep specialists, 6 well-known school and clinical psychologists, and 2 well-known measurement and statistics experts, 1 from Columbia University who has written a textbook on how to develop high-quality, accurate screening inventories, questionnaires and assessment tools.[6, 15, 84]

This validation sample of 821 children and teens is reflective of the U.S. Census Demographics in 2000 and 2010 (and probably also 2020, although we do not have those statistics at the time of this publication). This is important if a questionnaire is used nationwide. No other sleep inventory in the United States has this demographic representation.

This report with graph provides raw scores, standard t-scores, percentiles and three risk levels of having a sleep disorder (normal sleep, caution range and high-risk range). If a person scores in the caution or high-risk range of having one of these five major sleep disorders, the report will define this possible sleep disorder for the parents and professional, explain how it can negatively impact daytime performance, learning or health, and explain a variety of treatment options to be considered. It is important to note that this screening is *not* making a diagnosis but merely providing the probability of the person having one of the major sleep disorders for which it screens.

At the end of the report, a link to AASM-certified sleep clinics and sleep specialists is provided to parents and professionals that they can contact if a child/teen has a higher-than-normal risk of having a sleep disorder. The SDIS, and now the SDIS-R, is being used by professionals at hospitals, clinics, private practices and schools nationwide as well as in several countries internationally.

The SDIS-R questions can be viewed in this chapter's appendices (see Appendix 1 and Appendix 2). All statistical data, journal articles and the sleep inventories can be accessed at www .SleepInventory.com.

19.9 CONCLUSIONS

The quality and quantity of sleep have a greater impact on an individual's life and success than almost any other factors, except maybe the influences of nutrition and family love/support. We now have an abundance of research confirming that there are six major pediatric sleep disorders (i.e., SRBDs, PLMD, RLS, BIC/DSPS and narcolepsy), which if left unidentified and untreated can impair cognition, learning, behaviors, moods and/or health. The effects of these sleep disorders become accumulative the longer they go unidentified, causing increasing behavior problems and delays to academics, frequently resulting in special education placement,[6, 46] and eventually they may jeopardize graduation[24, 29, 43] and/or post–high school education/career training.[81] If these sleep disorders persist into adulthood, many of these adults are subjected to severe personal, career and health consequences, including higher rates of early death.

Despite these harmful consequences of unidentified and untreated sleep disorders, most professionals, even pediatric professionals, do not use a validated sleep screening instrument and process to identify these children and adolescents and help them obtain the proper treatment. If they do use a sleep screening tool, they usually use one that has not been normed and validated properly in a national study using all 11 recommended psychometric steps of validation. This can result in many false positives or false negatives. As a result of poor screening or no screening, they are often making diagnoses or prescribing medications or special education programs that would often not be necessary if these sleep disorders were corrected early.

One solution to resolving this dilemma is using the Sleep Disorders Inventory for Students-Revised (SDIS-R), which has undergone the most thorough and extensive validation process of any sleep screening inventory in the United States. It not only has high sensitivity and specificity for a quick, easy sleep screener, but it can be accessed online by both professionals and parents. The earlier these children with a major sleep disorder are identified and treated, the more successful and healthier they will be, and the greater the cost savings will be to our educational systems, insurance companies, and government agencies. Only after these major sleep disorders are ruled out should professionals proceed to other assessments and diagnoses with confidence.

REFERENCES

1. Byars, K.C., K. Yolton, J. Rausch, B. Lanphear, and D.W. Beebe. 2012. Prevalence, patterns, and persistence of sleep problems in the first 3 years of life. *Pediatrics*, 129(2):276–84.
2. Fricke-Oerkermann, L., J. Pluck, M. Schredl, K. Heinz, A. Mitschke, A. Wiater, and G. Lehmkuhl. 2007. Prevalence and course of sleep problems in childhood. *Sleep*, 30(10):1371–77.
3. Lam, P., H. Hiscock, and M. Wake. 2003. Outcomes of infant sleep problems: A longitudinal study of sleep, behavior, and maternal well-being. *Pediatrics*, 111(3):203–7.
4. Mindell, J.A., J.A. Owens, and M.A. Carskadon. 1999. Developmental features of sleep. *Child and Adolescent Psychiatric Clinics of North America*, 108(4):695–725.
5. Mindell J.A., and J.A. Owens. 2003. *A Clinical Guide to Pediatric Sleep: Diagnosis and Management of Sleep Problems*. Philadelphia: Lippincott Williams & Wilkins.
6. Luginbuehl, M.L. 2004. *The Initial Development and Validation Study of the Sleep Disorders Inventory For Students*. Diss. *Abstrs International Sect. A: Humanities & Soc Sci*, 64(12-A):4376.
7. Chervin, R.D., K.H. Archbold, J.E. Dillon, P. Panahi, K.J. Pituch, R.E. Dahl, and C. Guilleminault. 2002. Inattention, hyperactivity, and symptoms of sleep-disordered breathing. *Pediatrics*, 109(3):449–56.
8. Chervin, R.D., J.E. Dillon, C. Bassetti, D.A. Ganoczy, and K.J. Pituch. 1997. Symptoms of sleep disorders, inattention, and hyperactivity in children. *Sleep*, 20(12):1185–92.
9. Crabtree, V.M., J.W. Varni, and D. Gozal. 2004. Health-related quality of life and depressive symptoms in children with suspected sleep-disordered breathing. *Sleep*, 27(6):1131–38.

10. Worley, S.L. 2018. The extraordinary importance of sleep: The detrimental effects of inadequate sleep on health and public safety drive an explosion of sleep research. *P & T: A Peer-Reviewed Journal for Formulary Management*, 43(12):758–63.

11. Friedman, B.C., A. Hendeles-Amitai, and E. Kozminsky. 2003. Adenotonsillectomy improves neuro-cognitive functioning in children with obstructive sleep apnea syndrome. *Sleep*, 26(8):999–1005.

12. Mantua, J., and G. Simonelli. 2019. Sleep duration and cognition: Is there an ideal amount? *Sleep*, 42(3):zsz010. https://doi.org/10.1093/sleep/zsz010

13. Gozal, D. 1998. Sleep-disordered breathing and school performance in children. *Pediatrics*, 102:616–20.

14. Ivanenko, A., M.E. Barnes, V.M. Crabtree, and D. Gozal. 2004. Psychiatric symptoms in 490 children with insomnia referred to a pediatric sleep medicine center. *Sleep Medicine*, 5(3):253–59.

15. Luginbuehl, M.L., K.L. Bradley-Klug, J. Ferron, W.M. Anderson, and S.R. Benbadis. 2008. Pediatric sleep disorders: Validation of the sleep disorders inventory for students. *School Psychology Review*, 37(3):409–31.

16. Astill, R.G., K.B. Van der Heijden, M.H. Van Ijzendoorn, and E.J.W. Van Someren. 2012. Sleep, cognition, and behavioral problems in school-aged children: A century of research meta-analyzed. *Psychological Bulletin*, 138(6):1109–38.

17. Chaput, J.P., C.E. Gray, V.J. Poitras, V. Carson, R. Gruber, and T. Olds. 2016. Systematic review of the relationships between sleep duration and health indicators in school-aged children and youth. *Applied Physiology, Nutrition, and Metabolism*, 41(6, Suppl. 3):S266–S82.

18. Montgomery-Downs, H.E., V.M. Crabtree, and D. Gozal. 2005. Cognition, sleep and respiration in at-risk children treated for obstructive sleep apnoea. *European Respiratory Journal*, 25:336–42.

19. Taras, H., and W. Potts-Datema. 2005. Sleep and student performance at school. *Journal of School Health*, 75:248–54.

20. Urschitz M.S., S. Eitner, A. Guenther, E. Eggebrecht, J. Wolff, and P.M. Urschitz-Duprat. 2003. Habitual snoring, intermittent hypoxia, and impaired behavior in primary school children. *Pediatrics*, 114(4):1041–8. pmid:15466103.

21. Billiard, M., A. Besset, and J. Cadilhac. 1983. The clinical and polygraphic development of narco-lepsy. In *Sleep/Wake Disorders: Natural History, Epidemiology, and Long-term Evolution*, eds. C. Guilleminault, and E. Lugaresi, 171–85. New York: Raven Press.

22. Rosen, R.C., R. Zozula, E.G. Jahn, and J.L. Carson. 2001. Low rates of recognition of sleep disorders in pri-mary care: Comparison of a community-based versus clinical academic setting. *Sleep Medicine*, 2(1):47–55.

23. Beebe, D.W., M.D. Ris, M.E. Kramer, E. Long, and R. Amin. 2010. The association between sleep disor-dered breathing, academic grades, and cognitive and behavioral functioning among overweight subjects during middle to late childhood. *Sleep*, 33:1447–56.

24. Broughton, R., Q. Ghanem, Y. Hishikawa, Y. Sugita, S. Nevsimalova, and B. Roth. 1981. Life effects of narcolepsy in 180 patients from North America, Asia, and Europe compared to matched controls. *Canadian Journal of Neurological Science*, 8:299–304.

25. Gozal, D., O.S. Capdevila, and L. Kheirandish-Gozal. 2008. Metabolic alterations and systemic inflam-mation in obstructive sleep apnea among non-obese and obese pre-pubertal children. *American Journal of Respiratory Critical Care Medicine*, 177:1142–9.

26. Marcus, C.L. 2001. Sleep disordered breathing in children. *American Journal of Respiratory Critical Care Medicine*, 164:16–30.

27. Picchietti, D.L., S.J. England, A.S. Walters, K. Willis, and T. Verrico. 1998. Periodic limb movement disorder and restless legs syndrome in children with attention-deficit hyperactivity disorder. *Journal of Child Neurology*, 13:588–94.

28. Wise, M.S. 1998. Childhood narcolepsy. *Neurology*, 50:37–42.

29. Wolfson, A.R., and M.A. Carskadon. 2003. Understanding adolescents' sleep patterns and school per-formance: A critical appraisal. *Sleep Medicine Review*, 7(6):491–506.

30. *American Heritage Dictionary*. 2001. 4th ed. Boston: Houghton Mifflin.

31. Pediatric Pulmonology Subcommittee on Obstructive Sleep Apnea Syndrome, American Academy of Pediatrics. 2002. Clinical practice guideline: Diagnosis and management of childhood obstructive sleep apnea syndrome. *Pediatrics*, 109:704–12.

32. American Academy of Sleep Medicine. 2014. *International Classification of Sleep Disorders*. 3rd ed. Darien, IL: American Academy of Sleep Medicine.

33. Lumeng, J.C., and R.D. Chervin. 2008. Epidemiology of pediatric obstructive sleep apnea. *Proceedings of the American Thoracic Society*, 5(2):242–52.

34. Johnson, E.O., and T. Roth. 2006. An epidemiologic study of sleep disordered breathing symptoms adolescents. *Sleep*, 29(9):1135–42.

35. Marcus, C.L., T.L. Keens, D.B. Bautista, W.S. von Pechann, and S.L. Davidson-Ward. 1991. Sleep Apnea in children with Down syndrome. *Pediatrics*, 88:132–9.
36. Rosen, C.L. 1999. Clinical features of obstructive sleep apnea hypoventilation syndrome in otherwise healthy children. *Pediatric Pulmonology*, 27(6):403–9.
37. Carroll, J.L., and G.M. Loughlin. 1995. Obstructive sleep apnea syndrome in infants and children: Clinical features and pathophysiology. In *Principles and Practice of Sleep Medicine in the Child*, ed. R. Ferber, and M. Kryger, 163–91. Philadelphia: W.B. Saunders.
38. Carroll, J.L., and G.M. Loughlin. 1992. Diagnostic criteria for obstructive sleep apnea syndrome in children. *Pediatric Pulmonology*, 14:71–4.
39. Witte R. 2007. The relationship between sleep disorders, behaviors, and pre-academic skills in pre-kindergartners. PhD diss., University of South Florida, Tampa (FL).
40. French R. 2008. Health and behavioral problems associated with symptoms of pediatric sleep disorders. PhD diss., University of South Florida, Tampa (FL).
41. Wilhelm, I., A. Prehn-Kristensen, and J. Born. 2012. Sleep-dependent memory consolidation: What can be learnt from children? *Neuroscience & Biobehavioral Reviews*, 36:1718–28.
42. Ax, E.A. 2006. Effect of sleep disorders on school behavior, academic performance and quality of life. PhD diss., University of South Florida, Tampa (FL).
43. Hysing, M., A.G. Harvey, S.J. Linton, K.G. Askeland, and B. Sivertsen. 2016. Sleep and academic performance in later adolescence: Results from a large population-based study. *Journal of Sleep Research*, 25(3):318–24.
44. Bourke, R.S., V. Anderson, J.S. Yang, A.R. Jackman, A. Killedar, et al. 2011. Neurobehavioral function is impaired in children with all severities of sleep disordered breathing. *Sleep Medicine*, 12:222–9.
45. Popkave K.M. 2007. The relationship between parent-identified sleep problems, internalizing behaviors, externalizing behaviors, and adaptive functioning in a pediatric population. Educational spec. thesis, University of South Florida, Tampa (FL).
46. Bonuck, K., T. Rao, and L. Xu. 2012. Pediatric Sleep Disorders and Special Education Needs at 9: A Population-Based Cohort Study. *Pediatrics*, 130(4):634–642; DOI: https://doi.org/10.1542/peds.2012-0392
47. Findley L.J., and P.M. Suratt. 2001. Serious motor vehicle crashes: The cost of untreated sleep apnoea. *Thorax*, 56(7):505.
48. Arens, R., and H. Muzumdar. 2010. Childhood obesity and obstructive sleep apnea syndrome. *Journal of Applied Physiology*, 108:436–44.
49. Arens, R., S. Sin, K. Nandalike, J. Rieder, U.I. Khan, et al. 2011. Upper airway structure and body fat composition in obese children with obstructive sleep apnea syndrome. *American Journal of Respiratory Critical Care Medicine*, 183:782–7.
50. Horne, R.S., J.S. Yang, L.M. Walter, H.L. Richardson, D.M. O'Driscoll, A.M. Foster, S. Wong, M.L. Ng, F. Bashir, R. Patterson, G.M. Nixon, D. Jolley, A.M. Walker, V. Anderson, J. Trinder, M.J. Davey. 2011. Elevated blood pressure during sleep and wake in children with sleep-disordered breathing. *Pediatrics*, 128:e85–92.
51. Lindberg, E., J. Theorell-Haglow, M. Svensson, T. Gislason, C. Berne, and C. Janson. 2012. Sleep apnea and glucose metabolism: A long-term follow-up in a community-based sample. *Chest*, 142:935–42.
52. O'Driscoll, D.M., A.M. Foster, M.L. Ng, J.S. Yang, F. Bashir, S. Wong, G.M. Nixon, M.J. Davey, V. Anderson, A.M. Walker, J. Trinder, and R.S. Horne. 2009. Central apnoeas have significant effects on blood pressure and heart rate in children. *Journal of Sleep Research*, 18:415–21.
53. Bhattacharjee, R., J. Kim, W.H. Alotaibi, L. Kheirandish-Gozal, O.S. Capdevila, and D. Gozal. 2012. Endothelial dysfunction in children without hypertension: Potential contributions of obesity and obstructive sleep apnea. *Chest*, 141:682–91.
54. Yousefian, J., and M. Brown. 2019. Reduction in orthopedic conditions through teledontic treatment of pharyngorofacial disorders. In *Metabolic Therapies in Orthopedics*, ed. Kohlstadt I., and K. Cintron. Boca Raton: CRC Press/Taylor & Francis.
55. Yoon, A., S. Zaghi, R. Weitzman, et al. 2017. Toward a functional definition of ankyloglossia: Validating current grading scales for lingual frenulum length and tongue mobility in 1052 subjects. *Sleep Breath*, 21:767–75.
56. Schoenwolf, G., S. Bley, P.R. Brauer, and P.H. Francis-West. 2015. *Larsen's Human Embryology*. 5th ed. Philadelphia, PA: Elsevier.
57. Srinivasan B., and A.B. Chitharanjan. 2013. Skeletal and dental characteristics in subjects with ankyloglossia. *Progress in Orthodontics*, 14(1):1–7.
58. Meenakshi S., and N. Jagannathan. 2014. Assessment of lingual frenulum lengths in skeletal malocclusion. *Journal of Clinical and Diagnostic Research: JCDR*, 8(3):202.

59. Guilleminault, C. 2013. Pediatric obstructive sleep apnea and the critical role of oral-facial growth: Evidences. *Frontiers in Neurology*, 3:184.

60. Martins, D.L.L., L.F.S.C. Lima, V.S. de Farias Sales, V.F. Demeda, Â.R.S. de Oliveira, F.M. de Oliveira, and S.B.F. Lima. 2014. The mouth breathing syndrome: Prevalence, causes, consequences and treatments. A literature review. *Journal of Surgical and Clinical Research*, 5(1):47–55.

61. Boyd, K.L., and S.H. Sheldon. 2014. Chapter 34—childhood sleep-disorder breathing: A dental perspective. In *Principles and Practice of Pediatric Sleep Medicine*, 273–279. Elsevier Health Sciences.

62. Fitzpatrick, M.F., H. McLean, A.M. Urton, A. Tan, and D. O'Donnell, et al. 2003. Effect of nasal or oral breathing route on upper airway resistance during sleep. *European Respiratory Journal*, 22:827–32.

63. Lee, S.Y., C. Guilleminault, H.Y. Chiu, and S.S. Sullivan. 2015. Mouth breathing, nasal 'dis-use and sleep- disordered-breathing. *Sleep-Breath*. (in press)

64. Mahowald, M.W., and M.J. Thorpy. 1995. Nonarousal parasomnias in the child. In *Principles and Practice of Sleep Medicine in the Child*, ed. R. Ferber, and M. Kryger, 115–23. Philadelphia: W.B. Saunders Company.

65. Montplaisir, J., Godbout, R., Pelletier, G., & Warnes, H. (1994). Restless legs syndrome and periodic limb movements during sleep. In *Principles and Practice of Sleep Medicine*, ed. M.H. Kryger, T. Roth, and W.C. Dement, 589–97. Philadelphia: W.B. Saunders Company.

66. Scofield, H., T. Roth, and C. Drake. 2008. Periodic limb movements during sleep: Population prevalence, clinical correlates, and racial differences. *Sleep*, 31(9):1221–27.

67. Earley, C.J., R.P. Allen, and W. Hening. 2021. Restless legs syndrome and periodic leg movements in sleep. In *Handbook of Clinical Neurology*, ed. Aminoff, M.J., F. Boller, and D.F. Swaab, 913–48. Elsevier B.V.

68. Kotagal, S., and M.H. Silber. 2004. Childhood-onset restless legs syndrome. *Annals of Neurology*, 56:803–7.

69. Delrosso, L., and O. Bruni. 2019. Treatment of pediatric restless legs syndrome. In *Advances in Pharmacology*, ed. Clemens S., and I. Ghorayeb, 84, 237–53. Elsevier B.V.

70. Lowenfeld, L. 1902. Ueber narkolepsie. *Münchener Medizinische Wochenschrift*, 49:1041–45.

71. Dement, W.C., M. Carskadon, and R. Ley. 1973. The prevalence of narcolepsy. II [abstract]. *Sleep Research*, 2:147.

72. Carskadon, M.A., K. Harvey, and W.C. Dement. 1981. Multiple sleep latency tests during the development of narcolepsy. *The Western Journal of Medicine*, 135(5):414–8.

73. Mitler, M.M., J. Van den Hoed, M.A. Carskadon, G. Richardson, R. Park, C. Guilleminault, and W.C. Dement. 1979. REM sleep episodes during the multiple sleep latency test in narcoleptic patients. *Electroencephalography and Clinical Neurophysiology*, 46(4):479–81.

74. Weitzman, E.D., C.A. Czeisler, R.M. Coleman, W.C. Dement, and C. Pollak. 1979. Delayed sleep phase syndrome: A biological rhythm disorder. *Sleep Research*, 8:221.

75. Mindell, J.A., A.M., A. Sadeh, R. Kwon, and D.Y. Goh. 2015. Bedtime routines for young children: A dose-dependent association with sleep outcomes. *Sleep*, 38(5):717–22.

76. Thorpy, M.J., E. Korman, A.J. Spielman, and P.B. Klovinsky. 1988. Delayed sleep phase syndrome in adolescents. *Journal of Adolescent Health*, 9:22.

77. Mindell, J.A., and J. Owens. 2010. *A Clinical Guide to Pediatric Sleep: Diagnosis and Management of Sleep Problems*. New York: Wolters Kluwer/Lippincott Williams & Wilkins.

78. Aronen, E.T., E.J. Paavonen, M. Fjällberg, M. Soininen, and J. Törrönen. 2000. Sleep in psychiatric symptoms in school-age children. *J Am Acad Child Adolesc Psychiatry*, 39(4):502–8.

79. Roth, T. 1995. Recognition of insomnias, their diagnosis and public health importance. *Sleep Research Abstracts*, 24A:361.

80. Roehrs, T., and T. Roth. 1994. Chronic insomnias associated with circadian rhythm disorders. In *Principles and Practice of Sleep Medicine*, ed. Kryger M.H., T. Roth, and W.C. Dement. 2nd ed., 477–81). Philadelphia: W.B. Saunders Company.

81. Gaultney, J. 2010. The prevalence of sleep disorders in college students: Impact on academic performance. *Journal of American College Health*, 59(2):91–7.

82. Luginbuehl, M.L. 2019a. New sleep disorders inventory for students: Revised and the sleep disorders inventory for adults. *Journal of Psychiatry & Mental Disorders*, 4(1):1009–11.

83. Luginbuehl, M.L. 2019b. Launch of the sleep disorders inventory for students-revised and the sleep disorders inventory for adults on a new digital platform. *Curr Trends in Otolaryngol Rhinol*, 2:128. DOI: 10.29011/CTOR-128.000028.

84. Chatterji, M. 2003. *Designing and Using Tools for Educational Assessment*. Boston: Allyn & Bacon/Pearson.

APPENDIX 1

Sleep Disorders Inventory for Students-Revised-Children's Form (SDIS-R-C): For ages 2 through 10 years

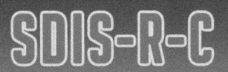

Sleep Disorders Inventory for Students-Revised-Children

Ages 2 through 10

WORKSHEET

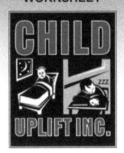

Thank you for agreeing to complete this inventory. It is important that you answer every question to the best of your abilities based on your child's behaviors over the last 3 months. If you are not sure how to mark some questions, observe your child sleep on two different nights for two hours, beginning approximately 1-2 hours after s/he falls asleep, and then again for 60 minutes around 4:00 or 5:00 A.M. If possible, rate your child's behaviors when s/he is not taking medication.

Please rate your child's behaviors based on the following rating scale:

NEVER — Your child never exhibits this behavior before evaluation.

RARELY — Your child exhibits this behavior maybe once every month or two.

OCCASIONALLY — Your child exhibits this behavior 3 to 4 times per month.

SOMETIMES — Your child exhibits this behavior several times per week.

OFTEN — Your child exhibits this behavior on a daily basis before the evaluation.

ALMOST ALWAYS — Your child exhibits this behavior multiple times per day or night.

ALWAYS — Your child exhibits this behavior multiple times per hour daily or nightly.

Behavior Questions

1   Child stops breathing for 5 or more seconds while sleeping
☐ NEVER ☐ RARELY ☐ OCCASIONALLY ☐ SOMETIMES ☐ OFTEN ☐ ALMOST ALWAYS ☐ ALWAYS

2   Breathes through the mouth while awake
☐ NEVER ☐ RARELY ☐ OCCASIONALLY ☐ SOMETIMES ☐ OFTEN ☐ ALMOST ALWAYS ☐ ALWAYS

3   Breathes through the mouth while asleep
☐ NEVER ☐ RARELY ☐ OCCASIONALLY ☐ SOMETIMES ☐ OFTEN ☐ ALMOST ALWAYS ☐ ALWAYS

4   Appears sleepy more often in daytime than other children of the same age
☐ NEVER ☐ RARELY ☐ OCCASIONALLY ☐ SOMETIMES ☐ OFTEN ☐ ALMOST ALWAYS ☐ ALWAYS

5   Makes repeated leg or arm jerking movements during sleep
☐ NEVER ☐ RARELY ☐ OCCASIONALLY ☐ SOMETIMES ☐ OFTEN ☐ ALMOST ALWAYS ☐ ALWAYS

6   Child has raspy breathing or snores lightly at night
☐ NEVER ☐ RARELY ☐ OCCASIONALLY ☐ SOMETIMES ☐ OFTEN ☐ ALMOST ALWAYS ☐ ALWAYS

7   Snores loudly at night
☐ NEVER ☐ RARELY ☐ OCCASIONALLY ☐ SOMETIMES ☐ OFTEN ☐ ALMOST ALWAYS ☐ ALWAYS

8   Shows confusion or disorientation when awakened
☐ NEVER ☐ RARELY ☐ OCCASIONALLY ☐ SOMETIMES ☐ OFTEN ☐ ALMOST ALWAYS ☐ ALWAYS

9   Child rolls or moves around the bed when sleeping
☐ NEVER ☐ RARELY ☐ OCCASIONALLY ☐ SOMETIMES ☐ OFTEN ☐ ALMOST ALWAYS ☐ ALWAYS

10 Gasps, snorts or chokes for breath during sleep
☐ NEVER ☐ RARELY ☐ OCCASIONALLY ☐ SOMETIMES ☐ OFTEN ☐ ALMOST ALWAYS ☐ ALWAYS

11 Sweats a lot while asleep
☐ NEVER ☐ RARELY ☐ OCCASIONALLY ☐ SOMETIMES ☐ OFTEN ☐ ALMOST ALWAYS ☐ ALWAYS

12 Is irritable
☐ NEVER ☐ RARELY ☐ OCCASIONALLY ☐ SOMETIMES ☐ OFTEN ☐ ALMOST ALWAYS ☐ ALWAYS

13 Child is very tired during the morning in school between 8:00 and 12:00 noon, but alert in the afternoon and evening (Check with teachers if unsure)
☐ NEVER ☐ RARELY ☐ OCCASIONALLY ☐ SOMETIMES ☐ OFTEN ☐ ALMOST ALWAYS ☐ ALWAYS

14 Sleeps in strange positions such as cocking the head backwards or sleeping while sitting upright on pillows or kneeling
☐ NEVER ☐ RARELY ☐ OCCASIONALLY ☐ SOMETIMES ☐ OFTEN ☐ ALMOST ALWAYS ☐ ALWAYS

15 Exhibits heavy breathing without exercising
☐ NEVER ☐ RARELY ☐ OCCASIONALLY ☐ SOMETIMES ☐ OFTEN ☐ ALMOST ALWAYS ☐ ALWAYS

16 Wakes up during the night
☐ NEVER ☐ RARELY ☐ OCCASIONALLY ☐ SOMETIMES ☐ OFTEN ☐ ALMOST ALWAYS ☐ ALWAYS

17 Seems tired after getting plenty of sleep
☐ NEVER ☐ RARELY ☐ OCCASIONALLY ☐ SOMETIMES ☐ OFTEN ☐ ALMOST ALWAYS ☐ ALWAYS

18 Takes more than 30 minutes to fall asleep once child is in bed and attemps to sleep
☐ NEVER ☐ RARELY ☐ OCCASIONALLY ☐ SOMETIMES ☐ OFTEN ☐ ALMOST ALWAYS ☐ ALWAYS

19 Child's attempts to change bedtime from a post-midnight to a pre-midnight pattern on school nights are unsuccessful because the student is unable to fall asleep earlier
☐ NEVER ☐ RARELY ☐ OCCASIONALLY ☐ SOMETIMES ☐ OFTEN ☐ ALMOST ALWAYS ☐ ALWAYS

20 Falls asleep more during the daytime than other children of the same age
☐ NEVER ☐ RARELY ☐ OCCASIONALLY ☐ SOMETIMES ☐ OFTEN ☐ ALMOST ALWAYS ☐ ALWAYS

21 Has a high activity level and has difficulty sitting still
☐ NEVER ☐ RARELY ☐ OCCASIONALLY ☐ SOMETIMES ☐ OFTEN ☐ ALMOST ALWAYS ☐ ALWAYS

22 Child is often touchy or loses temper
☐ NEVER ☐ RARELY ☐ OCCASIONALLY ☐ SOMETIMES ☐ OFTEN ☐ ALMOST ALWAYS ☐ ALWAYS

23 Actively defies or refuses to comply with adults' requests
☐ NEVER ☐ RARELY ☐ OCCASIONALLY ☐ SOMETIMES ☐ OFTEN ☐ ALMOST ALWAYS ☐ ALWAYS

24 Has difficulty falling asleep on school nights before
☐ No Dificulty ☐ 10:00 p.m. ☐ 11:00 p.m. ☐ 12:00 midn ☐ 1:30 a.m. ☐ 3:00 a.m. ☐ 4:00 a.m.

25 Has difficulty falling asleep on weekend nights before

☐ No Dificulty ☐ 10:00 p.m. ☐ 11:00 p.m. ☐ 12:00 midn ☐ 1:30 a.m. ☐ 3:00 a.m. ☐ 4:00 a.m.

26 Does child grind teeth while sleeping?

☐ NEVER ☐ RARELY ☐ OCCASIONALLY ☐ SOMETIMES ☐ OFTEN ☐ ALMOST ALWAYS ☐ ALWAYS

27 Does child sleep-walk?

☐ NEVER ☐ RARELY ☐ OCCASIONALLY ☐ SOMETIMES ☐ OFTEN ☐ ALMOST ALWAYS ☐ ALWAYS

28 Does child talk in sleep?

☐ NEVER ☐ RARELY ☐ OCCASIONALLY ☐ SOMETIMES ☐ OFTEN ☐ ALMOST ALWAYS ☐ ALWAYS

29 Does child awake with night terrors (wild-eyed, crying or screaming; unresponsive to parent comforting and cannot remember the night terror the following morning)?

☐ NEVER ☐ RARELY ☐ OCCASIONALLY ☐ SOMETIMES ☐ OFTEN ☐ ALMOST ALWAYS ☐ ALWAYS

30 Does child have bed-wetting episodes?

☐ NEVER ☐ RARELY ☐ OCCASIONALLY ☐ SOMETIMES ☐ OFTEN ☐ ALMOST ALWAYS ☐ ALWAYS

Medical History Questions

1 Did your child's birth occur within the due date range?

☐ Yes ☐ No

If no, check the answer below that is the most accurate

☐ Two weeks past the due date
☐ 3-4 weeks past due date
☐ 3-4 weeks prematurely (too early)
☐ 5-6 weeks prematurely
☐ 2 months prematurely
☐ Birth occurred 3 or more months prematurely

2 Did your child experience any difficulties during delivery?

☐ Yes ☐ No

If yes, check any problem(s) you had

☐ Induced labor delivery
☐ Epidural anesthesia (an anesthesia given to block pain in the lower half of the body)
☐ Extended or prolonged labor beyond 18-20 hours
☐ Caesarian (C-Section) delivery
☐ Delivery with Forceps
☐ Birth assisted with a Vacuum
☐ Manual Rotation (turning baby around in womb)
☐ Umbilical cord wrapped around neck
☐ Placenta Previa (placenta lies low in the uterus and partially or completely covers the cervix)
☐ Breech (baby was born bottom first instead of head first)
☐ Had to be cared for in neonatal intensive care after birth

3 Did your child breathe spontaneously (naturally) at birth?

☐ Yes ☐ No

If no, please check any of the following that happened

☐ Turned blue during/after birth
☐ Did not start breathing immediately after birth and had to be resuscitated (revived)
☐ Needed to be given oxygen after birth

4 Check any answer/s below that best describe your child's milk drinking behaviors during infancy:

☐ Able to latch on and breastfeed immediately after birth and only breastfed
☐ Breast fed with some supplements of a bottle
☐ Only bottle fed
☐ Intolerant of most baby formulas
☐ Only tube-fed the first four-to-six months due to very poor sucking ability
☐ Some tube-feeding due to very poor sucking ability with some supplements from a bottle

5 Has your child ever had any oral sucking habits mentioned below?

☐ Yes ☐ No

If yes, please check the ones you had

☐ Thumb or finger sucking
☐ Lip sucking
☐ Blanket sucking
☐ Pacifier
☐ Toy sucking

6 Please check any of the descriptions of this child's muscle tone that may apply:

☐ Normal muscle tone
☐ Was delayed as an infant or toddler in gross motor skills such as sitting up, crawling or walking
☐ Has floppy or limp muscle tone now

☐ Has stiffness of the muscles and limbs now, or there is resistance when the arms or legs are being stretched out during rest
☐ Gets tired more easily now than same-aged peers when doing physical activities
☐ Needs a walker or is wheelchair bound

7   Check the image below that is closest to your child's face profile:

☐   ☐   ☐

8   Choose the image below that best represents your child's body posture

☐   ☐   ☐

9   Does your child have any daytime breathing problems?

☐ Yes   ☐ No

If yes, please check any of these problems that you exhibit

☐ Open-mouth breathing
☐ Blocked or stuffy nose often
☐ Noisy breathing
☐ Small, narrow, or asymmetric (uneven) nostrils (nose openings)
☐ Breathing with the chest instead of the belly

10 Click the image below that best represents the size and shape of the youth's nostrils:

☐   ☐   ☐   ☐   ☐   ☐   ☐

11 Has your child had any of the following speech problems?

☐ Yes   ☐ No

If yes, please check any issues

☐ Tongue- or lip-tied
☐ Stuttering
☐ Lisping
☐ Difficulty forming words or speaking
☐ Delayed speech

12 Did your child ever have difficulty swallowing or does your child now have difficulty swallowing?

☐ Yes   ☐ No

If yes, please check any issues

☐ Liquids
☐ Soft foods
☐ Solid foods
☐ Pills / Vitamins

13 Check if your child has any of the dental problems below:

☐ Yes   ☐ No

If yes, please check any issues

☐ Over-bite (the upper teeth overlap the bottom teeth excessively)
☐ Under-bite (the lower teeth project beyond the upper teeth)
☐ Cross-bite (One or more teeth may be tilted toward the cheek or toward the tongue when compared to the tooth above or below it)
☐ Too much space between some teeth
☐ Narrow jaw
☐ Large or protruding tongue
☐ NO Problems Noticed

14 Has your child ever had vision problems?

☐ Yes   ☐ No

15 Has your child ever had hearing problems?

☐ Yes   ☐ No

16 Was your child underweight as an infant or preschool-aged child?

☐ Yes ☐ No

17 Is your child overweight now?

☐ Yes ☐ No

18 Does your child have multiple ear infections per year?

☐ Yes ☐ No

19 Does your child have multiple respiratory infections per year?

☐ Yes ☐ No

20 Has a physician ever reported that your child has large tonsils?

☐ Yes ☐ No

21 Has your child's tonsils been removed?

☐ Yes ☐ No

22 Has a physician ever reported that your child has enlarged adenoids?

☐ Yes ☐ No

23 Has your child's adenoids been removed?

☐ Yes ☐ No

24 If your child is between kindergarten and 8th grade, please check the academic grades that your child typically receives:

☐ Child is younger than kindergarten age and does not receive formal grades
☐ Child is home-schooled and does not receive formal grades
☐ Mostly A's and B's or grades of "Excellent" or "Superior"
☐ Mostly C's or grades of "Average" or "Satisfactory"
☐ Mostly D's or grades of "Below Average" or "Needs Improvement"
☐ Mostly F's or grades of "Unsatisfactory"

APPENDIX 2

Sleep Disorders Inventory for Students-Revised: Adolescent Form (SDIS-R-A): For ages 11 through 18 years

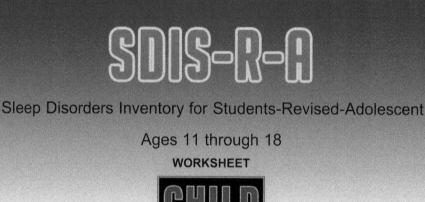

Sleep Disorders Inventory for Students-Revised-Adolescent

Ages 11 through 18

WORKSHEET

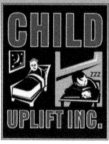

Thank you for agreeing to complete this inventory. It is important that you answer every question to the best of your abilities based on your adolescent's behaviors over the last 3 months. If you are not sure how to mark some questions, observe your adolescent sleep on two different nights for two hours, beginning approximately 1-2 hours after s/he falls asleep, and then again for 60 minutes around 4:00 or 5:00 A.M. If possible, rate your adolescent's behaviors when s/he is not taking medication.

Please rate your teen's behaviors based on the following rating scale:

NEVER	Your student never exhibits this behavior before evaluation.
RARELY	Your student exhibits this behavior maybe once every month or two.
OCCASIONALLY	Your student exhibits the behavior 3 to 4 times per month.
SOMETIMES	Your student exhibits the behavior several times per week.
OFTEN	Your studetn exhibits this behavior on a daily basis before the evaluation.
ALMOST ALWAYS	Your student exhibits this behavior multiple times per day or night.
ALWAYS	Your student exhibits this behavior multiple times per hour daily or nightly.

Behavior Questions

1 Student stops breathing for 5 or more seconds while sleeping
  ☐ NEVER ☐ RARELY ☐ OCCASIONALLY ☐ SOMETIMES ☐ OFTEN ☐ ALMOST ALWAYS ☐ ALWAYS

2 Breathes through the mouth while awake
  ☐ NEVER ☐ RARELY ☐ OCCASIONALLY ☐ SOMETIMES ☐ OFTEN ☐ ALMOST ALWAYS ☐ ALWAYS

3 Appears sleepy more often in daytime than other students of the same age
  ☐ NEVER ☐ RARELY ☐ OCCASIONALLY ☐ SOMETIMES ☐ OFTEN ☐ ALMOST ALWAYS ☐ ALWAYS

4 When student is awakened on school days by parent or alarm clock, s/he takes longer than 5-10 minutes to arise and begin the daily routine
  ☐ NEVER ☐ RARELY ☐ OCCASIONALLY ☐ SOMETIMES ☐ OFTEN ☐ ALMOST ALWAYS ☐ ALWAYS

5 Is unable to talk or move for seconds to minutes when awakened by parent
  ☐ NEVER ☐ RARELY ☐ OCCASIONALLY ☐ SOMETIMES ☐ OFTEN ☐ ALMOST ALWAYS ☐ ALWAYS

6 Makes repeated leg or arm jerking movements during sleep
  ☐ NEVER ☐ RARELY ☐ OCCASIONALLY ☐ SOMETIMES ☐ OFTEN ☐ ALMOST ALWAYS ☐ ALWAYS

7 Student has raspy breathing or snores lightly at night
  ☐ NEVER ☐ RARELY ☐ OCCASIONALLY ☐ SOMETIMES ☐ OFTEN ☐ ALMOST ALWAYS ☐ ALWAYS

8 Snores loudly at night
  ☐ NEVER ☐ RARELY ☐ OCCASIONALLY ☐ SOMETIMES ☐ OFTEN ☐ ALMOST ALWAYS ☐ ALWAYS

9 Shows confusion or disorientation when awakened
  ☐ NEVER ☐ RARELY ☐ OCCASIONALLY ☐ SOMETIMES ☐ OFTEN ☐ ALMOST ALWAYS ☐ ALWAYS

10 Stays up past 1:00 a.m. on school nights (playing video/computer games, watching T.V., talking on the phone or partying with friends)
  ☐ NEVER ☐ RARELY ☐ OCCASIONALLY ☐ SOMETIMES ☐ OFTEN ☐ ALMOST ALWAYS ☐ ALWAYS

11 Gasps, snorts or chokes for breath during sleep
  ☐ NEVER ☐ RARELY ☐ OCCASIONALLY ☐ SOMETIMES ☐ OFTEN ☐ ALMOST ALWAYS ☐ ALWAYS

12 Is irritable
  ☐ NEVER ☐ RARELY ☐ OCCASIONALLY ☐ SOMETIMES ☐ OFTEN ☐ ALMOST ALWAYS ☐ ALWAYS

13 Student reports an urge to move legs or an uncomfortable crawling feeling in legs or arms when resting or laying down to sleep
  ☐ NEVER ☐ RARELY ☐ OCCASIONALLY ☐ SOMETIMES ☐ OFTEN ☐ ALMOST ALWAYS ☐ ALWAYS

14 Student is very tired during the morning in school between 8:00 and 12:00 noon, but alert in the afternoon and evening (Check with teachers if unsure)
  ☐ NEVER ☐ RARELY ☐ OCCASIONALLY ☐ SOMETIMES ☐ OFTEN ☐ ALMOST ALWAYS ☐ ALWAYS

15 Sleeps in strange positions such as cocking the head backwards or sleeping while sitting upright on pillows or kneeling
  ☐ NEVER ☐ RARELY ☐ OCCASIONALLY ☐ SOMETIMES ☐ OFTEN ☐ ALMOST ALWAYS ☐ ALWAYS

16 Has attacks of extreme muscular weakness or loss of muscle function (such as limpness in the neck, knees or limbs, inability to speak clearly and/or falling down) that occurs only when laughing, surprised, fearful or angry
  ☐ NEVER ☐ RARELY ☐ OCCASIONALLY ☐ SOMETIMES ☐ OFTEN ☐ ALMOST ALWAYS ☐ ALWAYS

17 Wakes up during the night
  ☐ NEVER ☐ RARELY ☐ OCCASIONALLY ☐ SOMETIMES ☐ OFTEN ☐ ALMOST ALWAYS ☐ ALWAYS

18 Seems tired after getting plenty of sleep
  ☐ NEVER ☐ RARELY ☐ OCCASIONALLY ☐ SOMETIMES ☐ OFTEN ☐ ALMOST ALWAYS ☐ ALWAYS

19 Student has complained of vivid, often frightening dreams or hallucinations when drifting into sleep or awakening
  ☐ NEVER ☐ RARELY ☐ OCCASIONALLY ☐ SOMETIMES ☐ OFTEN ☐ ALMOST ALWAYS ☐ ALWAYS

20 Skips or is late for early classes due to difficulty waking up (check report card for attendance if unsure).
  ☐ NEVER ☐ RARELY ☐ OCCASIONALLY ☐ SOMETIMES ☐ OFTEN ☐ ALMOST ALWAYS ☐ ALWAYS

21 Takes more than 30 minutes to fall asleep once child is in bed and attempts to sleep
  ☐ NEVER ☐ RARELY ☐ OCCASIONALLY ☐ SOMETIMES ☐ OFTEN ☐ ALMOST ALWAYS ☐ ALWAYS

22 Falls asleep while talking to others or while standing up
  ☐ NEVER ☐ RARELY ☐ OCCASIONALLY ☐ SOMETIMES ☐ OFTEN ☐ ALMOST ALWAYS ☐ ALWAYS

23 Student's attempts to change bedtime from a post-midnight to a pre-midnight pattern on school nights are unsuccessful because the student is unable to fall asleep earlier
  ☐ NEVER ☐ RARELY ☐ OCCASIONALLY ☐ SOMETIMES ☐ OFTEN ☐ ALMOST ALWAYS ☐ ALWAYS

24 Performs some strange automatic behaviors (i.e., like putting a jacket in the refrigerator), and does not remember doing them
  ☐ NEVER ☐ RARELY ☐ OCCASIONALLY ☐ SOMETIMES ☐ OFTEN ☐ ALMOST ALWAYS ☐ ALWAYS

25   Falls asleep more during the daytime than other students of the same age

☐ NEVER   ☐ RARELY   ☐ OCCASIONALLY   ☐ SOMETIMES   ☐ OFTEN   ☐ ALMOST ALWAYS   ☐ ALWAYS

26   Student is often touchy or loses temper

☐ NEVER   ☐ RARELY   ☐ OCCASIONALLY   ☐ SOMETIMES   ☐ OFTEN   ☐ ALMOST ALWAYS   ☐ ALWAYS

27   Actively defies or refuses to comply with adults' requests

☐ NEVER   ☐ RARELY   ☐ OCCASIONALLY   ☐ SOMETIMES   ☐ OFTEN   ☐ ALMOST ALWAYS   ☐ ALWAYS

28   Has difficulty falling asleep on school nights before

☐ No Difficulty   ☐ 10:00 p.m.   ☐ 11:00 p.m.   ☐ 12:00 midn   ☐ 1:30 a.m.   ☐ 3:00 a.m.   ☐ 4:00 a.m.

29   Has difficulty falling asleep on weekend nights before

☐ No Difficulty   ☐ 10:00 p.m.   ☐ 11:00 p.m.   ☐ 12:00 midn   ☐ 1:30 a.m.   ☐ 3:00 a.m.   ☐ 4:00 a.m.

30   Check the average amount of time your child takes daytime naps:

☐ No Naps   ☐ Naps 2-3 times/wk.   ☐ 30 min./day   ☐ 1 hr/day   ☐ 1 1/2 hrs/day   ☐ 2 hrs/day   ☐ 3+ hrs/day

31   Does adolescent grind teeth while sleeping?

☐ NEVER   ☐ RARELY   ☐ OCCASIONALLY   ☐ SOMETIMES   ☐ OFTEN   ☐ ALMOST ALWAYS   ☐ ALWAYS

32   Does adolescent sleep-walk?

☐ NEVER   ☐ RARELY   ☐ OCCASIONALLY   ☐ SOMETIMES   ☐ OFTEN   ☐ ALMOST ALWAYS   ☐ ALWAYS

33   Does adolescent talk in sleep?

☐ NEVER   ☐ RARELY   ☐ OCCASIONALLY   ☐ SOMETIMES   ☐ OFTEN   ☐ ALMOST ALWAYS   ☐ ALWAYS

34   Does adolescent awake with night terrors (wild-eyed, crying or screaming; unresponsive to parent comforting and cannot remember the night terror the following morning)?

☐ NEVER   ☐ RARELY   ☐ OCCASIONALLY   ☐ SOMETIMES   ☐ OFTEN   ☐ ALMOST ALWAYS   ☐ ALWAYS

35   Does adolescent have bed-wetting episodes?

☐ NEVER   ☐ RARELY   ☐ OCCASIONALLY   ☐ SOMETIMES   ☐ OFTEN   ☐ ALMOST ALWAYS   ☐ ALWAYS

Medical History Questions

1   Did this youth's birth occur within the due date range?

☐ Yes   ☐ No   ☐ Don't Know (DK)

If no, check the answer below that is the most accurate

☐ Two weeks past the due date
☐ 3-4 weeks past due date
☐ 3-4 weeks prematurely (too early)
☐ 5-6 weeks prematurely
☐ 2 months prematurely
☐ Birth occurred 3 or more months prematurely

2   Did he or she experience any difficulties during delivery?

☐ Yes   ☐ No   ☐ Don't Know (DK)

If yes, check any problem(s) you had

☐ Induced labor delivery
☐ Epidural anesthesia (an anesthesia given to block pain in the lower half of the body)
☐ Extended or prolonged labor beyond 18-20 hours
☐ Caesarian (C-Section) delivery
☐ Delivery with Forceps
☐ Birth assisted with a Vacuum
☐ Manual Rotation (turning baby around in womb)
☐ Umbilical cord wrapped around neck
☐ Placenta Previa (placenta lies low in the uterus and partially or completely covers the cervix)
☐ Breech (baby was born bottom first instead of head first)
☐ Had to be cared for in neonatal intensive care after birth

3   Did he or she breathe spontaneously (naturally) at birth?

☐ Yes   ☐ No   ☐ Don't Know (DK)

If no, please check any of the following that happened

☐ Turned blue during/after birth
☐ Did not start breathing immediately after birth and had to be resuscitated (revived)
☐ Needed to be given oxygen after birth

4   Check any answer/s below that best describe your adolescent's milk drinking behaviors during infancy:

☐ Don't know
☐ Able to latch on and breastfeed immediately after birth and only breastfed
☐ Breast fed with some supplements of a bottle
☐ Only bottle fed

☐ Intolerant of most baby formulas
☐ Only tube-fed the first four-to-six months due to very poor sucking ability
☐ Some tube-feeding due to very poor sucking ability with some supplements from a bottle

5   Has he or she ever had any oral sucking habits mentioned below?

☐ Yes   ☐ No   ☐ Don't Know (DK)

If yes, please check the ones you had

☐ Thumb or finger sucking
☐ Lip sucking
☐ Blanket sucking
☐ Pacifier
☐ Toy sucking

6   Please check any of the descriptions of this person's muscle tone that may apply:

☐ Normal muscle tone
☐ Was delayed as an infant or toddler in gross motor skills such as sitting up, crawling or walking
☐ Has floppy or limp muscle tone now
☐ Has stiffness of the muscles and limbs now, or there is resistance when the arms or legs are being stretched out during rest
☐ Gets tired more easily now than same-aged peers when doing physical activities
☐ Needs a walker or is wheelchair bound

7   Click onto the image below that is closest to this youth's face profile:

☐   ☐   ☐

8   Click onto the image below that best represents the youth's posture:

☐   ☐   ☐

9   Does he or she have any daytime breathing problems now?

☐ Yes   ☐ No

If yes, please check any of these problems that you exhibit

☐ Open-mouth breathing
☐ Blocked or stuffy nose often
☐ Noisy breathing
☐ Small, narrow, or asymmetric (uneven) nostrils (nose openings)
☐ Breathing with the chest instead of the belly

10 Click the image below that best represents the size and shape of the youth's nostrils:

☐   ☐   ☐   ☐   ☐   ☐   ☐

11 Has he or she had any of the following speech problems?

☐ Yes   ☐ No   ☐ Don't Know (DK)

If yes, please check any issues

☐ Tongue- or lip-tied
☐ Stuttering
☐ Lisping
☐ Difficulty forming words or speaking
☐ Delayed speech

12 Did your student ever have difficulty swallowing or does your student now have difficulty swallowing?

☐ Yes   ☐ No

If yes, please check any issues

☐ Liquids
☐ Soft foods
☐ Solid foods
☐ Pills / Vitamins

13 Check any of the dental problems below:

☐ Over-bite (the upper teeth overlap the bottom teeth excessively)
☐ Under-bite (the lower teeth project beyond the upper teeth)
☐ Cross-bite (One or more teeth may be tilted toward the cheek or toward the tongue when compared to the tooth above or below it)
☐ Too much space between some teeth
☐ Narrow jaw
☐ Large or protruding tongue
☐ NO Problems Noticed

14 Has this youth ever had vision problems?

☐ Yes   ☐ No   ☐ Don't Know (DK)

15 Has this youth ever had hearing problems?

☐ Yes   ☐ No   ☐ Don't Know (DK)

16 Was he or she underweight as an infant or child?

☐ Yes   ☐ No   ☐ Don't Know (DK)

   If yes, please select one

      ☐ Mildly Underweight   ☐ Moderately   ☐ Severely

17 Is this youth overweight now?

☐ Yes   ☐ No

   If yes, please select one

      ☐ Mildly Overweight   ☐ Moderately   ☐ Severely

18 Does he or she have multiple ear infections each year?

☐ Yes   ☐ No

19 Does he or she have multiple respiratory infections each year?

☐ Yes   ☐ No

20 Has a physician ever reported that this youth has large tonsils?

☐ Yes   ☐ No   ☐ Don't Know (DK)

21 Has his/her tonsils ever been removed?

☐ Yes   ☐ No   ☐ Don't Know (DK)

22 Has a physician ever reported that this youth has enlarged adenoids?

☐ Yes   ☐ No   ☐ Don't Know (DK)

23 Has his/her adenoids ever been removed?

☐ Yes   ☐ No   ☐ Don't Know (DK)

24 Please check the academic grades that this student typically receives:

☐ Student is home-schooled and does not receive formal grades
☐ Student mostly receives A's and B's or grades of 'Excellent' or 'Superior'
☐ Mostly receives C's or grades of 'Average' or 'Satisfactory'
☐ Mostly receives D's or grades of 'Below Average' or 'Needs Improvement'
☐ Mostly receives F's or grades of 'Unsatisfactory'

20 Circadian and Mitochondrial Effects of Light

Joshua Rosenthal

CONTENTS

20.1 INTRODUCTION

Circadian biology will eventually become woven into the threads of all modalities of healing. It has yet to be appreciated to the extent that is needed to merge with current management for all forms of therapeutics. Circadian rhythms are present in all organisms and intimately connected to health and disease (Abbott & Zee, 2019). From gastrointestinal health, the microbiome, metabolism and cardiovascular health to immunity, circadian rhythms are found to be connected to normal physiologic function and disease states (Katya Frazier, 2017; Panda, 2016; Portaluppi et al., 2012; Voigt et al., 2019; Waggoner, 2020). Expansion of the circadian connections to physiology and pathophysiology are made almost every day. A greater understanding of the circadian mechanism and how its disturbance is created will allow more comprehensive treatments in all specialties. Besides considerations of therapy to adjust the rhythm back to normal, even drug and treatment administration have an optimal time (Sulli et al., 2017). Treatment of the actual circadian rhythm is now being considered as the therapeutic target (Ruan et al., 2021). Given its deep connection to health and disease, a holistic approach to healing must incorporate circadian approaches in the treatment plan.

20.2 CIRCADIAN BIOLOGY

Sleep and circadian rhythms are linked as they apply to health. Hormones, classically defined as chemicals that are secreted into the bloodstream to act on distant tissues, often in a regulatory function, are seemingly well understood in the field of medicine. They are measured as sufficient or deficient and corrected biochemically to achieve the clinical improvements that come with balance. Hormone regulation connects to cell and organ optimal functioning and requires proper sleep

DOI: 10.1201/b23304-22

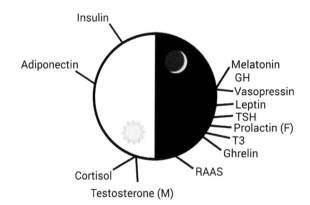

FIGURE 20.1   Time of day at which circulating levels of key endocrine factors peak in humans. GH, growth hormone; TSH, thyroid stimulating hormone; T3, triiodothyronine; RAAS, renin–angiotensin–aldosterone system; (F), females only; (M), males only. (Adapted from Gamble, K.L. et al., *Nat. Rev. Endocrinol.*, 10, 466–475, 2015.)

(Morris et al., 2012). Best studied are the fluctuating levels of biochemicals produced by the hypothalamic–pituitary axis, such as cortisol, growth hormone (GH), prolactin (PRL), thyroid hormone via thyroid stimulating hormone (TSH), and the sex hormones (Brambilla et al., 2009; Nokin et al., 1972; Sun et al., 2020; Weitzman, 1975) (Figure 20.1).

Other hormones and endocrine factors, such as insulin and adiponectin, have diurnal variation under light-dark control mechanisms (Scheer et al., 2010; Whichelow et al., 1974). Beside endocrine control of digestion, the vast expression of genes and secreted molecules involved in all aspects of metabolism appears to be under circadian gene control (Panda, 2016) (Figure 20.2).

There is almost always an interplay of hormones and related signaling molecules with the clock mechanism.

Sleep is the most obvious vital sign of circadian biology. In fact, the author believes it should be measured and trended as all the other vital signs are in medicine. When sleep is optimal, regeneration and systemic hormonal balance are achieved. When sleep is dysfunctional, small disparities can slowly accumulate and eventually result in disease. Any disruptions in sleep, such as reduction of sleep time, night shift work or inappropriate nighttime exposure to light, has been associated with obesity and diabetes (Sridhar & Sanjana, 2016). There is no better explanation of sleep's integral role in all human physiology than its direct connections to longevity and mortality. This association has been shown in a large meta-analysis where long and short sleep duration was associated with all-cause mortality (Cappuccio et al., 2011; Gallicchio & Kalesan, 2009). It remains when comparing the sleep duration of diabetics and non-diabetics, with the comorbidity increasing the effect of short and long sleep (Wang et al., 2020) (Figure 20.3).

Short sleep duration, usually defined as less than or equal to 5–6 hours per night, is associated with obesity, reduced leptin, increased ghrelin, diabetes, hypertension, atrial fibrillation and cancer (Ayas et al., 2003; Cappuccio et al., 2007; Genuardi et al., 2019; Kakizaki et al., 2008; Mallon et al., 2005; Taheri et al., 2004). Long sleep duration, generally defined as more than 8 hours per night, has also been associated with similar poor outcomes (Ayas et al., 2003; Buxton & Marcelli, 2010; Ma et al., 2016). Research has been devoted to identify biomarkers associated with these two conditions to better define the pathophysiology of this connection (Williams et al., 2007). The author believes that short sleep duration can be pathophysiologic in those without any other reason to have disease and that long sleep duration defines those with preexisting circadian disruption and poor-quality sleep, creating the drive for more sleep. In this way, short sleepers create the hormonal and gene expression abnormalities because of inadequate sleep time for their production, while long sleepers already have a broken system for which they are trying to compensate.

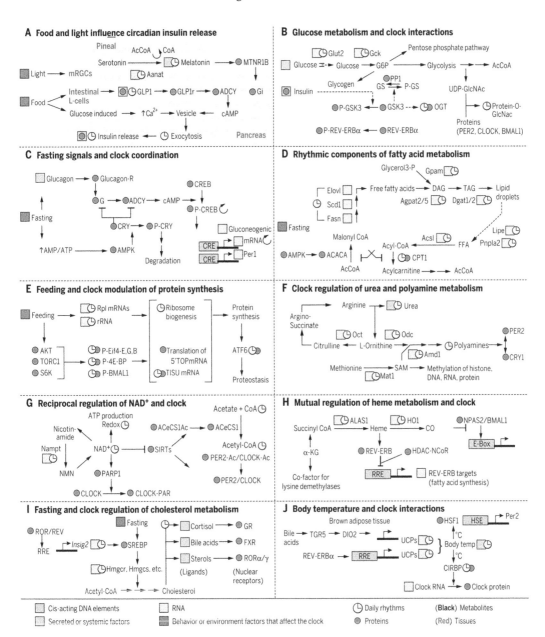

FIGURE 20.2 Examples of circadian regulation of metabolic pathways and metabolic pathways affecting clock components. Cis-acting DNA elements are in green, RNA in blue, proteins in orange; metabolites are shown in black letters, and tissues are underlined. Any RNA, protein or metabolite (other than clock components) known to show daily rhythms is marked with ☾. Secreted or systemic factors are highlighted in yellow, and behavior or environment factors that can affect the clock are highlighted in gray. (A) Light and food intake can interact through multiple tissues to modulate insulin release from pancreatic islet cells. (B) Feeding-induced glucose metabolism in the liver affects clock components. (C) During fasting, activation of glucagon receptor and AMPK impinges on clock components. (D) Fatty acid synthesis and degradation are under feeding-fasting and circadian regulation. (E) Circadian clock and feeding signals act together to produce a daily rhythm in protein synthesis. (F) Circadian regulation of urea cycle, SAM synthesis and polyamine production. Polyamines affect interaction between PER2 and CRY1. (G) Reciprocal regulation between circadian clock and NAD production. (H) Circadian production of heme and CO affects the function of core circadian clock components. (I) Fasting and circadian clock regulate cholesterol metabolism and production of several ligands for nuclear hormone receptors. (J) Reciprocal regulation between circadian clock and body-temperature rhythm. (From Panda, S., *Physiol. Behav.*, 176, 139–148, 2016.)

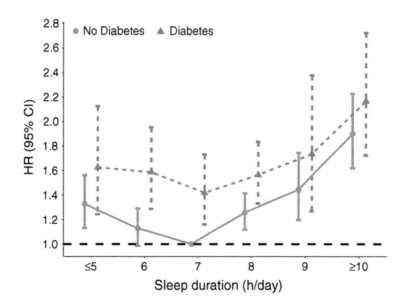

FIGURE 20.3 Adjusted mortality risk according to sleep duration stratified by type 2 diabetes. (From Wang, Y. et al., *Diabetologia*, 63, 2292–2304, 2020.)

Furthermore, the connection of sleep and the immune system may drive an understanding of the root cause of all inflammation. These have a bidirectional connection, whereby poor sleep weakens the immune system, and significant immune system activation worsens sleep (Besedovsky et al., 2019). Circadian rhythms control hormones, which of course, also interconnect back to the immune system. Sex hormones even have demonstrated photic feedback to the suprachiasmatic nucleus (SCN), which explains some sex differences seen in sleep and circadian rhythms (Mong et al., 2011). This further illustrates the bidirectional coupled nature of hormones and sleep-wake cycles. The linkage even connects further down to the gears of immunity, implicating etiologies for autoimmunity as well. Interleukin (IL)-17-producing T helper (Th17) cells are key immune cells that help clear pathogens and are associated with inflammatory diseases, but are also involved in autoimmune diseases such as multiple sclerosis, psoriasis, rheumatoid arthritis, inflammatory bowel disease, systemic lupus erythematosus and asthma (Bedoya et al., 2013). The cytokine production of these cells is pathogenic, and they remain future targets of treatments for autoimmune diseases (Yamagata et al., 2015). Th17 cell development varies diurnally and is linked to the circadian mechanism via the nuclear receptor Rev-erb α (Yu et al., 2013). Also, CD4+ T cells themselves contain circadian oscillators that drive their immune function via gene expression (Bollinger et al., 2011). All these links may explain the circadian symptomatology of many immunologic diseases and possible behavioral therapies aimed at restoring proper clock rhythms and sleep. Regardless, it is evident that sleep and the coupled circadian gene expressions are required for optimal health. By design, it seems that no physiologic system is immune to control by light-dark cycles and sleep in some fashion. When considering the clock regulation of hormones, the predominant hormone system coupled to light and dark is melatonin and cortisol.

20.3 MELATONIN

Melatonin, an *N*-[2-(5-methoxy-1*H*-indol-3-yl)ethyl]acetamide, was first discovered by dermatologist Aaron Lerner and colleagues in 1958 as a pineal gland factor that could lighten skin color and inhibited melanocyte stimulating hormone (MSH) (Lerner et al., 1958). While not successful as a treatment for diseases of pigmentation, melatonin was found to affect the brain and neuroendocrine system (Reiter et al., 1978). After further research on this chemical, it became evident that it was in fact connected to the neuroendocrine system but regulated by light-dark cycles (Wurtman, 1985). Melatonin secretion is also the chemical transduction of the photoperiod, globalized by the SCN in a circadian and circannual fashion (Reiter, 1991; Wehr, 1991). The action spectrum of melatonin in different monochromatic light shows a unique short wavelength–specific suppression, worse with increasing irradiance, which is highest in blue frequencies and decreasing in the green frequencies, a result that is not consistent with the action spectra of scotopic and photopic visual systems (Thapan et al., 2001) Figure 20.4.

The pineal gland's melatonin release is highly sensitive to low lighting intensities and driven by the non-visual photopigment of intrinsically photosensitive retinal ganglion cells (ipRGCs) via melanopsin (Prayag et al., 2019). However, melatonin in not just produced in the pineal gland; its production has been verified in the brain, retina, cochlea, airway epithelium, skin, gastrointestinal tract, liver, kidney, thyroid, pancreas, thymus, spleen, immune system cells and reproductive tract as well as in almost all biologic fluids (Acuña-Castroviejo et al., 2014). There is a subcellular

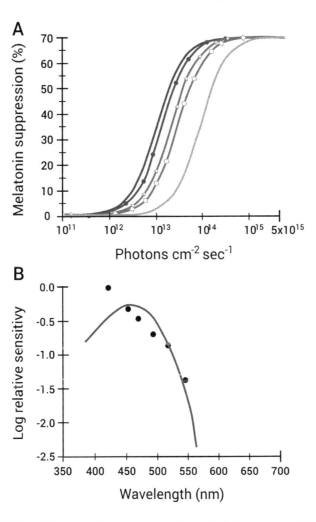

FIGURE 20.4 Sensitivity of plasma melatonin to monochromatic light exposure. (A) Percentage melatonin suppression at irradiance response curves for 424 (dark line), 472 (triangles), 496 (triangles), 520 (diamonds) and 548 nm (pale line). (B) Action spectrum for melatonin corrected for lens filtering (•), which best fits a rhodopsin template with λ_{max} 459 nm ($r^2 = 0.74$). (Adapted from Thapan, K. et al., *J. Physiol.*, *535*, 261–267, 2001.)

Metabolic Regulation

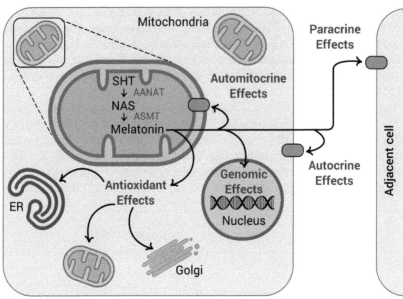

FIGURE 20.5 The mitochondria produce melatonin. Unlike pinealocytes, which release melatonin into the cerebrospinal fluid and blood, non-pinealocyte cells make local mitochondria-synthesized melatonin for metabolic regulation, which is not released into the systemic circulation. Surgical pinealectomy significantly reduces concentrations of melatonin in the blood but has no impact on the much greater concentrations of melatonin in mitochondria. Melatonin, in addition to its functions inside this organelle, diffuses out of the mitochondria, where it feeds back onto melatonin receptors with automitocrine effects in the mitochondrial membrane as well as impacting the nuclear genome. Melatonin also likely has autocrine and paracrine effects after diffusing into the intracellular space. AANAT, arylalkylamine *N*-acetyltransferase; ASMT, acetylserotonin methyltransferase. (Adapted from Reiter, R. et al., *J. Pineal Res.*, 0–1, 2020.)

production of melatonin, as is clearly shown by localization of the required enzymatic machinery in the mitochondria (Kerényi et al., 1975; Tan et al., 2016) (Figure 20.5).

In this way, melatonin is universally used as a direct connection to the environment to create the appropriate physiologic response inside every cell, including its many other beneficial biochemical and biophysical properties.

While melatonin is well understood as a hormone of darkness, its connection to circadian biology should implicate connection with its production and daytime processes. In fact, morning tryptophan intake with sunlight has been shown to increase nighttime melatonin secretion (Fukushige et al., 2014). Breakfast intake of the serotonin precursors tryptophan and vitamin B6 with morning sunlight has also been shown to improve morning chronotype when compared with intake without sunlight (Nakade et al., 2012). In this way, melatonin production is coupled to both day and nighttime signals, with its precursor building blocks being further activated during daytime and its nighttime secretion and globalization coupled to lack of appropriate light frequencies during nighttime.

Melatonin's effects extend beyond its direct circadian control. Research has shown melatonin to reduce acute and chronic inflammation with multiple targets of inactivating the inflammasome (Tarocco et al., 2019) (Figure 20.6).

Wellness is nothing more than decreasing the damage of daily living, also known as inflammation. One of the more important aspects of melatonin on health is its antioxidant properties. Melatonin can function as a direct free radical scavenger, stimulate synthesis of glutathione, promote antioxidative enzymes, augment other antioxidants and optimize mitochondrial electron

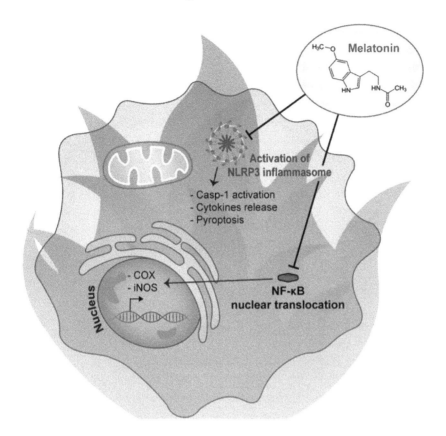

FIGURE 20.6 Anti-inflammatory effects of melatonin. Melatonin is mainly reported to possess anti-inflammatory properties by inhibiting inflammasome activation, thus inhibiting caspase-1 activation, release of cytokines, and pyroptosis. In addition, melatonin can also inhibit the expression of the cyclooxygenase (COX) and inducible nitric oxide synthase (iNOS) by inhibiting nuclear NF-κB translocation. (From Tarocco, A. et al., *Cell Death Dis., 10,* 2019.)

chain transport, further lowering free radical production (Reiter et al., 2003). Its free radical scavenging ability has been shown to be more powerful than that of vitamin E, a comparison made because of its effective lipid-soluble antioxidant properties (Pieri et al., 1994). Melatonin is highly permeable to cell membranes and can cross the blood–brain barrier as well as affecting autophagy and modulating apoptosis via the mitochondrial permeability transition pore (Tarocco et al., 2019). This role in regeneration should be emphasized when trying to improve or reverse any disease state (Figure 20.7).

A less appreciated consequence of melatonin is its induction of mitophagy, allowing improved bioenergetics, which are required for proper cellular functioning. Understanding the importance of circadian rhythms and mitochondrial bioenergetics can be seen in many ways. Mothers with preeclampsia have abnormal melatonin levels and abnormal circadian variation of blood pressure as well as adverse outcomes (Bouchlariotou et al., 2014). It has been shown that the appropriate circadian rhythm and melatonin levels stabilize the physiology of mother and fetus (Reiter et al., 2014). In these ways, melatonin controls circadian rhythms, regulates local/regional inflammation and induces mitochondrial repair to improve cellular bioenergetics, making it one of the most important chemicals for generating optimal health. The correlation of all artificial lighting source frequencies to this action spectrum should raise concern after understanding how intimately health is connected to this physiology.

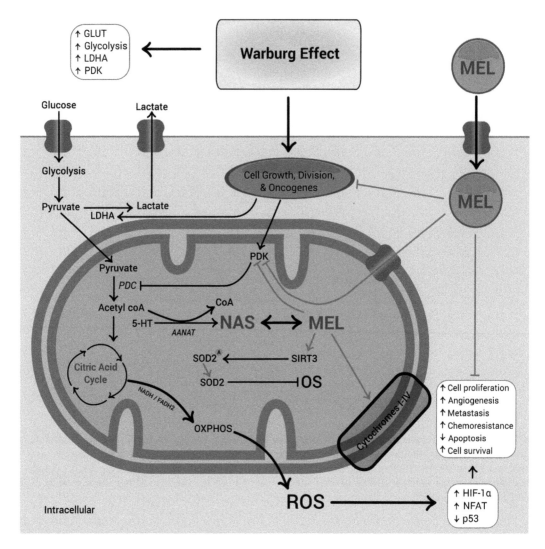

FIGURE 20.7 Summary of the interactions of melatonin with mitochondrial physiology in normal and cancerous cells. In normal cells, glucose enters the cytosol via the glucose transporter (GLUT), where it is metabolized to pyruvate, which is mostly translocated into the mitochondria, where under the action of pyruvate dehydrogenase complex (PDC), it is metabolized to acetyl-CoA. Acetyl-CoA enters the citric acid cycle, which supports oxidative phosphorylation (OXPHOS) in the inner mitochondrial membrane. Acetyl-CoA is also a required co-factor/substrate for the rate-limiting enzyme in melatonin synthesis, arylalkylamine N-acetyltransferase (AANAT), which converts serotonin (5-HT) to the melatonin precursor, N-acetylserotonin (NAS), which is transformed into melatonin. Melatonin also can be reverse-metabolized back to NAS. Melatonin and NAS directly scavenge partially reduced reactive oxygen species (ROS) generated during OXPHOS. Additionally, melatonin stimulates sirtuin 3 (SIRT3), allowing the deacetylation of superoxide dismutase 2 (SOD2), leading to its activation, thereby reducing oxidative stress (OS). Pyruvate, rather than being shunted into the mitochondria normally, can be diverted by solid tumor cells and instead metabolized to lactate with the aid of the enzyme lactate dehydrogenase A (LDHA); lactate is then released in large quantities into the blood. Pyruvate does not enter mitochondria, since PDC is inhibited by the gatekeeper enzyme, pyruvate dehydrogenase kinase (PDK), which is upregulated in cancer cells. These metabolic changes that cancer cells undergo are often referred to as the Warburg effect, which provides tumor cells with advantages in terms of tumor biomass enlargement, invasiveness and metastasis. Additionally, since acetyl-CoA is not produced in cancer cell mitochondria, they may not be capable of producing their own melatonin. Blood-borne melatonin has several pathways to enter the cytosol and mitochondria, where it will presumably inhibit PDK, allowing the activation of PDC; melatonin thus reverses the Warburg effect and aids in halting cancer cell growth. Arrows indicate stimulation; blunt lines indicate inhibition. FADH$_2$, flavin adenine dinucleotide; HIF-1α, hypoxia inducible factor 1α; NFAT, nuclear factor of activated T cells. (Adapted from Reiter, R. et al., *J. Pineal Res.*, 0–1, 2020.)

20.4   CORTISOL

Cortisol is the counter hormone to melatonin, with an important role in circadian physiology as well. Just as melatonin, which peaks at night, can be considered the hormone to create sleep, cortisol has the function of driving the waking-up process with its morning secretion. The cortisol awakening response is a robust increase in free cortisol secretion within the first 30 minutes of waking up, a circadian-controlled representation of the hypothalamic–pituitary–adrenal axis function (Wüst et al., 2000). Too much or too little cortisol in the morning or at the wrong time is associated with poor clinical outcomes. Abnormal diurnal secretion of cortisol is associated with many clinical disorders, including increased pain, cardiovascular disease mortality, type 2 diabetes mellitus, obesity, depression and anxiety (Adam et al., 2011; Adam et al., 2014; Hackett et al., 2014; Kumari et al., 2010, 2011; Mayes et al., 2014). Chronic insomniacs have been found to have higher than normal adrenocorticotropic hormone (ACTH) and cortisol levels at night compared with controls (Basta et al., 2007). It should be noted that cortisol production from the adrenal glands is related to the production of corticotropin releasing factor (CRF) from the paraventricular nucleus (PVN) of the hypothalamus (Raux-Demay & Girard, 1985). The response of PVN cells is increased with light of increasing color temperature and decreased with light sources that have less blue-frequency light (Yokoyama et al., 2019). This connects artificial light, heavy in the blue frequency spectrum, to circadian dysregulation of both melatonin and cortisol. Also, cortisol synthesis occurs with production of pregnenolone from cholesterol and cortisol from 11-deoxycortisol occurring inside the mitochondria (Picard et al., 2018). With this information, it can be seen that adrenal fatigue actually begins with light stress in the eye, starting a physiologic response that is responsible for putting adrenal glands in overdrive, which can eventually lead to complete exhaustion if continued over a long time period.

20.5   CIRCADIAN OSCILLATORS

Timing of biologic processes is the function of circadian biology. The body has multiple rhythms, which are connected to the needs of the various physiologic systems. The term "circadian" originates from the Latin phrase "circa diem," which means "around a day." The field of chronobiology is dedicated to studying the timing and rhythm of biologic activities of living organisms. The rhythms include those shorter than a day but longer than an hour, such as ultradian rhythms, the circadian rhythm of a 24-hour day, and infradian rhythms, which extend for periods longer than a day. There are even circannual rhythms that span an entire year. Clock disorders are generally thought of as they relate to sleep. The American Academy of Sleep Medicine has published practice parameters on the treatment of "exogenous" circadian rhythm sleep disorders, such as shift work disorder and jet lag disorder, and "endogenous" circadian rhythm sleep disorders, such as advanced sleep phase disorder, delayed sleep phase disorder, irregular sleep-wake rhythm, and the non-24-hour sleep-wake syndrome or free-running disorder (Morgenthaler et al., 2007). These include recommendations on the medical evaluation and treatment of these conditions. While very helpful clinically, it should be noted that these recommendations address clock dysfunction on a central scale only. Circadian oscillations can act centrally from the main clock, the SCN in the brain, but also must be coordinated in peripheral clocks in the local cells of targeted tissues and organs themselves (Dibner et al., 2010). In this way, cellular clocks are able to drive rhythms of gene transcription through mRNA both globally and locally to create physiologic change when appropriate for health (Duffield et al., 2002; Panda et al., 2002).

However, for optimal functioning of an organism, the clocks must keep accurate timing centrally and peripherally in a way that is responsive to environmental signals that require appropriate physiologic adaptation. Even a transplanted SCN will maintain its rhythmicity in an organism (Ralph et al., 1990). It has also been shown in experimental models of peripherally attenuatable clocks that systemic central oscillators can maintain local gene expression even when the peripheral controllers are absent (Kornmann et al., 2007). Gene expression must be regulated to meet an organism's local and global needs, which can change in relationship to changes in temperature, photoperiod and seasonal availability of resources (Wehr, 2001; Wood & Loudon, 2014). Likely a vestige from our hibernating ancestors preparing for winter, humans have been shown to have weight changes based upon light timing and intensity (Reid et al., 2014). Many are aware of the recurrent depressive episodes of seasonal affective disorder created by the short photoperiod of winter, which despite this dysrhythmicity, still maintain normal winter-summer dexamethasone suppression testing (Rosenthal et al., 1984). Another well-known consequence of violating circadian rhythms consists of the psychomotor, sleep, gastrointestinal and mood disruptions seen when travelling across time zones, also known as "jet lag" (Rockwell, 1975). The circadian clock system is complex and interconnected, with varying robustness amongst individuals responsible for how well they can maintain optimal physiology in varying environments.

20.6   ZEITGEBERS AND MELANOPSIN

Defining human circadian oscillation starts by understanding the master clock or SCN, which takes light information via the retinohypothalamic tract from the eyes (Morin & Allen, 2006; Sadun et al., 1984). This clock runs at a time pace of just over 24 hours, 24.18 hours to be exact (Czeisler et al., 1999). To keep proper time, we must reset this clock daily so that we do not run over and eventually out of sync. This is performed by "Zeitgebers," directly translated as "time givers," or external cues that help to synchronize the biologic clock, a term coined by Jürgen Aschoff, a founder of the field of chronobiology. Of the many Zeitgebers, light appears to be the major entrainment cue, more so than food (Oishi et al., 2004; Refinetti, 2015). The human eye is extremely sensitive and has demonstrated the ability to perceive a single photon of light (Tinsley et al., 2016). Since there is already evidence that peripheral clocks utilize the central information, it should come as no surprise that even when food or other cues help to manage a rhythm, the main clock can modify this signal as necessary based on environmental information. When has become more important than what.

The most basic circadian mechanism of each cell is the clock genes. Clock genes have been well studied, with connections of physiologic processes being made every day. In an interview with Veronique Greenwood for *Quanta Magazine*, circadian researcher Satchin Panda said that "almost every cell in our body has a circadian clock." The foundation of molecular clock genetics is based on a transcriptional-translational feedback loop consisting of transcription factors CLOCK and BMAL, which promote *Per* and *Cry* gene transcription, which allows the corresponding protein products to inhibit CLOCK and BMAL activity (Cox & Takahashi, 2019) (Figure 20.8)).

Evidence has suggested that this genetic clock machinery is intimately linked to the nuclear receptor family of 48 human transcription factors (such as PPAR-γ, ROR, REV-ERB, RXR and VDR), many of which have currently targeted clinical therapeutic drugs (Zhao et al., 2014). These nuclear receptors are the molecular mechanism that hormones, including the steroids, retinoids, thyroid hormones and vitamin D3, as well as other orphan molecules, utilize to control nuclear transcription and gene regulation (Mangelsdorf et al., 1995). Many of these nuclear receptors, such as REV-ERB and the retinoic acid receptor, control physiologic processes and are pharmaceutical targets for treatment of diabetes, atherosclerosis, autoimmunity and cancer (Kojetin & Burris, 2014). With the significant number of already elucidated nuclear receptor pathways, control of health is additionally linked to the environmental light cues allowed, which instruct these molecular clock mechanisms.

When talking about time creation in the SCN, we must first begin in the eye. While the rods and cones in the retina translate color information into "images" that we see, there is another type of retinal cell, which functions to supply time information. The intrinsically photosensitive retinal ganglion cells (ipRGCs) play little role in the visual process dominated by rods and cones. Now, at least five subtypes of these ipRGCs have been found, with some of these cells'

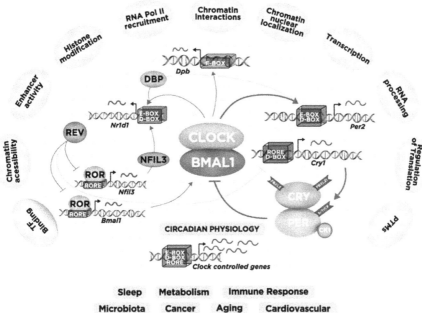

FIGURE 20.8 The circadian gene network and layers of genome-wide regulation in mammals. At the core of the network, the transcription factors CLOCK and BMAL1 activate the Per1, Per2, Cry1 and Cry2 genes (here, we show Per2 and Cry1 as examples), whose protein products (PER and CRY) repress their own transcription. The PER and CRY proteins are post-translationally regulated by parallel E3 ubiquitin ligase pathways (FBXL3 and FBXL21 for CRY and β-TrCP for PER), with PER levels being also regulated by CK1. CLOCK and BMAL1 also regulate the expression of the Nrld1/2 genes, which encode the nuclear receptors REV-ERBα/β, respectively. These nuclear receptors rhythmically repress the transcription of Bmal1 and Nfil3, two genes that are activated by retinoic acid-related orphan receptor-α/β (RORα/β). In turn, NFIL3 together with D-box binding protein (DBP), as well as CLOCK and BMAL1, regulates a rhythm in the REV-ERBα/β nuclear receptors. These three interlocked transcriptional feedback loops regulate the majority of cycling genes, leading to rhythms in various different physiological systems, from sleep to metabolism and aging (bottom of figure). Note that the E- and D-boxes and the RORE-binding regions are in cis upstream at the promoter; however, they are represented here as a stacked box for simplicity. Recent work has identified additional levels of regulation of circadian gene expression (outer layer of regulation in the figure), including rhythmic histone modifications, RNA polymerase II (Pol II) recruitment, circadian chromosomal conformation interactions and post-translational modifications (PTMs). (From Rijo-Ferreira, F. and Takahashi, J.S., *Genome Med.*, 11, 1–16, 2019.)

roles not yet defined (Sonoda & Schmidt, 2016). In 2000, a novel photosensitive pigment known as melanopsin was found, which can allow phototransduction of night and day for the SCN (Hattar et al., 2002; Provencio et al., 2000). This blue light chromophore has also been found in the skin, adipose tissue and blood vessels (Kusumoto et al., 2020; Ondrusova et al., 2017; Sikka et al., 2014). This is another way in which environmental cues are not only conveyed to our main clock but also to peripheral clocks, tightly coupling physiology to the signals that we live in. Before melanopsin, it was believed that frequencies of about 500 nm in the blue/green region were responsible for photoentrainment (Takahashi et al., 1984). After the discovery of melanopsin, ipRGCs were shown using this novel opsin, which connected directly to the SCN to help keep time (Hattar et al., 2002). In fact, these cells were shown to wire also to other locations in the brain involved in the pupillary light reflex (Gooley et al., 2001; Hattar et al., 2002). The spectral sensitivity after further research has shown a curve with a peak around 480 nm and covering around 30–40 nm of decreasing sensitivity on both sides of the peak (Panda et al., 2005; Wahl et al., 2019). (Figure 20.9).

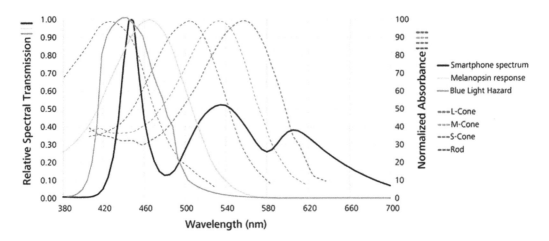

FIGURE 20.9 Irradiance of the blue light hazard function. The blue light hazard function, according to ISO 8980, represents the relative spectral sensitivity of the human eye to blue light hazards, based on the effectiveness of radiation to induce photoreversal of bleaching. The emission spectrum of an ordinary smartphone screen on maximum brightness shows a distinct overlap in the potentially harmful blue peak area, melanopsin sensitivity, and also image-forming-related S-cone and rod absorbance spectrum. Normalized absorbance spectra are depicted according to J. K. Bowmaker, H. J. Dartnall, *J. Physiol.* 1980, 298, 501. (From Wahl, S. et al., *J. Biophotonics*, 12, 1–14, 2019.)

Melanopsin works via a light activated G-protein signaling to mobilize calcium or regulate gene expression (Brown & Robinson, 2004) (Figure 20.10).

This opsin contains a light-sensing vitamin A–coupled chromophore, 11-cis-retinal, which is transformed to all-trans-retinal in response to light (Sonoda & Lee, 2016). It turns out that this opsin is bistable, and the all-trans-retinal can be converted back to 11-cis-retinal with long-wavelength light (Panda et al., 2005). In this way, the vitamin A cycle is linked back to the circadian mechanism and can be significantly disrupted with constant artificial blue light. However, it should be noted that increased all-trans-retinal can induce damage to the retina by reactive oxidative species (ROS), which is already implicated in age-related macular degeneration (Chen et al., 2012). Blue light–induced retinoid intermediates, including free all-trans-retinal, can cause toxicity, which may be manifested by plasma membrane permeability and mitochondrial oxidative stress–associated apoptosis (Maeda et al., 2009). Also, delayed clearance of all-trans-retinal leads to an increase of a condensation product, pyridinium bisretinoid A2E, which when further illuminated by 430 nm blue-frequency light, damages DNA proportionally to the light exposure (Sparrow et al., 2003). It has been further shown that all-trans-retinal-induced photoreceptor degeneration occurs via increased ferrous (Fe^{+2}) ion, decreased glutathione (GSH) and mitochondrial damage from a non-apoptotic cell death known as ferroptosis (Chen et al., 2021). Ferroptotic cell death is different from apoptosis, necrosis and autophagy, with iron-dependent accumulation of lipid ROS intimately involved in the mechanism of death (Dixon et al., 2012). The pathophysiologic processes of tumors, nervous system disease, ischemia-reperfusion injury, kidney injury and blood disease have been shown to be closely related to ferroptotic cell death (Li et al., 2020).

Ubiqinol, a reduced form of coenzyme Q10, found in the mitochondrial membranes can help control the lipid peroxidation that can trigger ferroptosis (Passegué, 2021). Q10 is a lipophilic molecule that plays a role in the mitochondrial membrane passing electrons down the respiratory chain, and its deficiency is associated with poor ATP production and increased ROS formation, which makes it an important target for potentially mitigating a variety of mitochondrial damage (Acosta et al., 2016). It has been previously shown that these potentially damaging aldehyde retinal isomers can bind to retinol-binding protein, but the resulting chromophore–protein created shows alterations in conformation and associated changes in the absorption spectrum (Horwitz & Heller, 1973). The

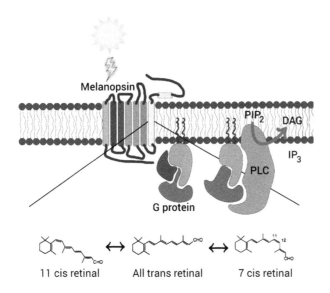

FIGURE 20.10   Melanopsin light transduction coupled to G-protein-coupled pathways. DAG, Diacylglycerol; IP3, Inositol 1,4,5-triphosphate; PIP2, PI4,5-biphosphate; PLC, Phospholipase C.

author suggests this as a mechanism of transporting any vitamin A aldehydes created by excessive blue light outside the cell. While most of the published research involves all-trans retinal-induced retinopathies, given melanopsin's additional presence in skin, adipose tissue and blood vessels, it could be suggested that further regional mitochondrial damage could be facilitated by free retinal release locally and also further downstream regionally via the bloodstream.

Artificial light can affect the circadian mechanism via melanopsin-mediated signal transduction, which leads to altered clock and timing functions of cells and chemical messengers. Excessive stimulation by the particular blue frequencies in artificial light sources can also create toxic vitamin A isomers, which can create further damage locally and regionally. These are the melanopsin pathologic mechanisms that underpin the hazards of excessive artificial blue light. International guidelines by the International Commission on Non-Ionizing Radiation Protection (ICNIRP) show the blue light hazard function of damage to the retina to be over 0.8 from wavelengths of 415 to 460 nm and over 0.1 from 400 to 500 nm (Ziegelberger, 2013). This is the definition of the spectrum of frequencies that are found in artificial light sources (see Figure 20.10), which are forever shining on the human melanopsin receptors by day and night. When will we start to recognize the effect of the frequencies of the electromagnetic spectrum that are allowed to change cellular functioning in these ways?

20.7   BIOPHYSICAL EVOLUTION

20.7.1   Mitochondrial Connection

The first mitochondrial DNA (mtDNA) originated in Africa approximately 200,000 years ago. This gave rise to variant mtDNA, which appeared slowly with the migration patterns of early humans moving across Africa, and then other variants moving into Europe, and again in Asia and the Americas (Wallace, 2013). It is a logical assumption that these mutations would be random; however, evolutionary pressure would help select variants that could facilitate the survival of environmentally optimized mitochondria. Over time, mitochondria accumulated specific epigenetic programming changes directly in their mtDNA engine makeup, known as haplotypes, which map geographically to this evolutionary migration of humans (Wallace, 2013) (Figure 20.11).

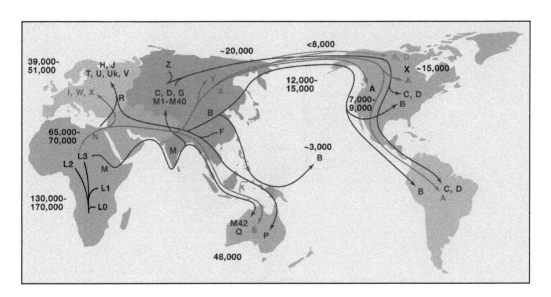

FIGURE 20.11 Regional radiation of human mtDNAs from their origin in Africa and colonization of Eurasia and the Americas implies that environmental selection constrained regional mtDNA variation. All African mtDNAs are subsumed under macrohaplogroup L and coalesce to a single origin about 130,000–170,000 YBP. African haplogroup L0 is the most ancient mtDNA lineage found in the Koi-San peoples, L1 and L2 in Pygmy populations. The M and N mtDNA lineages emerged from Sub-Saharan African L3 in northeastern Africa, and only derivatives of M and N mtDNAs successfully left Africa, giving rise to macrohaplogroups M and N. N haplogroups radiated into European and Asian indigenous populations, while M haplogroups were confined to Asia. Haplogroups A, C, and D became enriched in northeastern Siberia and were positioned to migrate across the Bering Land Bridge 20,000 YBP to found Native Americans. Additional Eurasian migrations brought to the Americas haplogroups B and X. Finally, haplogroup B colonized the Pacific Islands. (Figure reproduced from MITOMAP, 2015) (Wallace, D.C., *Cell*, 163, 33–38, 2015.)

From Doug Wallace's work, we know that we inherit our mitochondria from our mother (Giles et al., 1980). This should make sense from an epigenetic evolutionary perspective. Nature decided to have the mother, the deliverer of the progeny, be the most sensitive to the environmental signals. The eggs in the mother's body present at birth are a representation of the grandmother's environment, for the mother's original zygote cell accumulated exposure of the environment of her mother. Additionally, the mother's eggs, already carrying information from the grandmother's environment, are exposed to the life and environment of the mother, now accumulating information from this environment as well until fertilization. It is highly likely that egg selection occurs in a fashion that selects an egg which is best matched to the present environment. It is already established that maternal intraovarian systems are in place to remove eggs with the most severe mitochondrial defects, optimizing function based on mitochondrial–nuclear coupling interaction (Fan et al., 2008; Hill et al., 2014; Latorre-Pellicer et al., 2019). This is how transgenerational epigenetics proceeds, able to select eggs with mutations and modifications that will allow the progeny to thrive. This assumes that the electromagnetic information communicated to the mitochondria in the egg cells is truly representative of the environment and not artificially created (Figure 20.12).

While it is clear that the mitochondria are energy producers of the cells, what is not as clear is the role of bioenergetics in disease. Mitochondria "produce about 90% of cellular energy, regulate cellular redox status, produce ROS, maintain Ca^{2+} homeostasis, synthesize and degrade high-energy biochemical intermediates, and regulate cell death through activation of the mitochondrial permeability transition pore" (Wallace, 2013). Mitochondrial energetics are mostly determined by the state of the mitochondrial genome, which is present right in the mitochondrion itself. While some of its genome is present in the cell's nuclear DNA, 37 genes of its circular mtDNA are present directly

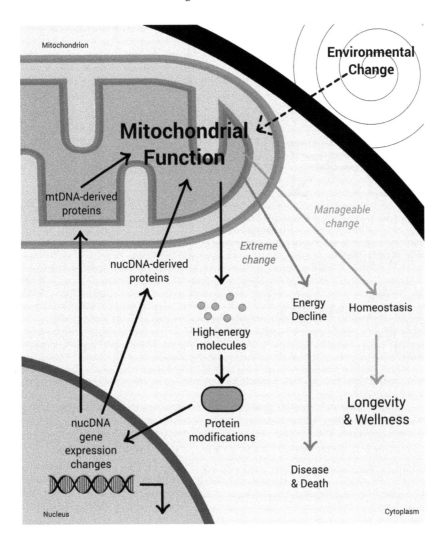

FIGURE 20.12 Mitochondrial function is directly influenced by environmental changes, so the mitochondrion must have a central role in translating the environmental to genomic responses. High-energy molecules and even reactive oxygen species act as signaling molecules, along with protein modifications that regulate nuclear DNA (nucDNA) expression. These changes modify gene expression, altering expression of nucDNA- and mtDNA-derived proteins that act in and on the mitochondria – creating feedback loops. When energetic homeostasis can be re-established, health and longevity are preserved. However, if genetic or environmental circumstances cannot be overcome, energy production declines, leading to disease and even death. (Adapted from Wallace, D.C., *Nature*, 535, 498–500, 2016.)

next to the electron transport chain itself. In this way, ROS that are created nearby can and will cause damage to the mitochondrial genes, which then can limit the mitochondrion's ability to create energy as efficiently. Therefore, a cell will have many mitochondria that are performing optimally and a varying degree with mtDNA mutations which are performing less optimally; this is called mitochondrial heteroplasmy (Figure 20.13).

The mitochondrial free radical theory of aging is linked to age-related disease expression bioenergetically, and when considered with the heteroplasmy inheritance pattern, elucidates a possible mechanism (Sanz & Stefanatos, 2008). Understanding mitochondrial epigenetic and bioenergetic functions may explain why we see diseases starting younger and younger via transgenerational changes. Transfer of mitochondrial DNA variants has shown the ability to cause systemic changes

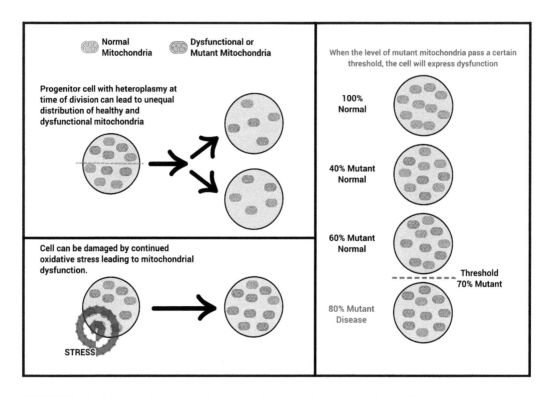

FIGURE 20.13 Mitochondrial heteroplasmy and disease. Although homoplasty with completely undamaged mitochondria would be the optimal normal state, different populations of normal and dysfunctional mitochondria may coexist in a cell, known as the state of heteroplasmy. Since division of the whole cell mitochondria during cellular replication is mostly random, daughter cells will have different ratios of normal to dysfunctional mitochondria compared with the parent cell. If the population of mutant mitochondria in a cell reaches a certain threshold (70% in this example, but this will be highly variable based on tissue and disease), then the cell expresses dysfunction, and symptoms or disease can appear. (Adapted from White, A.J., *Sex. Transm. Infect.*, 77, 158–173, 2001.)

in the transplanted organism from its original mitochondrial type (Wallace, 2016). These mtDNA mutations are passed down through the generations through inheritance as well as being shaped by selection, and have been associated with pathogenesis of human disease (Wei & Chinnery, 2020). The heteroplasmy rate increases when there are fewer mitochondria in the most energy-efficient state and many others with acquired defects causing decreased energy production. This means that at certain decreased cellular energetic levels, biochemical systems will stop working, and disease "appears." Hence, expected damage to mitochondria with decreased function is associated with aging (Chistiakov et al., 2014; Sanz & Stefanatos, 2008). This increased heteroplasmy of mitochondria is responsible for transcriptional gene changes, which have been shown to affect phenotype (Picard et al., 2014). The energy production of the mitochondrial electron transport chain produces oxidative stress, which essentially comprises instructions from the environment that create epigenetic change through histone posttranscriptional modifications (García-Giménez et al., 2021). These are the mechanisms of either health or disease for current and future generations.

The mitochondrion in its very design contains the ability to transform electron information into differing levels of biochemical components, with NAD+ and NADH levels being important in this signal transduction (Logan, 2003; Massudi et al., 2012; Yang & Sauve, 2016). This is one way in which the electron transport chain can be responsible for messengers encoding food and environmental signals. The appropriate transfer of electrons is also an energy used to create the electrochemical gradient across the mitochondrial membranes, just like a capacitor in electronics

(Rottenberg, 1998). Mitochondria as cellular organelles can act independently, but they can also oscillate together, aligning their inter-mitochondrial junctions, which have been shown to correlate to both high -energy output of active muscle tissue lines and low-energy output of cancer cell lines (Picard et al., 2015). The many folds of a mitochondrion provide a huge surface area for this electrical charge to be separated, which is used to create ATP via the ATPase spinning, which also by physics will create a magnetic field. This magnetism can further control and couple to the biochemistry in other ways. Since oxygen is paramagnetic, the mitochondrial components, when spinning, can magnetically attract oxygen as the final electron acceptor. It has already been shown that DNA information can be transduced through water with electromagnetic waves (Montagnier et al., 2015). Extremely low-frequency electromagnetic fields have been shown to interact with water and other biologic targets (Foletti et al., 2009). The mitochondrial cytochrome oxidase enzymes have been shown to emit light corresponding to a peak of 900 nm in the infrared range (Tuszyński & Dixon, 2001). Surrounded by water, this light release can form the high-density crystalline exclusion water that Gerald Pollack has described, "shrinking" water and bringing the electron chain transfer components closer together (Li & Pollack, 2020; Pollack et al., 2009). Shorter distances create lower-energy barriers that facilitate mitochondrial electron tunneling (Moser et al., 2006). Improved bioenergetics, again, means fewer ROS and improved cellular efficiency. In time, biophysics will be shown as the main controller of all the molecular genetic and proteomic studies being published today, with the mitochondria as the cellular electromagnetic conductor.

There is no doubt that mitochondria are intimately connected to health. As well as control of respiratory metabolism by the clock genes, there is also an interplay of oxidative phosphorylation controlling the clock genes themselves (Scrima et al., 2016). The mitochondria control the production of hormones and make melatonin, whose role in health is often underestimated. Controlling the energy dynamics of the cell and transforming environmental changes into signals to create favorable biochemistry should dictate the importance of these electromagnetic engines, whose full biophysical powers have yet to be discovered. Regardless, the preservation of function and strategies to repair and regenerate damaged mitochondria must be considered part of treating the root cause of disease.

20.8 DHA

Docosahexaenoic acid (DHA, C22:6) is the omega-3 polyunsaturated fatty acid (PUFA) provided from fish oil. The central nervous system has a high concentration of phospholipids, of which DHA is a major membrane component. This ancient nutrient has correlated with human evolution and expansion of cerebral function, with dietary access being needed, given poor endogenous synthesis ability (Bradbury, 2011). The impact of its presence brings antioxidant properties, memory function, neurogenesis, lipid raft signaling, inflammation balance and cardiovascular health (Hashimoto et al., 2017). A major structural component of the outer segment membranes of the retinal photoreceptors, DHA may also function in a protective fashion for vascular and neurologic pathology via production of the many bioactive molecules it interacts with, such as eicosanoids, angiogenic factors, matrix metalloproteins (MMP), ROS, neurotransmitters and cytokines (SanGiovanni & Chew, 2005). The molecule of DHA, in additional to its G-protein-coupled phototransduction cascade, has been shown to add fluidity to cell membranes, which can modulate permeability, transport, membrane-bound enzymatic activity and neurotransmission (Hashimoto et al., 2017; Gawrisch & Soubiasr, 2014). This essential fatty acid also can produce resolvins, protectins and maresins, all synthesized mediators that help resolve and modulate the inflammatory response in positive ways (Duvall & Levy, 1998; Serhan & Levy, 2018). These many factors contribute to its biochemical benefits in living organisms. It is also beneficial to mitochondrial energy production. Dietary supplementation of DHA has been shown to improve skeletal muscle mitochondrial function and endurance (Le Guen et al., 2016). Despite all these factors, one particular biophysical factor may be most important in why it is a fatty acid that has not been replaced in over 600 million years of animal evolution

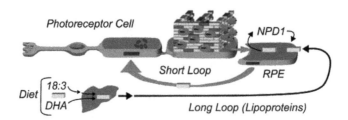

FIGURE 20.14 Extracellular trafficking of DHA and neuroprotectin D1 synthesis in retinal pigment epithelial cells. The liver-to-photoreceptor long loop is the transport of DHA through the bloodstream by lipoproteins. Yellow bricks depict DHA. Short loop retrieval of DHA through interphotoreceptor matrix after intermittent photoreceptor outer segment renewal. Wall in outer segment illustrates disc membranes; the red "fruit-like" structure represents rhodopsin molecules. (Modified and published with permission from Bazan, NG., *Trends Neurosci.*, 29, 263–271, 2006; Bazan, N.G., *Prostaglandins Leukot. Essent. Fatty Acids*, 81, 205–211, 2009.)

(Crawford et al., 2013). Crawford et al.'s publication (2013) explains DHA's quantum mechanical benefit for life on earth, which is the ability of its pi-electrons to function as a phototransducer of light-activated signals to electricity. This electrical signal is able to be conveyed through cytoskeletal elements of the cell as well as via the plasma membrane itself, creating a whole-body signaling network (Friesen et al., 2015; Shi et al., 2021; Wallace, 2010). DHA's association with the eye and the neurologic system makes greater sense when considering its quantum properties.

Unfortunately, the incorporation of DHA into the mitochondrial membrane has been shown to be susceptible to peroxidation by ROS (Malis et al., 1990). This susceptibility would be vulnerable to attack by previously described free all-trans-retinal from blue light in photoreceptors as well as by excessive free radical production in phospholipid membranes. Stress on the brain, proven in an experimental stroke model, was also shown to release DHA, likely for its various neuroprotective effects (Bazan et al., 2005). Given its importance in the bioenergetics of an organism described earlier, its destruction and loss can be seen as a bioenergetic problem, which can lead to disease. Nicholas Bazan has helped to elucidate the replacement of DHA via two mechanisms, a long and short loop (Bazan, 2009) (Figure 20.14).

The long loop involves proper liver function to take linoleic acid (18:3) and synthesize docosahexaenoic acid (22:3), which is then packaged in lipoproteins and returned to membranes in the brain and retina (Scott & Bazan, 1989). Photoreceptors themselves also have a short loop, whereby daily usage of DHA can be actively recycled back into use (Bazan et al., 1994). Understanding proper photoreceptor biology, the more blue light damage that is created, the more DHA should be supplemented to keep the circadian mechanism and cell signaling functioning optimally. The DHA molecule has a dipole moment from its π bonds, making it paramagnetic and therefore, attracted to magnetic fields such as those created by mitochondria (Alexander-north et al., 1994). Appropriate DHA intake is therefore necessary for the optimal bioenergetics of cell membranes, including mitochondria, and supplementation can be considered based upon suspicion of poor mitochondrial function and excessive blue light exposure.

20.9 BLUE LIGHT

The frequencies from 400 to 500 nm constitute light of blue frequencies. Blue frequencies are known to cause damage to the very retinal epithelium structures responsible for circadian light transduction (Pang et al., 1998; Seko et al., 2001). This blue light damage is caused by a variety of proposed mechanisms, including oxidative stress, photochemical damage, mitochondrial and inflammatory apoptosis, and mitochondrial DNA damage (Ouyang et al., 2020; Smick et al., 2013). Blue light exposure at 460 nm at night has been shown to increase EEG correlates of alertness as opposed to 555 nm green light (Rahman et al., 2014). These wavelength-dependent effects work to suppress melatonin, increase body temperature and increase heart rate to achieve their alerting response (Cajochen et al., 2005). Retinal photoreceptor apoptosis, which has been seen in age-related macular degeneration (AMD), pathologic myopia, retinal detachment, retinoblastoma and other eye disease, can be induced by blue light exposure (Katya Frazier, 2017; Seko et al., 2001; Wu et al., 1999). In AMD, the blue light–mediated cell death has been shown to work via vitamin A cycle free retinal production of the phototoxic compound A2E, which impairs the cytochrome oxidase function of the mitochondria (Shaban & Richter, 2002). DHA and negatively charged phospholipids protect from this A2E-mediated cell death (Bazan et al., 2011). As previously stated, DHA intake should be considered, based upon blue light toxicity, to facilitate and offset damage to the very structures needed for circadian phototransduction.

Godley et al. showed that after 3 hours of blue light exposure, mitochondrial DNA was shown to be damaged by ROS, while nuclear DNA was not affected. While some repair mechanisms were evident at 6 hours, there was still no improvement in the mitochondrial redox function of the cell at 9 hours, suggesting that this inefficient repair mechanism may further oxidative phosphorylation dysfunction, promoting more oxidative stress (Godley et al., 2005). Human beings were prepared for a small amount of damage protection, but not the current onslaught that artificial lighting technologies are producing daily.

20.10 TECHNOLOGY AND SCREENS

To understand the growing effect of excessive blue light, we must look at the societal changes towards technology in all aspects of daily living. The use of mobile technology such as smartphones, tablets and even older laptop/desktop computer technology is clearly on the rise in almost all age groups, with much published evidence of poor sleep and health associations (Christensen et al., 2016; Rosen et al., 2014; Stiglic & Viner, 2019). Use of this media relies greatly on light emitting diode (LED)-based screens and monitors that are heavy in blue light frequencies. Add the variety of social media platforms, video communications and gaming prospects to fill free time, and it is no wonder that there are new health problems arising. Most youth and adults spend little time outdoors with natural sunlight exposure (Espiritu et al., 1994; Savides et al., 1986). Besides the lack of time outdoors, indoor screen time has psychological consequences. With or without the American Psychiatric Association adding new diagnoses such as "Internet Gaming Disorder," it is obvious that there is an addictive psychology developed to keep consumers using blue light screens (Kuss & Griffiths, 2011; Kuss & Lopez-Fernandez, 2016). It is no surprise that the dopaminergic system relating to reward and addiction is controlled by circadian clock genes (Parekh et al., 2015). Studies have also shown fluorescent lighting exposure to decrease the amount of tyrosine hydroxylase–positive dopaminergic neurons in the substantia nigra, an alteration associated with aging and Parkinson's disease (Romeo et al., 2013). Does this imply that there is a physiologic addiction in addition to the psychologic addiction to technology?

While new energy-efficient lighting has no doubt saved many people from large energy bills, the excessive artificial light, both direct and indirect, is having a negative impact on human health (Irwin, 2018). It is evident from research that the amount of the earth's artificially lit surface is growing by 2.2% per year, and the total irradiance is growing by 1.8% (Kyba et al., 2017). Since the amount of lighting is increasing, not only is this causing increases in energy expenditure, but this light pollution is having an impact on ecological function and human health (Bennie et al., 2014). The lighting emission of these technologies, even when compared with similar color temperatures, contains very different spectral frequency information (Blume, 2019) (Figure 20.15).

All artificial light sources tend to have significant emission in the blue frequencies, which match the frequencies associated with the blue light hazard, as well as absence of the red light frequencies found in sunlight.

The sun's radiation is represented by about 43% of red and infrared light frequencies. This is a large proportion of the spectrum that finds its way to the earth and all the life found therein.

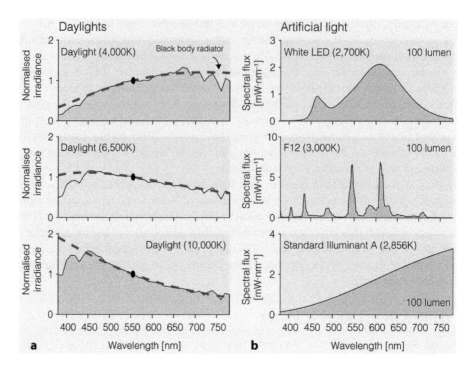

FIGURE 20.15 Spectral power distributions of common light sources in our environment. (a) Spectral power distributions of daylight at different correlated color temperatures (CCT; 4000 K; 6500 K; 10,000 K). Spectra are normalized to 555 nm. (b) Spectral power distributions of a white LED (top), a fluorescent source at 3000 K (middle) and an incandescent source (tungsten-filament; 2856 K, bottom). All three artificial sources have the same luminous flux (normalized to 100 lm),and approximately the same color temperature (2700–3000 K), but the spectra are very different in shape and scale (see y axis). (From Blume, C., *Somnologie*, 147–156, 2019.)

Nature's design follows this in that the red light frequencies are utilized in the mitochondria, such that the nanomotor ATPase head spins at near 100% efficiency with exposure to near-infrared light (Kinosita et al., 2000; Sommer et al., 2015). The frequencies from artificial sources and screens are strongest at suppressing melatonin and therefore, ruin sleep, hormones and health (Heo et al., 2017). Continued usage of these sources at night creates a chronic circadian disruption and even worse, mitochondrial DNA damage via excessive free radical signaling (Godley et al., 2005). The study of red light therapy, also known as low-level laser therapy (LLLT) or photobiomodulation (PBM), has clearly shown its anti-inflammatory properties (Cho, 2016). Natural sunset has very specific changes of the blue to red light ratio, which occur as the sun hits the horizon (Johnson et al., 1967). Understanding of melanopsin biology and red light's biophysical properties with water should allow inferences as to just how this changing information may be used by circadian rhythms to further fine-tune timing information centrally and peripherally. At the time much of this research was obtained, there was no understanding of melanopsin and the photopigment gears of the circadian clock, which make sense of these findings to further refine time in an organism. It should be no surprise that humans' technology addiction and light pollution with a loss of the natural light signal are significant contributors to the health crises of current times.

20.11   LIGHT AT NIGHT

Much scientific research has been published that shows the dangers of this blue light circadian disruption without ever mentioning "blue light." Artificial light at night (ALAN) is a term that generally represents any artificial source of light, which as already explained, is high in content of blue-frequency melanopsin-disturbing and melatonin- suppressing light. ALAN has been associated with obesity in women (Park et al., 2019). The most concerning associations of inappropriate light exposure at night are seen for cancer pathophysiology, which is associated with many of the dysfunctions that occur in the circadian phototransduction pathways (Jasser et al., 2006). This connection is further reinforced by epidemiologic studies of ambient environmental light at night. Increased risk of breast cancer due to such light has been shown in many studies (Hurley et al., 2014; James et al., 2017; Xiao et al., 2020). Additionally, outdoor ALAN has been associated with prostate cancer and colon cancer (Garcia-Saenz et al., 2018, 2020). The light at night theory has even been hypothesized as the etiology of melanoma (Kvaskoff & Weinstein, 2010). More recently, a positive increased risk of 55% thyroid cancer incidence was seen with ALAN (Zhang et al., 2021). Whether it be through melatonin suppression, melanopsin damage, ROS, mitochondrial dysfunction or chronic circadian phototransduction systemic defects, the association is clear. Break nature's circadian programming, and suffer from illness and disease.

20.12   BLOCKING THE BLUES

If artificial blue light is so damaging, and there is an endless supply of sources emitting these frequencies on humans all day and night, what can be done? From an evolutionary perspective of circadian health, simply not using any type of lighting or screens after sundown would suffice, as it has already been explained that melanopsin receptors for this type of light are present in the eyes and all over the body via skin, adipose tissue and blood vessels. As this may not be ideal for most modern-day humans, the next level of mitigation would be consideration of firelight sources such as candles or a fireplace, similar to human's first lighting exposures in history. Even these types of firelight, which are much more predominant in red-frequency spectral distribution, create a small amount of melatonin suppression (Morita & Tokura, 1998). Further improvements can be made to eliminate sources by the choice of artificial bulbs. As seen previously (see Figure 20.15), incandescent bulbs have much lower 400–500 nm frequency spectral emission than compact fluorescent or LED bulbs. An initial and foundational measure to prevent SCN clock disruption is to utilize blue-blocking glasses after sundown, which block 100% of all blue frequencies from 400 to 500 nm as well as some blockage up to 550 nm. This incorporates the melatonin action spectra to prevent the previously discussed damage (Brainard et al., 2001) (Figure 20.16).

This maneuver only addresses melanopsin dysfunction at the retina level, directing the SCN closer to central circadian harmony and helping to reestablish healthy melatonin rhythms. Peripheral clock damage can be further mitigated by clothing, preventing the signaling on skin and soft tissues.

While not often discussed clinically, there is significant scientific research behind the use of blue light blocking modalities. Much more of blue light's mechanism of damage has been discussed previously. Monochromatic blue light of 460 nm was shown to cause twice as much circadian phase delay and melatonin suppression as monochromatic light of 555 nm of equivalent photon density (Lockley et al., 2003). Amber blue light–blocking glasses used during nighttime light exposures prevented the melatonin suppression effects seen in controls (Kayumov et al., 2005). Multimedia screen–using teenagers wearing blue-blocking glasses showed less evening melatonin suppression and less alertness before bedtime compared with controls using clear lenses, even when polysomnographically scored sleep stages were unchanged following usage (Van Der Lely et al., 2015). Insomniacs undergoing cognitive behavioral therapy using blue-blocking glasses showed a statistically significant decrease in subjective time to fall asleep, increase in subjective total sleep time and decrease in subjective anxiety compared with controls (Janků et al., 2020). Adult males exposed to regular smartphones with LED screens or smartphones with suppressed blue light LED screen emission showed significantly decreased sleepiness as well as increased body temperature, and lower melatonin secretion at a later time (Heo et al., 2017). Insomniacs

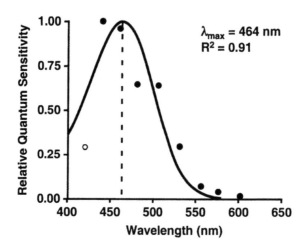

FIGURE 20.16   This graph demonstrates the action spectrum for percentage control-adjusted melatonin suppression in 72 healthy human subjects. The *filled circles* represent the half-saturation constants of eight wavelengths from 440 to 600 nm that were normalized to the maximum response and plotted as log relative sensitivity. The *open circle* represents the estimated half-saturation constant derived from the 420 nm data. The *solid curve* portrays the best-fit template for vitamin A1 retinaldehyde photopigments, which predicts a maximal spectral absorbance (λmax) of 464 nm (Partridge and De Grip, 1991). There is a high coefficient of correlation for fitting this opsin template to the melatonin suppression data ($R2 = 0.91$). (From Brainard, G.C. et al., *J. . Neurosci.*, 21, 6405–6412, 2001.)

using amber glasses showed increased working memory and processing speed from the blue light blockade (Zimmerman et al., 2019).

All this data should start to convince the reader of the merits of blue-blocking technologies; however, literature searches may reveal some studies with mixed results depending on the end parameters evaluated in the study. It should be noted that there is no standardization of how blue blocking is performed, the required frequencies to be blocked for optimal results, quantification of the artificial light environment, or exposure to natural frequencies, which also contribute to the circadian rhythmicity. Many of the studies evaluating blue light blocking techniques fail to evaluate the status of the circadian rhythm to begin with and therefore, also lack the ability to make clear conclusions from the data. Combine this with the robustness of the physiologic system to absorb short-term circadian stress, and it should be clear that proper evaluation of the published data requires evaluation of whether or not the study design is even appropriate to make any scientific conclusions. The readers of the chapter should have a foundational understanding of many shortcomings of already published research. Use of nighttime blue-blocking amber glasses is a noninvasive method of preserving circadian rhythmicity and melatonin secretion and avoiding free radical damage, and should be considered as a first-line modality in establishing holistic wellness.

Many have heard of sleep hygiene recommendations to facilitate quality sleeping conditions; however, it should be stressed that it is in fact the "light" that is allowed that creates the environment for appropriate health repair during sleep. Understanding what "light hygiene" really means defines those who are truly able to reestablish optimal circadian rhythms, thereby allowing regeneration and health to follow. Melatonin, blue light and melanopsin science has been well published but has not been widely understood by the mainstream or utilized for clinical outcomes. Protecting the eyes, skin and mitochondria from excessive damage is one of the single most important steps in any health journey. The ability to sustain appropriate cellular energy and signaling is required for any disease reversal attempt. Sleep and circadian rhythms are intimately connected to wellness and must be respected as a foundation of the optimal functioning of any human being.

20.13 CONCLUSION

Health and wellness can be seen as the byproduct of circadian rhythms, epigenetics and mitochondrial function. Anything that interrupts the circadian rhythm has systemic neuroendocrine effects that can change the organism's phenotype. When environmental factors that destroy the clock mechanism, such as constant unfettered blue light technology exposure, also cause damage to the bioenergetic creation system, the mitochondria, synergistic damage results. Silent electromagnetic toxicity from these environmental signals is therefore a major contributor to the healthcare crisis seen today. Lifestyle changes and awareness can reestablish balance and allow physiology to correct itself when these epigenetic signals are mitigated. Any healing modality attempting to improve disease or optimize health should include this consideration, or the therapy will only fail in the long run due to the persistent faulty environment that created the problem. In this way, no disease state can truly be fixed without first improving the toxic environment that created it.

While complex and interconnected, circadian and mitochondrial dynamics are non-linear by nature of their connection to the properties of light. Small changes in these environmental signals can have much larger effects than would normally be expected. Seeing the sunlight in the morning and getting into nature, as well as blocking and mitigating harmful artificial frequencies, is really not that hard. Practitioners and patients can utilize the information in this chapter to help achieve better health, often without significant additional expense. Nature's electromagnetics were responsible for human evolution, and if we are able to accept the antagonistic role modern living and technology play in disease, we have found a missing piece in the recipe for health. May wellness be found *in time* for those who are ready.

REFERENCES

Abbott, S. M., & Zee, P. C. (2019). Circadian rhythms: implications for health and disease. *Neurologic Clinics*, *37*(3), 601–613. https://doi.org/10.1016/j.ncl.2019.04.004

Acosta, M. J., Fonseca, L. V., Desbats, M. A., Cerqua, C., Zordan, R., Trevisson, E., & Salviati, L. (2016). Coenzyme Q biosynthesis in health and disease. *BBA: Bioenergetics*, *1857*(8), 1079–1085. https://doi .org/10.1016/j.bbabio.2016.03.036

Acuña-Castroviejo, D., Escames, G., Venegas, C., Díaz-Casado, M. E., Lima-Cabello, E., López, L. C., Rosales-Corral, S., Tan, D. X., & Reiter, R. J. (2014). Extrapineal melatonin: sources, regulation, and potential functions. *Cellular and Molecular Life Sciences*, *71*(16), 2997–3025. https://doi.org/10.1007/ s00018-014-1579-2

Adam, E. K., Doane, L. D., Zinbarg, R. E., Mineka, S., Craske, M. G., & Griffith, J. W. (2011). Prospective prediction of major depressive disorder from cortisol awakening responses in adolescence. *Psychoneuroendocrinology*, *35*(6), 921–931. https://doi.org/10.1016/j.psyneuen.2009.12.007.Prospective

Adam, E. K., Vrshek-Schallhorn, S., Kendall, A. D., Mineka, S., Zinbarg, R. E., & Craske, M. G. (2014). Prospective associations between the cortisol awakening response and first onsets of anxiety disorders over a six-year follow-up −2013 Curt Richter Award Winner. *Psychoneuroendocrinology*, *44*, 47–59. https://doi.org/10.1016/j.psyneuen.2014.02.014

Alexander-north, L. S., North, J. A., Kiminyo, K. P., Buettner, G. R., & Spector, A. A. (1994). Polyunsaturated fatty acids increase lipid radical formation induced by oxidant stress in endothelial cells. *Journal Lipid Research*, *35*(10), 1773–1785. https://doi.org/10.1016/S0022-2275(20)39772-8

Ayas, N. T., White, D. P., Manson, J. A. E., Stampfer, M. J., Speizer, F. E., Malhotra, A., & Hu, F. B. (2003). A prospective study of sleep duration and coronary heart disease in women. *Archives of Internal Medicine*, *163*(2), 205–209. https://doi.org/10.1001/archinte.163.2.205

Basta, M., Chrousos, G. P., Vela-Bueno, A., & Vgontzas, A. N. (2007). Chronic Insomnia and the Stress System. *Sleep Medicine Clinics*, *2*(2), 279–291. https://doi.org/10.1016/j.jsmc.2007.04.002

Bazan, N G, Rodriguez de Turco, E. B., & Gordon, W. C. (1994). Docosahexaenoic acid supply to the retina and its conservation in photoreceptor cells by active retinal pigment epithelium-mediated recycling. *World Review of Nutrition and Dietetics*, *75*, 120–123. https://doi.org/10.1159/000423564

Bazan, N. G. (2009). Cellular and molecular events mediated by docosahexaenoic acid-derived neuroprotectin D1 signaling in photoreceptor cell survival and brain protection. *Prostaglandins Leukotrienes and Essential Fatty Acids*, *81*(2–3), 205–211. https://doi.org/10.1016/j.plefa.2009.05.024

Bazan, N. G., Molina, M. F., & Gordon, W. C. (2011). Docosahexaenoic acid signalolipidomics in nutrition: significance in aging, neuroinflammation, macular degeneration, Alzheimer's, and other neurodegenerative diseases. *Annual Review of Nutrition, 31*, 321–351. https://doi.org/10.1146/annurev.nutr.012809 .104635

Bazan, N. G, Marcheselli, V. L., & Cole-Edwards, K. (2005). Brain response to injury and neurodegeneration: endogenous neuroprotective signaling. *Annals of the New York Academy of Sciences, 1053*, 137–147. https://doi.org/10.1196/annals.1344.011

Bedoya, S. K., Lam, B., Lau, K., & Iii, J. L. (2013). Th17 cells in immunity and autoimmunity. *Clinical and Developmental Immunology, 2013*.

Bennie, J. J., Duffy, J. P., Inger, R., & Gaston, K. J. (2014). Biogeography of time partitioning in mammals. *Proceedings of the National Academy of Sciences, 111*(38), 13727–13732. https://doi.org/10.1073/pnas .1216063110

Besedovsky, L., Lange, T., & Haack, M. (2019). The sleep-immune crosstalk in health and disease. *Physiological Reviews, 99*(3), 1325–1380. https://doi.org/10.1152/physrev.00010.2018

Blume, C. (2019). Effects of light on human circadian rhythms, sleep and mood. *Somnologie*, 147–156. https:// doi.org/10.1007/s11818-019-00215-x

Bollinger, T., Leutz, A., Leliavski, A., Skrum, L., Kovac, J., Bonacina, L., Oster, H., Solbach, W., Benedict, C., & Lange, T. (2011). Circadian clocks in mouse and human CD4 + T cells. *PLoS ONE, 6*(12), 1–11. https://doi.org/10.1371/journal.pone.0029801

Bouchlariotou, S., Liakopoulos, V., Giannopoulou, M., Arampatzis, S., Eleftheriadis, T., Mertens, P. R., Zintzaras, E., Messinis, I. E., & Stefanidis, I. (2014). Melatonin secretion is impaired in women with preeclampsia and an abnormal circadian blood pressure rhythm. *Renal Failure, 36*(7), 1001–1007. https://doi.org/10.3109/0886022X.2014.926216

Bradbury, J. (2011). Docosahexaenoic acid (DHA): an ancient nutrient for the modern human brain. *Nutrients, 3*(5), 529–554. https://doi.org/10.3390/nu3050529

Brainard, G. C., Hanifin, J. R., Greeson, J. M., Byrne, B., Glickman, G., Gerner, E., & Rollag, M. D. (2001). Action spectrum for melatonin regulation in humans: evidence for a novel circadian photoreceptor. *Journal of Neuroscience, 21*(16), 6405–6412. https://doi.org/10.1523/jneurosci.21-16-06405.2001

Brambilla, D. J., Matsumoto, A. M., Araujo, A. B., & McKinlay, J. B. (2009). The effect of diurnal variation on clinical measurement of serum testosterone and other sex hormone levels in men. *Journal of Clinical Endocrinology and Metabolism, 94*(3), 907–913. https://doi.org/10.1210/jc.2008-1902

Brown, R. L., & Robinson, P. R. (2004). Melanopsin - Shedding light on the elusive circadian photopigment. *Chronobiology International, 21*(2), 189–204. https://doi.org/10.1081/CBI-120037816

Buxton, O. M., & Marcelli, E. (2010). Short and long sleep are positively associated with obesity, diabetes, hypertension, and cardiovascular disease among adults in the United States. *Social Science & Medicine (1982), 71*(5), 1027–1036. https://doi.org/10.1016/j.socscimed.2010.05.041

Cajochen, C., Münch, M., Kobialka, S., Kräuchi, K., Steiner, R., Oelhafen, P., Orgül, S., & Wirz-Justice, A. (2005). High sensitivity of human melatonin, alertness, thermoregulation, and heart rate to short wavelength light. *Journal of Clinical Endocrinology and Metabolism, 90*(3), 1311–1316. https://doi.org/10 .1210/jc.2004-0957

Cappuccio, F. P., Cooper, D., Delia, L., Strazzullo, P., & Miller, M. A. (2011). Sleep duration predicts cardiovascular outcomes: a systematic review and meta-analysis of prospective studies. *European Heart Journal, 32*(12), 1484–1492. https://doi.org/10.1093/eurheartj/ehr007

Cappuccio, F. P., Stranges, S., Kandala, N. B., Miller, M. A., Taggart, F. M., Kumari, M., Ferrie, J. E., Shipley, M. J., Brunner, E. J., & Marmot, M. G. (2007). Gender-specific associations of short sleep duration with prevalent and incident hypertension: the whitehall II study. *Hypertension, 50*(4), 693–700. https://doi .org/10.1161/HYPERTENSIONAHA.107.095471

Chen, C., Chen, J., Wang, Y., Liu, Z., & Wu, Y. (2021). Ferroptosis drives photoreceptor degeneration in mice with defects in all-trans-retinal clearance. *Journal of Biological Chemistry, 296*(20), 100187. https://doi .org/10.1074/JBC.RA120.015779

Chen, Y., Okano, K., Maeda, T., Chauhan, V., Golczak, M., Maeda, A., & Palczewski, K. (2012). Mechanism of all-trans-retinal toxicity with implications for stargardt disease and age-related macular degeneration. *Journal of Biological Chemistry, 287*(7), 5059–5069. https://doi.org/10.1074/jbc.M111.315432

Chistiakov, D. A., Sobenin, I. A., Revin, V. V., Orekhov, A. N., & Bobryshev, Y. V. (2014). Mitochondrial aging and age-related dysfunction of mitochondria. *BioMed Research International, 2014*. https://doi .org/10.1155/2014/238463

Cho. (2016). Laser light therapy in inflammatory, musculoskeletal, and autoimmune disease. *Physiology & Behavior, 176*(1), 100–106. https://doi.org/10.1007/s11882-019-0869-z

Christensen, M. A., Bettencourt, L., Kaye, L., Moturu, S. T., Nguyen, K. T., Olgin, J. E., Pletcher, M. J., & Marcus, G. M. (2016). Direct measurements of smartphone screen-time: relationships with demographics and sleep. *PLoS ONE*, *11*(11), 1–14. https://doi.org/10.1371/journal.pone.0165331

Cox, K. H., & Takahashi, J. S. (2019). Circadian clock genes and the transcriptional architecture of the clock mechanism. *Journal of Molecular Endocrinology*, *63*(4), 93–102. https://doi.org/10.1530/JME-19-0153

Crawford, M. A., Leigh Broadhurst, C., Guest, M., Nagar, A., Wang, Y., Ghebremeskel, K., & Schmidt, W. F. (2013). A quantum theory for the irreplaceable role of docosahexaenoic acid in neural cell signalling throughout evolution. *Prostaglandins Leukotrienes and Essential Fatty Acids*, *88*(1), 5–13. https://doi.org/10.1016/j.plefa.2012.08.005

Czeisler, C. A., Duffy, J. F., Shanahan, T. L., Brown, E. N., Mitchell, J. F., Rimmer, D. W., Ronda, J. M., Silva, E. J., Allan, J. S., Emens, J. S., Dijk, D. J., & Kronauer, R. E. (1999). Stability, precision, and near-24-hour period of the human circadian pacemaker. *Science*, *284*(5423), 2177–2181. https://doi.org/10.1126/science.284.5423.2177

Dibner, C., Schibler, U., & Albrecht, U. (2010). The mammalian circadian timing system: organization and coordination of central and peripheral clocks. *Annual Review of Physiology*, *72*, 517–549. https://doi.org/10.1146/annurev-physiol-021909-135821

Dixon, S. J., Lemberg, K. M., Lamprecht, M. R., Skouta, R., Zaitsev, E. M., Gleason, C. E., Patel, D. N., Bauer, A. J., Cantley, A. M., Yang, W. S., Morrison, B., & Stockwell, B. R. (2012). Ferroptosis: an iron-dependent form of nonapoptotic cell death. *Cell*, *149*(5), 1060–1072. https://doi.org/10.1016/j.cell.2012.03.042

Duffield, G. E., Best, J. D., Meurers, B. H., Bittner, A., Loros, J. J., & Dunlap, J. C. (2002). Circadian programs of transcriptional activation, signaling, and protein turnover revealed by microarray analysis of mammalian cells. *Current Biology*, *12*(7), 551–557. https://doi.org/10.1016/S0960-9822(02)00765-0

Duvall, M. G., & Levy, B. D. (1998). DHA- and EPA-derived resolvins, protectins, and maresins in airway inflammation. *Chest*, *114*(4), 290S. https://doi.org/10.1378/chest.114.4_supplement.290s

Espiritu, R. C., Kripke, D. F., Ancoli-Israel, S., Mowen, M. A., Mason, W. J., Fell, R. L., Klauber, M. R., & Kaplan, O. J. (1994). Low illumination experienced by San Diego adults: association with atypical depressive symptoms. *Biological Psychiatry*, *35*(6), 403–407. https://doi.org/10.1016/0006-3223(94)90007-8

Fan, W., Waymire, K. G., Narula, N., Li, P., Rocher, C., Coskun, P. E., Vannan, M. A., Narula, J., MacGregor, G. R., & Wallace, D. C. (2008). A mouse model of mitochondrial disease reveals germline selection against severe mtDNA mutations. *Science*, *319*(5865), 958–962. https://doi.org/10.1126/science.1147786

Foletti, A., Lisi, A., Ledda, M., de Carlo, F., & Grimaldi, S. (2009). Cellular ELF signals as a possible tool in informative medicine. *Electromagnetic Biology and Medicine*, *28*(1), 71–79. https://doi.org/10.1080/15368370802708801

Friesen, D. E., Craddock, T. J. A., Kalra, A. P., & Tuszynski, J. A. (2015). Biological wires, communication systems, and implications for disease. *Bio Systems*, *127*, 14–27. https://doi.org/10.1016/j.biosystems.2014.10.006

Fukushige, H., Fukuda, Y., Tanaka, M., Inami, K., Wada, K., Tsumura, Y., Kondo, M., Harada, T., Wakamura, T., & Morita, T. (2014). Effects of tryptophan-rich breakfast and light exposure during the daytime on melatonin secretion at night. *Journal of Physiological Anthropology*, *33*(1), 1–9. https://doi.org/10.1186/1880-6805-33-33

Gallicchio, L., & Kalesan, B. (2009). Sleep duration and mortality: a systematic review and meta-analysis. *Journal of Sleep Research*, *18*(2), 148–158. https://doi.org/10.1111/j.1365-2869.2008.00732.x

Gamble, K. L., Berry, R., Frank, S. J., & Young, M. E. (2015). Circadian clock control of endocrine factors. *Nature Reviews Endocrinology*, *10*(8), 466–475. https://doi.org/10.1038/nrendo.2014.78

García-Giménez, J.-L., Garcés, C., Romá-Mateo, C., & Pallardó, F. V. (2021). Oxidative stress-mediated alterations in histone post-translational modifications. *Free Radical Biology & Medicine*, *170*, 6–18. https://doi.org/10.1016/j.freeradbiomed.2021.02.027

Garcia-Saenz, A., De Miguel, A. S., Espinosa, A., Costas, L., Aragonés, N., Tonne, C., Moreno, V., Pérez-Gómez, B., Valentin, A., Pollán, M., Castaño-Vinyals, G., Aubé, M., & Kogevinas, M. (2020). Association between outdoor light-at-night exposure and colorectal cancer in Spain. *Epidemiology*, *31*(5), 718–727. https://doi.org/10.1097/EDE.0000000000001226

Garcia-Saenz, A., de Miguel, A. S., Espinosa, A., Valentin, A., Aragonés, N., Llorca, J., Amiano, P., Sánchez, V. M., Guevara, M., Capelo, R., Tardón, A., Peiró-Perez, R., Jiménez-Moleón, J. J., Roca-Barceló, A., Pérez-Gómez, B., Dierssen-Sotos, T., Fernández-Villa, T., Moreno-Iribas, C., Moreno, V., … & Kogevinas, M. (2018). Evaluating the association between artificial light-at-night exposure and breast and prostate cancer risk in Spain (Mcc-spain study). *Environmental Health Perspectives*, *126*(4), 1–11. https://doi.org/10.1289/EHP1837

Gawrisch, K., & Soubiasr, O. (2014). Structure and dynamics of polyunsaturated hydrocarbon chains in lipid bilayers: significance for GPCR function. *Bone*, *23*(1), 1–7. https://www.ncbi.nlm.nih.gov/pmc/articles/PMC3624763/pdf/nihms412728.pdf

Genuardi, M. V., Ogilvie, R. P., Saand, A. R., DeSensi, R. S., Saul, M. I., Magnani, J. W., & Patel, S. R. (2019). Association of short sleep duration and atrial fibrillation. *Chest*, *156*(3), 544–552. https://doi.org/10.1016/j.chest.2019.01.033

Giles, R. E., Blanc, H., Cann, H. M., & Wallace, D. C. (1980). Maternal inheritance of human mitochondrial DNA. *Proceedings of the National Academy of Sciences of the United States of America*, *77*(11 I), 6715–6719. https://doi.org/10.1073/pnas.77.11.6715

Godley, B. F., Shamsi, F. A., Liang, F. Q., Jarrett, S. G., Davies, S., & Boulton, M. (2005). Blue light induces mitochondrial DNA damage and free radical production in epithelial cells. *Journal of Biological Chemistry*, *280*(22), 21061–21066. https://doi.org/10.1074/jbc.M502194200

Gooley, J. J., Lu, J., Chou, T. C., Scammell, T. E., & Saper, C. B. (2001). Melanopsin in cells of origin of the retinohypothalamic tract. *Nature Neuroscience*, *4*(12), 1165. https://doi.org/10.1038/nn768

Hackett, R. A., Steptoe, A., & Kumari, M. (2014). Association of diurnal patterns in salivary cortisol with type 2 diabetes in the Whitehall II study. *Journal of Clinical Endocrinology and Metabolism*, *99*(12), 4625–4631. https://doi.org/10.1210/jc.2014-2459

Hashimoto, M., Hossain, S., Al Mamun, A., Matsuzaki, K., & Arai, H. (2017). Docosahexaenoic acid: one molecule diverse functions. *Critical Reviews in Biotechnology*, *37*(5), 579–597. https://doi.org/10.1080/07388551.2016.1207153

Hattar, S., Liao, H. W., Takao, M., Berson, D. M., & Yau, K. W. (2002). Melanopsin-containing retinal ganglion cells: architecture, projections, and intrinsic photosensitivity. *Science*, *295*(5557), 1065–1070. https://doi.org/10.1126/science.1069609

Heo, J.-Y., Kim, K., Fava, M., Mischoulon, D., Papakostas, G. I., Kim, M.-J., Kim, D. J., Chang, K.-A. J., Oh, Y., Yu, B.-H., & Jeon, H. J. (2017). Effects of smartphone use with and without blue light at night in healthy adults: a randomized, double-blind, cross-over, placebo-controlled comparison. *Journal of Psychiatric Research*, *87*, 61–70. https://doi.org/10.1016/j.jpsychires.2016.12.010

Hill, J. H., Chen, Z., & Xu, H. (2014). Selective propagation of functional mitochondrial DNA during oogenesis restricts the transmission of a deleterious mitochondrial variant. *Nature Genetics*, *46*(4), 389–392. https://doi.org/10.1038/ng.2920

Horwitz, J., & Heller, J. (1973). Interactions of all-trans-, 9-, 1 l-, and 13-&-retinal, all-trans- retinyl acetate, and retinoic acid with human retinol-binding protein and prealbumin. *Journal of Biological Chemistry*, *248*(18), 6317–6324. https://doi.org/10.1016/S0021-9258(19)43450-9

Hurley, S., Goldberg, D., Nelson, D., Hertz, A., Horn-Ross, P. L., Bernstein, L., & Reynolds, P. (2014). Light at night and breast cancer risk among california teachers. *Epidemiology*, *25*(5), 697–706. https://doi.org/10.1097/EDE.0000000000000137

Irwin, A. (2018). The dark side of light. *Nature*, *553*, 268–270.

James, P., Bertrand, K. A., Hart, J. E., Schernhammer, E. S., Tamimi, R. M., & Laden, F. (2017). Outdoor light at night and breast cancer incidence in the nurses' health study II. *Environmental Health Perspectives*, *125*(8). https://doi.org/10.1289/EHP935

Janků, K., Šmotek, M., Fárková, E., & Kopřivová, J. (2020). Block the light and sleep well: evening blue light filtration as a part of cognitive behavioral therapy for insomnia. *Chronobiology International*, *37*(2), 248–259. https://doi.org/10.1080/07420528.2019.1692859

Jasser, S. A., Blask, D. E., & Brainard, G. C. (2006). Light during darkness and cancer: relationships in circadian photoreception and tumor biology. *Cancer Causes and Control*, *17*(4), 515–523. https://doi.org/10.1007/s10552-005-9013-6

Johnson, T. B., Salisbury, F. B., & Connor, G. I. (1967). Ratio of blue to red light: a brief increase following sunset. *Science*, *155*(3770), 1663–1665. https://doi.org/10.1126/science.155.3770.1663

Kakizaki, M., Kuriyama, S., Sone, T., Ohmori-Matsuda, K., Hozawa, A., Nakaya, N., Fukudo, S., & Tsuji, I. (2008). Sleep duration and the risk of breast cancer: the Ohsaki Cohort Study. *British Journal of Cancer*, *99*(9), 1502–1505. https://doi.org/10.1038/sj.bjc.6604684

Katya Frazier, E. B. C. (2017). Intersection of the gut microbiome and circadian rhythms in metabolism. *Physiology & Behavior*, *176*(3), 139–148. https://doi.org/10.1016/j.tem.2019.08.013.Intersection

Kayumov, L., Casper, R. F., Hawa, R. J., Perelman, B., Chung, S. A., Sokalsky, S., & Shapiro, C. M. (2005). Blocking low-wavelength light prevents nocturnal melatonin suppression with no adverse effect on performance during simulated shift work. *Journal of Clinical Endocrinology and Metabolism*, *90*(5), 2755–2761. https://doi.org/10.1210/jc.2004-2062

Kerényi, N. A., Sótonyi, P., & Somogyi, E. (1975). Localizing acethyl-serotonin transferase by electron microscopy. *Histochemistry*, *46*(1), 77–80. https://doi.org/10.1007/BF02463562

Kinosita, K., Yasuda, R., Noji, H., & Adachi, K. (2000). A rotary molecular motor that can work at near 100% efficiency. *Philosophical Transactions of the Royal Society B: Biological Sciences*, *355*(1396), 473–489. https://doi.org/10.1098/rstb.2000.0589

Kojetin, D. J., & Burris, T. P. (2014). REV-ERB and ROR nuclear receptors as drug targets. *Nature Reviews Drug Discovery*, *13*(3), 197–216. https://doi.org/10.1038/nrd4100.REV-ERB

Kornmann, B., Schaad, O., Bujard, H., Takahashi, J. S., & Schibler, U. (2007). System-driven and oscillator-dependent circadian transcription in mice with a conditionally active liver clock. *PLoS Biology*, *5*(2), 0179–0189. https://doi.org/10.1371/journal.pbio.0050034

Kumari, M., Chandola, T., Brunner, E., & Kivimaki, M. (2010). A nonlinear relationship of generalized and central obesity with diurnal cortisol secretion in the Whitehall II study. *Journal of Clinical Endocrinology and Metabolism*, *95*(9), 4415–4423. https://doi.org/10.1210/jc.2009-2105

Kumari, M., Shipley, M., Stafford, M., & Kivimaki, M. (2011). Association of diurnal patterns in salivary cortisol with all-cause and cardiovascular mortality: findings from the Whitehall II study. *Journal of Clinical Endocrinology and Metabolism*, *96*(5), 1478–1485. https://doi.org/10.1210/jc.2010-2137

Kuss, D. J., & Griffiths, M. D. (2011). Online social networking and addiction: a review of the psychological literature. *International Journal of Environmental Research and Public Health*, *8*(9), 3528–3552. https://doi.org/10.3390/ijerph8093528

Kuss, D. J., & Lopez-Fernandez, O. (2016). Internet addiction and problematic Internet use: a systematic review of clinical research. *World Journal of Psychiatry*, *6*(1), 143. https://doi.org/10.5498/wjp.v6.i1.143

Kusumoto, J., Takeo, M., Hashikawa, K., Komori, T., Tsuji, T., Terashi, H., & Sakakibara, S. (2020). OPN4 belongs to the photosensitive system of the human skin. *Genes to Cells*, *25*(3), 215–225. https://doi.org/10.1111/gtc.12751

Kvaskoff, M., & Weinstein, P. (2010). Are some melanomas caused by artificial light? *Medical Hypotheses*, *75*(3), 305–311. https://doi.org/10.1016/j.mehy.2010.03.010

Kyba, C. C. M., Kuester, T., Miguel De, A. S., Baugh, K., Jechow, A., Hölker, F., Bennie, J., Elvidge, C. D., Gaston, K. J., & Guanter, L. (2017). Artificially lit surface of Earth at night increasing in radiance and extent. *Science Advances*, *3*, November, 1–9, e1701528.

Latorre-Pellicer, A., Lechuga-Vieco, A. V., Johnston, I. G., Hämäläinen, R. H., Pellico, J., Justo-Méndez, R., Fernández-Toro, J. M., Clavería, C., Guaras, A., Sierra, R., Llop, J., Torres, M., Criado, L. M., Suomalainen, A., Jones, N. S., Ruíz-Cabello, J., & Enríquez, J. A. (2019). Regulation of mother-to-offspring transmission of mtDNA heteroplasmy. *Cell Metabolism*, *30*(6), 1120-1130.e5. https://doi.org/10.1016/j.cmet.2019.09.007

Le Guen, M., Chaté, V., Hininger-Favier, I., Laillet, B., Morio, B., Pieroni, G., Schlattner, U., Pison, C., & Dubouchaud, H. (2016). A 9-wk docosahexaenoic acid-enriched supplementation improves endurance exercise capacity and skeletal muscle mitochondrial function in adult rats. *American Journal of Physiology: Endocrinology and Metabolism*, *310*(3), E213–E224. https://doi.org/10.1152/ajpendo.00468.2014

Lerner, A. B., Case, J. D., Takahashi, Y., Lee, T. H., & Mori, W. (1958). Isolation of melatonin, the pineal gland factor that lightens melanocytes1. *Journal of the American Chemical Society*, *80*(10), 2587. https://doi.org/10.1021/ja01543a060

Li, J., Cao, F., Yin, H. L., Huang, Z. J., Lin, Z. T., Mao, N., Sun, B., & Wang, G. (2020). Ferroptosis: past, present and future. *Cell Death and Disease*, *11*(2). https://doi.org/10.1038/s41419-020-2298-2

Li, Z., & Pollack, G. H. (2020). Surface-induced flow: A natural microscopic engine using infrared energy as fuel. *Science Advances*, *6*(19), eaba0941. https://doi.org/10.1126/sciadv.aba0941

Lockley, S. W., Brainard, G. C., & Czeisler, C. A. (2003). High sensitivity of the human circadian melatonin rhythm to resetting by short wavelength light. *Journal of Clinical Endocrinology and Metabolism*, *88*(9), 4502–4505. https://doi.org/10.1210/jc.2003-030570

Logan, D. C. (2003). Mitochondrial dynamics. *New Phytologist*, *160*(3), 463–478. https://doi.org/10.1046/j.1469-8137.2003.00918.x

Ma, Q.-Q., Yao, Q., Lin, L., Chen, G.-C., & Yu, J.-B. (2016). Sleep duration and total cancer mortality: a meta-analysis of prospective studies. *Sleep Medicine*, *27–28*, 39–44. https://doi.org/10.1016/j.sleep.2016.06.036

Maeda, A., Maeda, T., Golczak, M., Chou, S., Desai, A., Hoppel, C. L., Matsuyama, S., & Palczewski, K. (2009). Involvement of all-trans-retinal in acute light-induced retinopathy of mice. *Journal of Biological Chemistry*, *284*(22), 15173–15183. https://doi.org/10.1074/jbc.M900322200

Malis, C. D., Weber, P. C., Leaf, A., & Bonventre, J. V. (1990). Incorporation of marine lipids into mitochondrial membranes increases susceptibility to damage by calcium and reactive oxygen species: evidence for enhanced activation of phospholipase A2 in mitochondria enriched with n-3 fatty acids. *Proceedings of the National Academy of Sciences of the United States of America, 87*(22), 8845–8849. https://doi.org /10.1073/pnas.87.22.8845

Mallon, L., Broman, J. E., & Hetta, J. (2005). High incidence of diabetes in men with sleep complaints or short sleep duration: a 12-year follow-up study of a middle-aged population. *Diabetes Care, 28*(11), 2762–2767. https://doi.org/10.2337/diacare.28.11.2762

Mangelsdorf, D. J., Thummel, C., Beato, M., Herrlich, P., Schiitq, G., Umesono, K., Blumberg, B., Kastner, P., Mark, M., Chambon, P., & Evan, R. M. (1995). The nuclear receptor superfamily: the second decade. *Cell, 83*, 835–839.

Massudi, H., Grant, R., Guillemin, G. J., & Braidy, N. (2012). NAD + metabolism and oxidative stress: the golden nucleotide on a crown of thorns. *Redox Report, 17*(1), 28–46. https://doi.org/10.1179/1351000212Y .0000000001

Mayes, L. A., McGuire, L., Page, G. G., Goodin, B. R., Edwards, R. R., & Haythornthwaite, J. (2014). The association of the cortisol awakening response with experimental pain ratings. *Bone, 23*(1), 1–7. https:// doi.org/10.1016/j.psyneuen.2009.03.008

MITOMAP. (2015). https://www.mitomap.org/foswiki/pub/MITOMAP/MitomapFigures/WorldMigrations2012. pdf

Mong, J. A., Baker, F. C., Mahoney, M. M., Paul, K. N., Schwartz, M. D., Semba, K., & Silver, R. (2011). Sleep, rhythms, and the endocrine brain: influence of sex and gonadal hormones. *Journal of Neuroscience, 31*(45), 16107–16116. https://doi.org/10.1523/JNEUROSCI.4175-11.2011

Montagnier, L., Del Giudice, E., Aïssa, J., Lavallee, C., Motschwiller, S., Capolupo, A., Polcari, A., Romano, P., Tedeschi, A., & Vitiello, G. (2015). Transduction of DNA information through water and electromagnetic waves. *Electromagnetic Biology and Medicine, 34*(2), 106–112. https://doi.org/10.3109/15368378 .2015.1036072

Morgenthaler, T. I., Lee-Chiong, T., Alessi, C., Friedman, L., Aurora, R. N., Boehlecke, B., Brown, T., Chesson, A. L., Kapur, V., Maganti, R., Owens, J., Pancer, J., Swick, T. J., & Zak, R. (2007). Practice parameters for the clinical evaluation and treatment of circadian rhythm sleep disorders: an American Academy of Sleep Medicine report. *Sleep, 30*(11), 1445–1459. https://doi.org/10.1093 /sleep/30.11.1445

Morin, L. P., & Allen, C. N. (2006). The circadian visual system, 2005. *Brain Research Reviews, 51*(1), 1–60. https://doi.org/10.1016/j.brainresrev.2005.08.003

Morita, T., & Tokura, H. (1998). The influence of different wavelengths of light on human biological rhythms. *Applied Human Science: Journal of Physiological Anthropology, 17*(3), 91–96. https://doi.org/10.2114 /jpa.17.91

Morris, C. J., Aeschbach, D., & Scheer, F. A. J. L. (2012). Circadian system, sleep and endocrinology. *Molecular and Cellular Endocrinology, 349*(1), 91–104. https://doi.org/10.1016/j.mce.2011.09.003.Circadian

Moser, C. C., Farid, T. A., Chobot, S. E., & Dutton, P. L. (2006). Electron tunneling chains of mitochondria. *Biochimica et Biophysica Acta (BBA)-Bioenergetic, 1757*, 1096–1109. https://doi.org/10.1016/j.bbabio .2006.04.015

Nakade, M., Akimitsu, O., Wada, K., Krejci, M., Noji, T., Taniwaki, N., & Takeuchi, H. (2012). Can breakfast tryptophan and vitamin B6 intake and morning exposure to sunlight promote morning-typology in young children aged 2 to 6 years? *Journal of Physiological Anthropology, 31*, Article number 11. https:// doi.org/10.1186/1880-6805-31-11.

Nokin, J., Vekemans, M., L'hermite, M., & Robyn, C. (1972). Circadian periodicity of serum prolactin concentration in man. *British Medical Journal, 3*(5826), 561–562. https://doi.org/10.1136/bmj.3.5826.561

Oishi, K., Shiota, M., Sakamoto, K., Kasamatsu, M., & Ishida, N. (2004). Feeding is not a more potent Zeitgeber than the light-dark cycle in Drosophila. *Neuroreport, 15*(4), 739–743. https://doi.org/10.1097 /00001756-200403220-00034

Ondrusova, K., Fatehi, M., Barr, A., Czarnecka, Z., Long, W., Suzuki, K., Campbell, S., Philippaert, K., Hubert, M., Kwan, P., Touret, N., Wabitsch, M., Lee, K. Y., & Light, P. E. (2017). Subcutaneous white adipocytes express a light sensitive signaling pathway mediated via a melanopsin / TRPC channel axis. *Scientific Reports, October*, 1–9. https://doi.org/10.1038/s41598-017-16689-4

Ouyang, X., Yang, J., Hong, Z., Wu, Y., Xie, Y., & Wang, G. (2020). Mechanisms of blue light-induced eye hazard and protective measures: a review. *Biomedicine & Pharmacotherapy, 130*(June), 110577. https:// doi.org/10.1016/j.biopha.2020.110577

Panda, S., Antoch, M. P., Miller, B. H., Su, A. I., Schook, A. B., Straume, M., Schultz, P. G., Kay, S. A., Takahashi, J. S., & Hogenesch, J. B. (2002). Coordinated transcription of key pathways in the mouse by the circadian clock. *Cell*, *109*(3), 307–320. https://doi.org/10.1016/S0092-8674(02)00722-5

Panda, S., Nayak, S. K., Campo, B., Walker, J. R., Hogenesch, J. B., & Jegla, T. (2005). Illumination of the melanopsin signaling pathway. *Science*, *307*(5709), 600–604. https://doi.org/10.1126/science.1105121

Panda, S. (2016). Circadian physiology of metabolism. *Physiology & Behavior*, *176*(12), 139–148. https://doi.org/10.1126/science.aah4967

Pang, J., Seko, Y., Tokoro, T., Ichinose, S., & Yamamoto, H. (1998). Observation of ultrastructural changes in cultured retinal pigment epithelium following exposure to blue light. *Graefe's Archive for Clinical and Experimental Ophthalmology*, *236*(9), 696–701. https://doi.org/10.1007/s004170050143

Parekh, P. K., Ozburn, A. R., & McClung, C. A. (2015). Circadian clock genes: effects on dopamine, reward and addiction. *Alcohol*, *49*(4), 341–349. https://doi.org/10.1016/j.alcohol.2014.09.034

Park, Y. M. M., White, A. J., Jackson, C. L., Weinberg, C. R., & Sandler, D. P. (2019). Association of exposure to artificial light at night while sleeping with risk of obesity in women. *JAMA Internal Medicine*, *179*(8), 1061–1071. https://doi.org/10.1001/jamainternmed.2019.0571

Partridge, J. C., De Grip, W. J. (1991) A new template for rhodopsin (vitamin A1 based) visual pigments. *Vision Research 31*, 619–630.

Passegué, E. (2021). Mitochondrial gatekeeper of cell death by ferroptosis. *News & Views*, *593*, 514–515.

Picard, M., Mcewen, B. S., Epel, E. S., & Sandi, C. (2018). An energetic view of stress: focus on mitochondria. *Frontiers in Neuroendocrinology, 49*(January), 72–85. https://doi.org/10.1016/j.yfrne.2018.01.001

Picard, M., McManus, M. J., Csordás, G., Várnai, P., Dorn, G. W., Williams, D., Hajnóczky, G., & Wallace, D. C. (2015). Trans-mitochondrial coordination of cristae at regulated membrane junctions. *Nature Communications*, *6*, 4–11. https://doi.org/10.1038/ncomms7259

Picard, M., Zhang, J., Hancock, S., Derbeneva, O., Golhar, R., Golik, P., O'Hearn, S., Levy, S., Potluri, P., Lvova, M., Davila, A., Lin, C. S., Perin, J. C., Rappaport, E. F., Hakonarson, H., Trounce, I. A., Procaccio, V., & Wallace, D. C. (2014). Progressive increase in mtDNA 3243 A G heteroplasmy causes abrupt transcriptional reprogramming. *Proceedings of the National Academy of Sciences of the United States of America*, *111*(38), E4033–E4042. https://doi.org/10.1073/pnas.1414028111

Pieri, C., Marra, M., Moroni, F., Recchioni, R., & Marcheselli, F. (1994). Melatonin: a peroxyl radical scavenger more effective than vitamin E. *Life Sciences*, *55*(15), 271–276. https://doi.org/10.1016/0024-3205(94)00666-0

Pollack, G. H., Figueroa, X., & Zhao, Q. (2009). Molecules, water, and radiant energy: new clues for the origin of life. *International Journal of Molecular Sciences*, *10*(4), 1419–1429. https://doi.org/10.3390/ijms10041419

Portaluppi, F., Tiseo, R., Smolensky, M. H., Hermida, R. C., Ayala, D. E., & Fabbian, F. (2012). Circadian rhythms and cardiovascular health. *Sleep Medicine Reviews*, *16*(2), 151–166. https://doi.org/10.1016/j.smrv.2011.04.003

Prayag, A. S., Najjar, R. P., & Gronfier, C. (2019). Melatonin suppression is exquisitely sensitive to light and primarily driven by melanopsin in humans. *Journal of Pineal Research*, *66*(4), 1–8. https://doi.org/10.1111/jpi.12562

Provencio, I., Rodriguez, I. R., Jiang, G., Hayes, W. P., Moreira, E. F., & Rollag, M. D. (2000). A novel human opsin in the inner retina. *Journal of Neuroscience*, *20*(2), 600–605. https://doi.org/10.1523/jneurosci.20-02-00600.2000

Rahman, S. A., Flynn-Evans, E. E., Aeschbach, D., Brainard, G. C., Czeisler, C. A., & Lockley, S. W. (2014). Diurnal spectral sensitivity of the acute alerting effects of light. *Sleep*, *37*(2), 271–281. https://doi.org/10.5665/sleep.3396

Ralph, M. R., Foster, R. G., Davis, F. C., & Menaker, M. (1990). Transplanted suprachiasmatic nucleus determines circadian period. *Science*, *247*(4945), 975–978. https://doi.org/10.1126/science.2305266

Raux-Demay, M.-C., & Girard, F. (1985). The physiology of corticotropin-releasing factor (CRF). *Reproduction Nutrition Development*, *25*(5), 931–943. https://doi.org/10.1051/rnd:19850709

Refinetti, R. (2015). Comparison of light, food, and temperature as environmental synchronizers of the circadian rhythm of activity in mice. *The Journal of Physiological Sciences*, 359–366. https://doi.org/10.1007/s12576-015-0374-7

Reid, K. J., Santostasi, G., Baron, K. G., Wilson, J., Kang, J., & Zee, P. C. (2014). Timing and intensity of light correlate with body weight in adults. *PLoS ONE*, *9*(4). https://doi.org/10.1371/journal.pone.0092251

Reiter, R., Sharma, R., & Ma, Q. (2020). Switching diseased cells from cytosolic aerobic glycolysis to mitochondrial oxidative phosphorylation: a metabolic rhythm regulated by melatonin? *Journal of Pineal Research*, 0–1. https://doi.org/10.1111/jpi.12677

Reiter, R J, Rollag, M. D., Panke, E. S., & Banks, A. F. (1978). *Melatonin: Reproductive Effects* (I. Nir, R. J. Reiter, & R. J. Wurtman (eds.), pp. 209–223). Springer.

Reiter, R. J. (1991). Melatonin: the chemical expression of darkness. *Molecular and Cellular Endocrinology*, *79*(1–3). https://doi.org/10.1016/0303-7207(91)90087-9

Reiter, R. J., Ma, Q., & Sharma, R. (2020). Melatonin in mitochondria: mitigating clear and present dangers. *Physiology*, *35*(2), 86–95. https://doi.org/10.1152/physiol.00034.2019

Reiter, R. J., Tan, D. X., Korkmaz, A., & Rosales-Corral, S. A. (2014). Melatonin and stable circadian rhythms optimize maternal, placental and fetal physiology. *Human Reproduction Update*, *20*(2), 293–307. https://doi.org/10.1093/humupd/dmt054

Reiter, R. J., Tan, D. X., Mayo, J. C., Sainz, R. M., Leon, J., & Czarnocki, Z. (2003). Melatonin as an anti-oxidant: biochemical mechanisms and pathophysiological implications in humans. *Acta Biochimica Polonica*, *50*(4), 1129–1146. https://doi.org/10.18388/abp.2003_3637

Rijo-Ferreira, F., & Takahashi, J. S. (2019). Genomics of circadian rhythms in health and disease. *Genome Medicine*, *11*(1), 1–16. https://doi.org/10.1186/s13073-019-0704-0

Rockwell, D. A. (1975). The jet lag syndrome. *Recenti Progressi in Medicina*, *90*(1), 1–3.

Romeo, S., Viaggi, C., Di Camillo, D., Willis, A. W., Lozzi, L., Rocchi, C., Capannolo, M., Aloisi, G., Vaglini, F., MacCarone, R., Caleo, M., Missale, C., Racette, B. A., Corsini, G. U., & Maggio, R. (2013). Bright light exposure reduces TH-positive dopamine neurons: implications of light pollution in Parkinson's disease epidemiology. *Scientific Reports*, *3*(3), 1–9. https://doi.org/10.1038/srep01395

Rosen, L. D., Lim, A. F., Felt, J., Carrier, L. M., Cheever, N. A., Lara-Ruiz, J. M., Mendoza, J. S., & Rokkum, J. (2014). Media and technology use predicts ill-being among children, preteens and teenagers independent of the negative health impacts of exercise and eating habits. *Bone*, *23*(1), 1–7. https://doi.org/10.1016/j.chb.2014.01.036.Media

Rosenthal, N. E., Sack, D. A., Gillin, J. C., Lewy, A. J., Frederick, K., Davenport, Y., Mueller, P. S., Newsome, D. A., & Wehr, T. A. (1984). Seasonal affective disorder. *Arch Gen Psychiatry*, *41*(January), 72–80.

Rottenberg, H. (1998). The generation of proton electrochemical potential gradient by cytochrome c oxidase.

Ruan, W., Yuan, X., & Eltzschig, H. K. (2021). Circadian rhythm as a therapeutic target. *Nature Reviews. Drug Discovery*, *20*(4), 287–307. https://doi.org/10.1038/s41573-020-00109-w

Sadun, A. A., Schaechter, J. D., & Smith, L. E. (1984). A retinohypothalamic pathway in man: light mediation of circadian rhythms. *Brain Research*, *302*(2), 371–377. https://doi.org/10.1016/0006-8993(84)90252-x

SanGiovanni, J. P., & Chew, E. Y. (2005). The role of omega-3 long-chain polyunsaturated fatty acids in health and disease of the retina. *Progress in Retinal and Eye Research*, *24*(1), 87–138. https://doi.org/10.1016/j.preteyeres.2004.06.002

Sanz, A., & Stefanatos, R. K. A. (2008). The mitochondrial free radical theory of aging: a critical view. *Current Aging Science*, *1*(1), 10–21. https://doi.org/10.2174/1874609810801010010

Savides, T. J., Messin, S., Senger, C., & Kripke, D. F. (1986). Natural light exposure of young adults. *Physiology & Behavior*, *38*(4), 571–574. https://doi.org/10.1016/0031-9384(86)90427-0

Scheer, F. A. J. L., Chan, J. L., & Fargnoli, J. (2010). Day/night variations of high-molecular-weight adiponectin and lipocalin-2 in healthy men studied under fed and fasted conditions. *Diabetologia*, *53*(11), 2401–2405. https://doi.org/10.1007/s00125-010-1869-7

Scott, B. L., & Bazan, N. G. (1989). Membrane docosahexaenoate is supplied to the developing brain and retina by the liver. *Proceedings of the National Academy of Sciences of the United States of America*, *86*(8), 2903–2907. https://doi.org/10.1073/pnas.86.8.2903

Scrima, R., Cela, O., Merla, G., Augello, B., Rubino, R., Quarato, G., Fugetto, S., Menga, M., Fuhr, L., Relógio, A., Piccoli, C., Mazzoccoli, G., & Capitanio, N. (2016). Clock-genes and mitochondrial respiratory activity: evidence of a reciprocal interplay. *BBA - Bioenergetics*, *1857*(8), 1344–1351. https://doi.org/10.1016/j.bbabio.2016.03.035

Seko, Y., Pang, J., Tokoro, T., Ichinose, S., & Mochizuki, M. (2001). Blue light-induced apoptosis in cultured retinal pigment epithelium cells of the rat. *Graefe's Archive for Clinical and Experimental Ophthalmology*, *239*(1), 47–52. https://doi.org/10.1007/s004170000220

Serhan, C. N., & Levy, B. D. (2018). Resolvins in inflammation: emergence of the pro-resolving superfamily of mediators. *Journal of Clinical Investigation*, *128*(7), 2657–2669. https://doi.org/10.1172/JCI97943

Shaban, H., & Richter, C. (2002). A2E and blue light in the retina: the paradigm of age-related macular degeneration. *Biol. Chem*, *383*, 537–545.

Shi, W., Yang, Y., Gao, M., Wu, J., Tao, N., & Wang, S. (2021). Optical imaging of electrical and mechanical couplings between cells. *ACS Sensors*, *6*(2), 508–512. https://doi.org/10.1021/acssensors.0c02058

Sikka, G., Hussmann, G. P., Pandey, D., Cao, S., Hori, D., Park, J. T., Steppan, J., Kim, J. H., Barodka, V., Myers, A. C., Santhanam, L., Nyhan, D., Halushka, M. K., Koehler, R. C., Snyder, S. H., Shimoda, L. A., & Berkowitz, D. E. (2014). Melanopsin mediates light-dependent relaxation in blood vessels. *Proceedings of the National Academy of Sciences of the United States of America*, *111*(50), 17977–17982. https://doi.org/10.1073/pnas.1420258111

Smick, K., Villette, T., Boulton, M. E., Brainard, G. C., Jones, W., Karpecki, P., Melton, R., Thomas, R., Sliney, D. H., Shechtman, D. L., & Grayson, M. (2013). Blue light hazard: new knowledge, new approaches to maintaining ocular health. *Report of a Roundtable (Essilor of Americas)*, 1–12.

Sommer, A. P., Haddad, M. K., & Fecht, H. J. (2015). Light effect on water viscosity: implication for ATP biosynthesis. *Scientific Reports*, *5*, 1–6. https://doi.org/10.1038/srep12029

Sonoda, T., & Lee, S. K. (2016). A novel role for the visual retinoid cycle in melanopsin chromophore regeneration. *Journal of Neuroscience*, *36*(35), 9016–9018. https://doi.org/10.1523/JNEUROSCI.1883-16.2016

Sonoda, T., & Schmidt, T. M. (2016). Re-evaluating the role of intrinsically photosensitive retinal ganglion cells: new roles in image-forming functions. *Integrative and Comparative Biology*, *56*(5), 834–841. https://doi.org/10.1093/icb/icw066

Sparrow, J. R., Zhou, J., & Cai, B. (2003). DNA is a target of the photodynamic effects elicited in A2E-laden RPE by blue-light illumination. *Investigative Ophthalmology and Visual Science*, *44*(5), 2245–2251. https://doi.org/10.1167/iovs.02-0746

Sridhar, G. R., & Sanjana, N. S. N. (2016). Sleep, circadian dysrhythmia, obesity and diabetes. *World Journal of Diabetes*, *7*(19), 515. https://doi.org/10.4239/wjd.v7.i19.515

Stiglic, N., & Viner, R. M. (2019). Effects of screentime on the health and well-being of children and adolescents: a systematic review of reviews. *BMJ Open*, *9*(1). https://doi.org/10.1136/bmjopen-2018-023191

Sulli, G., Manoogian, E. N., Taub, P. R., & Panda, S. (2017). Training the circadian clock, clocking the drugs and drugging the clock to prevent, manage and treat chronic diseases. *Physiology & Behavior*, *176*(5), 139–148. https://doi.org/10.1016/j.tips.2018.07.003

Sun, Q., Avallone, L., Stolze, B., Araque, K. A., Özarda, Y., Jonklaas, J., Parikh, T., Welsh, K., Masika, L., & Soldin, S. J. (2020). Demonstration of reciprocal diurnal variation in human serum T3 and rT3 concentration demonstrated by mass spectrometric analysis and establishment of thyroid hormone reference intervals. *Therapeutic Advances in Endocrinology and Metabolism*, *11*, 1–7. https://doi.org/10.1177/2042018820922688

Taheri, S., Lin, L., Austin, D., Young, T., & Mignot, E. (2004). Short sleep duration is associated with reduced leptin, elevated ghrelin, and increased body mass index. *PLoS Medicine*, *1*(3), 210–217. https://doi.org/10.1371/journal.pmed.0010062

Takahashi, J. S., DeCoursey, P. J., Bauman, L., & Menaker, M. (1984). Spectral sensitivity of a novel photoreceptive system mediating entrainment of mammalian circadian rhythms. *Nature*, *308*(5955), 186–188. https://doi.org/10.1038/308186a0

Tan, D. X., Manchester, L. C., Qin, L., & Reiter, R. J. (2016). Melatonin: a mitochondrial targeting molecule involving mitochondrial protection and dynamics. *International Journal of Molecular Sciences*, *17*(12). https://doi.org/10.3390/ijms17122124

Tarocco, A., Caroccia, N., Morciano, G., Wieckowski, M. R., Ancora, G., Garani, G., & Pinton, P. (2019). Melatonin as a master regulator of cell death and inflammation: molecular mechanisms and clinical implications for newborn care. *Cell Death and Disease*, *10*(4). https://doi.org/10.1038/s41419-019-1556-7

Thapan, K., Arendt, J., & Skene, D. J. (2001). An action spectrum for melatonin suppression: evidence for a novel non-rod, non-cone photoreceptor system in humans. *Journal of Physiology*, *535*(1), 261–267. https://doi.org/10.1111/j.1469-7793.2001.t01-1-00261.x

Tinsley, J. N., Molodtsov, M. I., Prevedel, R., Wartmann, D., Espigulé-Pons, J., Lauwers, M., & Vaziri, A. (2016). Direct detection of a single photon by humans. *Nature Communications*, *7*. https://doi.org/10.1038/ncomms12172

Tuszyński, J. A., & Dixon, J. M. (2001). Quantitative analysis of the frequency spectrum of the radiation emitted by cytochrome oxidase enzymes. *Physical Review. E, Statistical, Nonlinear, and Soft Matter Physics*, *64*(5 Pt 1), 51915. https://doi.org/10.1103/PhysRevE.64.051915

Van Der Lely, S., Frey, S., Garbazza, C., Wirz-Justice, A., Jenni, O. G., Steiner, R., Wolf, S., Cajochen, C., Bromundt, V., & Schmidt, C. (2015). Blue blocker glasses as a countermeasure for alerting effects of evening light-emitting diode screen exposure in male teenagers. *Journal of Adolescent Health*, *56*(1), 113–119. https://doi.org/10.1016/j.jadohealth.2014.08.002

Voigt, R. M., Forsyth, C. B., & Keshavarzian, A. (2019). Circadian rhythms: a regulator of gastrointestinal health and dysfunction. *Expert Review of Gastroenterology and Hepatology*, *13*(5), 411–424. https://doi.org/10.1080/17474124.2019.1595588

Waggoner, S. N. (2020). Circadian rhythms in immunity. *Current Allergy and Asthma Reports*, *20*(1), 1–11. https://doi.org/10.1007/s11882-020-0896-9

Wahl, S., Engelhardt, M., Schaupp, P., Lappe, C., & Ivanov, I. V. (2019). The inner clock: blue light sets the human rhythm. *Journal of Biophotonics*, *12*(12), 1–14. https://doi.org/10.1002/jbio.201900102

Wallace, D. C. (2013). A mitochondrial bioenergetic etiology of disease. *Journal of Clinical Investigation*, *123*(4), 1405–1412. https://doi.org/10.1172/JCI61398

Wallace, D. C. (2015). Mitochondrial DNA variation in human radiation and disease. *Cell*, *163*(1), 33–38. https://doi.org/10.1016/j.cell.2015.08.067

Wallace, D. C. (2016). Mitochondrial DNA in evolution and disease. *Nature*, *535*, 498–500.

Wallace, R. (2010). Neural membrane signaling platforms. *International Journal of Molecular Sciences*, *11*(6), 2421–2442. https://doi.org/10.3390/ijms11062421

Wang, Y., Huang, W., Neil, A. O., Lan, Y., Aune, D., Wang, W., Yu, C., & Chen, X. (2020). Association between sleep duration and mortality risk among adults with type 2 diabetes: a prospective cohort study. *Diabetologia*, *63*(11), 2292–2304.

Wehr, T. A. (2001). Photoperiodism in humans and other primates: evidence and implications. *Journal of Biological Rhythms*, *16*(4), 348–364. https://doi.org/10.1177/074873001129002060

Wehr, T. A. (1991). The durations of human melatonin secretion and sleep respond to changes in daylength (photoperiod). *Journal of Clinical Endocrinology and Metabolism*, *73*(6), 1276–1280. https://doi.org/10.1210/jcem-73-6-1276

Wei, W., & Chinnery, P. F. (2020). Inheritance of mitochondrial DNA in humans: implications for rare and common diseases. *Journal of Internal Medicine*, *287*(6), 634–644. https://doi.org/10.1111/joim.13047

Weitzman, E. D. (1975). Neuro-endocrine pattern of secretion during the sleep–wake cycle of man. In W. H. Gispen, T. B. van Wimersma Greidanus, B. Bohus, & D. B. T.-P. in B. R. de Wied (Eds.), *Hormones, Homeostasis and the Brain* (Vol. 42, pp. 93–102). Elsevier. https://doi.org/10.1016/S0079-6123(08)63648-1

Whichelow, M. J., Sturge, R. A., Keen, H., Jarrett, R. J., Stimmler, L., & Grainger, S. (1974). *Diurnal Variation in Response to Intravenous Glucose*. March, 488–491.

White, A. J. (2001). Mitochondrial toxicity and HIV therapy. *Sexually Transmitted Infections*, *77*(3), 158–173. https://doi.org/10.1136/sti.77.3.158

Williams, C. J., Hu, F. B., Patel, S. R., & Mantzoros, C. S. (2007). Sleep duration and snoring in relation to biomarkers of cardiovascular disease risk among women with type 2 diabetes. *Diabetes Care*, *30*(5), 1233–1240. https://doi.org/10.2337/dc06-2107

Wood, S., & Loudon, A. (2014). Clocks for all seasons: unwinding the roles and mechanisms of circadian and interval timers in the hypothalamus and pituitary. *Journal of Endocrinology*, *222*(2). https://doi.org/10.1530/JOE-14-0141

Wu, J., Seregard, S., Spångberg, B., Oskarsson, M., & Chen, E. (1999). Blue light induced apoptosis in rat retina. *Eye*, *13*(4), 577–583. https://doi.org/10.1038/eye.1999.142

Wurtman, R. J. (1985). Melatonin as a hormone in humans: a history. *Yale Journal of Biology and Medicine*, *58*(6), 547–552.

Wüst, S., Wolf, J., Hellhammer, D. H., Federenko, I., Schommer, N., & Kirschbaum, C. (2000). The cortisol awakening response: normal values and confounds. *Noise & Health*, *2*(7), 79–88. http://www.ncbi.nlm.nih.gov/pubmed/12689474

Xiao, Q., James, P., Breheny, P., Jia, P., Park, Y., Zhang, D., Fisher, J. A., Ward, M. H., & Jones, R. R. (2020). Outdoor light at night and postmenopausal breast cancer risk in the NIH-AARP diet and health study. *International Journal of Cancer*, *147*(9), 2363–2372. https://doi.org/10.1002/ijc.33016

Yamagata, T., Skepner, J., & Yang, J. (2015). Targeting Th17 effector cytokines for the treatment of autoimmune diseases. *Archivum Immunologiae et Therapiae Experimentalis*, *63*(6), 405–414. https://doi.org/10.1007/s00005-015-0362-x

Yang, Y., & Sauve, A. A. (2016). NAD+ metabolism: bioenergetics, signaling and manipulation for therapy. *Biochimica et Biophysica Acta - Proteins and Proteomics*, *1864*(12), 1787–1800. https://doi.org/10.1016/j.bbapap.2016.06.014

Yokoyama, M., Chang, H., Anzai, H., & Kato, M. (2019). Effects of different light sources on neural activity of the paraventricular nucleus in the hypothalamus. *Medicina*, *55*(11). https://doi.org/10.3390/medicina55110732

Yu, X., Rollins, D., Ruhn, K. A., Stubblefield, J. J., Green, C. B., Kashiwada, M., Rothman, P. B., Takahashi, J. S., & Hooper, L. V. (2013). TH17 cell differentiation is regulated by the circadian clock. *Science*, *342*(6159), 727–730. https://doi.org/10.1126/science.1243884

Zhang, D., Jones, R. R., James, P., Kitahara, C. M., & Xiao, Q. (2021). Associations between artificial light at night and risk for thyroid cancer: a large US cohort study. *Cancer, 127*(9), 1448–1458. https://doi.org/10.1002/cncr.33392

Zhao, X., Cho, H., Yu, R. T., Atkins, A. R., Downes, M., & Evans, R. M. (2014). Nuclear receptors rock around the clock. *EMBO Reports, 15*(5), 518–528.

Ziegelberger, G. (2013). ICNIRP guidelines on limits of exposure to incoherent visible and infrared radiation. *Health Physics, 105*(1), 74–96. https://doi.org/10.1097/HP.0b013e318289a611

Zimmerman, M. E., Kim, M. B., Hale, C., Westwood, A. J., Brickman, A. M., & Shechter, A. (2019). Neuropsychological function response to nocturnal blue light blockage in individuals with symptoms of insomnia: a pilot randomized controlled study. *Journal of the International Neuropsychological Society, 25*(7), 668–677. https://doi.org/10.1097/00152192-200505002-00087

21 COVID-19

Pathogenesis and Nutritional Support for Prophylaxis and Symptom De-Escalation

Chris Newton

CONTENTS

DOI: 10.1201/b23304-23

21.1 INTRODUCTION

In December 2019, an increasing number of patients with pneumonia of unknown origin were reported in the City of Wuhan, China. On January 7, 2020, Chinese authorities indicated that the causal agent was a coronavirus, and by January 10, the same authorities provided a full sequence analysis. Electron microscopy of clinical samples indicated a virus of between 60 and 140 nm in diameter and with characteristic corona spikes. Further sequence analysis was conducted by several laboratories, apparently confirming a positive strand RNA virus with a total sequence length of around 29.8 kilobases. The genome organization was published in late January 2020.[1] The viral genome encodes a series of non-structural proteins, an RNA-dependent polymerase, a spike (S) glycoprotein, a membrane (M) glycoprotein, an envelope (E) glycoprotein and a nucleocapsid (N) protein.

21.2 PROXIMAL ORIGIN OF VIRUS

The infective origin of the virus was originally suggested to be the Huanan Seafood market. However, the first documented case was not linked to the market. The assertion that the proximal origin of the virus is bat with the intermediate carrier being pangolin is also problematic, as 1) the overall nucleotide and amino acid sequence homology for the closest (to SARS-CoV-2) coronavirus from pangolin is less than for the closest coronavirus from bat and 2) no virus isolated so far from bat or pangolin has the unique polybasic furin cleavage site of SARS-CoV-2.[2]

Sequence analysis has also demonstrated very high similarity from different patients, much greater than the 85.5% to 92.4% sequence similarity to the pangolin virus.[3] This implies that either the human virus evolved extremely rapidly or the virus had been in the human population for some considerable time. Studies on epitope mapping for T-cell reactivity are consistent with the assertion that we were exposed to something similar to SARS-CoV-2 some time before the current outbreak.[4] The fact that SARS-CoV-2 is so well adapted to humans has led to searching questions by a number of investigators as to the origin of the virus.[5–7] Given the sequence homology, the most likely proximal origin is a bat coronavirus, such as RaTG13.[7]

Since the original outbreak of SARS-CoV-2, the virus has gone through a series of mutations. At the time of the last update of this chapter, the European Centre for Disease Prevention and Control has listed Beta, Gamma, Delta and most recently (November 2021), Omicron as variants of concern. By far the largest number of mutations are apparent in the receptor binding domain (RBD) of the Omicron variant. Currently, this variant is proving to be highly infectious; however, the disease for most individuals is relatively mild.

21.3 MODE OF VIRUS ENTRY INTO HUMAN CELLS

The infectivity of SARS-CoV-2 for particular cells (tropism) is attributable in large part to the way the RBD of the spike protein trimer interacts with angiotensin converting enzyme 2 (ACE2) within the membrane of human cells. The original SARS-CoV of the 2003 outbreak also used the ACE2 protein as the receptor; however, RBD of SARS-CoV-2 is better adapted to binding the ACE2 protein.[8] Paradoxically, despite being better adapted, the affinity of the entire spike is actually similar to or less than that of SARS-CoV.[9] The reason for this is that the RBD is not fully exposed, and the spike requires a conformational change to allow the optimum binding of the RBD to ACE2. This conformational change is facilitated by proteolytic cleavage at the boundary between the S1 and S2 subunits of the spike.[9] The S1 subunit (N-terminal orientation) contains the RBD, whilst S2

(C-terminal orientation) contains the membrane fusion domain. Once cleaved at the S1/S2 interface, the RBD is optimally exposed, allowing strong interaction with ACE2 and also the further processing of the S2 subunit to form S2′. In this way the S2′ subunit is able to fuse with cell membranes, allowing uptake of the main body of the virus and the release of genomic material (RNA coding sequence).

Processing at the S1/S2 interface can be performed by three mechanisms. The first is dependent on the presence of the enzyme TMPRSS2, transmembrane protease serine 2. As the name suggests, this enzyme is present within cell membranes, and it can cleave the spike protein at the S1/S2 interface and also within S2 to produce S2′. The second mechanism is endosomal uptake of the virus. Once within endosomes, the virus must be released, and this is facilitated by cathepsin proteases. These cut the spike protein, allowing fusion with the endosome membrane and release of the virus genetic material into the infected cell. The third mechanism is arguably the most important, as it facilitates the pre-processing of the virus before cellular release. This relies on the presence of a polybasic furin cleavage site at the S1/S2 boundary. MERS-CoV and some other coronaviruses have furin cleavage sites, but this site was absent from SARS-CoV. Furin is a protease that cuts between the amino acids arginine and serine. However, to do so, the enzyme requires appropriate flanking amino acids. In the case of SARS-CoV-2, these are an 8–amino acid stretch, RRARSVAS. Whilst this is a core requirement, there is evidence from deletion mutants that amino acids flanking this sequence alter furin interaction and therefore, enzyme activity. This core region shares exact amino acid homology with the furin cleavage site of the ENaC, the human epithelial sodium channel α-subunit.[2] Three amino acids of this stretch plus proline (P) give PRRA, the SARS-CoV-2 sequence that is not found in any other coronavirus and certainly not in viruses associated with bat or pangolin.

Given the similarity of this site to that of the ENaCα, this author has performed analysis on the gene coding for the ENaCα. Whilst the amino acids RRARSVAS are the same, the proximal amino acids at the N-terminus side of this sequence are completely different. For the ENaCα sequence, these are PPHGA, as opposed to QTNSP for SARS-CoV-2. Also, the base coding across the whole sequence is dissimilar. These observations strongly indicate that the furin site of SARS-CoV-2 is not derived by recombination within a human cellular system (in vivo or in vitro).

More recently, a second furin cleavage site has been identified in SARS-CoV-2 within the S2 domain.[10] This site appears to be important for infection; however, the relative roles of these two sites will be cell and context dependent.

Based on observations that furin pre-processing decreases stability of the spike protein,[11] an intriguing hypothesis by Letarov et al[12] is that shedding of S1 as a consequence of furin pre-processing may allow more of the cellular ACE2 enzyme to be inhibited, increasing the pathological consequences of infection.

Whilst there appear to be three fundamental mechanisms for SARS-CoV-2 uptake, evidence from in vitro cell infection systems suggests that they operate together. The exception from the literature is the cell line Vero. These are kidney epithelial cells derived from the African green monkey. By passing clinical isolates of SARS-CoV-2 through several rounds of culture in these cells (passage), a number of investigators have noted the loss of the polybasic furin cleavage sequence within only a few passages. Sakaki et al.[13] were able to show that for Vero cells modified to express TMPRSS2, the polybasic site remained intact. In Vero cells lacking TMPRSS2, uptake of the mutated SARS-CoV-2 was achieved via the endosomal route alone. These observations beg the question as to the mechanism by which a loss of enzyme expression can induce a genetic change (the RNA of SARS-CoV-2 is both template for protein synthesis and genome for the organism).

21.4   ORGAN DISTRIBUTION OF ACE2

The initial route of entry of SARS-CoV-2 is via the nasal passages and mouth (mucosal surfaces). The human olfactory epithelium, relative to upper airway epithelial cells, has considerably higher

ACE2 expression.[14] This is likely the reason for one of the cardinal symptoms of COVID-19, namely, loss of smell. From the Human Protein Atlas (www.proteinatlas.org/), other tissues showing high levels of ACE2 protein expression are duodenum, gallbladder, kidney, small intestine and testes. Lower-level expression of ACE2 is observed in the adrenal gland, colon, rectum and seminal vesicles. Given that a major target for infection is the lungs, surprisingly, expression of ACE2 here is below the limit of detection. This finding is repeated for a number of tissues where there is a disconnect between the presence of virus (as determined by reverse transcription polymerase chain reaction [RT-PCR] or immunohistochemistry for viral RNA or protein) and ACE2 expression. In the gastrointestinal tract, peak viral loads are seen in the colon, whilst ACE2 expression is highest in the small intestine. It may be that a few ACE2 molecules are sufficient to cause a productive SARS-CoV-2 infection, and this may explain the mismatch.

21.5   COVID-19 STAGES, SYMPTOMS, TREATMENT APPROACH AND DISEASE CLASSIFICATION

From initial infection with SARS-CoV-2, one can assign four phases to COVID-19, as indicated in Figure 21.1. From the uptake of the virus as respiratory droplets or airborne virus, an asymptomatic *incubation period* (phase I) lasts typically around 3–5 days, but it may be longer (up to 14 days). At sites of virus uptake (nasal cavity/nasopharynx and oral cavity), viral replication very much depends on the activity of the local innate immune system. Secretion of low-affinity secreted IgA antibodies (sIgA) and antimicrobial peptides (AMPs) into mucins produced by nasal goblet cells provides one element of innate defense.[15, 16] Other components of the innate response are neutrophils, natural killer cells (NK cells), macrophages and plasmacytoid dendritic cells (pDCs). The latter cells secrete type I interferons in response to single stranded RNA from virus uptake.[17]

Logically, one would assume that symptoms and severity would depend on viral load. So far, publications using samples from the nasopharynx and oropharynx have not shown this. The viral

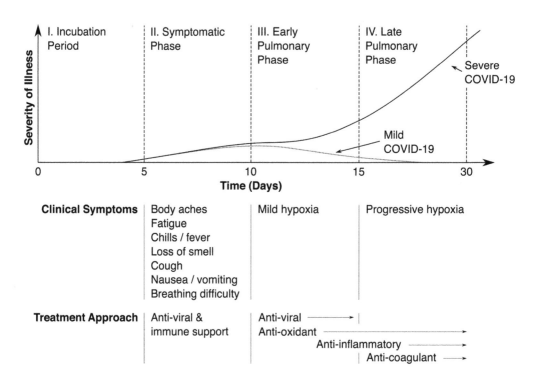

FIGURE 21.1   COVID-19 stages, symptoms and treatment approach.

load in asymptomatic and symptomatic patients reported in the studies by Ra et al. and Yilmaz et al.[18]was similar. One of the problems with RT-PCR used for determining viral load in these studies is that the method cannot distinguish between intact virus and fragments of viral RNA. A possible scenario is that asymptomatic individuals have higher local innate immune defenses (sIgA/AMPs/type I interferons), but virus RNA fragments remain. From ex vivo studies, Le Bert et al.[19]have shown that asymptomatic individuals, as evidenced by seroconversion, have a more robust adaptive immune response in comparison to symptomatic individuals. Production of cytokines representing T-helper 1 (Th1) lymphocytes is higher in asymptomatic than in symptomatic individuals, and this response is apparently balanced by the production of resolving cytokines, such as interleukin (IL)-10.

Following the incubation phase, the early *symptomatic phase* or viral phase (phase II) is characterized by chills/fever, dizziness ("spaced out"), muscle or body aches (including headache), skin sensitivity, extreme fatigue, loss of smell, dry cough and possibly, nausea or vomiting and diarrhea.[20]Toward the end of the symptomatic phase, some individuals may experience shortness of breath or dyspnea, and this may be associated with falling SpO_2[21]. Not all symptoms manifest in all individuals infected with SARS-CoV-2.

Falling SpO_2 signifies the transition to the *early pulmonary phase*, or stage III. This is a critical point, where the disease either progresses to a severe, life-threatening condition or resolves. At this stage, antiviral therapy must be complemented by agents that support antioxidant systems, that target immune cell activation and that target fibrosis, endothelial cell dysfunction and blood clotting. Figure 21.1 has suggested the timing of some of these therapies. The exact timing of the start of the pulmonary phase must be determined by clinical and if available, biochemical observations. For more information, the reader is referred to the work of Dr Shankara Chetty[21] and the FLCCC Alliance.[22]

In particular, Dr Chetty's work (and that of a growing number of other physicians) has revealed that it is vital to note precisely when dyspnea is first observed. At the time of the last update of this chapter, he has treated over 10,000 patients with no deaths. A particularly pertinent observation from this large cohort of patients is that COVID-19 is biphasic and therefore, a non-linear disease. Patients presenting with severe flu-like symptoms (typical of viral illness) over the first week do not necessarily transition into the pulmonary phase, and patients with more mild initial symptoms have been observed to transition. Of high significance is that following the start of the vaccination program for COVID-19, Dr Chetty has seen a considerable number of individuals who suffer *early pulmonary phase* symptoms without the early flu-like *symptomatic phase*. These observations and the treatment protocol[21] he uses for both infection and post-vaccine responses will be discussed in more detail in the last section of this chapter.

For the purpose of further discussion, disease classification of COVID-19 is as follows: 1) mild, where initial viral symptoms, independent of severity, resolve without transition or where transition occurs into *early pulmonary phase*, but symptoms are mild and resolve quickly; 2), moderate, with transition and often a prolonged period of lung and systemic inflammation (which encompasses Long COVID); and 3) severe (advanced COVID-19), with transition into *pulmonary phase*, accompanied by prolonged life-threatening hyper-inflammation and often Long COVID for those who survive.

21.6 THE "CYTOKINE STORM" (HYPER-INFLAMMATION) AND CYTOKINE PROFILES IN MODERATE AND SEVERE COVID-19

A cytokine storm is generally considered a response to infection where there is a large increase in inflammatory cytokines that are associated with a hyper-inflammatory state. Webb et al.[23] have performed a review on the clinical parameters of severe COVID-19 in comparison to hyper-inflammatory states, including macrophage activation syndrome (MAS), secondary hemophagocytic lymphohistiocytosis and cytokine release syndrome, and have come up with the term COVID-19-associated hyper-inflammatory syndrome (cHIS). The four parameters that characterized advanced COVID-19 most closely (leading to the separate classification of cHIS) were extremely low lymphocyte counts, extremely high D-dimer levels, extremely high fibrinogen levels and extremely high C-reactive protein (CRP). Whilst Webb et al.[23] described IL-6 as moderate to high, studies by Herold et al.[24] and Laguna-Goya et al.[25] have revealed this cytokine to be predictive of the need for mechanical ventilation, with optimal cut-off values of 80 pg/ml and 86 pg/ml, respectively (the concentration of IL-6 in control serum normally is 5 pg/ml or lower).

Numerous cell types, including macrophages and dendritic cells, produce IL-6, and this has major consequences for T-cell plasticity during antigen presentation. IL-6 can inhibit T-cell polarization to a T-helper1 (Th1) phenotype. Th1 lymphocytes provide support for CD8$^+$ cytotoxic T-cells, increasing their activity against virally infected cells. Sustained high levels of IL-6 also promote loss of endothelial cell barrier function,[26] and this is enhanced by co-produced tumor necrosis factor alpha (TNFα).[27] IL-6 is also involved in tissue repair and collagen secretion, and with transforming growth factor beta (TGF-β), it constitutes a major contributor to lung fibrosis,[28] one of the serious complications of SARS-CoV-2 infections and advanced COVID-19.[29] In this respect, vitamin D may have potent anti-fibrotic properties in COVID-19, as the ligand-bound vitamin D receptor interferes with Smad3, a transcription factor induced by TGF-β and involved in inducing an array of pro-fibrotic genes.[30, 31]

Binding of IL-6 to its receptor (IL-6Rα within the cell membrane or the soluble IL-6R via a trans-signaling mechanism, where IL-6-sIL-6Rα complex binds gp130 in any cell type) results in the transcriptional activation of STAT3.[32] By inducing Smad3, which has been shown to interact with STAT3, TGF-β can enhance transcription of IL-6-responsive genes.[33] The interaction between IL-6 and TGF-β may have high significance for the endothelial mesenchymal transition (EndMT) that occurs in severe COVID-19.[34] EndMT leads to the destruction of blood vessels, and both these cytokines appear to act in concert to induce such a transition.[35] Based on work with SARS-CoV-1 (SARS), it is possible that the nucleocapsid (N) protein of SARS-CoV-2 also modulates TGF-β signaling (Smad3) to block apoptosis of SARS-CoV-2-infected host cells whilst enhancing TGF-β-induced fibrosis.[36]

IL-6 is also a driver of CRP synthesis in the liver,[37] and CRP activates the antimicrobial complement cascade.[38] Sustained activation of the complement cascade can lead to tissue damage.[39]

By longitudinal profiling of cytokines in COVID-19, Lucas et al.[40] observed a core cluster of IL-1α, IL-1β, IL-17A, IL-12 p70 and interferon alpha (IFNα) common to all COVID-19 patients. Severe disease provoked a further set of cytokines, including thrombopoietin (TPO), IL-33, IL-16, IL-21, IL-23, IFNγ, eotaxin and eotaxin 3. Common to all severe COVID-19 and characteristic of a cytokine storm (with the exception of IL-10) were elevations of IL-1α, IL-1β, IL-6, IL-10, IL-18 and TNFα. These are fundamental cytokines of the innate immune system (except for IL-10, which is produced both by innate and adaptive immune cells) that are induced following inflammasome activation[41] by viral pathogen associated molecular patterns (PAMPs) binding to pattern recognition receptors (PRRs). Whilst the cytokine profiles noted by Lucas and colleagues[40] provide evidence of adaptive immune system activation (T-cell responses), patients with more severe COVID-19 show substantial losses of CD4$^+$ and CD8$^+$ T-cells. Indeed, lymphopenia has been a consistent finding, and it differentiates severe and moderate COVID-19.[42] The mechanism of lymphopenia may be similar to human immunodeficiency virus (HIV), as SARS-CoV-2 has been shown to infect T-cells by interacting with CD4.[43]

A particularly important finding from the study of Lucas and colleagues[40] was divergence that occurred after 6–10 days from symptom onset (DfSO) for those whose disease resolved in comparison to those who progressed to severe disease. Prior to this time point (combined measurements from 113 patients were made over time spans of 1–5, 6–10, 16–20 and 21–25 days), patients with moderate and severe disease displayed similar blood profiles, including the core cytokine profile referred to earlier. For moderate disease, these markers declined steadily after 6–10 DfSO, and resolving factors, such as epidermal growth factor (EGF), platelet-derived growth factor (PDGF) and vascular endothelial growth factor (VEGF), which are mediators of wound healing and tissue repair, were detected. In contrast, core signature markers remained elevated as disease progressed to severe, and additional correlations emerged with severe disease after 6–10 DfSO. Severe disease was particularly characterized by a large rise in neutrophil/lymphocyte ratio, a significant rise in eosinophils and evidence for the involvement of all Th arms of the adaptive immune system (Th1, Th2 and Th17), as well as strong activation of the innate immune system.

Paradoxically, a cytokine that is also characteristic of severe COVID-19 is IL-10.[44] Meta-analysis of non-severe and severe COVID-19 patients from 18 combined clinical studies has identified IL-6 and IL-10 as covariates that accurately predict disease severity.[45] This is surprising, as IL-10 is usually considered anti-inflammatory and part of the resolving phase of infection. Certainly, it has been suggested that IL-10 is fundamental to the optimal balance of the immune system in asymptomatic individuals.[19] From longitudinal profiling, Zhao et al.[46] have shown that IL-10 and IL-1RA (IL-1 receptor antagonist), both usually classed as anti-inflammatory cytokines, were increased within 1 week of symptom onset for patients who went on to severe disease (measurements were made on patient samples every 4–7 DfSO).

Also raised 4–7 DfSO was IP-10 (interferon gamma-induced protein 10, also known as CXCL10). It remained raised in severe disease whilst dropping to control levels in mild cases. IP-10 is a chemoattractant for a number of cell types, including macrophages and neutrophils, and its elevation is consistent with neutrophil influx into lungs with concomitant neutrophil extracellular trap (NET) formation[47] and blood clotting.[48]

A finding from the study of Zhao et al.,[46] consistent with the work of Le Bert et al.[19] on asymptomatic SARS-CoV-2-infected individuals (who seroconverted), was the observation of significantly raised RANTES in mild versus severe disease (the authors of this study noted that "patients with severe disease showed mild symptoms during weeks 1 and 2 and developed severe disease in weeks 3 to 4 after the onset of symptoms"). RANTES or CCL5 is a chemokine produced by a number of cells, including T-cells, epithelial cells, platelets and mast cells. It functions as an attractant for monocytes, T-cells, dendritic cells, NK cells and eosinophils. The authors of this study have suggested that elevation of CCL5 within the first week for those who after initial symptoms, went on to display mild disease in comparison to severe disease is due to production by virus-specific CD8[+] T-cells (cytotoxic T-cells).

Although associated with allergy, tissue-resident mast cells act as one of the primary sensors of environmental stressors.[49] One intriguing sensing mechanism is the extension of membranous projections into the lumen of blood vessels. Based on their innate sensing ability, an alternative explanation for the elevated production of CCL5 in mild in comparison to severe disease[46] is that tissue-resident mast cells produce this chemokine in response to virus recognition by the PRRs, such as toll-like receptor 3 (TLR3). In turn, CCL5 production may lead to recruitment of antigen-specific CD8[+] T-cells as a means to limit infection.

Neumann et al.[50] performed blood profiling and demonstrated markedly increased numbers of regulatory T-cells (Tregs) producing IL-10. However, this study failed to find evidence for a significant increase in effector CD4[+] T-cells (Th1, Th2 and Th17) in response to SARS-CoV-2 infection. Part of the reason for this may be lymphopenia, as SARS-CoV-2 would seem to infect CD4[+] T-cells, possibly using the CD4 protein as a docking site, allowing the spike protein to interact with ACE2 and be cleaved by the protease TMPRSS2.[43] Another explanation for the apparent lack of specific Th-cell response may involve methodology.

By performing studies on bronchoalveolar lavage fluid (BALF) samples, McGregor et al.[51] have shown that T-lymphocytes within these samples are Th1-skewed. In contrast, when they determined the T-cell distribution in peripheral blood mononuclear cells (PBMCs) obtained from whole blood, no significant differences in Th1, Th2 and Th17 lymphocyte types were apparent between control samples and COVID-19 samples. They suggested that "expression of the Th1 program is a specific feature of Th cells at the site of pulmonary inflammation where virus-specific T cells may be concentrated." In support of a T-cell response to SARS-CoV-2, Grifoni et al.[52] were able to detect T-cell responses to specific SARS-CoV-2 epitopes. Le Bert et al.[19] have shown a distinct Th1 response in response to ex vivo SARS-CoV-2 antigen stimulation. So in the unstimulated scenario, the inability to detect changes in Th-cell types probably represents the technical difficulty of detecting these cells amongst all other epitope-specific Th-cells in a sample of PBMCs isolated from whole blood.

The observation from the study of Lucas and colleagues,[40] that IL-33 (also known as an alarmin) is elevated, is in line with the proposal of Zizzo and Cohen[53] that when released from infected and damaged epithelial alveolar cells, it enhances TGFβ-mediated differentiation of Foxp3+ Treg-cells. In mild disease, where viral clearance has been successful, perhaps Tregs, via IL-10 production, drive the resolution phase of the disease, where alveolar macrophages transition to a scavenger and resolving (M2) phenotype,[54] producing factors such as EGF, FGF and VEGF[55] (as indicated in the blood profiling work of Lucas and colleagues[40]). Clearly, for individuals who progress to moderate and severe disease, the situation is rather different.

Returning to the early raised IL-10 (and perhaps increased abundance of Treg-cells) measured in the blood of advanced (severe) COVID-19 patients, a further strong possibility is that for infected cells, the N-protein of SARS-CoV-2 associates with the transcription factor Smad3, as was shown for SARS-CoV.[36, 56] The significance here is that during antigen priming of naive CD4+ T-cells (antigen presentation), Smad3 is induced by TGF-β, and Smad3 increases transcription of the Treg-specific factor Foxp3 (Forkhead box P3).[57] It is also possible that the drive to the Foxp3 pathway leads to an increase in Treg-cells by "overwriting" recently differentiated Th-cell phenotypes. The work on CD4+-facilitated SARS-CoV-2 uptake has certainly demonstrated that virally infected CD4+ T-cells increase production of IL-10,[43] a cytokine associated with Treg-cells.

Before leaving the Smad3 story for a while, Zhao et al.[36] further demonstrated that whilst the viral N-protein enhanced TGF-β-mediated effects in lung epithelial cells, it blocked Smad3-mediated apoptotic cell death. If this mechanism operates for SARS-CoV-2-infected CD4+ T-cells, viability may be maintained long enough to sustain several rounds of viral replication before the high cellular viral load perhaps induces cell death. Usually, virally infected cells of nearly all types are detected by CD8+ cytotoxic T-cells, and the infected cells are destroyed before extensive viral replication can take place. It would appear that a non-structural protein encoded by ORF8 of the SARS-CoV-2 genome potently downregulates MHC1 receptors,[58] thereby blocking cytotoxic T-cell recognition of infected CD4+ T-cells. This is a situation where NK cells should act as a "fail safe," as virally infected cells that lack MHC1 receptors provide a signal to activate NK cell cytotoxicity.

Whilst the described mechanisms may be involved in hyper-inflammation associated with COVID-19, clinical observations of Dr Shankara Chetty[21] (and others) suggest that the hyper-inflammatory phase of COVID-19 has its origin around 6–8 DfSO. This finding is reflected in the overview by Buszko et al.,[59] where it is stated that an "inflection point of illness occurs typically between days 5 and 7 of illness." They go on to suggest that "This interval is the time in which targeted immunomodulatory therapy will probably be most beneficial in lowering mortality."

So perhaps, increasing concentrations of viral fragments, together with increasing damage-associated molecular pattern (DAMP) concentrations (including alarmins like IL-33) and rising antibody production from plasma cells (initially IgM), act as a trigger for a hypersensitivity response.

Dr Chetty has suggested that this could be a type 1 response, where antigens interact with cognate IgE receptors that have become attached via Fc receptors (Fc-epsilon-RI) to mast cells in tissues surrounding and within blood vessel walls. Antigen binding to IgE induces cross-linking of rFc-epsilon-RI and mast cell degranulation, with the release of histamine and many other pro-inflammatory mediators (including IL-6). If so, this response is later in the disease time course than one would normally expect for a type 1 reaction.

Given the timing of the transition from symptomatic to early pulmonary phase, a type 2 or a type 3 hypersensitivity response (or both) might seem more likely. In the case of type 2, antibodies would be directed to a self-antigen. For type 3, insoluble immune complexes may be formed between antibodies and viral fragments attached to blood vessel walls, leading to vasculitis from complement activation and mast cell degranulation. One has to say that a rise in antibody titer sufficient to trigger a hypersensitivity response at around a week post symptom onset (and therefore, 10 days or so from infection) would suggest prior exposure to a similar coronavirus endowing a degree of immunological memory. Indeed, data on vaccination with a spike protein–expressing vector would suggests such a prior event, as IgG levels rise significantly 10 days post first vaccination.[60]

A further possibility is the direct activation of mast cells by virus components acting via the recently identified MRGPRX2 receptor.[61] This receptor can activate the high-affinity IgE receptor, Fc-epsilon-RI, in the absence of pre-formed IgE. If this is a mechanism for the transition from the symptomatic phase to the early pulmonary phase, then the rise in IL-6 that is noted for individuals who transition to the early pulmonary phase may reflect such a trigger. IL-6 is known to influence the polarization of the developing adaptive immune response away from a cell-mediated antiviral Th1 response and towards a humoral Th2 response. Using a rapid technique to determine the IgG antibody response in patients with mild, moderate and severe COVID-19, Deb et al.[62] have provided preliminary data to suggest that persons suffering severe disease do indeed have an immune response skewed towards a type 2 or Th2 phenotype.

Further discussion on the trigger events for the transition from the symptomatic to the early pulmonary phase will be presented in the overview discussion at the end of this chapter.

21.7 NUTRIENT TRANSFER, GUT MICROBIOME AND IMMUNITY

Whilst the stomach is essential for the initial processing of ingested food substances, most nutrient transfer occurs within the small and large intestine, and commensal microorganisms play a fundamental role in nutrient extraction.

21.7.1 GUT MICROBIOME AND GALT

It has been estimated that the colon harbors as many as a trillion bacteria per gram (microbiome) and this mass comprises more than 1000 different species of organism. In order to cope with this number of potentially invasive microorganisms, the gut has developed an efficient immune system. This defensive immune system is part of a wider group of tissues termed the GALT or gut-associated lymphoid tissue. These sites comprise a collection of multi-follicular structures, including tonsils, Peyer's patches, appendix, colonic and cecal patches, and a number of single follicular structures called isolated lymphoid follicles (ILF). These tissue structures are situated throughout the gastrointestinal tract, and with mesenteric lymph nodes (MLN), they help protect the host from infection following an epithelial barrier breach.

21.7.2 GUT MECHANISMS PREVENTING INFECTION

As a first line of defense, the gut lining (comprising different types of epithelial cells) must provide a barrier to prevent the bulk ingress of bacteria, components thereof and food components into the sub-epithelial spaces. Four major mechanisms are important here: 1) the secretion of AMPs into mucins produced by goblet cells, 2) the secretion of immunoglobulin A (IgA) antibodies (sIgA) from antigen-programmed plasma B lymphocytes and 3) regulation of the gap junctions between gut epithelial cells.[63] These three processes interact to limit incursion of microorganisms in a way that allows, on a strictly limited basis, the "sampling" of antigens from gut microorganisms. These antigens are "presented" to immune cells in the spaces behind the epithelial cell barrier, and in response, IgA antibodies are manufactured and secreted (sIgAs) into the lumen of the gut. These sIgA antibodies, together with mucins, help prevent the adherence of microorganisms to luminal surfaces and also help in the transport of microorganisms along the gut canal.[64]

21.7.3 INNATE AND ADAPTIVE IMMUNE SYSTEMS OF THE GALT

The sub-epithelial spaces of the gut, which comprise an element of the GALT, are populated by innate immune cells, such as macrophages and dendritic cells, B-cells, different types of CD4+

T-helper lymphocyte (Th-cells), CD4+ regulatory T-cells (Treg) and CD8+ cytotoxic T-cells. Some of these antigen-specific T-cells help in the production of secreted antibodies (Th2 cells), and some (Th1/Th17 and CD8+ cytotoxic T cells) help fight microorganisms that have managed to attach to the gut epithelium and then breach the gut barrier. It is the latter type of Th-cells and CD8+ cells, along with innate immune cells, that enhance the inflammatory response.

In addition to local gut effects, inflammatory Th-cells and cytotoxic T-cells can be carried via the systemic circulation to distant sites, where they can enhance an inflammatory response taking place due to damage or infection.[65] This non-local influence of the gut is also determined by the integrity of the gut barrier, and this decreases with age.[66]

21.7.4 The Gut–Lung Axis in Respiratory Infection

Severe COVID-19 is a virus-induced inflammatory disease, and as such, one might assume that the state of immune activation within the gut will have a bearing on the course of the disease. As indicated earlier, the immune state within areas of GALT is established as an interaction between food components and the gut microbiome, and this "inflammatory tone" is transferred not only within the GALT but also further afield. One area of the body first identified to be under this influence was the synovial cavity of the joint.[67]

Since the first ideas on the non-local influence of the GALT, much has been written on the gut–brain interaction, and now, literature is accumulating on the gut–lung axis.[68] This interaction is facilitated by the mesenteric lymphatic system. This system acts as a "drainage complex" where intact bacteria, their fragments, metabolites and gut-derived immune cells translocate across the intestinal barrier and from the mesenteric system, join the systemic circulation, and modulate the lung immune response.[69]

Age is associated with gut dysbiosis and as mentioned earlier, decreased barrier function.[66] As a consequence, translocation of gut-derived components and delivery to the lungs via the systemic circulation increases with age. This may establish a pro-inflammatory environment in the lungs that enhances the local cytokine response to SARS-CoV-2 and exacerbates COVID-19 in older people. One way of controlling this could be inclusion in the diet of sufficient fiber and probiotic bacteria capable of digesting fiber to produce short-chain fatty acids (SCFAs).

21.7.5 Gut-Derived SCFAs and Respiratory Virus Model

A paper published in 2018 on a mouse model of H1N1 infection[70] described how animals handled flu virus when fed a diet of high fiber (HFD) in comparison to low fiber. The results were astonishing. High fiber increased butyrate over 100-fold and had a large positive effect on survival. The authors found that although there was a small increase in viral load 5 days after infection, the high-fiber diet markedly reduced uptake of neutrophils into the lungs. These changes were reproduced by adding butyrate to drinking water 2 weeks prior to and during infection.

Further work revealed reduced expression by lung macrophages of the neutrophil chemokine CXCL1 in response to butyrate. This effect appeared to be due to butyrate shaping the phenotype of monocytes in bone marrow. On reaching the lungs, these cells differentiated into alternatively activated, IL-4- and IL-10-secreting macrophages (M2) with low inflammatory potential. In addition, butyrate increased antigen-specific CD8+ T-cells. The relevance of this study to COVID-19 is that a significant immune system response associated with lung damage is neutrophilia.[71]

In other cellular systems, butyrate would seem to impart a degree of trained immunity by increasing macrophage antimicrobial effects without increasing inflammatory potential.[72, 73]

In view of the earlier discussion on the downregulation of the antiviral response by IL-10-secreting cells, freeing a tissue of infection clearly requires an optimal balance between the degree of immune stimulation (inflammation) and the degree of immune suppression. Quite how this balance is achieved is not an easy question to answer.

21.7.6 Gut Microbiome Modification for Prophylaxis and Treatment of COVID-19

The gut microbiome has been shown to change during the course of COVID-19,[74] and given the influence of the gut microbiome on the lung, there have been calls for the use of prebiotics, probiotics, high fiber and indeed, butyrate in the treatment of COVID-19.[75, 76] Dr William Shaver[77] has used a combination of vitamin C, vitamin D and the prebiotic Kefir to successfully treat patients with early symptoms of COVID-19. Although not specifically related to COVID-19, Dr Shaver's work is supported by a wide literature[78] and in particular, an impressive study showing that a high–fermented food diet steadily increases microbiota (microbiome) diversity and decreases inflammatory markers.[79] Wischmeyer et al.[80] have demonstrated that daily *Lactobacillus rhamnosus* in a COVID-19 exposure setting resulted in prolonged time to development of COVID-19 and reduced symptoms.

21.8 FOOD GROUP COMPONENTS AND THE INFLAMMATORY TRIGGER SETTING

21.8.1 The Carbohydrate–Protein–Fat Balance and Inflammation

Much is currently written regarding the role of carbohydrate in the diet. Until some 5 years ago, the villain was fat, or more precisely, saturated fat. Now, this accolade is given to carbohydrates with a high glycemic index. Apart from the way they are metabolized, a fundamental difference between fats and "sugars" and indeed, proteins (amino acids) is the effect they have on autophagy. This is a "housekeeping process" whereby cellular components, both large (mitochondria) and small (macromolecules), are reprocessed using a combination of vesicle trafficking and lysosomal degradation. As for many processes, but particularly so for autophagy, its activity falls with age. Fatty acids have no direct effect on autophagy, but carbohydrates and amino acids decrease autophagic flux. The mechanism for this is that both increase the activity of mTORC1, a nutrient-responsive (glucose and amino acids) terminal kinase of the PI3K-AKT cascade. Through various signaling mechanisms, mTORC1 inhibits autophagy whilst increasing anabolic processes. Indeed, autophagy is at the heart of many life-extension programs involving selective nutrient deprivation.[81] The benefit of nutrient depravation may be due to the effect autophagy has on the inflammatory trigger setting of the body.

Autophagy and inflammatory pathways share some of the same components,[82] and this gives rise to a reciprocal relationship between the two processes. Autophagy is also associated with a primary trigger of immune activation, namely, the inflammasome.[83, 84]

The inflammasome is a multi-enzyme complex that is activated within cells by PAMPs and DAMPs and various other factors, such as oxidants. Following the activation of PRRs by PAMPs and/or DAMPs, the transcription factor NFκB is induced, and this upregulates the expression of inflammasome components. A second step, often involving reactive oxygen species (ROS), is necessary for full activation, resulting in the production of IL-1β and IL-18.[85]

Whilst no clinical studies have been undertaken, Hannan et al.[86] make a strong case for the benefit of calorie restriction to upregulate autophagy in COVID-19. However, evidence has been presented that the SARS-CoV-2 genome codes for a protease (PLpro) that degrades the serine-threonine kinase ULK1[87], a kinase regulating starvation-induced autophagy. If this is indeed so, then calorie restriction as a means to increase autophagic flux in SARS-CoV-2-infected cells may be rather ineffective unless PLpro can be inhibited.[88]

21.8.2 Dietary Polyunsaturated Fatty Acids and Control of Inflammation

Omega-3 fatty acids comprise α-linolenic acid, docosahexaenoic acid (DHA) and eicosapentaenoic acid (EPA). The latter two are fish oil associated, whilst α-linolenic acid is plant derived. As a component of membrane phospholipids, omega-3 polyunsaturated fatty acids (n3PUFAs) increase membrane fluidity[89] and by doing so, alter G-coupled receptor signaling processes, SH2 domain tyrosine kinase signal transduction and TLR4-mediated inflammatory signaling.[90] Also, the n3PUFA DHA binds to the peroxisome proliferator receptor gamma (PPAR-γ), a nuclear receptor that forms a heterodimer with the co-transcription factor PGC-1α. Together, they have multiple effects on metabolism.[91] DHA and EPA also bind to GRP120, and this has anti-inflammatory effects in macrophages and adipocytes, inhibiting both TLR and TNFα-activated pathways and decreasing insulin resistance.[92]

EPA and DHA also influence dendritic cell (DC) phenotype and function. DCs are critical to antigen presentation in lymph nodes near a site of infection. The type of helper T-cells generated very much depends on the co-stimulation that DCs received at the site of infection.

Whilst at the time of writing, there appear to be no reports of clinical trials involving PUFAs for COVID-19 prophylaxis or symptom de-escalation, evidence from sepsis and patients with acute respiratory distress syndrome (ARDS) have shown favorable results. Hosny et al.[93] considered the efficacy of 7 days' high-dose supplementation with DHA and EPA (9 g/d), along with 1 g/d ascorbic acid, 400 IU/12 h alpha-tocopherol (vitamin E) and 100 µg/d selenium, in patients with early-stage sepsis. Compared with the control group, the supplemented group exhibited lower levels of CRP, IL-6 and procalcitonin, a lower need/shorter duration for mechanical ventilation, and reduced development of severe sepsis. A recent Cochrane review of patients with ARDS receiving EPA and DHA supplementation revealed significant improvement in blood oxygenation, a reduced need for ventilation, less organ failure, shorter length of intensive care unit (ICU) occupancy and reduced mortality at 28 days.[94] Most reviews are now suggesting that appropriate supplementation with PUFAs such as EPA and DHA (4–6 g/day), under conditions where suitable antioxidant support is given, should be of benefit as a means of symptom de-escalation in COVID-19.[95, 96]

21.9 ANTIOXIDANT AND METABOLIC SUPPORT FOR COVID-19

21.9.1 Cellular Oxidative Stress and Infection

The generation of free radicals (oxidants) is an inherent consequence of aerobic metabolism, but infection places further demand on cellular antioxidant systems. Whilst SARS-CoV-2-encoded proteins may interfere with mitochondrial function,[97] leading to heightened mitochondrial oxidant generation, stress is often due to activation of oxidant-inducing pathways by infection-induced cytokines, particularly IL-6.

This cytokine is a powerful inducer of the cytosolic enzyme system NADPH oxidase, and activity of this enzyme results in the production of superoxide, which is further converted to the pro-oxidant H_2O_2. In the absence of sufficient catalase activity and/or glutathione/glutathione peroxidase, and in the presence of ferrous ions (Fe^{2+}), H_2O_2 is converted to the highly damaging hydroxyl radical. To counter this, the extracellular concentration of iron is maintained at a very low level by the iron binding protein lactoferrin. Early in the COVID pandemic, work was presented suggesting that SARS-CoV-2 could be taken up by erythrocytes by binding to CD147 and CD26 receptor proteins and release iron through interaction with hemoglobin (Hb).[98] This would not only swamp the iron binding capacity of lactoferrin; it would also result in anemia. The reduced oxygen-carrying ability of Hb could cause local tissue hypoxia, reducing mitochondrial function, and the free iron would induce cellular oxidative stress. These conditions could contribute to multi-organ failure, one of the outcomes of severe COVID-19. A further factor in this scenario is the ability of IL-6 to increase intracellular iron concentrations by inducing the synthesis of the intracellular iron binding protein ferritin.[99]

This pro-oxidant scenario is likely to play out through cytokine-induced clotting factors,[100, 101] in particular by SARS-CoV-2-induced NADPH oxidase following viral RNA activation of the toll-like receptor TLR-7.[102] The common link is that both IL-6 and SARS-CoV-2 infection induce NADPH oxidase, and subsequent oxidant generation induces NFκB and endothelial cell expression of tissue factor (TF), a primary trigger of coagulation.

21.9.2 Vitamin C (Ascorbic Acid) and Symptom De-escalation

Ascorbic acid (AA) is a water-soluble antioxidant. Since the 1950s, it has been known that infection places a huge burden on the pool of vitamin C within the human body.[103] This is now confirmed for SARS-CoV-2 infection. Xing et al.[104] reported that AA levels dropped from around 9.23 mg/l (50 µmol/l) in healthy volunteers to around 2.00 mg/l (11 µmol/l) in COVID-19 patients. This study also revealed that when provided intravenously (IV), vitamin C restored levels to around 13.46 mg/l (76 µmol/l). Such a fall may have severe consequences for various redox systems that depend on AA for regeneration. One of these is the glutathione/glutathione peroxidase system (see section to follow). Another system is nitric oxide synthase (NOS). The production of NO from L-arginine requires NADPH, (6R)-5,6,7,8-tetrahydrobiopterin (BH4), FAD, FMN, heme and Zn^{2+}. AA is required to maintain BH4 in its reduced form.[105] These findings and observations suggest that oral AA should be used for prophylaxis against SARS-CoV-2 infection and also administered IV, in the form of sodium ascorbate, for symptom de-escalation.[22, 106] Indeed, Dr Richard Cheng[107] has pioneered the use of IV vitamin C against COVID-19.

From work on pulmonary endothelial barrier function, it appears that IV vitamin C is particularly effective when used in combination with a corticosteroid.[108]Studies such as these have been the driving force for the work of Dr Paul Marik. He has used a combination of corticosteroids, vitamin C and thiamine for treating sepsis with good results.[109]

The mechanism for this successful combination has been explored by a number of authors.[110, 111] At the right dose, glucocorticoids are powerful anti-inflammatory agents, shutting down several arms of the immune system. However, the receptor to which they bind is negatively affected by oxidants.[112] This may be reversed by the administration of AA, which has been shown to restore glucocorticoid receptor function.[113] In addition to this, there is evidence that the cellular uptake of AA is mediated by the sodium-vitamin C transporter (SVCT2), and this is downregulated in inflammatory states.[114] Certainly, in a mouse cell culture model, Fujita et al.[115] have shown that the glucocorticoid dexamethasone induces expression of the SVCT2.

It is the work on sepsis that has provided a basis for treating advanced COVID-19. Dr Paul Marik, with other Critical Care Physicians, has formed the Front Line COVID-19 Critical Care Alliance.[22] They have developed the MATH+ protocol for advanced COVID-19, which includes methylprednisolone, IV vitamin C, thiamine, heparin and a list of other agents as indicated at their website. Their most recent addition is Ivermectin. The MATH+ protocol has so far been implemented in the treatment of COVID-19 patients at two hospitals in the United States: United Memorial Hospital in Houston, Texas and Norfolk General Hospital in Norfolk, Virginia. It has proved extremely successful, reducing mortality from 15–32% (worldwide ICU figures) to around 5%.

21.9.3 Vitamin E and COVID-19

Although there are eight fat-soluble isoforms of vitamin E, the body preferentially uses α-tocopherol. α-Tocopherol functions as a chain-breaking antioxidant, preventing the propagation of extremely damaging free radicals within lipid–protein structures of cell and organelle membranes. A further important role is preventing the oxidation of low-density lipoproteins, which in an oxidized state, are pro-inflammatory.[116] The paper by Soroki et al.[117] provides the rationale for protecting lipoproteins in COVID-19, as it suggests that lipoproteins with oxidized phospholipids and fatty acids could lead to virus-associated organ damage via over-activation of innate immune scavenger receptors. No studies are reported on vitamin E supplementation alone for COVID-19, but a clinical trial was described for a combination of vitamin E with vitamins A, C, D and B.[118] The results of this clinical trial were published in November 2021.[119] The trial involved 60 ICU patients with severe disease (30 control and 30 in the treatment group). The intervention included 300 IU twice daily of vitamin E, 25,000 IU daily of vitamin A, 500 mg four times daily of vitamin C, 600,000 IU vitamin D (one assumes cholecalciferol) once during the study, and one "amp" daily of B complex for 7 days.

Patients were monitored at baseline and after 7 days of supplementation. Overall, treatment substances were significantly raised in serum samples after 7 days. In response, inflammatory markers were significantly reduced in serum samples, as was severity of the disease. There were four deaths in the control group but none in the supplemented group.

21.9.4 Ascorbic Acid, L-Lysine and the "Bradykinin Storm"

A co-morbidity that increases the risk of severe COVID-19 is hypertension. In its extreme form, this condition is associated with damaged to major arteries, inflammation and vascular narrowing (atherosclerosis). Most of the current theories of atherosclerosis involve the interplay between endothelial dysfunction (inflammation) and cholesterol-containing lipoproteins.[120] An alternative view for the causation of atherosclerosis was presented in 1989 by Pauling and Rath.[121] This hypothesis proposed that damage to the artery wall was due to a shortage of vitamin C in the diet; in other words, a sub-clinical form of scurvy. The link with what might loosely be described as "the cholesterol hypothesis" was made by suggesting that insufficient AA leads to the deposition of a cholesterol transport lipoprotein, lipoprotein (a) (Lp(a)), within the vessel wall. Over time, Lp(a) becomes oxidized, leading to immune cell involvement and inflammation.[117] A fundamental aspect of this idea was that L-lysine could block Lp(a) binding to the arterial wall.

There is indeed evidence that Lp(a) has a lysine binding site that may contribute to fibrous plaque formation at the site of arterial damage.[122] So, L-lysine might act as a decoy, preventing Lp(a) binding to the arterial wall. This may have implications for the vascular damage and clotting that is seen in severe cases of COVID-19.[117, 123] L-lysine may also have a significant role in modulating the nitric oxide (NO) system that is activated after SARS-CoV-2 infection.

NO is a vasodilatory substance that counteracts the vasoconstricting effects of substances like angiotensin II (A2). A2 is part of the renin–angiotensin system (RAS). Its effect is diminished by the enzyme ACE2, which acts as the receptor for SARS-CoV-2 entry into cells. ACE2 converts angiotensin to Ang_{1-9} and Ang_{1-7} (the latter in cooperation with ACE, as A2 is converted to Ang_{1-7} by ACE2). So, under physiological circumstances, a balance is established between ACE (producing A2) and ACE2. Whilst the expression of ACE2 is rather low in lung tissue, work on bronchoalveolar lavage (BAL) samples from SARS-CoV-2-infected individuals has demonstrated a very large upregulation of ACE-2 (around 200-fold).[124] A significant effect of Ang_{1-7} and Ang_{1-9} is the induction of NO production.[125] Whilst beneficial under physiological circumstances, under conditions of oxidative stress (for example, IL-6-induced superoxide (O_2^-) overproduction), the presence of NO leads to the production of the peroxynitrite ($ONOO^-$) radical. Peroxynitrite is implicated in sepsis and ARDS,[126] and it is also overproduced in the advanced stages of COVID-19. NO production is dependent on cellular uptake of L-arginine, and this is competitively inhibited by L-lysine.[127]

An aspect of COVID-19 pathogenesis not so far discussed is the so-called "bradykinin storm." This was the subject of the paper by Garvin et al.[124] discussed earlier with reference to ACE2 in BAL samples from COVID-19 patients. Their work demonstrated that the RAS system was severely dysregulated in lung tissue infected by SARS-CoV-2. ACE expression in cells from BAL samples was decreased, whilst ACE2 expression was markedly increased. The overall effect will be a swing toward the production of Ang_{1-9} and bradykinin (BK). BK, like Ang_{1-9}, induces vasodilation. Indeed, Ang_{1-9} appears to sensitize the BKB2R form of the bradykinin receptor to BK, and this is associated with vasodilation, sodium retention and hypotension. Overall, these changes cause vascular dilation, hyperpermeability and vascular inflammation. In addition, hyaluronic acid was highly over-expressed in BAL samples,[124] and this would explain the presence of a viscous hydrogel-like substance that accumulates in lung alveoli of patients with advanced COVID-19, preventing gas exchange.

A fundamental aspect of Ang_{1-9} acting via AT2 receptors and BK acting via BKB2R receptors is the intracellular production of NO.[125, 128] Under conditions of an associated cytokine storm, the peroxynitrite radical will be formed, leading to further tissue damage.

Returning to L-lysine, this amino acid has been shown to decrease the synthesis of NO,[127] and so in combination with IV vitamin C (as sodium ascorbate), L-lysine administration may provide a means of reducing vascular hyperpermeability and vascular inflammation in advanced COVID-19. L-Lysine has also been suggested to have antiviral properties.[129]

21.9.5 N-ACETYLCYSTEINE (NAC) SUPPORT FOR GLUTATHIONE SYNTHESIS AND RECYCLING

NAC is a thiol antioxidant, and via deacetylation, it is converted to cysteine, the precursor of gluta-thione (GSH), one of the most important cellular antioxidants. NAC has an advantage over cysteine, as it more readily crosses cell membranes. In addition to its GSH-precursor role, it also induces Nrf2 (nuclear factor erythroid 2–related factor 2). Nrf2 binds to an antioxidant response element (ARE) in the promoter region of genes of antioxidant enzymes and phase 2 detoxifying enzymes, leading to their transcription. Antioxidant enzymes and their support enzymes induced by Nrf2 include super-oxide dismutase (SOD), glutathione peroxidase (GPx) and glutathione reductase. The last of these is particularly important, as it is responsible for recycling GSH.[130] GSH is oxidized by enzymatic systems, such as glutathione peroxidase, and also by redox coupling with the oxidized form of AA. As a water-soluble antioxidant, AA is converted to dehydroascorbate, which is recycled back to AA using GSH. If AA is to be used in the treatment of COVID-19 (late symptomatic phase onwards), then it is essential to include NAC in the protocol to maintain vitamin C in its reduced form.

Shi and Puyo[131] have reviewed the evidence regarding the use of NAC for respiratory infections and COVID-19, and have suggested a strategy whereby on first exposure to SARS-CoV-2, 600 mg NAC should be administered orally twice a day (BID). With symptoms, this dose is increased to 1200 mg BID. On ICU admission, patients should receive 100–150 mg/kg/day NAC by an IV route.

21.10 MELATONIN

Melatonin is a hormone synthesized from serotonin in the pineal gland. The terminal enzyme in its synthetic pathway is rate limiting and sensitive to light-dark cycles. It is also produced in the gonads, the retina, immune cells such as macrophages, and the gut, where it may alter the micro-biota and enhance goblet cell mucin production and antibacterial peptide synthesis.[132]

Despite endogenous synthesis, it is included in this review for reasons that have high significance for SARS-CoV-2 infection and COVID-19. Firstly, after 50 years of age, the diurnal rhythm of mela-tonin (blood concentrations peak around 1–2 a.m.) is lost, and this is strongly reflected by a reduc-tion in the total antioxidant capacity of serum.[133] This is significant for COVID-19, as the infection fatality rate (IFR) for SARS-CoV-2 increases with age.[134] Secondly, melatonin is unique among hormones in that it is a powerful antioxidant that targets mitochondria to support the glutathione/glutathione peroxidase system. In studies where endotoxin was used to induce protein and lipid oxi-dation, melatonin was more effective than the mitochondrial targeting antioxidant MitoQ.[135]

Unlike the pineal gland, where the activation of NFκB by PAMPS and/or DAMPS shuts down melatonin synthesis, in macrophages, NFκB induces melatonin synthesis.[136] So, infection induces melatonin production in macrophages, and melatonin, acting in an autocrine fashion, reduces inflammasome activation, possibly via Nrf2.[137] This will have the effect of dampening the inflam-matory response and provides a rationale for its inclusion in a therapeutic regime for advanced COVID-19.

Using system biology combined with artificial intelligence, Artigas et al.[138] have identified mela-tonin in combination with pirfenidone as a promising candidate therapy to reduce SARS-CoV-2 infection and to mitigate the cytokine storm of severe COVID-19. Pirfenidone is an antifibrotic agent with clinical utility for lung fibrosis.[139] It inhibits furin, a protease involved in TGF-β produc-tion and the cleavage of many protein sequences (often to activate the protein), including SARS-CoV-2 spike protein, where it cleaves at the S1/S2 site and in so doing, allows the spike protein to fuse with a cell membrane. Melatonin also appears to have a role in virus uptake, as two of its three membrane receptors, MTNR1A and MTNR1B, interact with GRP-78 (Glucose Regulated Protein 78), another protein associated with SARS-CoV-2 uptake by cells.[140] As noted earlier, melatonin may reduce inflammatory cytokines by decreasing NF-κB activation.[141]

Pirfenidone may therefore synergize with melatonin to reduce both TGF-β and IL-6, factors involved in lung inflammation and fibrosis, which characterize advanced COVID-19.

Melatonin is used as one of the fundamental components of the MATH+ protocol[22] for advanced COVID-19, and given its potential to block the entry of SARS-CoV-2 into cells and therefore infection, it might also be considered for prophylaxis.

In some countries, melatonin is a prescription-only compound. However, there are numerous natural sources.[142] Whilst the MATH+ protocol advocates the administration of 6–12 mg melatonin per day for hospitalized patients, levels in food sources are much lower. Despite this, blood concentrations can be increased significantly (140 pg/ml versus 32 pg/ml) by foods such as bananas.[143] Banana is estimated to contain around 1 μg/g melatonin. If bioavailability is anywhere near similar, one might assume that medical herbs such as St John's Wort (around 2000–4000 μg/g) and Feverfew (around 2000 μg/g) would raise blood concentrations considerably more.

21.11   B VITAMINS AND COVID-19

Thiamine (B1) has been included in therapies (see MATH+ protocol of FLCCC Alliance) because it is an essential cofactor for the enzyme pyruvate dehydrogenase, which converts pyruvate to acetyl-CoA for entry into the mitochondrial Krebs cycle.[144] Thiamine insufficiency reduces aerobic respiration, leading to a shift to less energetically efficient anaerobic pathway and a rise in tissue lactate. It also plays a role in metabolism of branched chain amino acids and in the pentose phosphate pathway that generates NADPH.

Niacin (B3) and its amide, nicotinamide, are precursors of NAD^+ and $NADP^+$ and therefore essential to mitochondrial and cytosolic energy transfer systems and for the production of reducing equivalents for pathways such as the pentose phosphate pathway. The latter is critical in the maintenance of GSH and the antioxidant status of cells, as indicated earlier. A hypothesis has been presented where NAD^+ deficiency in COVID-19 (which increases with age) enhances inflammation by reducing activation of SIRT1, an NAD^+-dependent deacylase.[145] SIRT1 activity plays a fundamental role in major metabolic processes, and it reduces inflammation.[146] A small clinical study has demonstrated dramatic improvement in the condition of several elderly COVID-19 patients treated with nicotinamide riboside.[147]

Folic acid (B9) is essential to supplying one-carbon or methyl groups for numerous metabolic reactions and for gene methylation.[148] Critical to what is known as the "folic acid cycle" is the enzyme 5,10-methylenetetrahydrofolic acid reductase (MTHFR). It is estimated that one-third of the world's population carry mutations in the MTHFR gene, and homozygous carriers have 20% of the normal enzyme activity. Acting within the folic acid cycle and in associated metabolic processes (methionine synthesis, methyl group donation and glutathione synthesis) are vitamins B6 (pyridoxal 5'-phosphate), B2 (riboflavin) and B12 (cobalamin). B3 is also critical for supplying reducing power in the form of NADPH for the MTHFR reaction, the product of which is 5-methyl-tetrahydrofolate (5-MTHF). Zinc also plays a critical role as cofactor in these enzymatic processes. Without sufficient MTHFR activity, folic acid is not helpful, and supplementation with 5-MTHF is required.[149]

A hypothesis regarding mutation of MTHFR (the common C677T polymorphism results in 50% of normal enzyme activity), involving the elevation in homocysteine as a consequence of low MTHFR activity in susceptible individuals, has been presented with regard to COVID-19.[150] Independently of MTHFR status, one should consider supplementing with 5-MTHF along with B12 (as methyl cobalamin, the active form) and the other B vitamins, particularly from the point of view of providing reducing equivalents to lower oxidative stress due to SARS-CoV-2 infection.[151]

B vitamins, along with Zn and Mg, are important for the synthesis of melatonin.[152]

21.12 MINERALS AND METABOLIC SUPPORT

Magnesium (Mg) is an essential mineral for mitochondrial ATP production. A deficiency in Mg has been linked to the release of cytochrome c (cyt c) into the cytoplasm of the cell, and this activates the apoptotic program. Studies from the United States show that intake of Mg has dropped from 450–485 mg/day in around 1900 to about 185–235 mg/day for large segments of the North American population.[153]

As part of a combination treatment with vitamin D (1000 IU/day) and vitamin B12 (500 µg/day), Mg (150 mg/day) reduced the proportion of clinically deteriorating COVID-19 patients and the requirement for oxygen support and/or intensive care support.[154]

Manganese (Mn) is an essential mineral required in many enzyme systems and metabolic processes. One of its best-known functions is as a component of mitochondrial superoxide dismutase (MnSOD), the enzyme that converts superoxide to H_2O_2 and then with the help of glutathione/glutathione peroxidase, to water.[155] Mn deficiency has been linked with a number of metabolic diseases, such as metabolic syndrome, type II diabetes (T2D), obesity, atherosclerosis and fatty liver syndrome. The commonality between these conditions is metabolic stress, particularly oxidative stress.[156] A higher intake of Mn was associated with reduced T2D along with lowered levels of inflammatory markers.[157]

Given its essential role in processes that reduce oxidative stress, Mn should be included in symptom de-escalation protocols for COVID-19.

Selenium (Se) plays a fundamental role in metabolic processes. Two of the essential requirements for Se are as a component of the antioxidant enzyme glutathione peroxidase and iodothyronine deiodinase, the enzyme that converts inactive thyroid hormone, T4, to the active hormone, T3.[158]

Early in the COVID-19 outbreak in China, a link between Se deficiency and disease severity was reported.[159] Since then, articles have appeared suggesting the same,[160] and it has been hypothesized that Se may prevent infection with SARS-CoV-2.[161]

Zinc (Zn) is the second most abundant mineral in the body. However, unlike iron, the most abundant mineral, there is no identified storage mechanism. Conditions related to Zn deficiency were first identified in the early 1960s.[162] Since then, Zn is recognized as essential in aspects of cell physiology such as folic acid metabolism, thyroid hormone metabolism and action,[163] and an array of other endocrine systems.[164] It is an essential component of tissue remodeling enzymes known as metalloproteinases[165] and also serves a critical function in the immune system.[166] Zn also appears to be required for the transcriptional function of Nrf2.[167]

A hypothesis regarding Zn deficiency in COVID-19 was presented in June 2020, where a number of known attributes of Zn were listed.[168] These included inhibition of SARS-CoV RNA-dependent RNA polymerase (RdRp) and synergism with hydroxychloroquine (HCQ). Numerous studies have shown efficacy of HCQ for COVID-19, and synergism with Zn is possibly due to HCQ acting as a Zn ionophore.[169] Benefits of zinc for COVID-19 prophylaxis and therapy have been further elaborated in a review article by Pal et al.[170] Ivermectin, which is now being used for COVID-19 therapy, also acts as an ionophore for Zn.[171]

21.13 VITAMIN D AND COVID-19

Unlike vitamin C, strictly, vitamin D is not a vitamin, as it is synthesized within the body from 7-dehydrocholesterol. The pathway involves UVB irradiation of skin to form pre-vitamin D in outer skin layers and then a non-enzymatic conversion to form cholecalciferol (D_3) in deeper layers of the skin. Cholecalciferol is taken up by the liver and converted to 25-hydroxyvitamin D3 (25-OHD) by the enzyme CYP2R1 and then in the kidney to the active form, 1,25-dihydroxyvitamin-D3 (1,25-OHD), by the enzyme CYP27B1.[172]

The majority of 25-OHD and indeed, the active form 1,25-OHD is transported in the circulation bound to D binding protein (DBP) or albumin, and less than 1% is free. Whilst parathyroid hormone regulates calcium uptake from the gut by increasing the activity of CYP27B1, it is the non-hormonal, immune cell metabolism of 25-OHD, and the response to 1,25-OHD in an autocrine/paracrine fashion, that is relevant to the situation of SARS-CoV-2 infection. Vitamin D, or strictly 1,25-OHD, interacts with a member of the superfamily of nuclear hormone receptors,[173] namely, the vitamin D receptor (VDR).

21.13.1 ANTIMICROBIAL EFFECTS OF VITAMIN D BINDING TO THE VDR

Over the past 10 to 15 years, the emphasis of investigations has moved from hormone to autocrine/paracrine effects of vitamin D; specifically, extra-renal synthesis of 1,25-OHD in cells of the immune system, especially macrophages and T-cells. The immune response to 1,25-OHD is one of both immune stimulation and inhibition. When concentrations of 1,25-OHD are sufficient, the VDR, which is mainly located in the nucleus, heterodimerizes with RXR (retinoid X receptor). This heterodimer binds to VDRE (vitamin D response element) in the promoter region of vitamin D–responsive genes and induces their transcription. The liganded VDR also interferes with the transcription of a number of genes either directly or through epigenetic mechanisms. Major targets for positive regulation by the VDR heterodimer are genes coding for AMPs such as cathelicidin and defensins.[174]In this important respect, the active form of cathelicidin, LL-37, has been shown to inhibit the binding of the SARS-CoV-2 spike protein to ACE2 on target cells.[175]

A critical aspect for AMP production is that CYP27B1 is induced following activation of PRRs (TLR1/2/4 and others) by PAMPs provided by the infective agent. This allows serum concentrations of 25-OHD from around 20 ng/ml (50 nmolar) to begin driving 1,25-OHD production within macrophages and in turn, AMP production. Using human donor monocytes in an ex vivo model, Adams et al.[176] found that concentrations of 25-OHD required for optimal AMP production varied with the age of the donors. In a cohort of older subjects, a twofold increase in monocyte cathelicidin levels required serum 25-OHD levels of around 80 ng/ml (200 nmolar). By contrast, monocytes from younger donors required 25-OHD levels of only 40 ng/ml (100 nmolar). The conclusion was that vitamin D functions as a "rheostatic regulator" of macrophage AMP production following TLR activation, where the magnitude of the effect is entirely dependent on the 25-OHD status of the individual.

Whilst the induction of CYP27B1 might appear specific to the PAMP and therefore, the type of PRR activated, a common element is the induction of NFκB, a factor essential to inflammasome activation and the production of IL-1β, IL-18 and IL-15.[177] The last molecule has been shown to induce CYP27B1 and the VDR.[178] Also known to induce IL-15 are type 1 interferons, such as virally induced IFNα.[179]

In the context of cooperation between the innate (macrophage) and adaptive immune system (Th-cells), PAMP-activation of PRRs (TLRs) leads to the upregulation of NFκB within macrophages and increased production of IL-15 (and the inflammasome-products IL-1β and IL-18). This circuit is amplified by IL-15 and IL-1β-driven Th1-cell proliferation[180, 181] and the paracrine influence of Th1-cell-produced IFN-γ (an interferon responsive to IL-18), which via the transcription factor, STAT-1, increases NFκB signaling in macrophages. The net result is more IL-15 and IFN-γ-induced CYP27B1, more IL-15-induced VDR expression, increased AMP expression, elevated antimicrobial autophagy with enhanced antigen presentation, and an overall increase in capacity for viral elimination. These pathways are outlined in Figure 21.2.

21.13.2 ANTI-INFLAMMATORY AND INFLAMMATORY EFFECTS OF VITAMIN D

The scheme shown in Figure 21.2 suggests that 1,25-OHD binding to the VDR reduces proliferation of Th1 lymphocytes. This is indeed a mechanism whereby the strong feedforward activation of the VDR by the cooperation between the innate (macrophage) and adaptive immune system (Th1 lymphocytes) produces enough 1,25-OHD to spill over in a paracrine fashion and bind to the

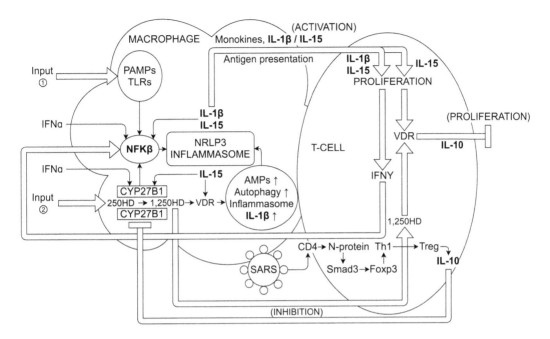

FIGURE 21.2 Pathways for the regulation of macrophage–T-cell interaction and the modulatory effect of vitamin D and SARS-CoV-2 infection (see main text for explanation).

VDR within Th1-skewed lymphocytes to reduce their proliferation. As mentioned earlier in this chapter, McGregor et al.[51] have shown that CD4+ T-cells from BALF of patients with COVID-19 are indeed Th1 skewed. They have also demonstrated that VDR activation induces IL-10 production, and that this cytokine is part of the shut-down process whereby T-lymphocyte proliferation is decreased.

Whilst macrophage collaboration with Th1-cells has evolved as a system to enhance pathogen elimination, SARS-CoV-2 may use part of the shut-down process to reduce antiviral effectiveness of recently differentiated Th1-cells that return from lymph nodes to the site of infection. This may occur within a SARS-CoV-2-target tissue (as suggested earlier) via a mechanism where after T-cell infection, the viral N-protein, by interacting with Smad3,[36] increases Foxp3 expression, thereby establishing a transcriptional program for overwriting early differentiated (still relatively plastic) antigen-specific Th1-cells, converting them to a Treg phenotype. These cells secrete IL-10, and this cytokine reduces the aggressiveness of macrophage function. Also, IL-10 may inhibit the conversion of 25-OHD to 1,25-OHD and thereby reduce the VDR-induced drive to the antimicrobial system.

Not so far explained in the pathway diagram of Figure 21.2 is the arrow suggesting that VDR activation increases IL-1β synthesis and so, inflammasome activation. Studies on *Mycobacterium tuberculosis* infection have shown that the human IL-1β gene has a VDRE and that vitamin D induces IL-1β secretion.[182] This response was apparent for all non-human primates but not for the mouse, rabbit or guinea pig, and so, the many experiments conducted on mouse cellular systems are not valid for human extrapolation. Vitamin D has also been shown to enhance IL-1β production from macrophages in response to the PAMP lipopolysaccharide.[183]

It would appear that IL-1β expression and protein secretion are dependent on the two-step process of NLRP3 inflammasome *priming* and *activation*. Kelly et al.[85] have described the process in detail. Through signal transduction pathways, IL-1β, TNFα and PAMPs/DAMPs activate NFκB, and this factor induces transcription of the gene for pro-IL-1β (and also IL-18) and the genes for inflammasome components. This is the *priming* step. The second step of *activation* is facilitated by a wide range of stimuli, including viral RNA, viroporins, ionic flux, mitochondrial dysfunction, lysosomal damage and oxidants.[184]

The ability of the activated VDR to induce the expression of IL-1β is likely a means of enhancing the antimicrobial response by driving antigen-specific Th1-cell proliferation. It may also be a means by which vitamin D can maintain a degree of antimicrobial defenses through neutrophil, NK cell and macrophage activation even if SARS-CoV-2 disables CD4$^+$ Th1-lymphocyte function, thereby impairing support for cytotoxic CD8$^+$ T-cells.[185]

Before returning to lymphocyte infection, the observation that mitochondrial dysfunction facilitates the activation step of the inflammasome,[184] together with the observations on the activation of autophagy as a means of disposing of dysfunctional mitochondria (mitophagy), suggests that the activation of the inflammasome and autophagy are linked. It is likely that the VDR has a role in activating both the inflammasome and the autophagic process.[186] The mechanism for this association most likely involves NFκB, IL-1β and the protein p62 (also called SQSTM1). In a similar vein to the way activation of the VDR by 1,25-OHD amplifies the magnitude of the AMP response to PRR activation, it is likely that the VDR serves to amplify the production of IL-1β in response to PAMPs/DAMPs. Transcription of the human IL-1β gene is induced by NFκB and also the VDR. A feedback loop is established, as the activation of NFκB is sensitive to signaling induced by IL-1β. So, 1,25-OHD will enhance NFκB activation and the transcription of genes sensitive to this transcription factor. One of these genes codes for p62. This protein can specifically bind to dysfunctional mitochondria that have been tagged for autophagic destruction (mitophagy) by Parkin-induced poly-ubiquitination. These dysfunctional, oxidant-generating mitochondria are processed by mitophagy. and in so doing, oxidative stress is diminished, moderating inflammasome activation.[187]

With regard to lymphocyte infection by SARS-CoV-2, after a period of viral replication within CD4$^+$ T-cells,[43] possibly facilitated by an escape from CD8$^+$ cytotoxic T-cell recognition of viral infection due to downregulation of MHC1 receptors[58] as discussed earlier, increased cellular viral load may eventually cause T-cell death.[188]. (Also see discussion to follow on viroporin and monocyte cell death.) Cells of the innate immune system will then be freed from virus-induced IL-10 suppression. Although their phenotype may have changed under the influence of IL-10, they will now come under the influence of inflammatory factors produced by epithelial cells and endothelial cells exposed to increased concentrations of virus and cellular fragments from lymphocyte cell death. This will again expand their inflammatory potential. Despite what seems to be self-limiting inflammasome activation in response to mitochondrial dysfunction (leading to mitophagy and reduced mitochondrial oxidant generation), in the presence of excessive intracellular oxidant generation (e.g. IL-6-induced superoxide in presence of NO, leading to peroxynitrite formation), an increase in lymphocyte cell death may signal a point in the disease at which vitamin D could enhance inflammation due to its potential to induce IL-1β expression.[182, 183] For this reason, close attention should be paid to blood concentrations of IL-6, lymphocyte counts and oxygen requirements 5–10 DfSO. These parameters may herald transition to the pulmonary phase and poor prognosis. At this stage, it is vital that vitamin D supplementation is supported by antioxidant provision to moderate inflammasome activation[184, 189] that otherwise could become unregulated.

The preceding discussion has linked vitamin D to enhanced antimicrobial effectiveness by way of increasing macrophage inflammasome activation, antigen presentation and AMP expression and also limiting the overshoot in the inflammatory process. Vitamin D may also be involved in mitigating the initial effect of CD4$^+$ T-cell infection by SARS-CoV-2. As discussed earlier, the N-protein of the virus, by activating the Smad3[36]/Foxp3 pathway, may lead to conversion of recently differentiated Th1-cells to IL-10-secreting cells (certainly, infection increases output of IL-10 from Th1-cells[43]), and this will impose an early block on the antiviral effectiveness of the macrophage–Th-lymphocyte system. However, the ligand-activated VDR has been shown to interfere with Smad3 transcriptional function.[30, 31] Vitamin D may therefore block a virus-induced change in T-cell phenotype. Also, in an environment rich in IL-6 (a cytokine that increases again at the transition between the symptomatic and the pulmonary phase[21]), Smad3 would be expected to recruit

STAT3 (a transcription factor driven by IL-6) to the promotor region of the RORγt gene, a master regulator of the Th17 phenotype.[190] Work by McGregor et al.[51] has demonstrated that in the absence of vitamin D, IL-6 added to Th-cells induces IL-17, whereas in the presence of vitamin D, IL-10 is produced. Further to this, these investigators demonstrated that STAT3 was involved in the response to IL-6 in the presence of vitamin D.[51]

Based on all this, it would appear most likely that sufficient dietary provision of vitamin D (to provide 25-OHD in the range 40–60 ng/ml) will prevent the subversion of the macrophage–Th1-lymphocyte antimicrobial system by SARS-CoV-2. In the presence of vitamin D, the macrophage–Th1-lymphocyte system will maintain its full antiviral activity, and so, the low level of viral infection of CD4+ cells will be insufficient to block MHCI expression, preserving the ability of CD8+ cytotoxic T-cells to seek out and kill infected CD4+ lymphocytes. 1,25-OHD will therefore be able to drive the shut-down process to limit inflammation (with the production of IL-10) when the virus has been eradicated.

This scenario concerning the role of vitamin D in cooperation between the innate and adaptive immune system, combined with numerous other findings, suggests that the concentration of 25-OHD within the blood of SARS-CoV-2-infected individuals will be one of the major determinants of the course of COVID-19. The clinical evidence for this assertion will now be briefly summarized.

21.13.3 Vitamin D Deficiency, SARS-CoV-2 Infection and COVID-19 Severity

It is widely accepted that in northern latitudes, vitamin D deficiency, defined as 25-OHD levels of 20 ng/ml (50 nmolar) and below, is highly prevalent. Surprisingly, vitamin D status is also poor in Middle Eastern countries.[191] Within these regions, ethnicity, obesity, age and institutionalization further contribute to low vitamin D status.[192, 193] From a global perspective, vitamin D is recognized as being effective in protecting against respiratory infection.[194]

Although only a statistical correlation, solar irradiation shows an inverse relationship with SARS-CoV-2 infection and COVID-19 severity.[195] This work is now corroborated by a multitude of studies showing that vitamin D status (measured as 25-OHD) correlates with SARS-CoV-2 positivity, inflammatory markers and COVID-19 disease severity. Indeed, the evidence base is now so extensive that only a few representative studies can be mentioned here:

- The SHADE study has demonstrated that a high proportion of asymptomatic or mildly positive PCR "cases" turn negative on short-term, high-dose supplementation (60,000 IU of cholecalciferol for 7 days) vitamin D.[196]
- Vitamin D status with 25-OHD in excess of 40 ng/ml (100 nmolar) is associated with a large reduction in PAMP-induced IL-6, TNFα and IP10,[197] and vitamin D deficiency is associated with an increase in inflammatory markers and disease severity.[198]
- 25-OHD level at admission to hospital is associated with disease severity and mortality,[199] and vitamin D deficiency is inversely associated with COVID-19 incidence and disease severity in Chinese people.[200].
- Serum concentrations of 25-OHD when determined from records over the months preceding illness show a strong correlation with COVID-19 severity.[201]
- Estimates suggests that nine out of ten COVID-19 deaths could be accounted for by vitamin D deficiency, defined as <20 ng/ml or 50 nmolar.[202]
- Numerous clinical trials are completed or ongoing on vitamin D supplementation. The study of Annweiler et al.[203] in frail elderly COVID-19 patients demonstrated that vitamin D supplementation improved outcomes when provided over a period of months before COVID-19 was diagnosed.
- At the time of the final update to this chapter, meta-analysis conducted on 207 treatment studies suggests a highly significant positive effect of vitamin D for both early and later

treatment (but particularly early) and a highly significant effect of vitamin D status on survival.[204] The greatest positive responses have been observed with the use of calcifediol. This meta-analysis is being continuously updated as studies are published.

Doctors' groups have been advocating the use of vitamin D since mid-2020.[205–207] Many are of the opinion that there is nothing to lose and everything to be gained by supplementing those at risk of infection (front line staff), the elderly and those with co-morbidities. Dosing regimes must realize 25-OHD levels of at least 30 ng/ml (75 nmolar) and preferably, in the region from 40 to 60 ng/ml (100 to 150 nmolar). In order to achieve this, most individuals will require a loading dose of at least 10,000–12,000 IU/day of cholecalciferol for 3 weeks (possibly considerably longer in some cases), after which a maintenance dose of around 4000–5000 IU/day should be taken.[208] Wherever possible, dosing regimens should be monitored by measuring blood levels of 25-OHD. For symptomatic individuals who have not previously dosed with vitamin D, one must take into account that conversion of cholecalciferol to 25-OHD is determined by initial dose. Vitamin D3 (cholecalciferol), when given as a very large dose (100,000–500,000 IU) as in many studies, is stored in adipose tissue and released slowly to provide 25-OHD. For therapy, it is more efficient to provide cholecalciferol in smaller divided doses, for example 12,000 to 24,000 IU/day.[209] Much preferred in the hospital setting is oral supplementation with 25-OHD (calcifediol).[22]

21.14 PHYTONUTRIENTS

These constitute a vast array of plant-derived compounds, and their properties with respect to SARS-CoV-2 inhibition and potential COVID-19 therapy have been reviewed early in 2020.[210] For the purpose of this chapter, the specific focus will be on two flavonoids, quercetin and epigallocatechin gallate (EGCG), the tetracyclic alkaloid berberine, the polyphenol resveratrol, and artemisia annua.

21.14.1 QUERCETIN

Found in a variety of fruits, vegetables, seeds, nuts, flowers, barks and leaves, quercetin is a polyphenolic compound with wide-ranging attributes in biological systems. These include protective roles in cancer, atherosclerosis and neurodegeneration as well as antibacterial and antiviral properties. Whilst the polyphenolic nature of quercetin endows the compound with oxidant-scavenging ability, many of the biological protective effects of quercetin may derive from an ability to activate Nrf2, a master transcriptional regulator of antioxidant enzyme systems. Indeed, as an oxidant scavenger, quercetin may act as a local pro-oxidant, and this may facilitate the canonical mechanism by which Nrf2 is activated.[211] Also of high significance is the finding that Nrf2 supports mitochondrial function by ARE-mediated induction of nuclear respiratory factor 1 (NRF1).[212] NRF1 is a transcriptional regulator of mitochondrial biogenesis that stimulates expression of nuclear-encoded mitochondrial transcription factor A (Tfam). Tfam helps regulate mammalian mtDNA copy number.[213]

It may be that the ability of quercetin to reduce oxidant formation is the reason for reports suggesting that quercetin inhibits inflammasome-induced IL-1β production and also IL-6.[214]

In addition to oxidant and metabolic control, quercetin has been shown to have direct antiviral effects by way of blockade of viral entry and inhibition of viral proteases and RNA-dependent RNA polymerase (RdRp).[215]

Combination with vitamin C has been suggested to be particularly effective in limiting SARS-CoV-2 replication,[216] and a combination of 500 mg quercetin with 500 mg vitamin C has been found effective as prophylaxis.[217]

Extensive studies on quercetin and EGCG have revealed that both compounds act as zinc ionophores.[218] These findings are of particular significance, as zinc inhibits viral RdRp,[219] and the combination of quercetin or EGCG with zinc may increase intracellular zinc sufficiently to block SARS-CoV-2 replication.

A further interesting possibility was suggested from in silico studies where quercetin and vitamin D were a potent combination to reduce the expression of multiple SARS-CoV-2 targets. This response was further enhanced by the addition of estradiol.[220]

Again, from in silico supercomputer studies, quercetin has been shown to dock with the ACE2 SARS-CoV-2 receptor protein,[221] and this has been confirmed in real-world biochemical studies.[222]

From clinical practice, Dr David Moskowitz has been treating patients with quercetin since April 2020 with extremely good outcomes. It should be noted that quercetin is a mast cell stabilizer (see discussion on mast cells to follow).

21.14.2 EPIGALLOCATECHIN GALLATE

Whilst quercetin is showing promise for prophylaxis and symptom de-escalation for SARS-CoV-2 infection, EGCG, a catechin flavonoid, may be similarly effective, with perhaps additional benefits in advanced disease. EGCG is the major ingredient in green tea and accounts for 50% to 80% of a brewed cup of green tea. As mentioned earlier, EGCG also acts as a zinc ionophore, and being water soluble (in comparison to quercetin, which is rather insoluble in an aqueous environment), may access different tissue compartments.

Whilst the combination with Zn may inhibit viral replication by inhibiting RdRp, another target is the viral main proteinase (Mpro), also called 3CL protease (3CLPro). This protease controls the activities of the coronavirus replication complex and is absolutely essential for virus propagation.[223] EGCG has been shown to inhibit 3CLpro, and so too have black tea–derived theaflavins,[224] suggesting that these compounds have a role in prophylaxis and the early stages of SARS-CoV-2 infection.

In addition to antiviral activity, positive effects of EGCG have been observed in a range of autoimmune conditions that involve over-activation of the innate and adaptive immune systems. Menegazzi et al.[225] have convincingly outlined benefits of EGCG in rheumatoid arthritis, Sjogren's syndrome, multiple sclerosis and inflammatory bowel diseases. The responses observed could not be ascribed to the antioxidant capacity of EGCG alone but rather, to inhibition/activation of specific cellular pathways: Specifically, the inhibition of JAK/STAT-mediated pathways and as for quercetin, the activation of the Nrf2/ARE pathway. Menegazzi et al.[225] make a strong case for the use of EGCG in COVID-19 as both an antiviral agent and one that may reduce hyper-inflammation and lung fibrosis in advanced COVID-19. Of particular importance is the suggestion that the sepsis-like overproduction of the alarmins, S100A8/A9 and HMGB1, which contribute to a condition similar to disseminated intravascular coagulation (DIC) often seen in advanced COVID-19, might be reduced by EGCG. An overall conclusion reached by Menegazzi and colleagues was that "timely administration of EGCG to COVID-19 patients is most likely crucial, we suggest administering EGCG, orally, at the dosage of 600–900 mg/day, once the symptoms aggravate and/or the blood C-reactive protein, or other markers of inflammation (e.g. IL-6), increase."

21.14.3 BERBERINE AND RESVERATROL

Berberine is a quaternary ammonium salt of the group of benzylisoquinoline alkaloids derived from plants such as the evergreen shrub Berberis. Resveratrol is a stilbenol and natural phenol produced by plants under stress. It is best known as a compound found in grape skins and indeed, many purple fruits. Berberine activates 5' AMP-activated protein kinase (AMPK), an enzyme that responds to nutrient deprivation, suppresses anabolic processes, activates autophagy, increases mitochondrial biogenesis and improves fitness by activating mitophagy.[226] Resveratrol activates the deacetylase SIRT1, and deacetylation activates PGC-1α, a master regulator of mitochondrial biogenesis. PGC-1α acts as a co-activator of nuclear respiratory factors NRF1 and NRF2 (SIRT1 has been discussed previously in relation to vitamin B3 deficiency, PGC-1α has been discussed in relation to PUFAs, and NRF1 has been discussed in relation to quercetin). PGC-1α is also activated by AMPK, and so, it is likely that berberine and resveratrol will synergize to increase mitochondrial function.[227, 228]

The significance of these findings for immunological control in relation to infection is that metabolism in recently differentiated and activated effector T-cells (such as Th1 and Th17) is skewed somewhat away from mitochondrial ATP generation and toward glycolysis. This is particularly pronounced for Th17 cells, where glycolysis is driven by hypoxia-inducible factor (HIF)-1α.[229, 230] Pharmacological blockade of glycolysis was shown to direct cells away from Th17 differentiation towards Treg-cells.[229]

Whilst these metabolic changes are clearly important to the early adaptive immune response to infection, they also provide a target for therapeutic manipulation. Caslin et al.[231] have demonstrated increased glucose uptake, glycolysis and mitochondrial oxidative phosphorylation by mast cells in response to IL-33 and that reducing glycolysis with 2-deoxyglucose decreased IL-6 and TNF production. In addition, they demonstrated that metformin, which is known to increase AMPK activity,[232] significantly decreased IL-6 production from mast cells in response to IL-33. They were also able to show that a synthetic SIRT1 agonist decreased IL-6 production.

Collectively, these observations provide a rationale for using a combination of berberine (AMPK activator) and resveratrol (SIRT1 activator) towards the end of the symptomatic phase of COVID-19. At this time point in the disease, it is likely that virus-damaged cells release IL-33 (amongst other DAMPs and alarmins), which increases the reactivity of mast cells to degranulating stimuli with the release of numerous pro-inflammatory and pro-fibrotic factors.

It may be no coincidence that a co-morbidity for COVID-19 is diabetes, and various agents directed to the activation of AMPK, SIRT1 and indeed, Nrf2 are of significance in reducing insulin resistance.[233] So, the link between diabetes and a more severe outcome following SARS-CoV-2 infection is likely to be dysregulated immuno-metabolic signaling.

21.14.4 Sweet Wormwood

Artemisia annua, often referred to as sweet wormwood, is a plant native to temperate Asia. It is used widely in Traditional Chinese Medicine for the treatment of malaria, particularly in many African countries. Artemisinin, a sesquiterpene lactone, appears to be a principal active compound in sweet wormwood. The derivatives, artesunate and artemether, apparently exhibit improved pharmacokinetic properties, and they are key ingredients of WHO-recommended anti-malaria combination therapies.

In vitro experimentation has demonstrated potency of wormwood extracts, artemisinin, artesunate and artemether against SARS-CoV-2.[234] A further study has indicated that potency against SARS-CoV-2 replication may also be due to unexplored compounds in sweet wormwood extracts.[235] This study, in particular, suggests that extracts of wormwood have promise as antiviral therapy throughout the symptomatic phase of COVID-19.

21.15 OVERVIEW DISCUSSION AND CONSENSUS NUTRITIONAL RECOMMENDATIONS (CONSENSUS-COVID)

Clinical observations since the start of the pandemic rather firmly indicate that COVID-19 is in fact two diseases with a common cause, namely, infection with SARS-CoV-2. Whilst Figure 21.1 provides a generic outline of the disease progression, with suggested staging of therapy, clinical observations, particularly by Chetty,[21] reveal that there is a distinct change in disease characteristics after about the first week of symptoms. Some patients who have more or less recovered from the symptomatic phase report the return of body aches, followed by dyspnea and falling SpO_2. This time point corresponds to the changes seen in the longitudinal cell and cytokine profiling described by Lucas et al.,[40] as discussed earlier.

Also apparent from Dr Chetty's work is that the severity of the somewhat confusingly assigned *symptomatic phase* is not a predictor of transition to the more serious *pulmonary phase*, where symptoms are more extreme. His observations reveal that individuals with severe initial symptoms often fail to transition, whilst those with more moderate initial symptoms can transition. He has formulated the clinical opinion that this transition is due to type 1 hypersensitivity.[21] By treating patients (10,000 and counting) at the first signs of transition with the corticosteroid prednisone, the antihistamine promethazine, and the leukotriene receptor antagonist montelukast,[21] he has not lost a single person. Most recently, his protocol has been modified to use an antihistamine, like promethazine and montelukast, at the first signs of transition and then to follow up (if necessary) with methylprednisolone (see: https://gig.regenerise.com/).

COVID-19 is therefore an eminently treatable disease, but the timing of treatment is critical.

In view of the success of Dr Chetty's therapeutic regimen, the requirement for ICU therapy must be considered a failure to provide timely early therapy. Indeed, many healthcare systems have abandoned individuals to their fate, and interaction has only occurred when individuals transition to the pulmonary phase. As a result, and particularly in 2020, COVID-19 has become synonymous with the hyper-inflammatory phase, and the most critical time at which treatment should be applied was, and still is in some cases, entirely missed.

With respect to hypersensitivity, McMillan et al.[236] have provided a review of current evidence and the role they consider antibodies raised to soluble ACE2[237] play in this response. Their view is that other types of hypersensitivity may also have a significant role in disease progression. Before discussing other types of hypersensitivity, it is appropriate to consider flu vaccines that induce an IgE response.[238] If a person is vaccinated and then later exposed to the same strain of flu to which the vaccine was raised, the course of the flu can be significantly worse, and the cytokine storm, in severe cases, is likely to be a combination event caused by infection and an allergic reaction. Death following flu infection in susceptible individuals is often wrongly characterized as septic shock. A more likely reason is anaphylactic shock caused by type 1 hypersensitivity.[239] This scenario is somewhat similar to COVID-19, except that for a type 1 response, the reaction in COVID-19 is rather delayed. An intriguing connection between flu vaccination and COVID-19 is that flu vaccines are generated using chicken eggs, and chicken eggs are contaminated with coronaviruses.[238] Chicken egg proteins have high homology to SARS-CoV-2.[238] One possibility for why some individuals suffer severe early symptoms is prior vaccination for flu and their viral symptoms being exacerbated by an allergic response.

As an alternative to an early (in symptomatic phase) type 1 hypersensitivity response, a delayed response could be a mechanism for transition if genetically susceptible individuals, who have previously been sensitized to a related coronavirus under a Th2-skewing environment (see discussion to follow on breaking tolerance), respond to a particular component of the virus, the concentration of which only reaches the required threshold around 6 to 8 DfSO. This component could be the spike protein (see later discussion on vaccines).

Returning to the other classes of hypersensitivity, McMillan et al.[236] have explored types 2 to 4 and conclude that all these may be involved in the hyper-inflammatory phase. In particular, and based on their earlier theory of an immune reaction to a chimera between soluble ACE2 and the spike protein ACE2 binding site,[237] they suggest that type 2 could result in an initial IgM-mediated complement activation (fixation) and vascular damage (vasculitis). This could then be followed by an IgG-mediated response some days later. A type 3 hypersensitivity response would manifest as insoluble immune complexes formed between IgG antibodies and viral debris. The trigger would be the increasing amount of viral antigens and a threshold concentration of IgG. The timing of the rise in detectable IgG may be compatible with the clinical observation of Dr Shankara Chetty,[21] particularly for those who have been previously infected with a similar virus, giving rise to cross-reactive memory B-cells. A type 4 hypersensitivity response is T-cell driven. It is a typical response to viral infection and involves Th1-cells and CD8+ cytotoxic T-cells. However, when targeted to self-antigens, it is considered an autoimmune response. Coeliac disease is an example of CD8+-mediated cellular damage.[240]

Appearing in 2020, around the same time as the paper by Chetty,[21] Sanchez-Gonzalez et al.[241] published a theoretical paper that also explored the role of hypersensitivity. These authors suggested that COVID-19 demonstrated many of the disease characteristics of a hypersensitivity pneumonitis. They proposed a therapeutic strategy very similar to that most successfully used by Chetty.[21]

A further informative finding from the work of Dr Shankara Chetty is that transition from the *viral* to the *early pulmonary* phase is apparent from measurement of IL-6 and CRP, which can increase many times above normal at around 7 to 10 DfSO. This finding is most consistent with a hypersensitivity response of types 1, 2 and 3, as each of these processes involves mast cell activation/degranulation. Whilst mast cells have large quantities of stored histamine, they are also able to synthesize IL-6 in response to degranulating stimuli provided by antigen-induced IgE-bound Fc receptor cross-linking [242] or in response to complement protein fragments in the form of anaphylatoxins such as C5a.[243, 244]

Rather than an origin due to mast cell degranulation as a result of a hypersensitivity reaction, the rise in blood concentrations of IL-6 at the end of the symptomatic phase, when body aches return, might reflect an event that precedes mast cell degranulation. This might be the primary trigger event. Such a situation might arise from accumulation of a critical threshold number of viroporin ion channels formed by ORF3a-encoded proteins and from the SARS-CoV-2 E proteins after successive rounds of viral replication. Viroporins have been shown to induce NLRP3 inflammasome activation (second step in inflammasome activation; see Kelley et al.[85] and Nieto-Torres et al.[245]) and also pyroptotic cell death.[246] Although lymphopenia has already been discussed in terms of viral infection via CD4+ and cell death, monocyte cell death has also been reported via inflammasome-dependent pyroptosis following SARS-CoV-2 infection.[247] It is therefore possible that the secondary rise in IL-6 is due to simultaneous pyroptosis of populations of virally infected cells. The release of viral PAMPs and cellular DAMPs will activate inflammasomes of surviving immune and tissue cells, and these will release a range of inflammatory cytokines, including IL-1β and IL-6. In this respect, the N-protein of SARS-CoV-2 has been shown to interact with the NLRP3 inflammasome to increase its activity.[248] This would enhance PAMP- and DAMP-induced inflammasome activation of virally infected cells.

DAMPs will include alarmins, of which IL-33 is a known activator of mast cells as well as acting as a co-stimulus for TGF-β in driving Treg formation. For individuals who transition to the early pulmonary phase, it has been suggested by Zizzo and Cohen[53] that the IL-33 pathway is over-activated, possibly by a combination of raised IL-33 and polymorphisms in ST2, the receptor for IL-33. They propose that with TGF-β, this leads to "increased expression of the canonical Th2 transcription factor GATA-binding factor 3 (GATA3), which impairs the suppressive function of Treg cells." They further suggest that "the dysregulation of GATA3+ Foxp3+ Treg cells might result in impaired immunological tolerance and increased secretion of type 2 cytokines, thus promoting autoinflammatory lung disease." GATA3 is the transcriptional regulator for IL-4, IL-5 and IL-13. The last cytokine has been shown to enhance production of the eosinophil chemotactic factor eotaxin.[249] Eosinophilia in lung tissue is indeed observed in COVID-19.[40]

The proposal of Zizzo and Cohen[53] also ties in with work presented earlier on the N-protein of SARS-CoV increasing Smad3 transcriptional activity.[36] Smad3 is a transcription factor that responds to TGF-β, a pathway that increases Foxp3 transcription.[57] So, infection of CD4+ lymphocytes within the lung may synergize with IL-33 released from damaged cells (monocytes, lung alveolar epithelial cells and others) to subvert Treg-cells, endowing them with a Th2-like phenotype.

To re-iterate, the initial trigger for the transition from *symptomatic phase* to *early pulmonary phase* may occur at a point where virus-induced viroporin ion channels activate the NLRP3 inflammasome to an extent sufficient to induce pyroptotic cell death of immune and tissue cells. These cells will release numerous DAMPs and alarmins such as HMGB-1, ATP, DNA, IL-1α, S-100 proteins and also IL-33. The last is intimately involved in mast cell activation,[231, 250] and it may enhance mast cell degranulation provoked by viral components (particularly the N-protein) binding to the MRGPRX2 receptor, a receptor specific to mast cells.[61] This receptor activates the high-affinity Fc-epsilonRI in the absence of pre-formed IgE. Against this background, susceptible individuals may react at this time to the release of the spike protein. This may give rise to what might be considered "the perfect storm," where in addition to the generalized response outlined earlier, the release of this protein induces the cross-linking of IgE bound to mast cells (see discussion to follow on vaccine and spike toxicity). Spike protein may be released due to cell death or more specifically, by an increase in furin protease expression, which may occur around this time in response to virus-enhanced TGF-β signaling.[36, 251] As mentioned near the beginning of this chapter, furin is a protease that promotes pre-processing of the virus spike, but this reduces the stability of the spike, allowing shedding of the S1 subunit.[11]

Whilst these various scenarios may provide the initiating event in the transition from *symptomatic* to *early pulmonary phase*, subsequent inflammatory responses, as discussed throughout this chapter, are likely to follow. The severity of these events most probably depends on environmental factors (e.g., nutrition), co-morbidities, and epigenetic and genetic factors.

In light of the preceding discussion, the provision of nutritional supplements for COVID-19 should be considered with respect to 1), likelihood of limiting infection and viral replication at an early stage, 2) downgrading symptoms and 3) their effects as adjuvants to pharmaceutical agents, such as steroids, antihistamines and leukotriene receptor blockers (for details of compounds used, see Chetty[21]) to prevent transition to the pulmonary phase.

Of all the nutritional agents discussed in this chapter, it is the author's conviction that a sufficient blood concentration of 25-OHD of between 40 and 60 ng/ml (100 and 150 nmolar) is paramount for prophylaxis and early disease control. The seven short rapid responses to the editor of *BMJ* entitled "Sixty seconds on vitamin D"[252]echo this conviction. In the era of the highly infectious Omicron variant, it is highly unlikely that vitamin D will prevent infection in all cases. However, by increasing the effectiveness of the innate immune response and the early cooperation between the innate and adaptive immune system (e.g., macrophage Th-cell system), it is highly likely that vitamin D will reduce viral load. This will not only reduce initial symptoms; it will also decrease the potential for transition to the *pulmonary phase*.

A confounding observation of relevance here is that individuals who seemingly have mild viral disease (initial symptoms) can suffer falling SpO_2 around 6–8 DfSO and transition to the pulmonary phase. This begs the question as to what determines the initial symptoms. Unfortunately, due to the way the COVID-19 pandemic has been managed in many countries around the world, we still have little information on the immunological changes in the early to mid-symptomatic phase of COVID-19.

The closest approach to this problem may be to consider flu virus infection. Of the so-called early cytokines produced at the site of infection, IFNα, TNFα, IL-1β, IL-6, the neutrophil chemoattractant IL-8 and monocyte-attracting chemokines are elevated.[253] These cytokines are produced as part of the innate immune response to infection, and one assumes that a similar response (perhaps with the exception of a weaker type 1 interferon response) will be apparent during the early symptomatic phase of COVID-19.

It is likely that symptom severity of the *viral phase* (or *symptomatic phase*) of COVID-19 is dependent on the response of the upper respiratory tract to virus in terms of cytokine production. The response is not necessarily a function of the amount of virus, as viral load between asymptomatic and symptomatic individuals is not so different.[18 13]From studies on asymptomatic individuals,[19] it would also seem that the adaptive immune response is stronger than in symptomatic individuals. Perhaps coupled with more efficient type 1 interferon response and robust NK cell activation, this would allow the virus to be cleared without provoking the production of inflammatory cytokines and chemokines to an extent that induces symptoms (of various degrees). This idea is perhaps borne out by studies showing that cold symptoms, for individuals infected with rhinovirus, are dependent on the degree to which the innate immune system is activated.[254] This unique study demonstrated that individuals suffering chronic stress were more prone to developing a cold due to glucocorticoid resistance. This resistance reduced negative regulation by the glucocorticoid-activated glucocorticoid receptor on virus-induced cytokine production. The take-home message here is that symptoms result from a reaction of the immune system to the virus rather than a direct effect of the virus on cellular systems.

Of significance with respect to cell death and potential therapy targeted to the transition from the symptomatic to the pulmonary phase of COVID-19 are observations on glycine. Since the pioneering work on modes of cell death beginning in the 1970s, studies have shown how the amino acid glycine is able to prevent necrosis. In 1987, it was reported that necrosis can be a regulated process and that glycine induces cytoprotection.[255] This cytoprotection would appear to be due to the ability of glycine to inhibit the membrane-associated changes that are induced during pyroptotic cell death. Given that SARS-CoV-2 induces NLRP3 inflammasome activation (through mechanisms discussed earlier) and that over-activation of the NLRP3 inflammasome initiates pyroptosis,[247] glycine may have a role in therapy for COVID-19. If, as suggested earlier in this discussion, transition from the *symptomatic phase* to the *early pulmonary phase* is marked by simultaneous cell death events, dietary inclusion of glycine as suggested by Li,[256] at an amount corresponding to 0.5–1.0 g/kg/day, may block transition. Also, where early therapy has not been provided, glycine may protect lung tissue later in the disease process.

Returning to vitamin D, what is clear from clinical experience is that its use in COVID-19 is by no means infallible. Individuals treated with vitamin D can still suffer disease, and on occasion, this can be serious. A fundamental consideration here is how long an optimal concentration of 25-OHD is maintained prior to and after SARS-CoV-2 exposure. Despite this caveat, all the currently available information on vitamin D suggests that it reduces the odds of progressive infection and serious disease.[204] For reasons given earlier, vitamin D may also have an important role in preventing fibrosis that occurs after transition to the pulmonary phase, and it may reduce the cleavage of the S1 subunit of the spike protein at this transition point. Both these effects could be due to the role that vitamin D might play in reducing TGF-β pathway activation,[31] as TGF-β induces expression of furin,[251] the enzyme that cleaves the spike protein at the S1/S2 region.

Based on what has been presented in this chapter, Table 21.1 provides a list of supplements to support vitamin D for prophylaxis and early-stage COVID-19. The core regime comprises vitamin C, vitamin D, zinc, magnesium, selenium and B vitamins. The last can be provided as high-dose multi-vitamin B supplements. Here, individual B doses should be chosen that approach those of Table 21.1. These core agents (shaded regions in Table 21.1) have been selected based on their known antiviral effects and an ability to provide immune support.

For early-stage symptomatic COVID-19, the dose of vitamin D should be increased to 24,000 IU/day with the addition of quercetin whilst keeping the other supplements as per prophylaxis. For the later symptomatic stage (6–8 DfSO), possibly with signs of transition to the early pulmonary phase (as evidenced by rising IL-6 and CRP and falling SpO$_2$), high-dose vitamin D (24,000 IU/day) should be provided with further antioxidant support by way of NAC, nicotinamide, omega-3 fatty acids, vitamin E, quercetin, EGCG and melatonin. These compounds are especially important to complement pharmaceutical agents such as antihistamines, leukotriene receptor blockers, and glucocorticoids such as methylprednisolone.[21] It is also recommended that berberine and resveratrol are provided at this stage to limit mast cell activation by IL-33.[231]

In the clinic or outpatient setting, it would be preferable to provide vitamin D as calcifediol (25-OHD). A suitable dose might be 20,000 IU on day 1 followed by daily doses of 4000 IU. This will avoid problems of conversion of cholecalciferol to 25-OHD.

Some of the compounds presented in Table 21.1, particularly quercetin and EGCG, have mixed activity in terms of antiviral and antioxidant effects. This poses a dilemma, as during the early stage of symptomatic COVID-19, the antiviral effect of inflammasome activation should be maintained for maximal antiviral effectiveness. There is evidence that compounds like quercetin increase Nrf2,[211] and this transcription factor increases antioxidant enzyme expression. This may reduce the antiviral effectiveness of the innate immune system by reducing inflammasome activation. Despite this, it is considered that the ionophore effects of quercetin to deliver Zn to the intracellular environment (and hence, antiviral effectiveness) may outweigh these considerations, and it is recommended that quercetin is used relatively early in the symptomatic phase. Perhaps of even greater importance (see following discussion) is the finding that quercetin is a mast cell stabilizer that acts

TABLE 21.1

Consensus Nutritional Supplements for COVID-19 Prophylaxis and Early and Late-Stage Symptomatic COVID-19 (Consensus-COVID)

Compound category	Compound formulation	Prophylaxis/early-stage symptomatic	Later symptomatic (days 5–7)/ early pulmonary phase/hospital admission
Vitamin C	Ascorbic acid	**Prophylaxis:** 1 g/day **Symptoms:** 0.5–2 g three times/day	0.5–2 g three times/day
Vitamin D	Cholecalciferol	**Prophylaxis:** Loading dose of 12,000 IU/day for 3 weeks followed by 4000 IU/day**Early symptomatic:** 24,000 IU/day for duration of symptoms, then 4000 IU/day	At least 24,000 IU/day for duration of symptoms, then maintenance dose of 4000 IU/dayIn hospital setting, preference is calcifediol 20,000 IU day 1, followed by 4000 IU/day
Zinc	Zinc sulphate	**Prophylaxis:** 50 mg**Early symptomatic:** 50 mg BID	50 mg BID
Quercetin		**Early symptomatic:** 500 mg BID	1000 mg BID
EGCG			600–900 mg/day
Berberine			500 mg/day
Resveratrol			500 mg/day
N-acetylcysteine (NAC)			1000 mg/BID
Vitamin E			800 IU/day
Vitamin B3	Nicotinamide	1000 mg/day	1000 mg/day
Omega-3 fatty acids	DHA and EPA		4 g/day combined DHA/EPA
Magnesium		200–500 mg/day	500 mg/day
Manganese			10 mg/day
Selenium		200 µg/day	200 µg/day
Melatonin			12 mg/day
Vitamin B12	Methylcobalamin	250–500 µg/day	500 µg/day
Vitamin B6	Pyridoxine	25–100 mg/day	100 mg/day
Vitamin B1	Thiamine	100 mg/day	200 mg/BID
Folic acid	Preferred, methyltetrahydrofolate	250–1000 µg/day	1000 µg/day

to reduce the release of histamine, leukotrienes and inflammatory cytokines, such as IL-6, from mast cells.[257, 258] For this reason, the dose of quercetin should be increased to 1 g twice a day at any sign of lowered SpO_2 or breathing difficulty. Other agents, such as EGCG, are restricted to the later symptomatic phase to provide additional antiviral activity and antioxidant support (and to act as mast cell stabilizers).

The same consideration is appropriate for L-lysine. It is likely that this amino acid plays a role in downgrading oxidative stress caused by virally induced bradykinin and cytokine storms. L-lysine has also been proposed as an antiviral agent.[129] Whilst based on the evidence this appears possible, it is perhaps more appropriate that L-lysine is used to treat more advanced COVID-19 in order to mitigate vascular hyperpermeability and vascular inflammation.[124]

As evidence is growing that the transition from the symptomatic to the pulmonary phase involves mast cell degranulation[241, 259, 260] triggered by the release of PAMPs, DAMPs and viral antigens from infected cells, nutritional supplements that stabilize mast cells should be considered. Vitamin C,[261] vitamin D,[262] quercetin[61] and EGCG [263]may be particularly important in this respect, especially in combination. In light of higher glycolytic activity of mast cells stimulated by IL-33,[231] it is important to note that the transcriptional regulator of glycolysis, HIF-1α, is a substrate for prolyl hydroxylase, and when hydroxylated, HIF-1α is marked for ubiquitinylation and proteosomal degradation. A co-substrate for prolyl hydroxylase is ascorbic acid (vitamin C).[264]

Mast cell activation syndrome (MCAS), a condition where mast cells are hypersensitive to activating stimuli, could greatly contribute to the transition from late symptomatic phase to early pulmonary phase of COVID-19, and MCAS may also have a significant part to play in the lingering symptoms of Long COVID.[265]

Another particularly important consideration regarding mast cell activation is the functional state of the glucocorticoid receptor (GR) under conditions of rising oxidative stress. It has been noted that at transition between the late symptomatic and early pulmonary phase, IL-6 begins to rise, and as indicated in the section on antioxidants, this cytokine induces NADPH oxidase, an enzyme that catalyzes the production of superoxide. In the presence of superoxide dismutase and Fe^{2+}, superoxide is converted to the highly damaging hydroxyl radical, a powerful oxidant that has been shown to reduce the transcriptional activation of the GR.[112] As glucocorticoids such as prednisolone and methylprednisolone are important therapeutic agents at transition,[21] GR function must be supported in particular by vitamin C and the thiol antioxidant and glutathione precursor N-acetylcysteine.

Further to the specific effect of glucocorticoid damping on mast cell activation, the ability of the hypothalamus–pituitary–adrenal system (HPA) to respond to pro-inflammatory cytokines (PICs) like IL-6, by producing sufficient cortisol and catecholamines (CAs, adrenaline and noradrenaline) to moderate inflammation,[266] is an important factor not so far considered for COVID-19. As part of the stress response to infection, CAs produced from sympathetic nerve endings and the adrenal medulla (in response to PICs) increase the concentration of cAMP, and this signaling molecule activates protein kinase A (PKA). Pace et al.[267] have demonstrated that the transcriptional activity of the GR is increased by PKA, and so both cortisol and CAs are required for the full transcriptional activation of the GR.

The clinical consequence of a strong adrenal response to the severe stress of infection was realized during Ebola virus disease (EBOV) outbreaks in West Africa from 2001 onwards. Leroy et al.[268] noted that individuals who survived Ebola infection were able to mount a much stronger adrenal response and produced more cortisol. Around 7 days after Ebola infection, survivors produced two to four times as much cortisol (morning cortisol up to 1 μM) as those who died. The HPA was apparently able to respond to the high levels of PICs and produce enough cortisol (and also adrenaline) to moderate the hyper-inflammatory response whilst maintaining the production of anti-inflammatory cytokines, such as IL-10.[269]

Whilst no studies can be found in the literature regarding the cortisol response at the beginning of the early pulmonary phase, significantly lower morning cortisol concentrations were found in hospitalized patients.[270] Whilst adrenal insufficiency may indeed be a factor in more advanced COVID-19,[271] of greater importance to progression of COVID-19 is how the HPA responds to rising PICs at transition from the late symptomatic to the early pulmonary phase. This is when it is most important to support adrenal function, and supplements suggested in Table 21.1 are most suitable in this respect. A specific example is that AA is a cofactor for CA synthesis,[272] and it has been shown that adrenocorticotropic hormone (ACTH), which drives adrenal cortisol synthesis and secretion, also causes the secretion of AA from the adrenal gland.[273]

It is clear from Table 21.1 that no recommendations have been made for advanced, life-threatening disease (advanced pulmonary phase). This stage of the disease requires specialist care, and the reader is again referred to the MATH+ protocol of the FLCCC Alliance.[22] Their protocol[274] is designed for hospitalized patients in both the early pulmonary and late pulmonary phases (the latter requiring ICU admission). One of the critical elements of the MATH+ protocol is the provision of IV methylprednisolone dependent on oxygen requirement or abnormal chest X-ray.

Earlier, ivermectin was mentioned as part of the MATH+ protocol.[22] The evidence for the benefit of ivermectin throughout the clinical course of COVID-19 is cited in Chaccour et al. (2021), Lawrie (2021) and Kory et al. (2021).[275–277]

Given the number of people infected worldwide, this chapter would be incomplete without expanding a little on Long COVID. A cohort study from Wuhan[278] of 1733 patients following hospitalization for COVID-19 (half younger than 57 years) revealed that 6 months after infection, 63% of those who had recovered suffered from fatigue or muscle weakness, 26% suffered sleep disturbances, and 23% suffered anxiety and/or depression. Patients who survived severe COVID-19 had a lingering impairment of pulmonary diffusion capacity and abnormal chest imaging. Many of these long-term effects may be due to continuing disturbance of the immune system. Ex vivo stimulation of PBMCs from patients recovering from severe disease (with SARS-CoV-2 antigens) has shown a greatly enhanced response of innate immune cells.[19] This indicates that symptoms of Long COVID could be due to a low-level inflammatory response, either as a constitutive response to unspecific activators or due to the continuing presence of viral fragments or even pockets of live virus. Of high significance here is the work of Patterson et al.[279] showing that the S1 component of the spike trimer is present in CD16+ monocytes of individuals up to 15 months after infection. This protein may be responsible for a continuing inflammatory response.

For these reasons, it is suggested that individuals suffering from Long COVID use the protocol suggested here for the late symptomatic phase of COVID-19 (Table 21.1). This protocol combines several elements, including antiviral, antioxidant and mast cell stabilization. MCAS has been suggested as one of the contributing factors for Long COVID syndrome.[265] A particularly important consideration might be that long-term inflammation through the acute phases of COVID-19 induces epigenetic changes in bone marrow monocyte progenitors. The phenotype of monocytes derived from stem cell progenitors may be altered by COVID-19 to give rise to more inflammatory macrophages.[19] Here, it may be particularly important to consider the role of vitamin D in combination with a plentiful supply of antioxidants, such as vitamin C,[280] as vitamin D is a known modulator of cellular epigenetic status.

At the time of the final update of this chapter, in April 2022, the vaccine program for COVID-19 has been running for well over a year in most countries around the world. Data from major reporting systems, such as the UK Health Security Agency (UKHSA), have suggested that the mRNA product from Pfizer-BioNTech, BNT162b2 (also known as COMIRNATY), the adenovirus vector-type vaccine from Oxford–AstraZeneca, AZD1222 (sold as Covishield and Vaxzevria), and the Moderna vaccine, mRNA-1273, sold under the brand name Spikevax, lead to reduced hospitalizations and deaths for people testing positive for SARS-CoV-2. Whilst the UKHSA Vaccine report to week 13[281] shows a reduction in hospitalizations and deaths, infection rates for the vaccinated are apparently higher than for the unvaccinated. These observations concerning infection are consistent with other countries, such as Israel, where the vaccinated appear to have a higher chance of becoming infected than the unvaccinated. If these observations represent a real effect, then the innate immune system, acting within the upper respiratory tract and mucosal surfaces, must be adversely affected by vaccination.

A strategy adopted to increase the stability of mRNA vaccines has been to replace uridine bases with N1-methylpseudouridine. This may have the unintended consequence of reducing the innate immune response to infection (in general). Toll-like receptors 3, 7 and 8 and also RIG-1 receptors are involved in recognizing RNA structures,[282], but they fail to recognize methyl and pseudouridine-modified RNAs.[283, 284] Depending on the tissue residence time of vaccinal mRNAs, the innate immune system may be partially blind to infection,[285] and this may have the effect of increasing infection rates in the vaccinated. A further unintended consequence may be the reactivation of latent viruses such as herpes zoster, HHV6/HHV7 (pityriasis rosea) and Epstein–Barr post mRNA vaccination.[286, 287] A loss of innate immune surveillance could also be problematic with respect to nascent cancer cell division and tumor growth. In vitro studies, the purpose of which were to look at antibody V(D)J recombination in B-cell immunity, have demonstrated that the spike protein of SARS-CoV-2 enters the nucleus. [288] Within the nucleus, the spike protein apparently impedes the recruitment of BRCA1 and 53BP1, reducing DNA damage repair. It should be noted that the mutated form of BRCA1 came to widespread attention as a hereditary risk factor for breast cancer. Presence of the mutated gene endows a 60% risk for developing breast cancer.

Whilst immunization with mRNA or adenovirus constructs does seem to produce strong IgG and IgA responses,[289] the choice of spike protein as antigen is problematic for a number of further reasons. From the clinical observations of Dr Shankara Chetty,[290] it is clear that vaccinated individuals often become ill with many of the symptoms of the early pulmonary phase. He describes this as "spike protein illness" and treats with the same protocol as for natural infection.[291] Many physicians and scientists now concur that the spike protein is indeed a toxin. Work conducted by the pathologists Professors Arne Burkhardt and Walter Lang have clearly demonstrated spike protein in the blood vessels of persons dying some months after vaccination. They performed detailed histopathology and immunohistochemistry and show spike protein associated with vascular endothelial cells together with marked lymphocyte infiltration and destruction of normal blood vessel architecture.[292] They also describe onion skin lesions or concentric circumvascular fibrosis in the spleen, a pathology seen in autoimmune conditions such as systemic lupus erythematosus. The presence of the spike protein, lymphocyte invasion and vascular destruction were found in the organs of deceased individuals, including, for example, the spleen, the heart, the liver, the kidney, the ovary, the thyroid gland, the salivary gland and the dura mater, some months after vaccination. These observations are consistent with an autoimmune attack on tissue structures.

Observations on spike protein toxicity from clinical practice and from post-mortem studies are supported by work showing that the RBD of the original Wuhan strain of SARS-CoV-2 is highly antigenic, much more so than the entire spike protein. [293] By subjecting the 3D structure of this region to epitope prediction, 9 sites were identified, 7 of which contained amino acids with sequence similarity to 12 pathogenic bacterial species, 2 malaria parasites and influenza virus A. Indeed, the 7 sites showed molecular similarity to 54 antigens from these bacteria, parasites and influenza virus. Particularly notable was that all seven sites showed antigenic similarity to *Mycobacterium tuberculosis* and *Plasmodium falciparum*. Also most intriguing was the antigenic similarity of four of these sites with *Borrelia burgdorferi*, the infective agent of Lyme disease. The author of this paper commented that

> most of the antigenic determinants found in pathogenic microorganisms were related to antigenic proteins having established function as toxin(s) and proven role in virulence and pathogenicity. Besides this, other antigenic determinants found similar to Mycobacterium antigens having role in persistence and survival of pathogen in host cells. Some antigenic determinants from HA and NP of influenza virus A were also in antigenic sites of SARS-CoV-2 and these antigens from influenza virus have role in assembly of newly budded virions in case of influenza virus A.

Although not undertaken in the study by Dakal,[293] as the variant had yet to be discovered, the author of the current chapter has considered the amino acid mutations in the Omicron variant.[294] Three of the seven sites identified as highly antigenic had mutations in Omicron that would probably reduce similarity to antigenic sites in all the identified bacteria, parasites and influenza virus A. The greatest change in antigenicity of Omicron is for antigens of the original Wuhan sequence that were shared with *Mycobacterium tuberculosis* and *Plasmodium falciparum*. These changes may go part way to explaining why the Omicron variant is less virulent than the previous variant of concern, the Delta. Also noted by the author of this chapter is that some versions of Omicron completely lack the polybasic furin cleavage site. This is very likely the reason for observations showing that cellular uptake of Omicron is by the endosomal pathway.[295]

In addition to similarity with antigenic determinants of microorganisms, the spike protein shows sequence similarity to a number of human proteins. Sorensen et al.[296] have indicated that 78.4% of the spike protein of SARS-CoV-2 has similarity with known human proteins. The authors of this paper suggest that "if all epitopes on the 1,255-amino acid long SARS-CoV-2 spike protein can be used by antibodies, then there will be 983 antibody binding sites which also could bind to epitopes on human proteins." As the engineered spike protein, delivered via mRNA transfection or adenovirus vector, is substantially similar to the wild type from SARS-CoV-2 infection, there is a high possibility for autoimmunity. These concerns have been shared by many, including Vojdani and Kharrazian[297] and Kanduc and Shoenfeld,[298] and they are realized in the post-mortem observations of Burkhardt and Lang.[292]

Of further significance with regard to toxicity of the spike protein is that in addition to the incorporation of N1-methylpseudouridine and an increase in the GC content of the engineered RNA sequence,[299] the mRNA codes for two substitute prolines in the S2 fusion domain at around 987 in the amino acid sequence.[300] This change was introduced to maintain the spike in an "open" configuration, preventing fusion with cell membranes but allowing attachment to ACE2. Translated spike protein that exits the cell will therefore bind to ACE2 of surrounding cells (or leave in extracellular vesicles, see later discussion) and remain attached without internalization. Suzuki et al. (2021)[301] and Suzuki and Gychka (2021)[302] have shown that the spike S1 subunit suppresses ACE2. Angiotensin II will not be so efficiently converted to Ang_{1-7}, and so, a large part of the damage inflicted by the spike protein may be due to oxidative stress, as angiotensin II is a potent inducer of NADPH oxidase.[303] These inhibitory effects on ACE2 are clearly at odds with the work presented earlier on bronchoalveolar lavage (BAL) samples.[124] This report revealed that expression of ACE2 was increased 200-fold in BAL samples from COVID-19 patients in comparison to non-COVID-19 samples. One can only assume that conditions in the lung during advanced disease give rise to a compensatory feedback loop that increases the expression of ACE2.

In addition to an ability to suppress ACE2 activity, the spike protein itself has been shown to induce angiotensin II type 1 receptor (AT1)–mediated signaling in endothelial cells, increasing the release of IL-6.[304] IL-6 also induces NADPH oxidase. Lei et al. (2021)[305] demonstrated that a pseudo virus with SARS-CoV-2 S1 protein caused inflammation of arteries and lungs of mice, and in endothelial cells, it reduced mitochondrial function and increased glycolysis. A significant finding was that the antioxidant and glutathione precursor, NAC, reversed these effects. These studies confirm that the spike protein, without the rest of SARS-CoV-2, is toxic for blood vessel endothelial cells and other cells expressing ACE2.

The finding on the apparent effect of the spike protein to activate the AT1 receptor can also explain the observed rise in IL-6 apparent for some individuals around a week after vaccination.[290] Also, for individuals who transition into the *early pulmonary phase*, around 6–10 days after symptom onset, the observations reported earlier reinforce the idea that there is a release of spike protein components from infected and damaged cells (see earlier discussion on viroporins and PAMP and DAMP release) at this time. The release of spike protein components is likely to be related to furin destabilization of the spike protein and the shedding of the S1 subunit.

Of concern for the longer-term effects of vaccination are prion-like elements within the spike protein. Prion-type proteins have characteristic glycine zipper motifs (GxxxG). They become toxic when α-helices misfold as β-sheets and the protein loses its normal membrane function.[306] The native amyloid protein, the amyloid-β precursor protein (APP), has four glycine zipper motifs. The SARS-CoV-2 spike glycoprotein has five. Tetz and Tetz[307] have suggested that the prion-like nature of the spike protein may enhance binding of the RBD to ACE2.

Adjacent to the RBD of the spike protein is a heparin binding site. This is thought essential for initial binding (anchoring) of the spike protein to cell membrane heparin sulphate glycocalyx polysaccharides. Initial anchoring allows more favorable interaction of the RBD with cellular ACE2.[308, 309] Whilst this may be the situation following infection with SARS-CoV-2 and where heparin administration may block binding of the virus to cell membranes, for the vaccine-derived spike protein, it is already in a configuration allowing more favorable binding of the RBD to ACE2. As such, the heparin sulphate binding site of the S1 region is exposed, allowing interaction with other heparin binding proteins. In this respect, Idrees and Kumar[310] have shown that "the SARS-CoV-2 S1 RBD binds to a number of aggregation-prone, heparin binding proteins including Aβ, α-synuclein, tau, prion, and TDP-43 RRM." This suggests that spike proteins that are expressed in or transported to the brain (perhaps by way of exosomes originating in other parts of the body[311]) could act as nuclei for the accumulation of toxic aggregates of misfolded brain proteins.

In addition to the long persistence of the S1 component in monocytes (15 months after infection),[279] the spike protein has been shown to be a component of extracellular vesicles (exosomes) 4 months after vaccination[312] These long residence times within the body raise the question as to whether the spike protein is continuously synthesized or whether its half-life is greatly extended under certain conditions. A group from MIT and Harvard University have conducted a series of experiments that suggest the SARS-CoV-2 RNA can be reverse transcribed and integrated into the human genome.[313] They found chimeric transcripts containing SARS-CoV-2 sequences in patients who recovered from COVID-19. Whether this could happen to transfected mRNA from vaccine preparations is a major question. In a study using the liver cell line Huh7, Aldén et al.[314] have demonstrated that mRNA from Pfizer-BioNtech BNT162b2 is taken up by these cells and is indeed reverse transcribed to DNA. The endogenous protein with reverse transcriptase capability responsible for this is likely to be long interspersed nuclear element-1 or LINE-1. Their work showed increased nuclear distribution of this enzyme after exposing cells to BNT162b2.

SINEs (short interspersed nuclear elements) and LINEs belong to a class of genetic elements called retrotransposomes. They can copy and paste DNA to new sites via RNA as an intermediate. In fact, nearly a third of the human genome comprises these mobile DNA elements. This may be particularly pertinent to sperm cells, as they express high levels of LINE 1, and testes are a site for vaccinal mRNA uptake. Sperm cells can reverse transcribe exogenous RNA to cDNA and deliver this as cDNA plasmids to fertilized eggs. Remarkably, these extrachromosomal structures survive to adulthood and can be passed to progeny as a template for protein synthesis.[315] LINE-1 is also expressed in cancer cells and in immune cells in autoimmune diseases, such as systemic lupus erythematosus, Sjogren's and psoriasis.[316]

As suggested earlier, the continued presence of spike protein after the acute symptoms of COVID-19 have abated most probably accounts for many of the symptoms of Long COVID. The symptoms of Long COVID cross over with those of post-vaccine illness, in particular, fatigue and exercise intolerance. It is most likely that the continuing presence of the spike protein is responsible for this too, and the spike-induced activation of stress-associated pathways alters metabolism, slewing it toward glycolysis and away from mitochondrial oxidative phosphorylation.

Based on studies of the effect of SARS-CoV-2 spike on cell signaling systems and on oxidative stress, a clear strategy for treatment of vaccine adverse effects would be to support antioxidant pathways. The compounds discussed in this article, such as ascorbic acid, NAC, quercetin, nicotinamide and melatonin (a powerful mitochondrial antioxidant), at the doses suggested in Table 21.1 (for the later symptomatic phase), would be most appropriate. It would also be appropriate to maintain 25OHD by supplementing daily with at least 4000 IU cholecalciferol and to maintain the concentrations of fundamental minerals and B vitamins, as suggested for the later *symptomatic phase*. Indeed, it would be wise to start supplementation before vaccination and to maintain for at least a month after vaccination. The dose of quercetin may be particularly important. It is recommended that 1 g is taken twice a day.

REFERENCES

1. Chan JF, Kok KH, Zhu Z et al. Genomic characterization of the 2019 novel human-pathogenic coronavirus isolated from a patient with atypical pneumonia after visiting Wuhan. *Emerg Microb Infect* 2020;9(1):221–236. https://doi.org/10.1080/22221751.2020.1719902
2. Anand P, Puranik A, Aravamudan M et al. Origin of virus SARS-CoV-2 strategically mimics proteolytic activation of human ENaC. *eLife* 2020;9:e58603 https://doi.org/10.7554/eLife.58603
3. Lam TTY, Jia N, Zhang YW. Identifying SARS-CoV-2-related coronaviruses in Malayan pangolins. *Nature* 2020;583:282–285. https://doi.org/10.1038/s41586-020-2169-0

4. Mateus J, Grifoni A, Tarke A et al. Selective and cross-reactive SARS-CoV-2 T cell epitopes in unexposed humans. *Science* 2020;370, Issue 6512, pp. 89–94 https://doi.org/10.1126/science.abd3871

5. Zhan SH, Deverman BE, Chan YA. SARS-CoV-2 is well adapted for humans. What does this mean for re-emergence? *bioRxiv* 2020.05.01.073262. https://doi.org/10.1101/2020.05.01.073262

6. Seyran M, Pizzol D, Adadi P et al. Questions concerning the proximal origin of SARS-CoV-2. *J Med Virol* 2020;1–3. https://doi.org/10.1002/jmv.26478

7. Latham J, Wilson A. *A Proposed Origin for SARS-CoV-2 and the COVID-19 Pandemic.* 2020 https://www.independentsciencenews.org/commentaries/a-proposed-origin-for-sars-cov-2-and-the-covid-19-pandemic

8. Piplani S, Singh PK, David A, Winkler DA and Petrovsky N. In silico comparison of SARS-CoV-2 spike protein-ACE2 binding affinities across species and implications for viral origin. https://arxiv.org/pdf/2005.06199.pdf

9. Shang J, Wan Y, Luo C et al. Cell entry mechanisms of SARS-CoV-2. *Proc Natl Acad Sci USA.* 2020;117(21):11727–11734. https://doi.org/10.1073/pnas.2003138117

10. Yue Zhang, Li Zhang, Jiajing Wu, Yuanling Yu, Shuo Liu, Tao Li, Qianqian Li, Ruxia Ding, Haixin Wang, Jianhui Nie, Zhimin Cui, Yulin Wang, Weijin Huang & Youchun Wang (2022) A second functional furin site in the SARS-CoV-2 spike protein, *Emerg Microb Infect.* 11(1):182–194. https://doi.org/10.1080/22221751.2021.2014284

11. Peacock TP, Goldhill DH, Zhou J et al. The furin cleavage site in the SARS-CoV-2 spike protein is required for transmission in ferrets. *Nat Microbiol.* 2021 Jul;6(7):899–909. https://doi.org/10.1038/s41564-021-00908-w

12. Letarov AV, Babenko VV, Kulikov EE. Free SARS-CoV-2 spike protein S1 particles may play a role in the pathogenesis of COVID-19 infection. *Biochemistry.* 2021 Mar;86(3):257–261. https://doi.org/10.1134/S0006297921030032

13. Sasaki M, Uemura K, Sato A et al. SARS-CoV-2 variants with mutations at the S1/S2 cleavage site are generated in vitro during propagation in TMPRSS2-deficient cells. *PLoS Pathog.* 2021 Jan 21;17(1):e1009233. https://doi.org/10.1371/journal.ppat.1009233

14. Chen M, Shen W, Rowan NR et al. Elevated ACE-2 expression in the olfactory neuroepithelium: Implications for anosmia and upper respiratory SARS-CoV-2 entry and replication. *European Respiratory Journal.* 2020;56:2001948. https://doi.org/10.1183/13993003.01948-2020

15. Travis CR. As plain as the nose on your face: The case for a nasal (mucosal) route of vaccine administration for covid-19 disease prevention. *Front. Immunol.* 30 September 2020. https://doi.org/10.3389/fimmu.2020.591897

16. West NP, Pyne DB, Renshaw G and Cripps AW. Antimicrobial peptides and proteins, exercise and innate mucosal immunity. *Immunol Med Microbiol.* 2006 Dec;48(3):293–304. https://doi.org/10.1111/j.1574-695X.2006.00132.x

17. Saitoh SI, Abe F, Kanno A et al. TLR7 mediated viral recognition results in focal type I interferon secretion by dendritic cells. *Nat Commun.* 2017;8:1592. https://doi.org/10.1038/s41467-017-01687-x

18. Ra SH, Lim JS, Kim G et al. Upper respiratory viral load in asymptomatic individuals and mildly symptomatic patients with SARS-CoV-2 infection. *Thorax* 2021;76:61–63; Yilmaz A, Marklund, E Maria Andersson M, et al. Respiratory Tract Levels of Severe Acute Respiratory Syndrome Coronavirus 2 RNA and Duration of Viral RNA Shedding Do Not Differ Between Patients With Mild and Severe/Critical Coronavirus Disease 2019.The Journal of Infectious Diseases 2020; Volume 223(1):15–18. https://academic.oup.com/jid/advance-article/doi/10.1093/infdis/jiaa632/5918189

19. Le Bert N, Clapham HE, Tan AT et al. Highly functional virus-specific cellular immune response in asymptomatic SARS-CoV-2 infection. *J Exp Med* 3 May 2021;218 (5): E20202617. https://doi.org/10.1084/jem.20202617

20. CDC. https://www.cdc.gov/coronavirus/2019-ncov/symptoms-testing/symptoms.html

21. Chetty S. Elucidating the pathogenesis and Rx of COVID reveals a missing element. *Modern Med* 2020;3:50–53.

22. FLCCC Alliance. https://covid19criticalcare.com/

23. Webb BJ, Peltan ID, Paul Jensen P et al. Criteria for COVID-19-associated hyperinflammatory syndrome: A cohort study. 2020; September 29. https://doi.org/10.1016/S2665-9913(20)30343-X

24. Herold T, Jurinovic V, Arnreich C, et al. Elevated levels of IL-6 and CRP predict the need for mechanical ventilation in COVID-19. *J Allergy Clin Immunol.* 2020;146(1):128-136.e4. https://doi.org/10.1016/j.jaci.2020.05.008

25. Laguna-Goya R, Utrero-Rico A, Talayero P et al. IL-6-based mortality risk model for hospitalized patients with COVID-19. *J Allergy Clin Immunol.* 2020;146(4):799-807.e9. https://doi.org/10.1016/j.jaci.2020.07.009

26. Alsaffar H, Martino N, Garrett JP and Adam AP. Interleukin-6 promotes a sustained loss of endothelial barrier function via Janus kinase-mediated STAT3 phosphorylation and de novo protein synthesis. *Am J Physiol Cell Physiol*. 2018 May 1;314(5):C589–C602. https://doi.org/10.1152/ajpcell.00235.2017

27. Lee J, Lee S, Zhang H, Hill MA, Zhang C, Park Y (2017) Interaction of IL-6 and TNF-α contributes to endothelial dysfunction in type 2 diabetic mouse hearts. *PLoS ONE* 12(11): E0187189. https://doi.org/10.1371/journal.pone.0187189

28. Wynn TA, Vannella KM. Macrophages in tissue repair, regeneration, and fibrosis. *Immunity*. 2016;44(3):450–462. https://doi.org/10.1016/j.immuni.2016.02.015

29. George PM, Wells AU, Jenkins RG. Pulmonary fibrosis and COVID-19: The potential role for antifibrotic therapy. *Lancet Respir Med*. 2020 Aug;8(8):807–815. https://doi.org/10.1016/S2213-2600(20)30225-3

30. Ding N, Yu RT, Subramaniam N et al. A vitamin D receptor/SMAD genomic circuit gates hepatic fibrotic response. *Cell*. 2013;153(3):601–613. https://doi.org/10.1016/j.cell.2013.03.028

31. Evans RM, Lippman SM. Shining light on the COVID-19 pandemic: A vitamin D receptor checkpoint in defence of unregulated wound healing. *Cell Metab*. 2020 Nov 3;32(5):704–709. https://doi.org/10.1016/j.cmet.2020.09.007

32. Ray S, Ju X, Sun H et al. The IL-6 trans-signaling-STAT3 pathway mediates ECM and cellular proliferation in fibroblasts from hypertrophic scar. *J Invest Dermatol*. 2013;133(5):1212–1220. https://doi.org/10.1038/jid.2012.499

33. Yamamoto T, Matsuda T, Muraguchi A et al. Cross-talk between IL-6 and TGF-β signaling in hepatoma cells. *FEBS Lett*. 2001;492(3):247–253. https://doi.org/10.1016/S0014-5793(01)02258-X

34. Eapen MS, Lu W, Gaikwad AV et al. Endothelial to mesenchymal transition (EndMT): A precursor to post-SARS-CoV-2 infection (COVID-19) interstitial pulmonary fibrosis and vascular obliteration? *Resp J*. Jan 2020;2003167. https://doi.org/10.1183/13993003.03167-2020

35. Yamada D, Kobayashi S, Wada H et al. Role of crosstalk between interleukin-6 and transforming growth factor-beta 1 in epithelial–mesenchymal transition and chemoresistance in biliary tract cancer. *Journal of Cancer* 2013;49(7) May 2013:1725–1740. https://doi.org/10.1016/j.ejca.2012.12.002

36. Zhao X, Nicholls JM, Chen Y-G. Severe acute respiratory syndrome-associated coronavirus nucleocapsid protein interacts with Smad3 and modulates transforming growth factor-β signaling. *J Biol Chem*. 2008;283(6):3272–3280. https://doi.org/10.1074/jbc.M708033200

37. Schmidt-Arras D, Rose-John S. IL-6 pathway in the liver: From physiopathology to therapy. *J Hepatol*. 2016 Jun;64(6):1403–15. https://doi.org/10.1016/j.jhep.2016.02.004. Epub 2016 Feb 8. PMID:26867490

38. Sproston NR, Ashworth JJ. Role of C-reactive protein at sites of inflammation and infection. *Front Immunol*. 2018;9:754. Published 2018 Apr 13. https://doi.org/10.3389/fimmu.2018.00754

39. Ram Kumar Pandian S, Arunachalam S, Deepak V et al. Targeting complement cascade: An alternative strategy for COVID-19. *3 Biotech 10*. 2020:479. https://doi.org/10.1007/s13205-020-02464-2

40. Lucas C, Wong P, Klein J et al. Longitudinal analyses reveal immunological misfiring in severe COVID-19. *Nature*. 2020;584:463–469. https://doi.org/10.1038/s41586-020-2588-y

41. Kelley N, Jeltema D, Duan Y, He Y. The NLRP3 inflammasome: An overview of mechanisms of activation and regulation. *Int J Mol Sci*. 2019;20(13):3328. Published 2019 Jul 6. https://doi.org/10.3390/ijms20133328

42. Tan L, Wang Q, Zhang D et al. Lymphopenia predicts disease severity of COVID-19: A descriptive and predictive study. *Sig Transduct Target Ther*. 2020;5:33. https://doi.org/10.1038/s41392-020-0148-4

43. Davanzo GG, Codo AC, Natalia S et al. *SARS-CoV-2 uses CD4 to Infect T Helper Lymphocytes 2020.09.25.20200329*. https://doi.org/10.1101/2020.09.25.20200329

44. Rojas JM, Avia M, Martín V, and Sevilla N. IL-10: A multifunctional cytokine in viral infections *J Immunological Research*. 2017:6104054. https://doi.org/10.1155/2017/6104054.

45. Dhar SK, Vishnupriyan K, Damodar S et al. IL-6 and IL-10 as predictors of disease severity in COVID 19 patients: Results from meta-analysis and regression. 2020.08.15.20175844. https://doi.org/10.1101/2020.08.15.20175844

46. Zhao Y, Qin L, Zhang P et al. Longitudinal COVID-19 profiling associates IL-1RA and IL-10 with disease severity and RANTES with mild disease. *JCI Insight*. 2020 Jul 9;5(13):e139834. https://doi.org/10.1172/jci.insight.139834

47. Hidalgo A. A NET-thrombosis axis in COVID-19. *Blood*. 2020;136 (10):1118–1119. https://doi.org/10.1182/blood.2020007951

48. Middleton EA, He XY, Denorme F et al. Neutrophil extracellular traps contribute to immunothrombosis in COVID-19 acute respiratory distress syndrome. *Blood*. 2020 Sep 3;136(10):1169–1179. https://doi.org/10.1182/blood.2020007008

49. Cruse G, Bradding P. Mast cells in airway diseases and interstitial lung disease. *Eur J Pharmacol.* 2016;778:125–138. https://doi.org/10.1016/j.ejphar.2015.04.046

50. Neumann J, Prezzemolo T, Vanderbeke L et al. Increased IL-10-producing regulatory T cells are characteristic of severe cases of COVID-19. *Clin. Transl. Immunol.* 2020:9:e1204. https://doi.org/10.1002/cti2.1204

51. McGregor R, Chauss D, Freiwald T et al. An autocrine vitamin D-driven Th1 shutdown program can be exploited for COVID-19. Preprint. *bioRxiv.* 2020;2020.07.18.210161. Published 2020 Jul 19. https://doi.org/10.1101/2020.07.18.210161

52. Grifoni A, Weiskopf D, Ramirez SI et al. Targets of T cell responses to SARS-CoV-2 coronavirus in humans with COVID-19 disease and unexposed individuals. *Cell.* 2020;181(7):1489–1501.e15. https://doi.org/10.1016/j.cell.2020.05.015

53. Zizzo G, Cohen PL. Imperfect storm: Is interleukin-33 the Achilles heel of COVID-19? *Lancet Rheumatol.* 2020 Dec;2(12):e779–e790. https://doi.org/10.1016/S2665-9913(20)30340-4

54. Tiemessen MM, Jagger AL, Evans HG, et al. CD4+CD25+Foxp3+ regulatory T cells induce alternative activation of human monocytes/macrophages. *Proc Natl Acad Sci USA* 2007;104:19446–51. https://doi.org/10.1073/pnas.0706832104

55. Liao M, Liu Y, Yuan J. et al. Single-cell landscape of bronchoalveolar immune cells in patients with COVID-19. *Nat Med* 2020;26:842–844 https://doi.org/10.1038/s41591-020-0901-9

56. SARS coronavirus 2 interactome. https://viralzone.expasy.org/9077

57. Xu L, Kitani A, Strober W. Molecular mechanisms regulating TGF-beta-induced Foxp3 expression. *Mucosal Immunol.* 2010;3(3):230–238. https://doi.org/10.1038/mi.2010.7

58. Zhang Y, Zhang J, Chen Y et al. The ORF8 protein of SARS-CoV-2 mediates immune evasion through potently downregulating MHC-I. *bioRxiv* 2020.05.24.111823. https://doi.org/10.1101/2020.05.24.111823

59. Buszko, M., Park, JH., Verthelyi, D et al. The dynamic changes in cytokine responses in COVID-19: A snapshot of the current state of knowledge. *Nat Immunol.* 2020;21:1146–1151. https://doi.org/10.1038/s41590-020-0779-1

60. Wei J, Stoesser N, Matthews PC et al. Antibody responses to SARS-CoV-2 vaccines in 45,965 adults from the general population of the United Kingdom. *Nat Microbiol.* 2021. https://doi.org/10.1038/s41564-021-00947-3

61. Moskowitz DW, Sanchez-Gonzalez MA, Marinelli ER et al. Quercetin for COVID19? *Diabetes Complications.* 2020;4(2);1–2. https://cannabiscancersite.wordpress.com/2021/12/03/dr-david-moskowitz-has-successfully-treated-covid-with-quercetin-since-april-2020/

62. Deb C, Salinas AN, Zheng T et al. A 1-minute blood test detects decreased immune function and increased clinical risk in COVID-19 patients. *Sci Rep.* 2021;11(1):23491. https://doi.org/10.1038/s41598-021-02863-2

63. Chairatana P, Nolan EM. Defensins, lectins, mucins, and secretory immunoglobulin A: Microbe-binding biomolecules that contribute to mucosal immunity in the human gut. *Crit Rev Biochem Mol Biol.* 2017;52(1):45–56. https://doi.org/10.1080/10409238.2016.1243654

64. Cerutti A, Rescigno M. The biology of intestinal immunoglobulin A responses. *Immunity* 2008;28(6):740–750

65. Scher JU, Abramson SB. The microbiome and rheumatoid arthritis. *Rheumatol* 2011 Aug 23;7(10):569–78. https://doi.org/10.1038/nrrheum.2011.121

66. Newton CJ (2017) Gut reactions (revisited): Breaking the barrier. https://www.linkedin.com/pulse/gut-reactions-revisited-breaking-barrier-chris-newton/

67. Jacques P, Elewaut D. Joint expedition: Linking gut inflammation to arthritis. *Mucosal Immunol.* 2008;1:364–371. https://doi.org/10.1038/mi.2008.24

68. Enaud R, Prevel R, Ciarlo E, et al. The gut-lung axis in health and respiratory diseases: A place for inter-organ and inter-kingdom crosstalks. *Front Cell Infect Microbiol.* 2020;10:9. Published 2020 Feb 19. https://doi.org/10.3389/fcimb.2020.00009

69. Ma Y, Yang X, Chatterjee V et al. The gut-lung axis in systemic inflammation. Role of mesenteric lymph as a conduit. *Respir Cell Mol Biol.* 2021 Jan;64(1):19–28. https://doi.org/10.1165/rcmb.2020-0196TR

70. Trompette A, Gollwitzer ES, Pattaroni C et al. Dietary fiber confers protection against flu by shaping Ly6c- patrolling monocyte hematopoiesis and CD8+ T cell metabolism. *Immunity.* 2018 May 15;48(5):992-1005.e8. https://doi.org/10.1016/j.immuni.2018.04.022

71. Narasaraju T, Tang BM, Martin Herrmann M et al. Neutrophilia and NETopathy as key pathologic drivers of progressive lung impairment in patients with COVID-19. *Front. Pharmacol.* 05 June 2020. https://doi.org/10.3389/fphar.2020.00870

72. Schulthess J, Pandey S, Capitani M et al. The short chain fatty acid butyrate imprints an antimicrobial program in macrophages. *Immunity.* 2019 Feb 19;50(2):432-445.e7. https://doi.org/10.1016/j.immuni .2018.12.018

73. Watt R, Parkin K, Martino D. The potential effects of short-chain fatty acids on the epigenetic regulation of innate immune memory. *Challenges.* 2020;11(2):25. https://doi.org/10.3390/challe11020025

74. Zuo T, Zhang F, Lui GCY et al. Alterations in gut microbiota of patients with COVID-19 during time of hospitalization. *Gastroenterology.* 2020 Sep;159(3):944-955.e8. https://doi.org/10.1053/j.gastro.2020.05 .048

75. Dhar D, Mohanty A. Gut microbiota and Covid-19- possible link and implications, *Virus Research.* 2020;285:198018. https://doi.org/10.1016/j.virusres.2020.198018

76. Archer DL, Kramer DC. The use of microbial accessible and fermentable carbohydrates and/or butyrate as supportive treatment for patients with coronavirus SARS-CoV-2 infection. *Front Med (Lausanne).* 2020;7:292

77. Shaver W. Vitamin C, vitamin D and Kefir for early treatment of COVID-19. https://www.william-shavermd.com/quick-treat-antiviral-regimen/

78. Peluzio M, Dias M, Martinez A and Milagro FI. Kefir and intestinal microbiota modulation: Implications in human health. *Front. Nutr.* 22 February 2021. https://doi.org/10.3389/fnut.2021.638740

79. Wastyk HC, Fragiadakis GK, Perelman D et al. Gut-microbiota-targeted diets modulate human immune status. *Cell.* 2021;184(16): P4137–4153.

80. Wischmeyer PE, Tang H, Ren Yi et al. Daily lactobacillus probiotic versus placebo in COVID-19-exposed household contacts (PROTECT-EHC): A randomized clinical trial. *medRxiv 2022.01.04.21268275.* https://doi.org/10.1101/2022.01.04.21268275

81. Barbosa MC, Grosso RA, Claudio Marcelo Fader CM. Hallmarks of aging: An autophagic perspective. *Endocrinol.* 09 January 2019. https://doi.org/10.3389/fendo.2018.00790

82. Lee H-M, Shin D-M, Yuk J-M et al. Autophagy negatively regulates keratinocyte inflammatory responses via scaffolding protein p62/SQSTM1. *J Immunol.* January 15, 2011;186 (2) 1248–1258. https://doi.org/10.4049/jimmunol.1001954

83. Abderrazak A, El Hadri K, Bosc E et al. Inhibition of the inflammasome NLRP3 by arglabin attenuates inflammation, protects pancreatic β-cells from apoptosis, and prevents type 2 diabetes mellitus development in ApoE2Ki mice on a chronic high-fat diet. *J Pharmacol Exp Ther.* 2016 Jun;357(3):487–94. https://doi.org/10.1124/jpet.116.232934

84. Biasizzo M, Kopitar-Jerala N. Interplay between NLRP3 inflammasome and autophagy. *Front. Immunol.* 09 October 2020. https://doi.org/10.3389/fimmu.2020.591803

85. Kelley N, Jeltema D, Duan Y, He Y. The NLRP3 inflammasome: An overview of mechanisms of activation and regulation. *Int J Mol Sci.* 2019;20(13):3328. Published 2019 Jul 6. https://doi.org/10.3390/ijms20133328

86. Hannan MA, Rahman MA, Rahman MS, et al. Intermittent fasting, a possible priming tool for host defense against SARS-CoV-2 infection: Crosstalk among calorie restriction, autophagy and immune response. *Immunol Lett.* 2020;226:38–45. https://doi.org/10.1016/j.imlet.2020.07.001

87. Mohamud Y, Xue YC, Liu, H et al. The papain-like protease of coronaviruses cleaves ULK1 to disrupt host autophagy. *Biochem Biophys Res Commun.* 2021;540:75–82. https://doi.org/10.1016/j.bbrc.2020.12 .091

88. Goswami D, Kumar M, Ghosh SK. Natural product compounds in Alpinia officinarum and ginger are potent SARS-CoV-2 papain-like protease inhibitors. *ChemRxiv.* 2020 Preprint. https://doi.org/10.26434/chemrxiv.12071997.v1

89. Carughi A, Huynh LT, Perelman D. Effect of omega-3 fatty acid supplementation on indicators of membrane fluidity. *FASEB J.* 2010;24:939.12–939.12. https://doi.org/10.1096/fasebj.24.1_supplement.939.12

90. Sunshine H, Iruela-Arispe ML. Membrane lipids and cell signaling. *Opin Lipidol.* 2017 Oct;28(5):408–413. https://doi.org/10.1097/MOL.0000000000000443

91. Liang H, Ward WF. PGC-1α: A key regulator of energy metabolism. *Adv Physiol Educ.* 2006;30:145–151. https://doi.org/10.1152/advan.00052.2006

92. Oh DY, Talukdar S, Bae EJ et al. GPR120 is an omega-3 fatty acid receptor mediating potent anti-inflammatory and insulin-sensitizing effects. *Cell.* 2010;142(5):687–698. https://doi.org/10.1016/j.cell .2010.07.041

93. Hosny M, Nahas R, Ali S and Elshafei SA. Khaled H. Impact of oral omega-3 fatty acids supplementation in early sepsis on clinical outcome and immunomodulation, *Egypt. J. Crit. Care Med.* 2013;1:119–126. https://doi.org/10.1016/j.ejccm.2013.11.002

94. Dushianthan A, Cusack R, Burgess VA et al. Immunonutrition for acute respiratory distress syndrome (ARDS) in adults. *Cochrane Database Syst. Rev.* 2019;1:CD012041. https://doi.org/10.1002/14651858 .CD012041.pub2

95. Bistrian BR Parenteral fish-oil emulsions in critically Ill COVID-19 emulsions. *J Parent Ent Nutrition.* 2020;44:1168–1168. https://doi.org/10.1002/jpen.1871

96. Calder PC. Nutrition, immunity and COVID-19. *BMJ Nutrition Prevent Health.* 2020; bmjnph-2020-000085. https://doi.org/10.1136/bmjnph-2020-000085

97. Burtscher J, Cappellano G, Omori A et al. Mitochondria: In the cross fire of SARS-CoV-2 and immunity. *iSience.* 2020;23(10):101631. https://doi.org/10.1016/j.isci.2020.101631

98. Cavezzi A, Troiani E, Corrao S. COVID-19: Hemoglobin, iron, and hypoxia beyond inflammation. A narrative review. *Clin Pract.* 2020 May 28;10(2):1271. https://doi.org/10.4081/cp.2020.1271

99. Edeas M, Saleh J, Peyssonnaux C. Iron: Innocent bystander or vicious culprit in COVID-19 pathogenesis? *Int J Infect Dis.* 2020 Aug;97:303–305. https://doi.org/10.1016/j.ijid.2020.05.110

100. Stojkovic S, Kaun C, Basilio J et al. Tissue factor is induced by interleukin-33 in human endothelial cells: A new link between coagulation and inflammation. *Sci Rep.* 2016 May 4;6:25171. https://doi.org /10.1038/srep25171

101. Zhang D, Zhou X, Yan S et al. Correlation between cytokines and coagulation-related parameters in patients with coronavirus disease 2019 admitted to ICU. *Clinica Chimica Acta.* 2020;510:47–53. https:// doi.org/10.1016/j.cca.2020.07.002.

102. DiNicolantonio JJ, McCarty M. Thrombotic complications of COVID-19 may reflect an upregulation of endothelial tissue factor expression that is contingent on activation of endosomal NADPH oxidase. *Open Heart* 2020;7:e001337. https://doi.org/10.1136/openhrt-2020-001337

103. Chakrabarti B, Banerjee S. Dehydroascorbic acid level in blood of patients suffering from various infectious diseases. *Proc Soc Experiment Biol Med.* 1955;88:581–583.

104. Xing Y, Zhao B, Yin L et al. Vitamin C supplementation is necessary for patients with coronavirus disease: An ultra-high-performance liquid chromatography-tandem mass spectrometry finding. *J Pharm Biomed Anal.* 2021 Mar 20;196:113927. https://doi.org/10.1016/j.jpba.2021.113927.

105. d'Uscio LV, Milstien, S, Richardson D et al. Long-term vitamin C treatment increases vascular tetrahydrobiopterin levels and nitric oxide synthase activity. *Circulation Res.* 2002;92:88–95.

106. Boretti A, Banik BK. Intravenous vitamin C for reduction of cytokines storm in acute respiratory distress syndrome. *PharmaNutrition.* 2020;12:100190. https://doi.org/10.1016/j.phanu.2020.100190

107. Cheng RZ. Can early and high intravenous dose of vitamin C prevent and treat coronavirus disease 2019 (COVID-19)? *Med Drug Discov.* 2020;5:100028. https://doi.org/10.1016/j.medidd.2020.100028

108. Barabutis N, Khangoora V, Marik PE and Catravas JD. Hydrocortisone and ascorbic acid synergistically prevent and repair lipopolysaccharide-induced pulmonary endothelial barrier dysfunction. *Chest.* 2017 Nov;152(5):954–962. https://doi.org/10.1016/j.chest.2017.07.014

109. Marik PE, Khangoora V, Rivera R et al. Hydrocortisone, vitamin C, and thiamine for the treatment of severe sepsis and septic shock: A retrospective before-after study. *Chest.* 2017 Jun;151(6):1229–1238. https://doi.org/10.1016/j.chest.2016.11.036

110. Moskowitz A, Andersen L W, Huang D T et al. Ascorbic acid, corticosteroids, and thiamine in sepsis: A review of the biologic rationale and the present state of clinical evaluation. *Crit Care.* 2018;22(1):283. https://doi.org/10.1186/s13054-018-2217-4

111. Marik PE. Hydrocortisone, ascorbic acid and thiamine (HAT Therapy) for the treatment of sepsis. Focus on ascorbic acid. *Nutrients.* 2018;10(11):1762.

112. Tanaka H, Makino Y, Okamoto K et al. Redox regulation of the glucocorticoid receptor. *Antioxid Redox Signal.* 1999 Winter;1(4):403–23. https://doi.org/10.1089/ars.1999.1.4-403

113. Okamoto K, Tanaka H, Makino Y and Makino I. Restoration of the glucocorticoid receptor function by the phosphodiester compound of vitamins C and E, EPC-K1 (L-ascorbic acid 2-[3,4-dihydro-2,5,7 ,8-tetramethyl-2-(4,8,12-trimethyltridecyl)-2H-1-benzopyran-6 -yl hydrogen phosphate] potassium salt), via a redox-dependent mechanism. *Biochem Pharmacol.* 1998;56(1):79–86. 10.1016/S0006-2952(98)00121-X.)(https://pubmed.ncbi.nlm.nih.gov/9698091/

114. Ludke AR, Sharma AK, Akolkar G et al. Downregulation of vitamin C transporter SVCT-2 in doxorubicin-induced cardiomyocyte injury. *Am J Physiol Cell Physiol.* 2012 Sep 15;303(6):C645–53. 10.1152/ ajpcell.00186.2012

115. Fujita I, Hirano J, Itoh N et al. Dexamethasone induces sodium-dependant vitamin C transporter in a mouse osteoblastic cell line MC3T3-E1. *Br J Nutr.* 2001 Aug;86(2):145–9. https://doi.org/10.1079/ bjn2001406

116. van Tits LJ, Stienstra R, van Lent PL et al. Oxidized LDL enhances pro-inflammatory responses of alternatively activated M2 macrophages: A crucial role for Krüppel-like factor 2. *Atherosclerosis.* 2011 Feb;214(2):345–9. https://doi.org/10.1016/j.atherosclerosis.2010.11.018

117. Sorokin AV, Karathanasis SK, Yang ZH et al. COVID-19-associated dyslipidemia: Implications for mechanism of impaired resolution and novel therapeutic approaches. *FASEB J.* 2020 Aug;34(8):9843–9853. https://doi.org/10.1096/fj.202001451

118. Beigmohammadi MT. Bitarafan S, Hoseindokht A et al. Impact of vitamins A, B, C, D, and E supplementation on improvement and mortality rate in ICU patients with coronavirus-19: A structured summary of a study protocol for a randomized controlled trial. *Trials.* 2020;21:614. https://doi.org/10.1186/s13063-020-04547-0

119. Beigmohammadi MT, Bitarafan S, Hoseindokht A, et al. The effect of supplementation with vitamins A, B, C, D, and E on disease severity and inflammatory responses in patients with COVID-19: A randomized clinical trial. *Trials.* 2021 Nov;22(1):802. https://doi.org/10.1186/s13063-021-05795-4

120. Mauricio D, Castelblanco E, Alonso N. Cholesterol and inflammation in atherosclerosis: An immune-metabolic hypothesis. *Nutrients.* 2020;12(8):2444. https://doi.org/10.3390/nu12082444

121. Rath M, Pauling L. Unified theory of human cardiovascular disease leading the way to the abolition of this disease as a cause for human mortality. *Atherosclerosis.* 1989;9:579–592

122. Xia J, May LF, Koschinsky ML. Characterization of the basis of lipoprotein [a] lysine-binding heterogeneity. *Journal of Lipid Research.* 2000;41(10):1578–1584

123. Weisel JW, Litvinov RI. Fibrin formation, structure and properties. *Subcell Biochem.* 2017;82:405–456. https://doi.org/10.1007/978-3-319-49674-0_13

124. Garvin MR, Alvarez C, Miller JI et al. A mechanistic model and therapeutic interventions for COVID-19 involving a RAS-mediated bradykinin storm. *eLife* 2020;9:e59177 https://doi.org/10.7554/eLife.59177

125. Mendoza-Torres E, Oyarzún A, Mondaca-Ruff D et al. ACE2 and vasoactive peptides: Novel players in cardiovascular/renal remodeling and hypertension. *Ther Adv Cardiovasc Dis.* 2015 Aug;9(4):217–37. https://doi.org/10.1177/1753944715597623

126. Fujiwara O, Fukuda S, Lopez E et al. Peroxynitrite decomposition catalyst reduces vasopressin requirement in ovine MRSA sepsis. *ICMx.* 2019;7(12). https://doi.org/10.1186/s40635-019-0227-4

127. Carter BW Jr, Chicoine LG, Nelin LD. L-lysine decreases nitric oxide production and increases vascular resistance in lungs isolated from lipopolysaccharide-treated neonatal pigs. *Pediatr Res.* 2004 Jun;55(6):979–87. https://doi.org/10.1203/01.pdr.0000127722.55965.b3

128. Gregnani MF, Hungaro TG, Martins-Silva L et al. Bradykinin B2 receptor signaling increases glucose uptake and oxidation: Evidence and open questions. *Front. Pharmacol.* 2020; 11:1162. DOI: 10.3389/fphar.2020.01162.

129. Kagan C, Chaihorsky A, Tal R and Karlicki B. *Lysine Therapy for SARS-CoV-2.* 2020.

130. Harvey CJ, Thimmulappa RK, Singh A et al Nrf2-regulated glutathione recycling independent of biosynthesis is critical for cell survival during oxidative stress. *Free Radic Biol Med.* 2009 Feb 15;46(4):443–53. https://doi.org/10.1016/j.freeradbiomed.2008.10.040.

131. Shi Z, Puyo CA. N-Acetylcysteine to combat COVID-19: An evidence review. *Ther Clin Risk Manag.* 2020;16:1047–1055. Published 2020 Nov 2. https://doi.org/10.2147/TCRM.S273700

132. Kim SW, Kim S, Son M et al. Melatonin controls microbiota in colitis by goblet cell differentiation and antimicrobial peptide production through Toll-like receptor 4 signalling. Sci Rep 2020;10:2232. https://doi.org/10.1038/s41598-020-59314-7

133. Benot S, Goberna R, Reiter RJ et al. Physiological levels of melatonin contribute to the antioxidant capacity of human serum. *J Pineal Res.* 1999;27:59–64.

134. Ioannidis J. Infection fatality rate of COVID-19 inferred from seroprevalence data. *Bulletin of the World Health Organization* 2020;99 (1):19 –33F. World Health Organization. https://doi.org/10.2471/BLT.20.265892

135. Lowes DA, Webster NR, Murphy MP, et. al. Antioxidants that protect mitochondria reduce interleukin- 6 and oxidative stress, improve mitochondrial function, and reduce biochemical markers of organ dysfunction in a rat model of acute sepsis. *Br J Anesth.* 2013;110:472–480.

136. Markus RP, Cecon E, Pires-Lapa MA. Immune-pineal axis: Nuclear factor κB (NF-kB) mediates the shift in the melatonin source from pinealocytes to immune competent cells. *Int J Mol Sci.* 2013 May 24;14(6):10979–97. https://doi.org/10.3390/ijms140610979

137. Arioz BI, Tastan B, Emre Tarakcioglu E et al. Melatonin attenuates LPS-induced acute depressive-like behaviors and microglial NLRP3 inflammasome activation through the SIRT1/Nrf2 pathway. *Front. Immunol.* 02 July 2019. https://doi.org/10.3389/fimmu.2019.01511

138. Artigas L, Coma M, Matos-Filipe P et al. In-silico drug repurposing study predicts the combination of pirfenidone and melatonin as a promising candidate therapy to reduce SARS-CoV-2 infection progression and respiratory distress caused by cytokine storm. *PLoS ONE*. 2020:15(10): E0240149. https://doi.org/10.1371/journal.pone.0240149

139. Maher TM, Corte TJ, Fischer A et al. Pirfenidone in patients with unclassifiable progressive fibrosing interstitial lung disease: Design of a double-blind, randomised, placebo-controlled phase II trial. *BMJ Open Respir Res*. 2018 Sep 4;5(1):e000289. https://doi.org/10.1136/bmjresp-2018-000289

140. Ibrahim IM, Abdelmalek DH, Elshahat ME and Elfiky AA. COVID-19 spike-host cell receptor GRP78 binding site prediction. *J Infect*. 2020; pmid:32169481

141. Huang SH, Liao CL, Chen SJ et al. Melatonin possesses an anti-influenza potential through its immune modulatory effect. *J Funct Foods*. 2019;58:189–198

142. Meng X, Li Y, Li S et al. Dietary sources and bioactivities of melatonin. *Nutrients*. 2017;9(4):367. Published 2017 Apr 7. https://doi.org/10.3390/nu9040367

143. Sae-Teaw M, Johns J, Johns NP and Subongkot S. Serum melatonin levels and antioxidant capacities after consumption of pineapple, orange, or banana by healthy male volunteers. *J Pineal Res*. 2013 Aug;55(1):58–64. https://doi.org/10.1111/jpi.12025

144. Bubber P, Ke ZJ, Gibson GE. Tricarboxylic acid cycle enzymes following thiamine deficiency. *Neurochem Int*. 2004 Dec;45(7):1021–8. https://doi.org/10.1016/j.neuint.2004.05.007. PMID:15337301.

145. Miller R, Wentzel AR, Richards GA. COVID-19: NAD$^+$ deficiency may predispose the aged, obese and type2 diabetics to mortality through its effect on SIRT1 activity. *Med Hypotheses*. 2020;144:110044. https://doi.org/10.1016/j.mehy.2020.110044

146. Xie J, Zhang X, Zhang Li. Negative regulation of inflammation by SIRT1. *Pharmacological Research*. 2013:67(1) 60–67. https://doi.org/10.1016/j.phrs.2012.10.010

147. Huizenga R. *Dramatic Clinical Improvement in Nine Consecutive Acutely Ill Elderly COVID-19 Patients Treated with a Nicotinamide Mononucleotide Cocktail: A Case* Series. 2020. https://ssrn.com/abstract=3677428

148. Kok DEG, Dhonukshe-Rutten RAM, Lute C et al. The effects of long-term daily folic acid and vitamin B12 supplementation on genome-wide DNA methylation in elderly subjects. *Clin Epigenet*. 2015;7:121. https://doi.org/10.1186/s13148-015-0154-5

149. Servy E, Menezo Y. The Tetrahydrofolate Reductase (MTHFR) isoform challenge. High doses of folic acid are not a suitable option compared to 5 Methyltetrahydrofolate treatment. Clin *Obstet Gynecol Reprod Med*. 2017 https://doi.org/10.15761/COGRM.1000204

150. Karst M, Hollenhorst J, Achenbach J. Life-threatening course in coronavirus disease 2019 (COVID-19): Is there a link to methylenetetrahydrofolic acid reductase (MTHFR) polymorphism and hyperhomocysteinemia? *Med Hypotheses*. 2020;144:110234. https://doi.org/10.1016/j.mehy.2020.110234

151. dos Santos LMJ. Can vitamin B12 be an adjuvant to COVID-19 treatment? *GSC Biol Pharmaceut Scie*. 2020;11(03):001–005. https://doi.org/https://doi.org/10.30574/gscbps.2020.11.3.0155

152. Peuhkuri K, Sihvola N, Korpela R. Dietary factors and fluctuating levels of melatonin. *Food Nutr Res*. 2012;56. https://doi.org/10.3402/fnr.v56i0.17252

153. Altura BM, Altura BT. Magnesium: Forgotten mineral in cardiovascular biology and atherogenesis. In: Nishizawa Y, Morii H, Durlach J. (eds) *New Perspectives in Magnesium Research*. Springer, London, 2007. https://doi.org/10.1007/978-1-84628-483-0_19

154. Tan CW, Ho LP, Kalimuddin S et al. A cohort study to evaluate the effect of vitamin D, magnesium, and vitamin B12 in combination on progression to severe outcomes in older patients with coronavirus (COVID-19). *Nutrition*. 2020;79–80:l 111017. https://doi.org/10.1016/j.nut.2020.111017

155. Holley AK, Bakthavatchalu V, Velez-Roman JM and St Clair DK. Manganese superoxide dismutase: Guardian of the powerhouse. *Int J Mol Sci*. 2011;12(10):7114–7162. https://doi.org/10.3390/ijms12107114

156. Li L, Yang X. The essential element manganese, oxidative stress, and metabolic diseases: Links and interactions. *Oxid Med Cell Longev*. 2018;2018:7580707. https://doi.org/10.1155/2018/7580707

157. Gong JH, Lo K, Liu Q et al. Dietary manganese, plasma markers of inflammation, and the development of type 2 diabetes in postmenopausal women: Findings from the women's health initiative care. Jun 2020;43 (6):1344–1351. https://doi.org/10.2337/dc20-0243

158. Wang N, Tan H-Y, Li S et al. Supplementation of micronutrient selenium in metabolic diseases: Its role as an antioxidant. *Oxidative Medicine and Cellular Longevity*. 2017;2017:7478523. https://doi.org/10.1155/2017/7478523

159. Zhang J, Taylor EW, Bennett K et al. Association between regional selenium status and reported outcome of COVID-19 cases in China. *Am J Clin Nutrition*. 2020;111(6):1297–1299. https://doi.org/10.1093/ajcn/nqaa095

160. Moghaddam A, Heller RA, Sun Q et al. Selenium Deficiency Is Associated with Mortality Risk from COVID-19. *Nutrients.* 2020 Jul 16;12(7):2098. https://doi.org/10.3390/nu12072098.

161. Kieliszek M, Lipinski B. Selenium supplementation in the prevention of coronavirus infections (COVID-19). *Medical Hypotheses* 2020;143:109878. https://doi.org/10.1016/j.mehy.2020.109878.

162. Prasad AS, Miale A, Farid Z et al. Zinc metabolism in patients with the syndrome of iron deficiency anemia, hepatosplenomegaly, dwarfism, and hypognadism. *J Lab Clin Med.* 1963;61:537–49

163. Severo JS, Morais JBS, de Freitas TEC et al. The role of zinc in thyroid hormones metabolism. *Int J Vitam Nutr Res.* 2019 Jul;89(1–2):80–88. https://doi.org/10.1024/0300-9831/a000262.

164. Baltaci AK, Mogulkoc R, Baltaci SB. The role of zinc in the endocrine system. *Pak. J. Pharm. Sci.* 2020;32(1):231–239

165. Nagase H, Visse R, Murphy G. Structure and function of matrix metalloproteinases and TIMPs, *Cardiovasc Res.* 2006;69(3):562–573. https://doi.org/10.1016/j.cardiores.2005.12.002

166. Maares M, Haase H. Zinc and immunity: An essential interrelation. *Arch Biochem Biophys.* 2016 Dec 1;611:58–65. https://doi.org/10.1016/j.abb.2016.03.022.

167. Li B, Cui W, Tan Y et al. Zinc is essential for the transcription function of Nrf2 in human renal tubule cells in vitro and mouse kidney in vivo under the diabetic condition. *J Cell Mol Med.* 2014 May;18(5):895–906. https://doi.org/10.1111/jcmm.12239

168. Mayor-Ibarguren A, Busca-Arenzana C, Robles-Marhuenda Á. A hypothesis for the possible role of zinc in the immunological pathways related to COVID-19 infection. *Front Immunol.* 2020 Jul 10;11:1736. https://doi.org/10.3389/fimmu.2020.01736

169. Xue J, Moyer A, Peng B et al. Chloroquine is a zinc ionophore. *PLoS One.* 2014;9(10): E109180. https://doi.org/10.1371/journal.pone.0109180

170. Pal A, Squitti R, Picozza M et al. Zinc and COVID-19: Basis of current clinical trials. *Biol Trace Elem Res* (2020). https://doi.org/10.1007/s12011-020-02437-9

171. Rizzo E. Ivermectin, antiviral properties and COVID-19: A possible new mechanism of action. *Naunyn-Schmiedeberg's archives of pharmacology.* 2020;393(7):1153–1156. https://doi.org/10.1007/s00210-020-01902-5

172. Mostafa WZ, Hegazy RA. Vitamin D and the skin: Focus on a complex relationship: A review. *Journal of Advanced Research.* 2015;6(6):793–804. https://doi.org/10.1016/j.jare.2014.01.011

173. Margolis RN, Christakos S. The nuclear receptor superfamily of steroid hormones and vitamin D gene regulation. An update. *Ann N Y Acad Sci.* 2010 Mar;1192:208–14. https://doi.org/10.1111/j.1749-6632.2009.05227.x. PMID:20392238

174. Campbell Y, Fantacone M L, Gombart A F. Regulation of antimicrobial peptide gene expression by nutrients and by-products of microbial metabolism. *Eur J Nutrition.* 2012;51(8):899–907

175. Roth A, Lütke S, Meinberger D et al. LL-37 fights SARS-CoV-2: The vitamin D-inducible peptide LL-37 inhibits binding of SARS-CoV-2 spike protein to its cellular receptor angiotensin converting enzyme 2 in vitro. *bioRxiv* 2020.12.02.408153. https://doi.org/10.1101/2020.12.02.408153

176. Adams JS, Ren S, Liu PT et al. D-directed rheostatic regulation of monocyte antibacterial responses. *J Immunol.* April 1, 2009;182 (7):4289–4295. https://doi.org/10.4049/jimmunol.0803736

177. Washizu J, Nishimura H, Nakamura N et al. The NF-kappaB binding site is essential for transcriptional activation of the IL-15 gene. *Immunogenetics.* 1998;48(1):1–7.

178. Krutzik S R, Hewison M, Liu P T et al. IL-15 links TLR2/1-induced macrophage differentiation to the vitamin D-dependent antimicrobial pathway. *J. Immunol.* 2008;181(10):7115–7120. https://doi.org/10.4049/jimmunol.181.10.7115

179. Azimi N, Shiramizu KM, Tagaya Y et al. Viral activation of interleukin-15 (IL-15): Characterization of a virus-inducible element in the IL-15 promoter region. *J Virol.* 2000;74(16):7338–7348.

180. Anthony S, Schluns KS. Emerging roles for IL-15 in the activation and function of T-cells during immune stimulation. *Res Rep Biol.* 2015;6:25–37. https://doi.org/10.2147/RRB.S57685

181. Ben-Sasson SZ, Hu-Li J, Quiel J, et al. IL-1 acts directly on CD4 T cells to enhance their antigen-driven expansion and differentiation. *Proc Natl Acad Sci USA.* 2009;106(17):7119–7124. https://doi.org/10.1073/pnas.0902745106

182. Verway M, Bouttier M, Wang T-T et al. Vitamin D induces interleukin-1ß expression: Paracrine macrophage epithelial signaling controls M. tuberculosis infection. *PLoS Pathog.* 2023:9(6): E1003407. https://doi.org/10.1371/journal.ppat.1003407

183. Chen L, Eapen M, Zosky G. Vitamin D both facilitates and attenuates the cellular response to lipopolysaccharide. *Sci Rep.* 2020;7:45172 . https://doi.org/10.1038/srep45172

184. Zhao C, Zhao W. NLRP3 inflammasome: A key player in antiviral responses. *Front. Immunol.*,18 February 2020. https://doi.org/10.3389/fimmu.2020.00211

185. Netea MG, Simon A, van de Veerdonk F et al. IL-1β processing in host defense: Beyond the inflammasomes. *PLoS Pathog.* 2010;6(2):e1000661. https://doi.org/10.1371/journal.ppat.1000661

186. Tavera-Mendoza LE, Westerling T, Libby E et al. VDR regulation of autophagy in mammary gland. *Proc Nat Acad Scie.* Mar 2017;114 (11) E2186–E2194. https://doi.org/10.1073/pnas.1615015114

187. Liu T, Zhang L, Joo D et al. NF-κB signaling in inflammation. *Sig Transduct Target Ther* 2. 2017;17023 https://doi.org/10.1038/sigtrans.2017.23

188. Razvi ES, Welsh RM. Programmed cell death of T lymphocytes during acute viral infection: A mechanism for virus-induced immune deficiency. *J Virol.* 1993;67(10):5754–5765. https://doi.org/10.1128/JVI.67.10.5754-5765.1993

189. Hennig P, Garstkiewicz M, Grossi S et al. The crosstalk between Nrf2 and inflammasomes. *Int. J. Mol. Sci.* 2018;19:562. https://doi.org/10.3390/ijms19020562

190. Itoh Y, Saitoh M, Miyazawa K, Smad3–STAT3 crosstalk in pathophysiological contexts. *Acta Biochim Biophys Sin.* 2018;50(1):82–90.

191. Lips P, Cashman KD, Lamberg-Allardt C et al. Current vitamin D status in European and Middle East countries and strategies to prevent vitamin D deficiency: A position statement of the European calcified tissue society. *J Endocrinol.* 2019;180:23–P54.

192. Griffin GG, Hewison M, Hopkin J et al. Vitamin D and COVID-19: Evidence and recommendations for supplementation. *R Soc Open Sci.* 2020;7201912. http://doi.org/10.1098/rsos.201912

193. Sutherland JP, Zhou A, Leach MJ and Hyppönen E. Differences and determinants of vitamin D deficiency among UK biobank participants: A cross-ethnic and socioeconomic study. *Nutrition.* November 24, 2020. https://doi.org/10.1016/j.clnu.2020.11.019

194. Martineau AR, Jolliffe DA, Hooper R et al. Vitamin D supplementation to prevent acute respiratory tract infections: Systematic review and meta-analysis of individual participant data *BMJ* 2017;356:i6583.

195. Isaia G, Diémoz H, Maluta F et al. Does solar ultraviolet radiation play a role in COVID-19 infection and deaths? An environmental ecological study in Italy. *Sci Total Environ.* 2021;757:143757. https://doi.org/10.1016/j.scitotenv.2020.143757

196. Rastogi A, Bhansali A, Khare N et al. Short term, high-dose vitamin D supplementation for COVID-19 disease: A randomised, placebo-controlled, study (SHADE study). *Postgraduate Med J.* 2020;0:1–4. https://doi.org/10.1136/postgradmedj-2020-139065

197. Ojaimi S, Skinner NA, Strauss BJ et al. Vitamin D deficiency impacts on expression of toll-like receptor-2 and cytokine profile: A pilot study. *Journal of Translational Medicine.* 2013;11:176. https://doi.org/10.1186/1479-5876-11-176

198. Jain A, Chaurasia R, Sengar NS et al. Analysis of vitamin D level among asymptomatic and critically ill COVID-19 patients and its correlation with inflammatory markers. *Sci Rep.* 2020;10:20191. https://doi.org/10.1038/s41598-020-77093-z

199. De Smet D, De Smet K, Herroelen P et al. Serum 25(OH)D level on hospital admission associated with COVID-19 stage and mortality. *Am J Clin Pathol.* 2020 Nov 25:aqaa252. https://doi.org/10.1093/ajcp/aqaa252

200. Luo X, Liao Q, Shen Y, et al. Vitamin D deficiency is inversely associated with COVID-19 incidence and disease severity in Chinese people. *J Nutrition.* 2021;151(1):98–103. https://doi.org/10.1093/jn/nxaa332

201. Dror AA, Morozov N, Daoud A et al. Pre-infection 25-hydroxyvitamin D3 levels and association with severity of COVID-19 illness. *PLoS One.* 2022;17(2):e0263069. Published 2022 Feb 3. https://doi.org/10.1371/journal.pone.0263069

202. Brenner H, Schöttker B. D insufficiency may account for almost nine of ten COVID-19 deaths: Time to act. Comment on: "Vitamin D deficiency and outcome of COVID-19 patients". *Nutrients.* 2020;12:2757.

203. Annweiler G, Corvaisier M, Gautier J, et al. Vitamin D supplementation associated to better survival in hospitalized frail elderly COVID-19 patients: The GERIA-COVID quasi-experimental study. *Nutrients.* 2020;12(11):3377.

204. Vitamin D is effective for COVID-19: Real-time meta analysis of 191 studies. April 5, 2022. https://vdmeta.com/

205. Over 200 Scientists & Doctors Call For Increased Vitamin D Use To Combat COVID-19 Scientific evidence indicates vitamin D reduces infections & deaths://vitamindforall.org/letter.html

206. McCartney DM, O'Shea PM, Faul JL et al. Vitamin D and SARS-CoV-2 infection: Evolution of evidence supporting clinical practice and policy development: A position statement from the Covit-D Consortium. *Ir J Med Sci.* 2020. https://doi.org/10.1007/s11845-020-02427-9

207. Newton CJ. Nutritional supplements for COVID-19 prophylaxis and symptom de-escalation. https://www.linkedin.com/pulse/nutritional-supplements-covid-19-prophylaxis-symptom-chris-newton/

208. Bleizgys A. Vitamin D and COVID-19: It is time to act. *Int J Clin Pract.* 2020;00:e13748. https://doi.org/10.1111/ijcp.13748

209. Heaney RP, Armas LA, Shary JR et al. 25-Hydroxylation of vitamin D3: Relation to circulating vitamin D3 under various input conditions. *Am J Clin Nutr.* 2008 Jun;87(6):1738–42. https://doi.org/10.1093/ajcn/87.6.1738

210. Mani JS, Johnson JB, Steel JC et al. Natural product-derived phytochemicals as potential agents against coronaviruses: A review. *Virus Res.* 2020;284:197989. https://doi.org/10.1016/j.virusres.2020.197989

211. Robledinos-Antón N, Fernández-Ginés R, Manda G and Cuadrado A. Activators and inhibitors of NRF2: A review of their potential for clinical development. *Oxidative Med Cell Longevity.* 2019:9372182. https://doi.org/10.1155/2019/9372182

212. Piantadosi CA, Carraway MS, Babiker A and Suliman HB. Heme oxygenase-1 regulates cardiac mitochondrial biogenesis via Nrf2-mediated transcriptional control of nuclear respiratory factor-1. *Circ Res.* 2008;103(11):1232–1240. https://doi.org 10.1161/01.RES.0000338597.71702.ad

213. Piantadosi CA, Suliman HB. Transcription factor A induction by redox activation of nuclear respiratory factor. *J Biol Chem.* 2006;281(1):324–333. https://doi.org/10.1074/jbc.M508805200

214. Tőzsér J, Benkő S. Natural compounds as regulators of NLRP3 inflammasome-mediated IL-1β production. *Mediators Inflamm.* 2016;2016:5460302. https://doi.org/10.1155/2016/5460302

215. Agrawal K, Agrawal C, Blunden G. Antiviral significance and possible COVID-19 integrative considerations. *Nat Prod Commun.* 2020;15(12):1–10 © https://doi.org/10.1177/1934578X20976293

216. Colunga-Biancatelli RML, Berrill M, Catravas JD and Marik PE. Quercetin and vitamin C: An experimental, synergistic therapy for the prevention and treatment of SARS-CoV-2 related disease (COVID-19). *Front Immunol.* 2020;11:1451. https://doi.org/10.3389/fimmu.2020.01451

217. Arslan B, Ergun NU, Topuz S et al. Synergistic effect of quercetin and vitamin C against COVID-19: Is a possible guard for front liners. *SSRN.* 2020. https://doi.org/10.2139/ssrn.3682517

218. Dabbagh-Bazarbachi H, Clergeaud G, Quesada IM et al. Zinc ionophore activity of quercetin and epigallocatechin-gallate: From hepa 1–6 cells to a liposome model. *Agric Food Chem.* 2014;62(32):8085–8093. https://doi.org/10.1021/jf5014633

219. teVelthuis AJW, van den Worm SHE, Sims AC et al. Zn^{2+} inhibits coronavirus and arterivirus RNA polymerase activity in vitro and zinc ionophores block the replication of these viruses in cell culture. *PLoS ONE.* November 4, 2010. https://doi.org/10.1371/journal.ppat.1001176

220. Glinsky GV. Tripartite combination of candidate pandemic mitigation agents: Vitamin D, quercetin, and estradiol manifest properties of medicinal agents for targeted mitigation of the COVID-19 pandemic defined by genomics-guided tracing of SARS-CoV-2 targets in human cells. *Biomedicines.* 2020 May 21;8(5):129. https://doi.org/10.3390/biomedicines8050129

221. Smith M, Smith JC. Repurposing therapeutics for COVID-19: Supercomputer-based docking to the SARS-CoV-2 viral spike protein and viral spike protein-human ACE2 interface. *ChemRxiv;*2020. https://doi.org/10.26434/chemrxiv.11871402.v3

222. Liu X, Raghuvanshi R, Ceylan FD, Bolling BW. Quercetin and its metabolites inhibit recombinant human angiotensin-converting enzyme 2 (ACE2) activity. *J Agric Food Chem.* 2020;68(47):13982–13989. https://doi.org/10.1021/acs.jafc.0c05064

223. Hegyi A and Ziebuhr J. Conservation of substrate specificities among coronavirus main proteases. *J Gen Virol.* 2002;83(3):595–599.

224. Jang M, Park Y-I, Cha Y-E et al. Tea polyphenols EGCG and theaflavin inhibit the activity of SARS-CoV-2 3CL-protease in vitro. *Evid Based Complement Altern Med.* 2020; Article ID 5630838. https://doi.org/10.1155/2020/5630838

225. Menegazzi M, Campagnari R, Bertoldi M et al. Protective effect of epigallocatechin-3-gallate (EGCG) in diseases with uncontrolled immune activation: Could such a scenario be helpful to counteract COVID-19? *Int J Mol Sci.* 2020;21(14):5171. https://doi.org/10.3390/ijms21145171

226. Herzig S, Shaw RJ. AMPK: Guardian of metabolism and mitochondrial homeostasis. *Nat Rev Mol Cell Biol.* 2018;19(2):121–135. https://doi.org/10.1038/nrm.2017.95

227. Ruderman NB, Xu XJ, Nelson L et al. AMPK and SIRT1: A long-standing partnership? *Am J Physiol Endocrinol Metabol.* 2010;298:4:E751–E760.

228. Price NL, Gomes AP, Ling AJ et al. SIRT1 is required for AMPK activation and the beneficial effects of resveratrol on mitochondrial function. *Cell Metab.* 2012;15(5):675–690. https://doi.org/10.1016/j.cmet.2012.04.003

229. Shi LZ, Wang R, Huang G et al. HIF1alpha-dependent glycolytic pathway orchestrates a metabolic checkpoint for the differentiation of TH17 and Treg cells. *J Exp Med.* 2011;208(7):1367–1376. https://doi.org/10.1084/jem.20110278

230. Dang EV, Barbi J, Yang HY et al. (2011) Control of T(H)17/T(reg) balance by hypoxia-inducible factor 1. *Cell* 146:773–784.

231. Caslin HL, Taruselli MT, Haque T et al. Inhibiting glycolysis and ATP production attenuates IL-33-mediated mast cell function and peritonitis. *Front Immunol.* 2018 Dec 18;9:3026. https://doi.org/10.3389/fimmu.2018.03026

232. Rena G, Hardie DG, Pearson, ER. The mechanisms of action of metformin. *Diabetologia.* 2017;60:1577–1585. https://doi.org/10.1007/s00125-017-4342-z

233. Bousquet J, Cristol JP, Czarlewski W et al. Nrf2-interacting nutrients and COVID-19: Time for research to develop adaptation strategies. *Clin Transl Allergy.* 2020;10:58. https://doi.org/10.1186/s13601-020-00362-7

234. Zhou Y, Gilmore K, Ramirez S et al. In vitro efficacy of artemisinin-based treatments against SARS-CoV-2. *Sci Rep* 2021;11:14571. https://doi.org/10.1038/s41598-021-93361-y

235. Nair MS, Huang Y, Fidock DA et al. Artemisia annua L. extracts inhibit the in vitro replication of SARS-CoV-2 and two of its variants. *J. Ethnopharmacol.* 2021;274:114016. https://doi.org/10.1016/j.jep.2021.114016.

236. McMillan P, Dexhiemer T, Neubig RR, Uhal BD. COVID-19: A theory of autoimmunity against ACE-2 explained. *Front. Immunol.* 23 March 2021. https://doi.org/10.3389/fimmu.2021.582166

237. McMillan P, Uhal BD. COVID-19-A theory of autoimmunity to ACE-2. *MOJ Immunol.* 2020;7(1):17–19.

238. Arumugham V. Proteins that contaminate influenza vaccines have high homology to SARS-CoV-2 proteins thus increasing risk of severe COVID-19 disease and mortality. https://zenodo.org/record/3997694#.YKGVe2ZKj-1

239. Arumugham V. 2018. https://www.bmj.com/content/360/bmj.k1378/rr-15

240. Newton CJ. A new model (hypothesis) for the aetiology of coeliac disease. https://www.linkedin.com/pulse/new-model-hypothesis-aetiology-coeliac-disease-chris-newton/

241. Sanchez-Gonzalez MA, Moskowitz D, Issuree PD et al. A pathophysiological perspective on COVID-19's lethal complication: From Viremia to hypersensitivity pneumonitis-like immune dysregulation. *Infect Chemother.* 2020 Sep;52(3):335–344. https://doi.org/10.3947/ic.2020.52.3.335

242. Kandere-Grzybowska K, Kempuraj D, Cao J, Cetrulo CL, Theoharides TC. Regulation of IL-1-induced selective IL-6 release from human mast cells and inhibition by quercetin. *Br J Pharmacol.* 2006;148(2):208–215. https://doi.org/10.1038/sj.bjp.0706695

243. Carvelli J, Demaria O, Vély F et al. Association of COVID-19 inflammation with activation of the C5a–C5aR1 axis. *Nature.* 2020;588:146–150. https://doi.org/10.1038/s41586-020-2600-6

244. de Vries MR, Wezel A, Schepers A et al. Complement factor C5a as mast cell activator mediates vascular remodelling in vein graft disease. *Cardiovasc Res.* 2013;97:311–320. https://doi.org/10.1093/cvr/cvs312

245. Nieto-Torres JL, Verdiá-Báguena C, Castaño-Rodriguez C et al. Relevance of viroporin ion channel activity on viral replication and pathogenesis. *Viruses.* 2015;7(7):3552–3573. https://doi.org/10.3390/v7072786

246. Cao Y, Yang R, Lee I et al. Characterization of the SARS-CoV-2 E protein: Sequence, structure, viroporin, and inhibitors. *Protein Sci.* 2021;30:1114–1130. https://doi.org/10.1002/pro.4075

247. Ferreira AC, Soares VC, de Azevedo-Quintanilha IG et al. SARS-CoV-2 induces inflammasome-dependent pyroptosis and downmodulation of HLA-DR in human monocytes medRxiv 2020.08.25.20182055. https://doi.org/10.1101/2020.08.25.20182055

248. Pan P, Shen M, Yu Z et al. SARS-CoV-2 N protein promotes NLRP3 inflammasome activation to induce hyperinflammation. *Nat Commun* 2021;12:4664. https://doi.org/10.1038/s41467-021-25015-6

249. Ito Y, Al Mubarak R, Roberts N et al. IL-13 induces periostin and eotaxin expression in human primary alveolar epithelial cells: Comparison with paired airway epithelial cells. *PLoS ONE.* 2018;13(4):e0196256. https://doi.org/10.1371/journal.pone.0196256

250. Jang TY, Kim YH. Interleukin-33 and mast cells bridge innate and adaptive immunity: From the allergologist's perspective. *Int Neurourol J.* 2015;19:142–150. https://doi.org/10.5213/inj.2015.19.3.142

251. Blanchette F, Rudd P, Grondin F et al. Involvement of smads in TGFbeta1-induced furin (fur) transcription. *J Cell Physiol.* 2001 Aug;188(2):264–73. https://doi.org/10.1002/jcp.1116

252. *BMJ* 2020;371:m3872

253. Van Reeth K. Cytokines in the pathogenesis of influenza. *Vet Microbiol.* 2000 May 22;74(1–2):109–16. https://doi.org/10.1016/s0378-1135(00)00171-1

254. Cohen S, Janicki-Deverts D, Doyle WJ et al. Chronic stress, glucocorticoid receptor resistance, inflammation, and disease risk. *Proc Natl Acad Sci USA.* 2012 Apr 17;109(16):5995–9. https://doi.org/10.1073/pnas.1118355109

255. Weinberg JM, Davis JA, Abarzua M, Rajan T. Cytoprotective effects of glycine and glutathione against hypoxic injury to renal tubules. *J Clin Invest.* 1987;80(5):1446–1454. https://doi.org/10.1172/JCI113224

256. Li C-Y. Can glycine mitigate COVID-19 associated tissue damage and cytokine storm? *Radiat Res.* 2020;194(3):199–201. https://doi.org/10.1667/RADE-20-00146.1

257. Weng Z, Zhang B, Asadi S, Sismanopoulos N. Quercetin is more effective than cromolyn in blocking human mast cell cytokine release and inhibits contact dermatitis and photosensitivity in humans. *PLoS One.* 2012;7(3):e33805. https://doi.org/10.1371/journal.pone.0033805

258. Raymond M, Ching-A-Sue G, Van Hecke O. Mast cell stabilisers, leukotriene antagonists and antihista-mines: A rapid review of the evidence for their use in COVID-19. https://www.cebm.net/covid-19/mast-cell -stabilisers-leukotriene-antagonists-and-antihistamines-a-rapid-review-of-effectiveness-in-covid-19/

259. Malone RW, Tisdall P, Fremont-Smith P, et al. COVID-19: Famotidine, histamine, mast cells, and mech-anisms. Preprint. *Res Sq.* 2020;rs.3.rs-30934. Published 2020 Jun 22. https://doi.org/10.21203/rs.3.rs -30934/v2

260. Sanchez-Gonzalez MA, Moskowitz D, Issuree PD et al. Pathophysiological perspective on COVID-19's lethal complication: From Viremia to hypersensitivity pneumonitis-like immune dysregulation. *Infect Chemother.* 2020 Sep;52(3):335–344. https://doi.org/10.3947/ic.2020.52.3.335

261. Yazdani Shaik BD, Conti P. Relationship between vitamin C, mast cells and inflammation. *J Nutr Food Sci* 2016;6:1. https://doi.org/10.4172/2155-9600.1000456

262. Liu ZQ, Li XX, Qiu SQ et al. Vitamin D contributes to mast cell stabilization. *Allergy Eur J Allergy Clin Immunol.* 2017;72(8):1184–92.

263. Inoue T, Suzuki Y, Ra C. Epigallocatechin-3-gallate inhibits mast cell degranulation, leukotri-ene C4 secretion, and calcium influx via mitochondrial calcium dysfunction. *Free Radic Biol Med.* 2010 Aug 15;49(4):632–40. https://doi.org/10.1016/j.freeradbiomed.2010.05.015. Epub 2010 May 25. PMID:20510351.

264. Osipyants AI, Poloznikov AA, Smirnova NA et al. L-ascorbic acid: A true substrate for HIF prolyl hydroxylase? *Biochimie.* 2018;147:46–54. https://doi.org/10.1016/j.biochi.2017.12.011

265. Afrin LB, Weinstock LB, Molderings GJ. Covid-19 hyperinflammation and post-Covid-19 illness may be rooted in mast cell activation syndrome. *Int J Infect Dis.* 2020;100:327–332. https://doi.org/10.1016/j .ijid.2020.09.016

266. Turnbull AV, River CL. Regulation of the hypothalamic-pituitary-adrenal axis by cytokines: Actions and mechanisms of action. *Pharmacol Rev.* 1999;79(1):1–71.

267. Pace TWW, Hu F, Miller AH. Activation of cAMP-protein kinase A abrogates STAT5- medi-ated inhibition of glucocorticoid receptor signalling by interferon-alpha. *Brain Behav Immunol.* 2011;25(8):1716–1724.

268. Leroy EM, Baize S, Debre P et al. Early immune response accompanying asymptomatic Ebola infec-tions. *Clin Exp Immunol.* 2001;124:453–460

269. Wauquier N, Becquart P, Padilla C et al. Human fatal Zaire Ebola virus infection is associated with an aberrant innate immunity and with massive lymphocyte apoptosis. *PLoS Neglect Trop Dis.* 2010;4(10):1–10.

270. Alzahrani AS, Mukhtar N, Aljomaiah A et al. The impact of COVID-19 viral infection on the hypotha-lamic-pituitary-adrenal axis. *Endocr Pract.* 2021;27(2):83–89. https://doi.org/10.1016/j.eprac.2020.10.014

271. Siejka A, Barabutis N. Adrenal insufficiency in the COVID-19 era. *Am J Physiol Endocrinol Metabol.* 2021;320:4:E784–E785.

272. May JM, Qu ZC, Nazarewicz R and Dikalov S. Ascorbic acid efficiency enhances neuronal synthesis of norepinephrine from dopamine. *Brain Res Bull.* 2013;90:35–42.

273. Padayatty SJ, Doppman JL, Chang R et al. Human adrenal glands secrete vitamin C in response to adrenocorticotrophic hormone. *Am J Clin Nutr.* 2007;86:145–149

274. Kory P, Meduri GU, Iglesias J, Varon J, Marik PE. Clinical and scientific rationale for the "MATH+" hospital treatment protocol for COVID-19. *J Intens Care Med.* 2021 Feb;36(2):135–156. https://doi.org /10.1177/0885066620973585

275. Chaccour C, Casellas A, Blanco-Di Matteo A et al. The effect of early treatment with ivermectin on viral load, symptoms and humoral response in patients with non-severe COVID-19: A pilot, double-blind, placebo-controlled, randomized clinical trial. *The Lancet.* 2021 January 19. https://doi.org/10 .1016/j.eclinm.2020.100720

276. Lawrie T. Ivermectin reduces the risk of death from COVID-19: A rapid review and meta-analysis in support of the recommendation of the front line COVID-19 critical care alliance. Evidence-Based Medicine Consultancy Ltd. 2021. https://b3d2650e-e929-4448-a527-4eeb59304c7f.filesusr.com/ugd /593c4f_8cb655bd21b1448ba6cf1f4c59f0d73d.pdf

277. Kory P, Umberto MG, Varon J et al. Review of the emerging evidence demonstrating the efficacy of ivermectin in the prophylaxis and treatment of COVID-19. *Am J Therap.* 2021;28(3):e299–e318. https://doi.org/10.1097/MJT.0000000000001377

278. Huang C, Huang L, Wang Y et al. 6-Month consequences of COVID-19 in patients discharged from hospital: A cohort study. *Lancet* 2021;397:220–232.

279. Patterson BK, Francisco EB, Yogendra R et al. Persistence of SARS CoV-2 S1 protein in CD16+ monocytes in post-acute sequelae of COVID-19 (PASC) up to 15 months post-infection. *bioRxiv* 2021.06.25.449905. https://doi.org/10.1101/2021.06.25.449905

280. Vollbracht C, Kraft K. Feasibility of vitamin C in the treatment of post viral fatigue with focus on long COVID, based on a systematic review of IV vitamin C on fatigue. *Nutrients.* 2021;13(4):1154. https://doi.org/10.3390/nu13041154

281. *UKHSA Vaccine Report.* https://assets.publishing.service.gov.uk/government/uploads/system/uploads/attachment_data/file/1057599/Vaccine_surveillance_report_-_week-8.pdf

282. Hart OM, Athie-Morales V, O'Connor GM, Gardiner CM. TLR7/8-mediated activation of human NK cells results in accessory cell-dependent IFN-gamma production. *J Immunol.* 2005 Aug 1;175(3):1636–42. https://doi.org/10.4049/jimmunol.175.3.1636. PMID:16034103

283. Karikó K, Buckstein M, Ni H, Weissman D. Suppression of RNA recognition by toll-like receptors: The impact of nucleoside modification and the evolutionary origin of RNA. *Immunity.* 2005;23(2):165–175

284. Karikó K, Weissman D. Naturally occurring nucleoside modifications suppress the immunostimulatory activity of RNA: Implication for therapeutic RNA development. *Curr Opin Drug Discov Devel.* 2007 Sep;10(5):523–32.

285. Liu J, Wang J, Xu J et al. Comprehensive investigations revealed consistent pathophysiological alterations after vaccination with COVID-19 vaccines. *Cell Discov.* 2021;7(1):99. https://doi.org/10.1038/s41421-021-00329-3

286. Furer V, Zisman D, Kibari A et al. Herpes zoster following BNT162b2 mRNA COVID-19 vaccination in patients with autoimmune inflammatory rheumatic diseases: A case series. *Rheumatology.* 2021;60(SI):SI90–SI95. https://doi.org/10.1093/rheumatology/keab345

287. Cyrenne BM, Al-Mohammedi F, DeKoven JG, Alhusayen R. Pityriasis rosea-like eruptions following vaccination with BNT162b2 mRNA COVID-19 Vaccine. *J Eur Acad Dermatol Venereol.* 2021;35(9):e546–e548. https://doi.org/10.1111/jdv.17342

288. Jiang H, Mei YF. SARS-CoV-2 spike impairs DNA damage repair and inhibits V(D)J recombination in vitro. *Viruses.* 2021;13(10):2056. https://doi.org/10.3390/v13102056

289. Wisnewski AV, Campillo Luna J, Redlich CA. Human IgG and IgA responses to COVID-19 mRNA vaccines. *PLoS One.* 2021;16(6):e0249499. Published 2021 Jun 16. https://doi.org/10.1371/journal.pone.0249499

290. Chetty S. 2021 Personal communication.

291. Chetty S. https://wonderland.org.za/2021/10/30/observations-treatment-of-covid19-missing-element/

292. http://pathologie-konferenz.de/en/

293. Dakal TC. Antigenic sites in SARS-CoV-2 spike RBD show molecular similarity with pathogenic antigenic determinants and harbors peptides for vaccine development. *Immunobiology.* 2021;226(5):152091. https://doi.org/10.1016/j.imbio.2021.152091

294. Kumar S, Thambiraja TS, Karuppanan K, Subramaniam G. Omicron and delta variant of SARS-CoV-2: A comparative computational study of spike protein. *J Med Virol.* 2021. https://doi.org/10.1002/jmv.27526

295. Dance A. Omicron's lingering mysteries. *Nature.* 2022. https://media.nature.com/original/magazine-assets/d41586-022-00428-5/d41586-022-00428-5.pdf

296. Sørensen B, Susrud A, Dalgleish A. Biovacc-19: A candidate vaccine for covid-19 (SARS-CoV-2) developed from analysis of its general method of action for infectivity. *QRB Disc.* 2020;1:E6. https://doi.org/10.1017/qrd.2020.8

297. Vojdani A, Kharrazian D. Potential antigenic cross-reactivity between SARS-CoV-2 and human tissue with a possible link to an increase in autoimmune diseases. *Clin Immunol.* 2020;217;108480.

298. Kanduc D, Shoenfeld Y. Molecular mimicry between SARS-CoV-2 spike glycoprotein and mammalian proteomes: Implications for the vaccine. *Immunol Res.* 2020;68:310–313. https://doi.org/10.1007/s12026-020-09152-6

299. McKernan K, Kyriakopoulos AM, McCullough PA. Differences in vaccine and SARS-CoV-2 replication derived mRNA: Implications for cell biology and future disease. https://doi.org/10.31219/osf.io/bcsa6

300. Jeong D-E, McCoy M, Artiles K et al. Assemblies of putative SARS-CoV2-spike-encoding mRNA sequences for vaccines BNT- 162b2 and mRNA-1273. https://www.semanticscholar.org/paper/Assemblies-of-putative-SARS-CoV2-spike-encoding-for-Jeong-McCoy/150b70589516b969ce20fe83b9808478dd6f0e72

301. Suzuki YJ, Nikolaienko SI. Dibrova VA et al. SARS-CoV-2 spike protein-mediated cell signaling in lung vascular cells. *Vasc Pharmacol* 2021;137:106823

302. Suzuki YJ, Gychka SG. SARS-CoV-2 spike protein elicits cell signaling in humanhost cells: Implications for possible consequences of COVID-19 vaccines. *Vaccines.* 2021;9:36

303. Wen H, Gwathmey JK, Xie LH. Oxidative stress-mediated effects of angiotensin II in the cardiovascular system. *World J Hypertens.* 2012;2(4):34–44. https://doi.org/10.5494/wjh.v2.i4.34

304. Patra T, Meyer K, Geerling L et al. SARS-CoV-2 spike protein promotes IL-6 trans-signaling by activation of angiotensin II receptor signaling in epithelial cells. *PLoS Pathog.* 2020 Dec 7;16(12):e1009128. https://doi.org/10.1371/journal.ppat.1009128

305. Lei Y, Zhang J, Schiavon CR et al. SARS-CoV-2 spike protein impairs endothelial function via down-regulation of ACE 2. *Circ Res.* 2021;128(9):1323–1326. https://doi.org/10.1161/CIRCRESAHA.121.318902

306. Kupfer L, Hinrichs W, Groschup MH. Prion protein misfolding. *Curr Mol Med.* 2009;9(7):826–835. https://doi.org/10.2174/156652409789105543

307. Tetz G, Tetz V. SARS-CoV-2 prion-like domains in spike proteins enable higher affinity to ACE2. *Preprints* 2020;2020030422. https://doi.org/10.20944/preprints202003.0422.v1

308. Kalra RS, Kandimalla R. Engaging the spikes: Heparan sulfate facilitates SARS-CoV-2 spike protein binding to ACE2 and potentiates viral infection. *Sig Transduct Target Ther.* 2021;6:39. https://doi.org/10.1038/s41392-021-00470-1

309. Clausen TM, Sandoval DR, Spliid CB et al. SARS-CoV-2 infection depends on cellular heparan sulfate and ACE2. *Cell.* 2020 Nov 12;183(4):1043-1057.e15. https://doi.org/10.1016/j.cell.2020.09.033

310. Idrees D, Kumar V. SARS-CoV-2 spike protein interactions with amyloidogenic proteins: Potential clues to neurodegeneration. *Biochem Biophys Res Commun.* 2021;554:94–98.

311. Liu S, Hossinger A, Gbbels S, Vorberga I M. Prions on the run: How extracellular vesicles serve as delivery vehicles for self-templating protein aggregates. *Prion.* 2017;11(2):98–112.

312. Bansal S, Perincheri S, Fleming T et al. Cutting edge: Circulating exosomes with COVID spike protein are induced by BNT162b2 (Pfizer-BioNTech) vaccination prior to development of antibodies: A novel mechanism for immune activation by mRNA vaccines. *J Immunol.* 2021 Nov 15;207(10):2405–2410. https://doi.org/10.4049/jimmunol.2100637

313. Zhang L, Richards A, Inmaculada Barrasa M et al. Reverse-transcribed SARS-CoV-2 RNA can integrate into the genome of cultured human cells and can be expressed in patient-derived tissues. *Proc Nat Acad Sci.* 2021;118 (21):e2105968118. https://doi.org/10.1073/pnas.2105968118

314. Aldén M, Olofsson Falla F, Yang D et al. Intracellular reverse transcription of Pfizer BioNTech COVID-19 mRNA vaccine BNT162b2 in vitro in human liver cell line. *Curr Issues Mol Biol.* 2022;44(3):1115–1126. https://doi.org/10.3390/cimb44030073

315. Spadafora C. A reverse transcriptase-dependent mechanism plays central roles in fundamental biological processes. *Syst Biol Reprod Med.* 2008;54(1):11–21. https://doi.org/10.1080/19396360701876815

316. Zhang X, Zhang R, Yu J. New understanding of the relevant role of LINE-1 retrotransposition in human disease and immune modulation. *Front Cell Dev Biol.* 2020. https://doi.org/10.3389/fcell.2020.00657

22 A Psychotherapeutic Approach to Living Life Forward
The Neuroplastic Synergy of Mindfulness and Intentionality

Martha Stark

CONTENTS

DOI: 10.1201/b23304-24

Life can only be understood backwards; but it must be lived forwards.

Soren Kierkegaard (Kierkegaard & Hannay 1996)

The author's Psychodynamic Synergy Paradigm (PSP) is an integrative approach to the psycho-therapy of patients with deeply embedded emotional injuries and relational scars resulting from unmastered traumatic experiences in their past, compromising the quality of their lives in the present, and undermining their dreams for the future. PSP is a method of treatment that aims to advance patients from psychological rigidity to psychological flexibility such that once they have come to understand their life backward, they can focus on living it forward.

22.1 INTRODUCTION: A SYNERGISTIC APPROACH TO MENTAL HEALTH

PSP (Stark 1999, 2016, 2017) was developed by the author, a psychoanalyst and integrative psychia-trist who has long been interested in both the complex interdependence of mind and body and the actual process by which psychotherapy patients (whatever their level of health or psychopathology) are released from the toxicity of their past and empowered to embrace love, work, and play to their greatest potential going forward.

Elaborated over the course of 30 years and drawing upon the finely honed wisdom of both long-term, in-depth treatments (most of which are psychodynamically informed) and short-term, inten-sive treatments (many of which use brain-based strategies), PSP features five models – the first four of which focus on the relationship between the past and the present, and the fifth of which focuses on the relationship between the present and the future.

Whereas Models 1–4 (representing, respectively, the classical psychoanalytic perspective, the self psychological perspective, the contemporary relational perspective, and the existential-human-istic perspective) are all in the tradition of understanding our history as our destiny (which we are condemned to repeat unless we can remember it), the author's freshly minted Model 5 focuses on our destiny as our choice (which is ours to create if in the present, we can take embodied ownership of our desire to extricate ourselves from the ties that bind us to our past and create a new narrative for ourselves going forward).

Whereas Models 1–4 focus on recognizing the entangled relationship between past and present and understanding, on the deepest of levels, all the ways in which the toxicity of the past is suffusing the essence of the present, Model 5 focuses on disentangling the past from the present, envisioning the possibility of an alternative, preferred reality for the future, and committing to action in align-ment with that vision going forward.

Put simply, whereas Models 1–4 require that we take ownership of our past, Model 5 requires that we take ownership of our future.

Finally, whereas Models 1–4 focus on ferreting out, and working through, early relational trau-mas, Model 5 focuses on challenging outdated, maladaptive narratives – constructed as a result of those early relational traumas – in order adaptively to update them.

For example, consider the case of a patient who resists venturing into new social situations for fear of being shamed. Models 1–4 would focus on exploring the origin of this irrational fear and would then incrementally work it through. Model 5, however, would highlight the fact of the patient's expectation of being shamed as maladaptive and outdated and would then, repeatedly and decisively, challenge this learned expectation in order to update it to a more adaptive, realistic, and appropriate expectation of being, say, accepted (Small 2015).

As will later be elaborated, in Model 5, adaptive updating of narratives and jumpstarting forward movement will be the result of ongoing and embodied challenging of preconceived, ill-founded expectations with new experiences (whether real or simply envisioned) that violate those expectations, thereby disconfirming the conditioned responses.

22.1.1 OLD BAD AND NEW GOOD PSYCHIC STRUCTURES

Despite their different lexicons, all five models involve transformation of psychological rigidity into psychological flexibility. Where Models 1–4 use the language of r*igid defenses* and *flexible adaptations*, Model 5 uses the language of *outdated narratives* and *updated narratives.*

Whatever the model being referenced, however, throughout this chapter, *old bad* and *new good* will be terms used to represent, respectively, psychic structures that are rigid, outdated, and growth-disrupting and psychic structures that are flexible, updated, and growth-promoting.

Parenthetically, it has been suggested that defenses are the lies we tell ourselves in order to avoid the pain in our lives, and adaptations are the things we come up with in order to make the best of bad situations.

22.1.2 A QUANTUM-NEUROSCIENTIFIC APPROACH TO HEALING

The author's Model 5 is a quantum-neuroscientific approach to healing. It is an action-oriented, solution-focused, future-directed model that conceives of the mind as holding infinite potential and of memory as dynamic and continuously updating itself on the basis of new experience.

More specifically, at the heart of the therapeutic action in Model 5 is the synergy of mindfulness (paying embodied attention) and intentionality (setting impassioned intention). Mindfulness asks of patients that they pay attention to the wisdom of their body in order to access the outdated, disempowering narratives fueling their inertia and thwarting their growth; intentionality asks of patients that they use their quantum mind to envision an alternative, preferred reality and then, going forward, that they set the intention to act in alignment with that vision so that they can overcome their inertia and jumpstart their growth.

Whereas Models 1–4 focus on our lives as predetermined, Model 5 is more uplifting and hopeful. Its focus is on envisioned possibilities, commitment to action, empowerment, personal agency, freedom, ownership of desire, realization of dreams, and actualization of potential.

An amusing aside: In *The Marvelous Mrs. Maisel* (a comedy-drama TV mini-series), Abe Weissman (played by Tony Shalhoub) – angry that the housekeeper has gone into his office to clean it – complains, "Just because there is a door, does not mean you use it! A door does not represent infinite possibilities. Leave that room the way it is!"

With respect to the quantum piece, as we shall see, the quantum mind can envision an infinite array of possibilities. By engaging the quantum mind, patients will become able to distance themselves from the maladaptive patterns of thinking, feeling, and acting that have become part of their identity. At the same time, they will be able to accept the possibility that, going forward, there are alternative perspectives and more adaptive ways of acting, reacting, and interacting. After all, thoughts are just thoughts and need not define who we are or how we behave; thoughts are no more powerful than we allow them to be (Hayes et al. 2016).

With respect to the neuroscientific piece, as we shall see, repeated embodied juxtaposition of *old bad* learned expectations with *new good* envisioned possibilities will create decisive – and potentially transformational – mismatch experiences. If these mismatch experiences are repeated often enough, forcefully enough, and dramatically enough within the critical time frame of 4 to 6 hours (dubbed the *reconsolidation window* by neuroscientists), then these ongoing violations of learned expectation will eventually trigger energetic decoupling of the patient's toxic past from her present and advancement of the patient from entrenched inaction to intentioned action as disempowering, growth-impeding narratives are replaced by empowering, growth-promoting ones.

Indeed, the freshly revitalized neuroplastic concept of memory reconsolidation (central to the therapeutic action in Model 5) is at the heart of learning and of how old memories – consolidated and stored in long-term memory – can be subsequently updated and reconsolidated in response to ongoing and embodied new experience. In essence, the brain is continuously modifying itself – structurally and functionally – at the level of the neural synapse in order to stay current and relevant. This reconstructive process (involving both the destruction of old neural networks and the construction of new ones) speaks to the adaptive capacity of the brain and the dynamic nature of memory.

Rewiring the brain (by reconfiguring its neural networks) and reprogramming the mind (by revamping the outdated narratives encoded by those networks) will create the possibility for deep, enduring psychotherapeutic change.

22.1.3   When One Door Closes, Another Door Opens

Disentangling the past from the present in order to eliminate its toxic impact necessarily involves not only dismantling old, negative, and disempowering narratives that had been constructed by the developing child in a desperate attempt to make meaning of her world but also crafting new and empowering narratives that will reframe, or recontextualize, those traumatic experiences in a more positive, self-compassionate, and reality-based light.

To the point here are the pithy words of the neuroscientist Iryna Ethell (2018), "To learn we must first forget."

And, the neuroscientist Joe Dispenza (2013) highlights the need to "break the habit of being yourself" in order to "reinvent a new self" and, more specifically, the need to "lose your mind" in order to "create a new one."

Indeed, one door closes and another door opens when old, outdated memories are deconsolidated and forgotten, and new, updated narratives – specifically designed to take their place – are reconsolidated and locked in.

22.1.4   The Narrative Changes but the Episodic Memory Remains

When therapeutic memory reconsolidation updates a traumatic memory, what exactly is it that changes, and what is it that remains the same? Importantly, the fact of the event underlying the traumatic memory will not change – the episodic memory itself will remain intact. What will change, however, will be the affective coloring of the experience, how the patient positions herself in relation to it, and the relational narrative she constructs about self, others, and the world as a result of it.

Again, the conscious memory of the actual event will remain, but the narrative constructed as a result of it will have changed, as will the patient's emotional relationship to it.

22.1.5   Maria Gains Perspective and Reframes Her Father's Abuse

By way of example, when Maria was a young girl, she had experienced frequent emotional abuse at the hands of her rageful, alcoholic father and, in a desperate attempt to make sense of that abuse, she had decided that it must have been she who was the bad one, she who was at fault.

But Maria, within the context of her secure attachment to a therapist who understood the transformational power of therapeutic memory reconsolidation, was fortunate enough to be offered a rapid-fire series of disconfirming experiences that repeatedly and forcefully challenged Maria's learned expectation of being always a victim.

These juxtaposition experiences took place in conjunction with reactivated memories of her father's abuse, such that Maria was eventually able to update her self-negating narrative. No longer did she experience herself as ever at risk of being abused. Instead, Maria came to realize that it was her alcoholic father who had been the victimizer and she who was innocent.

Importantly, despite now having an updated narrative that offered a fresh, more reality-based perspective, Maria still remembered the fact of her father's abusive rages, but she was no longer convinced that she had deserved the abuse and that the world was a dangerous, unsafe place. In essence, she was able to re-interpret the entire scenario as a story not about herself as ever vulnerable to being abused but about her father as an often out-of-control alcoholic who would periodically fly into irrational and unjustified rages.

22.1.6 ALLOYING THE PURE GOLD OF ANALYSIS

The author's recent addition of a fifth, quantum-neuroscientific model to her psychotherapy paradigm – almost 30 years after the first models were conceived – is in the tradition of Freud's (1919) eventual acknowledgement that, in order to broaden its range of applicability, the "pure gold of analysis" might well need to be "alloyed" with the "copper of direct suggestion … and hypnotic influence" (p. 168). Although the concept of creating an alloy might imply the creation of something inferior or debased, alloys are also associated with desirable qualities such as hardness, lightness, and strength.

Indeed, Model 5 is a problem-oriented, solution-focused, action-oriented, goal-directed, and future-focused model that directly targets the seemingly intractable stuckness of patients who refuse to take embodied ownership of their need to change. It is a no-nonsense model that insists upon commitment to action in order for transformational healing to take place. It explicitly privileges not just thinking and feeling differently but actually doing differently.

Furthermore, Model 5 becomes particularly relevant whenever Models 1–4 have been advancing psychodynamic awareness (that is, understanding life backward) but not providing sufficient impetus for empowered and goal-directed action (that is, living life forward).

22.1.7 BRIEF OVERVIEW OF THE FIVE MODES OF THERAPEUTIC ACTION

Briefly, Model 1 is the classical psychoanalytic perspective – an approach that involves *enhancement of knowledge*, emphasizes *interpretation,* and becomes relevant in those moments when the focus is on the patient's *neurotic conflictedness.*

Model 2 is the deficiency-compensation perspective of self psychology – an approach that involves *provision of experience*, emphasizes *empathic immersion,* and becomes relevant in those moments when the focus is on the patient's *narcissistic vulnerability* and *relentless pursuits.*

Model 3 is the intersubjective perspective of contemporary relational theory – an approach that involves *engagement in relationship*, emphasizes *authentic relatedness,* and becomes relevant in those moments when the focus is on the patient's *compulsive and unwitting re-enactments.*

Model 4 is the existential-humanistic perspective – an approach that involves *facilitation of surrender*, emphasizes a *holding environment,* and becomes relevant in those moments when the focus is on the patient's *schizoid retreat* and *psychic withdrawal.*

Model 5 is the quantum-neuroscientific perspective (and the primary focus of this chapter) – an approach that involves *envisioning of possibilities*, emphasizes *quantum consciousness* and *therapeutic memory reconsolidation*, and becomes relevant in those moments when the focus is on the patient's *implicitly held memories* and *deeply embedded relational expectations.*

22.1.8 UNDERSTANDING LIFE BACKWARD BUT LIVING LIFE FORWARD

It was only more recently that this psychoanalyst author, although a bit late to the game, came to appreciate that *going forward* was just as important as *looking backward*. Amusingly relevant here is a TV commercial about Kia's line-up of SUVs: "The problem with hanging on to the past is that when you're always looking back, you can't see what's coming."

With respect to the *looking backward* encouraged by Models 1–4: It is sometimes simply not enough that the patient become more aware of the price she has paid for her past (Model 1), more accepting of the heartbreak she has experienced along the way as a result (Model 2), more account-able for her often misguided attempts to engage in relationship with others (Model 3), and more accessible despite her longstanding, deep-seated fears (Model 4). Rather, it is critically important that the patient be encouraged to *look forward* – that she embrace her power to release herself from the ties that bind her to her past, take embodied ownership of her need to change, and commit to taking action to create her future going forward.

Echoing this sentiment are the evocative words of Joe Dispenza (2013): "The best way to predict your future is to create it."

Models 1–4, in keeping with the psychoanalytic tradition in which they are rooted, tend to focus on the patient as passively receiving and permanently retaining the cognitive-emotional-visceral imprint of her unmastered early relational experiences. Model 5, in the tradition of constructivist psychologies, tends to focus on the patient as a more active participant in constructing her world-view and in shaping the meaning she makes of her life as a result of all the early privations, depriva-tions, and insults sustained along the way.

Models 1–4 focus on the cumulative impact of relational traumas in the past and the patient's gaining of insight into their toxic impact on her life in the present. Model 5 focuses on outdated and maladaptive narratives as potentially able to be rewritten and interpreted anew – narratives constructed by the patient during her formative years in a desperate attempt to make sense of her world. Instead of sealing her fate, they are seen as holding the potential for reconfiguring her future.

Models 1–4 strive to facilitate, often by way of grieving, in-depth healing of emotional injuries and relational scars deriving from the patient's past. Model 5 aims to facilitate focused action spe-cifically designed to overcome the patient's inertia and actualize her potential.

Paraphrasing only slightly the words of the psychologist and coach Carol Kauffman (2006), "As a [psychodynamic] therapist, I follow the trail of tears to healing; as a coach, I follow the trail of dreams to actualization."

22.1.9 MEMORY INTEGRATION (MODELS 1–4) VERSUS MEMORY RECONSOLIDATION (MODEL 5)

Whereas the therapeutic action in Models 1–4 (understanding life backward) is subtle and gradual, as the patient slowly but steadily gains psychodynamic awareness and advances step by step from reflexive defense to reflective adaptation, the therapeutic action in Model 5 (living life forward) is abrupt and dramatic, as jolting mismatch experiences prompt the overriding of paralyzing inaction and thwarted potential by way of triggering committed action and decisive movement forward.

Parallel to this clinical distinction between therapeutic movement that is nuanced and under-stated and therapeutic movement that is more sudden and striking, cognitive neuroscientists have been making a similar and very exciting distinction between *memory integration* (the term they use to describe the *elaboration* and refinement of already existing mental schemas) (Gisquet-Verrier & Riccio 2019) and *memory reconsolidation* (the aforementioned term they use to describe the com-plete *eradication* of mental schemas and the locking in, or reconsolidation, of entirely new ones) (Schiller et al. 2010; Ecker et al. 2012, 2013).

In 2019, David Feinstein, an experienced clinician and eloquent advocate for this compelling clinical and neuroscientific distinction, writes, "Memory integration appears to be more applicable for new experiences that augment an earlier learning, leading to incremental changes. Memory reconsolidation appears to be more applicable when a new experience decisively contradicts an old learning at its emotional roots." Feinstein continues, "Both theories are supported by evidence, and further research will determine how they interact and the conditions under which each has greater explanatory power" (p. 346).

Memory integration (with its incremental integration of new meanings into already exist-ing and interrelated but long since outdated narratives – as happens in Models 1–4) and memory reconsolidation (with its precipitous and dramatic deleting of old programs and their replacement with new ones – as happens in Model 5) are therefore contrasting but complementary mechanisms whereby the brain is continuously being rewired and the mind continuously reprogrammed when optimally challenged with new information and experience.

22.1.10 DE NOVO PROTEIN SYNTHESIS

Of note is the fact that whereas refinement of already existing neural networks (memory integration) does not require the synthesis of new proteins (Gisquet-Verrier et al. 2015), erasure of outdated memories and their replacement by new, more updated memories (memory reconsolidation) does indeed appear to involve *de novo protein synthesis* (Nader et al. 2000; Alberini et al. 2006).

More specifically, just as the consolidation of labile, short-term memory into more stable, long-term memory (long-term potentiation) requires of the brain that it synthesize new proteins on the postsynaptic membranes of downstream neurons in order both to reinforce the fragile memory traces and to facilitate the transfer of these engrams from short-term storage in the hippocampus to long-term storage in distributed neocortical networks, so too, memory reconsolidation involves de novo synthesis of receptor proteins on the postsynaptic membranes of the downstream target cells (Alberini 2005; Gold 2008).

Not surprisingly, studies have confirmed that memory reconsolidation, like memory consolidation, is blocked by protein synthesis inhibitors, such as the antibiotic anisomycin (Nader et al. 2000). In other words, if protein synthesis is inhibited within a few hours after the new learning has occurred, then what had been newly learned never actually gets locked in, that is, gets neither consolidated nor reconsolidated, and is essentially forgotten.

This discovery that protein synthesis is required for the formation of memories was the result of laboratory experiments conducted in the 1990s on rodents that were then unable to reintegrate a learned fear when exposed to chemical agents that disrupted protein synthesis (Nader et al. 2000). "Because the learning could not be reintegrated, it was as if the fear had been permanently erased" (Feinstein 2019, p. 346).

Unfortunately, anisomycin is toxic to humans, which has obviously limited its usefulness in clinical trials, although the injection of anisomycin into the hippocampus (which plays such an important role in the consolidation of information from short-term to long-term memory) has been rather boldly proposed by several investigators (Wang et al. 2005) for selective removal of traumatic memories.

In any event, in contradistinction to this requirement for de novo protein synthesis when memories are being consolidated and reconsolidated, scientific research has demonstrated that protein synthesis inhibitors have no impact on memory integration. This makes sense, because when memory integration is involved (and not memory reconsolidation), no new memories are actually being formed, only elaboration and further refinement of already existing networks of mental schemas (Gisquet-Verrier et al. 2015).

22.1.11 INHIBITION OF MEMORY RECALL BY THE BETA-BLOCKER PROPRANOLOL

The drug most frequently used in humans to "reduce the saliency of emotional memories" is propranolol, a beta-adrenergic blocker that (peripherally) dampens the stress response and (centrally) inhibits protein synthesis.

In a landmark 1994 study, Cahill and his colleagues demonstrated that propranolol taken just prior to viewing an emotionally disturbing short story significantly impaired later recall of the story but did not affect recall of a closely matched, but more emotionally neutral, story (Cahill et al. 1994).

Since that time, many studies have replicated this finding that dampening stress-induced hyperarousal and inhibiting protein synthesis with propranolol will interfere with later recall of emotionally charged memories. Furthermore, because (as noted earlier) memory reconsolidation is essentially a recapitulation of memory consolidation, researchers have extended their studies to include the inhibitory impact of propranolol on the locking in of new memories in the place of old, emotionally arousing ones (Lonergan et al. 2013).

22.1.12 Optimal Stress within the Window of Tolerance

All five models, whatever their lexicon or particular focus, involve the judicious and ongoing use of *optimal stress* (Stark 2015) within a *window of tolerance* (Siegel 1999; Ogden et al. 2006). In other words, all five models involve the therapeutic use of just the right balance of challenge (to precipitate disruption) and support (to allow repair) within the context of secure attachment to a therapist whose finger is ever on the pulse of the patient's level of anxiety and capacity to tolerate further stress.

Like the three bowls of porridge sampled by Goldilocks – one too hot, one too cold, but one just right (which is the one that worked best for her) – so too the dose of stress provided by the therapist's interventions will be either too much, too little, or just right (which will be the one that works best for the patient).

The ultimate goal of optimally stressful PSP interventions is to facilitate advancement of the patient from mindless (defensive) reactivity to intentioned (adaptive) activity as outdated narratives that distort reality are replaced by updated narratives that are more accurate renderings of self, others, and the world. Simultaneously, the patient will advance from psychological rigidity and defensiveness to psychological flexibility and adaptability.

22.2 JUMPSTARTING ANALYSIS PARALYSIS

Models 1–4 are all informed by time-honored psychoanalytic concepts and focus on the working through of traumatic experiences that had once been overwhelming and therefore defended against but that can now, in the context of a solid therapeutic relationship characterized by empathic attunement and authentic engagement, be processed, integrated, and adapted to.

As we know, the goal in all four models is to help patients gain an in-depth and comprehensive understanding of how they have come to be as they are. The emphasis is on insight, awareness, understanding, knowledge – and not on action. Of course, the therapist's hope is that patients, inspired by all that they have come to know, will simply find themselves modifying their behavior and changing how they relate to self, others, and the world as an offshoot of their ever- evolving psychodynamic awareness. But if the psychodynamic therapist *needs* her patient to take action or *needs* her to get better, then the therapist will be faulted for having too much *therapeutic zeal* (Freud 1919).

So, what about patients who remain stuck and fundamentally unfulfilled in their lives despite having acquired deep insight into their inner workings (the goal in Model 1), despite having confronted and grieved heartbreaking truths about the objects of their desire and the futility of their relentless pursuits (the goal in Model 2), despite having taken ownership of the dysfunctional relational dynamics they compulsively re-enact on the stage of their lives (the goal in Model 3), and despite having dared to let themselves be found such that they can now experience at least occasional moments of meaningful and joyous connection with others (the goal in Model 4)?

22.2.1 Refractory Inertia and Thwarted Potential

It could be said that such patients are suffering from a form of *analysis paralysis*. They might indeed be now more aware (Model 1), more accepting (Model 2), more accountable (Model 3), and more accessible (Model 4) and, on some level, their lives might indeed be now working better for them as a result; but, on another level, they are not loving, working, or playing to their greatest capacity, realizing their dreams, or fulfilling their potential.

A prime example of thwarted potential was the young man this author saw in consultation a long time ago – a man who had been in a psychodynamic treatment (and on medication) for many years and had come to know himself deeply but was still very stuck in his life and desperately unhappy. He reported to the author that every single day after work, he would sit in the dark in his living room, hour after hour, doing nothing, his mind blank. By his side would be his stereo and a magnificent collection of his favorite classical music. The flick of a switch and he would feel better – and yet, night after night, overwhelmed with immobilizing despair, he would never once touch that switch.

It was this young man's story and the sobering stories of countless other therapy patients who have found themselves paralyzed in their efforts to move forward in their lives that prompted the author to expand her PSP to include a fifth mode of therapeutic action – one that would more explicitly address the importance of actual behavioral change for the promotion of overall well-being.

In the prophetic words of Lao Tzu – "If you do not change direction, you may end up where you are heading."

22.2.2 DOCUMENTED EFFECTIVENESS OF SHORT-TERM, INTENSIVE TREATMENTS

Further incentivizing was the fact that over the course of the past 10 to 15 years, the author has had the opportunity to broaden her therapeutic horizons by immersing herself in the study of a variety of short-term, intensive treatments, including Acceptance and Commitment Therapy (ACT) (Hayes et al. 2016), Eye Movement Desensitization and Reprocessing (EMDR) (Shapiro 2017), Intensive Short-Term Dynamic Psychotherapy (ISTDP) (Frederickson 2013; Coughlin 2016), Accelerated Experiential Dynamic Psychotherapy (AEDP) (Fosha 2000), Neuro-Linguistic Programming (NLP) (Bandler & Grinder 1982), Internal Family Systems (IFS) (Schwartz 1997), Somatic Experiencing (SE) (Levine 1997), Sensorimotor Psychotherapy (Ogden et al. 2006), Pesso Boyden System Psychomotor (PBSP) (Pesso 1969), Narrative Therapy (Schafer 1994), Motivational Interviewing (Miller & Rollnick 1992), Hypnotherapy (Braid 2019), Emotional Freedom Techniques (EFT)/ Meridian Tapping (Craig 2011), and Energy Psychology (Eden & Feinstein 2008) – all of which have had impressive and documented success in the relief of problematic symptoms and, more generally, in the treatment of psychological and physical disorders across a broad spectrum.

Patricia Coughlin (2004), a world-renowned mental health practitioner at the forefront of clinical research on the therapeutic process and its effectiveness, has asserted that the methods of time-limited treatments are the "gold standard of therapy" and enable patients to achieve dramatic results, often within weeks. She notes that the cost-effectiveness of brief treatments is a major advantage of these brain-based approaches.

Coughlin (2016) cites the 1986 meta-analytic research done by Howard (2009), who studied the relationship between length of treatment and patient benefit. Howard's data were based on more than 2,400 patients and spanned more than 30 years of research. Coughlin summarizes Howard's impressive findings as follows: 30% of the patients studied were early responders and improved by the second session; 60–65% experienced significant symptomatic relief within seven sessions; 70–75% within 6 months; and 85% after a year.

Additionally, with respect to the Intensive Short-Term Dynamic Psychotherapy (1977) approach originally developed by the Boston-trained psychoanalyst Habib Davanloo (a vocal proponent of fostering a collaborative therapeutic alliance in order to *unlock the unconscious*), Coughlin (2016) asserts, "ISTDP is a scientifically validated method of psychotherapy that dramatically accelerates the process of change, such that patients will see measurable results within weeks and months, rather than years."

Indeed, rather than the long-term, incremental, step-by-step psychodynamic process, with its ongoing cycles of disruption and repair as the patient gradually evolves from illness to wellness, the aforementioned time-limited, targeted treatments are more solution focused, action based, goal directed, and future oriented – and in the right hands, can indeed often produce rather dramatic and abrupt symptomatic relief and observable modification of behavior.

A number of neuroscientifically inclined clinicians (Ecker et al. 2012, 2013; Feinstein 2019) have advanced the hypothesis that most of the above-referenced short-term therapies rely upon *therapeutic memory reconsolidation* as the mechanism whereby the brain can update itself on the basis of new experience. Their contention is that this brain-based strategy is the organizing principle that transcends the theories and techniques of the different schools of psychotherapy and provides an overarching, unifying conceptual framework for understanding the therapeutic action of these time-limited, targeted approaches.

22.2.3 IMMEDIATE AND DRAMATIC RELIEF OF SYMPTOMS

The following two transformational vignettes had a profound impact on the author and further incentivized her to delve into the neuroscientific literature on learning and memory so that she would be able to broaden and deepen her understanding of how the brain can be rewired and the mind reprogrammed, thereby enabling her to expand her psychotherapy paradigm to be more inclusive. Both patients appear to have experienced immediate, seemingly miraculous relief of their symptoms as a result of having had their brains exposed to sudden, shocking jolts that the author hypothesizes must have triggered resynchronization of disturbed patterns of neural activity.

22.2.4 JUANITA'S MIND-BOGGLING EXPERIENCE WITH AN OPIOID

What follows is something that Juanita (a psychotherapy patient on whom the author did a consultation several years ago) shared with the author.

Juanita had been struggling to get over the pain of her grief about the loss of a man she had felt was the love of her life. Together for almost 10 years, she and Eduardo had shared what appeared to be almost a storybook life together – although her own, not yet fully processed history of having been sexually abused by her stepfather made her a reluctant sex partner, sadly for both Eduardo and her.

One day, Juanita accidentally discovered, to her absolute heartbreak, that Eduardo had been having an affair with one of his colleagues at work. This precipitated a series of major arguments and, ultimately, a breakup, with Eduardo finally moving out.

Juanita, not only overwhelmed with grief at the loss of Eduardo but also unable to forgive herself for the part she knew she had played in his straying because of her unresolved issues, then found herself experiencing such acute psychic distress that she became profoundly and immobilizingly depressed – and even found herself contemplating suicide as a possible escape from the pain of it all.

One evening, exhausted from the effort of having struggled through each and every day since their breakup, Juanita, someone who ordinarily shunned the idea of using recreational drugs and even medications prescribed by doctors, blindly reached for a few of the hydrocodone pills that she still had in her possession from the time when her wisdom teeth had been extracted. Her intent was not to kill herself but to find oblivion in reduced consciousness and sleep.

Fortunately, Juanita did not die. Instead, after becoming sedated, somewhat numbed, and a bit calmer, eventually fell into a deep, opioid-induced sleep. Upon awakening hours and hours later and more refreshed than she had felt in weeks, she suddenly realized – to her total amazement and delight – that the pills prescribed by her dentist to relieve physical pain had actually obliterated her psychic pain. As Juanita reported it to me, it was almost as if she, in discovering the possibility of living without deep psychic pain (by virtue of the opioid-induced numbing), was able to reframe her entire experience of loss as a manageable, albeit still heartbreakingly sad, way of living.

In any event, Juanita's mind-boggling experience of an opioid-induced repositioning of herself in relation to what had felt like unbearable grief is a dramatic demonstration of how changes in the state of the brain can impact mental health.

22.2.5 ALINA'S MIRACULOUS RELEASE FROM THE TYRANNY OF OBSESSIVE LOVE

Particularly distressing for Alina (a friend of the author's) was her obsessive love for Josh, a man she knew would not be right for her. Among other things, he was married. Although she and Josh had had very little actual contact, the several times they had run into each other had been extremely exciting for Alina, and she was finding herself becoming increasingly obsessed with fantasies about him and the possibility of having a future with him – despite the fact that there were no indications that his marriage was in trouble or that he was even all that interested in her.

A therapist herself and in a long-term psychodynamic therapy, Alina had come to understand that her intense longing for Josh was probably related, at least in part, to unresolved oedipal feelings that she still had in relation to her dad, a very seductive man with whom she had had a very intimate, albeit complicated, relationship.

But despite Alina's ever-evolving awareness that some of what she was experiencing in relation to Josh was fueled by unmastered yearnings for her dad, she remained tormented by her obsessive love for this inappropriate (for a whole mix of reasons) and unavailable man – fantasies that, although pleasurable and compelling, were also self-defeating and filled her with self-loathing and shame.

One day, Alina was unfortunately involved in a serious car accident and suffered a bad concussion. Although she recovered fairly quickly, she did sustain some permanent memory loss, most especially with respect to the events leading right up to the accident. Even though an investigation was done into the cause of the two-car accident, and the scene was reconstructed, Alina's retrograde amnesia persisted, and she herself was never able to retrieve the memory of the events preceding the crash, which made it more difficult to figure out the insurance piece and which driver had been at fault.

In any event, it was shortly thereafter that Alina, with mixed feelings of relief and disappointment, suddenly realized that after the car accident she had simply stopped obsessing about Josh! In fact, all thoughts of Josh had miraculously vanished – and it had happened through no conscious intent on her part!

As the author later came to formulate things, Alina was probably engaging in her favorite guilty pleasure, namely, fantasizing about Josh, as she was driving and right up to the moment of actual impact with the other car. The retrograde amnesia that she suffered as a result caused her to forget not only the pre-crash events but also her obsessive thoughts about Josh!

Alina's miraculous release from the tyranny of obsessive love as a result of her retrograde amnesia was something that prompted the author to think ever more seriously about including in her PSP a more brain-based approach to the therapeutic action – one that would take into consideration not just psychodynamic awareness but also the brain's microarchitecture and its complex synaptic web of neural circuits.

22.2.6   Retrograde Amnesia – Richard Rubin and His Team of Researchers

The idea that deeply entrenched traumatic memories could be erased if certain conditions were met was actually the result of a cleverly designed study conducted over 50 years ago by the behavior therapists Rubin, Fried, and Franks (1969) – all the more remarkable because, back in the 1960s, most neuroscientists still embraced the idea that once a deep emotional learning had been acquired, it was *forever*.

Although it was not appreciated at the time for the significance that it was later to assume, the experiment that Richard Rubin and his team of investigators devised is now being widely quoted by proponents of memory reconsolidation. Rubin and his group came up with the innovative idea of capitalizing upon the well-known retrograde amnesia "produced by the disruptive effect of electroconvulsive therapy (ECT) on memory trace consolidation" at the level of the memory trace's "structural encoding" (Rubin et al. 1969, p. 37).

Earlier studies involving the use of ECT had generally been conducted on subjects who were anesthetized and therefore unconscious during their treatments. But Rubin and his colleagues formulated the following, testable hypothesis: "If the patient's attention is strongly directed … to his most disturbing feelings and imagery … and if he is instantly given ECT (awake), there should result a significantly greater amelioration and reduction of symptoms than that obtained when ECT is given in the usual way" (Rubin et al. 1969, p. 39).

The investigators specifically selected subjects who were suffering from obsessions, delusions, and hallucinations. Then, in order to reactivate the neural mechanisms encoding the "psychopathological imagery" underlying these distorted perceptions of reality, the subjects were instructed to focus their attention on their symptoms. Rubin reasoned that having them focus their attention in this way would return the neural networks fueling the symptoms to a malleable state, which would render those circuits vulnerable to being disrupted. ECT was immediately administered with the subjects being kept awake throughout the treatment.

Of the 15 patients in Rubin's study, 7 had been previously treated anywhere from 5 to 28 times with routine ECT (and anesthesia) – but those treatments had been ineffective. These seven patients therefore served as their own controls.

Following a single treatment with ECT, all 15 of the patients "improved dramatically for periods of three months to three years [the duration of the study]. One relapsed after nine months but recovered after another treatment" (Rubin et al. 1969, p. 40). The authors go on to write, "The probability of the effectiveness of this treatment resulting from chance factors only is less than 0.1%. This estimate is based on the number of previous, ineffective treatments" (Rubin et al. 1969, p. 40). To calculate this percentage, they used Fisher's exact test, more accurate than the chi-square test and recommended when the total sample size is less than 1000.

Rubin and his team (Rubin et al. 1969) astutely concluded that their study was proof that, at least in principle, the mental schemas fueling the symptoms must have been entirely obliterated, because treatment with ECT prompted complete remission of symptoms only when those mental schemas were reactivated in subjects who were awake while given the electroconvulsive shock – and not when those mental schemas were lying dormant with the subjects unconscious.

Parenthetically, although Rubin's brilliantly conceived study appeared to demonstrate eradication of *old bad*, it did not specifically address the introduction of *new good*. In other words, although the subjects appeared to be released from the tyranny of their obsessions, delusions, and hallucinations, it was not clear what, if anything, got locked in, or reconsolidated, in the place of those pathological perceptions of reality.

That notwithstanding, Rubin's trailblazing experiment was ingenious and, although largely ignored by the neuroscientific community until the 1990s, laid the groundwork for future research efforts.

22.2.7   Interdependence of the Five Models

In order to optimize therapeutic effectiveness, the PSP therapist can shift back and forth from one model to the next based upon what she, in the moment, intuitively senses is the point of emotional urgency for the patient, that is, whether it is the patient's resistance to awareness (the classical psychoanalytic perspective of Model 1), her relentless pursuit of the unattainable (the self psychological perspective of Model 2), her re-enactment of unmastered early relational traumas (the contemporary relational perspective of Model 3), her relentless despair and retreat from the world (the existential-humanistic perspective of Model 4), or her refractory inertia, refusal to change, and relentless inaction (the quantum-neuroscientific perspective of Model 5).

PSP therefore involves the complex interplay of all five modes of therapeutic action, each gaining momentum by virtue of advancement in the other four. In essence, all five models are interdependent and, in order to bring about enduring, broad-ranging, characterological change, symptomatic relief, behavioral modification, and actualization of potential, all will come into play at various points in a serious, long-term treatment – as the therapeutic process evolves through healing cycles of destabilization and subsequent restabilization at ever higher levels of adaptive capacity, resilience, and psychological flexibility.

Furthermore, because for the most part the psychodynamically informed Models 1–4 encourage the patient to take the lead and to talk about whatever comes to mind for her, such treatments often run the risk of either getting bogged down or straying off course – and of then becoming "analysis paralysis" or, ultimately, "analysis interminable" (Freud 1937). It is when this happens that aspects of the more action-oriented and goal-directed Model 5 can be introduced into a longer-term, in-depth psychodynamic treatment in order to restore its focus, clarity, direction, and purpose.

Unlike Models 1–4, Model 5 does indeed spotlight vision, commitment, action, and results, that is, living life and not just understanding it.

An anonymous quote claimed by many captures the essence of Model 5: "Eyes forward. Mind focused. Heart ready. Game on, World."

22.3 THE DYNAMIC NATURE OF MEMORY: REWIRING THE BRAIN AND REPROGRAMMING THE MIND

Neuroscientists had long thought that once a new learning was consolidated in long-term memory, it would permanently installed. Perhaps, it could then be modified, or even eclipsed, by subsequent experiences, but it would nonetheless remain intact, lurking beneath the surface and ever vulnerable to being reactivated – and subsequently reinforced.

But, that has begun to change.

Over the course of the past two decades, a dedicated group of cognitive neuroscientists (Nader 2003; Verkhratsky & Butt 2007; Schiller et al. 2010; Dudai et al. 2015), ever intent upon teasing out the neural mechanisms underlying the dynamic nature of memory, have been using advanced neuroimaging techniques to deepen their understanding of how the brain continuously updates itself on the basis of new experience. Their interest is in understanding what actually happens, at the level of the neural synapse, when a thought is being thought, a feeling felt, or a memory remembered.

22.3.1 BRAIN IMAGING TECHNIQUES TO MAP BRAIN ACTIVITY

Advanced neuroimaging techniques, including functional magnetic resonance imaging, scanning microscopy, and optogenetics (a new technology that allows genetically modified neurons in the brain to be selectively turned on and off using an optical probe to deliver the light), are being used to map brain activity – and, as a result, to provide windows into the mind.

Indeed, researchers have made the groundbreaking discovery that when memories (traumatic and otherwise) are retrieved, the network of synapses encoding those memories will become unlocked for a time-limited period (Ecker et al. 2012, 2013; Lee et al. 2017; Feinstein 2019). This unlocking, or deconsolidation, signals the opening of the *reconsolidation window* – a brief window of opportunity when memories will become malleable, flexible, and therefore transiently sensitive to input from the outside. This time-limited reconsolidation window, which appears to last anywhere from 4 to 6 hours, must be utilized if there is to be major resculpting of the neural networks encoding those memories.

22.3.2 VIOLATION OF EXPECTATION

More specifically, for eradication of deeply embedded emotional memories to be permanent, neuroscientists hypothesize that *violation of expectation* (caused by the unanticipated introduction of something new that disconfirms the learned expectation of something old) must take place within this 4- to 6-hour reconsolidation window (Schiller et al. 2010). In the neuroscientific literature, this mismatch is referred to as a *prediction error* or *novelty detection* (Schlichting & Preston 2015; Wang 2018); in the clinical literature, it is referred to as a *juxtaposition experience* or *mismatch* (Ecker et al. 2012; Feinstein 2019; Armstrong 2019).

Broadly speaking, a prediction error or juxtaposition experience is a surprising and jolting mismatch between the learned, habitual expectation of *old bad* and the reality-based, present-focused, future-oriented experience of *new good* (be that experience real or simply envisioned). Intuitively, the idea that abruptly, rapidly, unexpectedly, and decisively introducing the element of surprise in order to provoke change certainly makes sense, as does the idea that when new information directly contradicting a previous learning is repeatedly juxtaposed with what had come to be expected, the old memory will eventually be forced adaptively to update itself.

Put simply, introducing an unanticipated (or even random) element or event will disrupt the brain's routine ways of organizing information, which will force the brain to reorganize itself in order to include the unexpected input, thereby altering neural patterns of connectivity.

22.3.3 Expansion and Contraction of Glial Cells

Neuroimaging studies demonstrate that opening the transient 4- to 6-hour window is initiated by the action of several types of glial cells (particularly astrocytes and microglia) – neuroimmune cells that reside in the brain's extracellular matrix (or interstitial space) and ensheathe the brain's neurons (Verkhratsky & Butt 2007).

Glial cells had long been known to nourish, protect, and support the nerve cells to which they were attached. More recently, however, brain imaging studies have been able to demonstrate that glial cells also play the critically important role of regulating synaptic connectivity, which they do by way of either their expansion or their contraction – alterations in size that result in either inhibitory or excitatory synaptic transmission.

More specifically, neuroimaging studies indicate that the swelling of glial cells inhibits the transmission of nerve impulses from the pre-synaptic to the post-synaptic membrane, whereas the shrinking of glial cells facilitates the propagation of nerve impulses across the synaptic cleft (Verkhratsky & Butt 2007).

22.3.4 The Introduction of Something New

When a memory is reactivated, the glial cells surrounding the synaptic junction will shrink in size, rendering the synapse transiently plastic (*synaptic plasticity*) – variously described as malleable, sensitive, fragile, and vulnerable to disruption by environmental input (Eroglu & Barres 2010; Rossouw 2014). In other words, when the glial cells contract, the network of synapses encoding the reactivated memory will become temporarily deconsolidated, or unlocked, such that something new can be introduced.

If the something new that is introduced is a positive experience that disconfirms the learned expectation of something negative, and if that mismatch is presented repeatedly enough and forcefully enough, then the new experience (and the fresh perspective to which it gives rise) will end up deleting the destabilized synapses and prompting the locking in, or reconsolidation, of new synapses encoding an updated, reality-based, growth-promoting, empowering narrative in the place of the old, outdated, maladaptive, growth-disrupting, disempowering one.

In other words, a more relevant narrative that reflects a fresh, more adaptive, healthier perspective will be constructed – a narrative that will then become incorporated into the intrinsic fabric of the patient's life and, going forward, will become the new filter through which the patient experiences self, others, and the world.

In essence, therapeutic memory reconsolidation will be taking place once the glial cells (appropriately named after the Greek word for *glue*) return to their swollen state and lock in, or reconsolidate, the new, more adaptive meaning in the place of the old, maladaptive one.

In the neuroscientific literature, it would seem that little specific attention is paid to whether the glial cells contract whenever a memory is being reactivated or if the glial cells contract only when a memory has been reactivated and, at the same time, a new experience is being presented – a new experience that mismatches the old one. This is a point of confusion in the literature and, quite frankly, glossed over by most researchers. In reading between the lines, however, this author has come to believe that reactivation of memory alone suffices to prompt glial cell contraction and destabilization of the synapses encoding the memory, thereby laying the groundwork for either therapeutic memory reconsolidation (if something new is presented) or simply reinforcement of the memory (if nothing new is presented).

22.3.5 EYE MOVEMENT DESENSITIZATION AND REPROCESSING (EMDR) THERAPY

A brain-based strategy designed to promote therapeutic memory reconsolidation is EMDR therapy, a highly effective psychotherapeutic method that, in order to recontextualize and detoxify traumatic memories, capitalizes upon the use of *bilateral alternating stimulation* to engage both sides of the brain, thereby bringing to bear the analytic wisdom of the present-focused left brain on the emotional knowledge harbored in the past-focused right brain (Shapiro 2017).

The patient is instructed to focus her mind's eye on a distressing and unmastered traumatic experience, memory, or image and to let herself re-experience whatever thoughts, feelings, and sensations are evoked as she dares to remember. Alternately, repetitively, and rhythmically, the clinician then stimulates both sides of the patient's brain (whether visually, auditorily, or tactilely) – left, right, left, right, left, right, and so on.

Activating both sides of the brain in this way will bring to bear the rationality and perspective of the more evolved left brain on the processing of the reactivated traumatic memory stored, unprocessed, in the patient's less evolved right brain, where it has been festering and fueling her maladaptive symptoms and dysfunctional behaviors.

The bilateral sensory stimulation can involve the eyes, the ears, or touch. Early research, however, suggests that movement of the eyes back and forth behind closed lids is particularly effective in evoking the desired retrieval of traumatic memories (Shapiro 2017).

Intuitively, this makes sense, inasmuch as taking a minute to close your eyes when you have misplaced your keys, say, or forgotten where you have parked your car will often make it easier to recover the memory. And when faced with a difficult task, people often spontaneously close their eyes or look away. Doing so appears to enhance visualization by minimizing distractions and facilitating focus. In fact, eye closure is described in the literature as an instinctive reaction designed to reduce *cognitive load* (Vredeveldt et al. 2011).

Once the traumatic memory has been reactivated, the window of opportunity will open for replacement of *old bad* with *new good*.

Indeed, as the patient is revisiting – visually, cognitively, emotionally, and somatically – the unprocessed traumatic experience, she is being continuously reminded by the clinician that she is now in the present. *That was then, and this is now.*

Prompting the patient to focus her attention on both the past (as the traumatic memory stored in her right brain, or body consciousness, is being reactivated) and the present (as the analytic wisdom of her left brain, or brain consciousness, is being brought to bear) is designed to capitalize upon the patient's capacity for *dual awareness*. In other words, dual awareness is being fostered when the patient is being asked to focus her attention on what she is experiencing in the moment at the same time as she is being encouraged to step back from that experience in order to detach herself from the traumatic memory, gain distance, and recover perspective.

As the bilateral alternating stimulation continues, the clinician is prompting the patient to assume a stance of detached compassion, repeatedly offering the patient such mesmerizing statements as:

> Imagine yourself watching it all on a movie screen or a TV. But it's in the past – it's old stuff. Just notice it and let it go. Imagine yourself riding on a train and the images, thoughts, and feelings that you are having are just scenery passing by – but it's over now and you're safe. It's history – just watch it go by. Imagine yourself driving in a tunnel – but just keep your foot on the pedal and keep moving forward. That's right. That's good.

The therapeutic action in EMDR (as in Model 5) involves helping the patient maintain this dual awareness so that the traumatic experience can be tamed, detoxified, and integrated as the patient moves toward a more adaptive resolution, one that no longer triggers cognitive, emotional, somatic, or behavioral reactions.

22.3.6   LAKISHA – FROM POWERLESS VICTIM TO EMPOWERED SURVIVOR

Lakisha presented to the author for a consultation. She reported that she was struggling to make her peace with a trauma that she had experienced years earlier when she had accepted a ride home from a party with an attractive man whom she had just met – a man who had then attempted to rape her. He had driven her into a secluded area in the woods and tried to force himself on her. By dint of her incredible determination and instinct for survival, however, Lakisha had managed to wrest herself free, to jump out of his truck, and to flee for safety. But, Lakisha was haunted by the memory of the attempted rape and was having difficulty forgiving herself for having allowed herself to be seduced into accepting a ride from this man whom she barely knew.

The author did one session of EMDR on Lakisha, which, in fairly short order and felicitously, enabled her to reposition herself in relation to the traumatic event, such that instead of experiencing shame because she had allowed herself to be seduced by this man, she came to feel good about herself, her survival skills, and her ability to outsmart him. By the end of the session, Lakisha still remembered what had happened in the woods that dark night, but it was no longer a source of excoriating pain and charged with emotion. Rather, she reported that she was now feeling a sense of pride – and empowerment – that she had managed to save herself from being abused by this seductive and dangerous man.

In essence, Lakisha, by tapping into the analytic wisdom of her brain consciousness, was able to get enough distance from the trauma (the internal record of which had been stored in her body consciousness) that she was then able to reprocess and detoxify the experience. In essence, she was able to desensitize the traumatic experience enough that she was able to update the narrative she had constructed of herself as gullible, vulnerable, and disempowered to one of herself as strong, determined, and empowered.

22.3.7   HEBBIAN THEORY AND ASSOCIATIVE LEARNING

When a memory is being reactivated, whether the new experience that gets introduced during the 4- to 6-hour reconsolidation window is in line with what had been expected or at odds with what had been expected, the updated memory that gets reconsolidated will conform to Donald Hebb's (2002) neuroscientific postulate that nerve cells firing together will wire together.

In order to demonstrate Hebbian theory in action, we return now to Lakisha. The EMDR session that was done enabled her to reposition herself in relation to the near-rape experience that had traumatized her years earlier, such that she was able to construct an updated narrative of herself as no longer a powerless victim but an empowered survivor.

How might Hebbian theory explain this transformation?

In response to instructions from the author (and after installing a safe place as a comforting backdrop for the more challenging work that was to follow), Lakisha reactivated the traumatic memory of her near-rape by continuously focusing, in her mind, on what had happened in the woods that fateful night and by simultaneously reliving, in her heart and in her body, the outrage, devastation, shame, and sick feeling in her gut that were accompanying the reawakened, and excruciatingly painful, memory.

Had there been no new cognitive-emotional-somatic experience introduced at this juncture, then reactivating the traumatic memory and having Lakisha simultaneously relive the horror of it all would simply have served to strengthen the intensity of the horrifically traumatizing memory.

Indeed, in accordance with Hebbian theory, revisiting a trauma over and over again – without at the same time introducing a fresh, new perspective that will reframe, or recontextualize, the traumatic experience – will simply reinforce the synaptic connection between the fact of the event and both the traumatizing emotions associated with it and the disempowering narrative to which that traumatizing experience had given rise.

After all, Hebb's postulate has it that nerve cells firing together will wire together.

But, this is not what happened for Lakisha during her EMDR session because, as a result of repeatedly and persistently tapping into the analytic wisdom of her left brain by way of stimulating, alternately, both sides of her brain, a fresh, new perspective was indeed being continuously introduced, such that the traumatic event of the near-rape was ultimately being reframed as a story not about Lakisha as a defeated victim but about Lakisha as a triumphant survivor.

Again, in accordance with Hebbian theory, the repetitive linking of the fact of an event with a more positive recontextualization of it will prompt the rewiring, and reconsolidation, of updated synaptic connections between the fact of the event and now more modulated emotions and a more empowering narrative.

After all, Hebb's postulate has it that nerve cells firing together will wire together – except that now, Hebb's postulate can be seen as providing support for the concept of synaptic plasticity and associative learning. In essence, Hebb's postulate lends further credence to the way in which the brain (and its synapses) can be rewired and the mind (and its narratives) reprogrammed, which is what happens with therapeutic memory reconsolidation – and in Model 5.

22.3.8   THE BRAIN'S NEUROPLASTICITY

In truth, the brain has a remarkable ability to adapt to changing conditions (Martin et al. 2000). Both memory integration and memory reconsolidation are complementary processes whereby the brain is continuously updating itself on the basis of contemporary information and experience – either incrementally through cycles of disruption (in reaction to challenge) and repair (in response to support) or more abruptly and decisively as a result of perceived mismatch between the envisioned experience of something *new* and *good* and the anticipated experience of something *old* and *bad*.

Admittedly, both memory integration and memory reconsolidation remain topics for much heated debate in the scientific literature. But, the dedicated group of neuroscientists who study learning and memory and the neuroscientifically inclined mental health practitioners who are similarly impassioned all agree that the brain must be doing something miraculous to be bringing itself continuously up to date on the basis of new experience.

Whether memory integration (with its incremental integration of new meanings into already existing and interrelated but long since outdated narratives) or memory reconsolidation (with its precipitous and dramatic deleting of old programs that have long since outlived their usefulness), the brain is continuously, and adaptively, updating itself in order to keep itself current and relevant.

Reference is here being made, of course, to the newly revitalized field of neuroplasticity, that is, reprogramming of the mind and rewiring of the brain – aptly described by the psychoanalyst Norman Doidge (2007) as "the brain that changes itself."

22.4   MODEL 5 QUANTUM DISENTANGLEMENT STATEMENTS

22.4.1   THE NEUROPLASTIC SYNERGY OF MINDFULNESS AND INTENTIONALITY

As noted repeatedly throughout this chapter, the author has come to appreciate the transformational power of therapeutic memory reconsolidation and believes that one way to capitalize upon this brain-based concept of replacing *old bad* with *new good* is by prompting the patient to pay embodied attention to *old bad* and to set impassioned intention for *new good* – such that juxtaposition of those two mismatched experiences will precipitate a rewiring of the brain (as a result of remodeled neural circuits) and simultaneously, a reprogramming of the mind (as a result of updated mental schemas).

The cutting edge of the therapeutic action in Model 5 will entail the therapist's targeting the emotional knowledge harbored in the patient's body consciousness – that is, the embodied emotional learnings and procedurally organized relational expectations underlying the patient's maladaptive symptoms and self-defeating behaviors – and then bringing to bear the analytic wisdom of the patient's brain consciousness.

More specifically, the internal cognitive-emotional-somatic tension created through the judicious and ongoing use of optimally stressful Model 5 interventions highlighting the dramatic contrast between *what has been* (accessed by way of mindfulness) and *what could be* (introduced by way of intentionality) will provide the impetus needed for reprogramming the patient's outdated mental schemas and rewiring the complex web of neural networks in the patient's corticolimbic system encoding them.

22.4.2 Mindfulness – Compassionate Witnessing of the Present Moment

Mindfulness refers to cultivating the practice of being a compassionate and nonjudgmental witness to the present moment of one's internal experience.

In the current context, mindfulness (paying attention to *old bad*) will allow the experiential emergence of implicit knowledge into explicit awareness. *Mindful awareness*, in conjunction with the hard-earned *psychodynamic awareness* achieved by way of the therapeutic action in Models 1–4, can then be used to inform intentionality (setting intention for *new good*) going forward.

22.4.3 Intentionality – Harnessing the Pluripotent Potential of Every Moment in Time

In the current context and borrowing from quantum theory, intentionality refers to recognizing that the quantum realm holds an infinite array of possibilities and that every moment in time holds limitless potential.

When we set an intention, we are directing our focused attention toward the expression of a positive outcome and the actualization of a preferred reality. More specifically, by way of our conscious intent, we are hoping to influence our subconscious mind to manifest a latent possibility, the potential for which was there all along, just waiting to be discovered.

Understanding the transformational power of intentionality requires an appreciation for, and even a reverence for, the impact of the energetic realm (which is physically imperceptible) on the material realm (which is physically perceptible). In other words, intentionality involves mind over matter – a mystical concept that, for some, is difficult to grasp and, for others, completely obvious.

Put simply, living your life without intention has been likened to getting into your car and having no destination in mind. But if you live your life with intention and purpose, then you get into your car and drive to your desired destination.

22.4.4 A Quantum Approach to Therapeutic Change

Model 5 is described as not only a neuroscientific approach to healing but also a quantum approach, because it capitalizes upon the quantum concepts of entanglement, disentanglement, and superposition. These constructs provide a coherent conceptual framework for understanding a critically important piece of the therapeutic action in Model 5, namely, (1) that the toxicity of the past, across time and space, is continuously and energetically infusing the present (quantum entanglement); (2) that this toxic past must be energetically decoupled from the present (quantum disentanglement); and (3) that every precious moment in time and space, once energetically disentangled from the past, holds infinite potential and hope for the future (quantum superposition).

22.4.5 From Determinism to Free Will

So, how exactly do the concepts of quantum entanglement, quantum disentanglement, and quantum superposition come into play in Model 5?

The *adhesiveness of the id* (fueled as it is by both libidinal and aggressive energies) was one of the constructs used by Freud to explain the tenacity with which patients, unwittingly, cling to their infantile attachments, their relentless pursuits, and their compulsive repetitions, that is, cling to the toxicity of their past (Erwin 2003).

The author's decision to develop a model that draws upon quantum theory was informed, at least in part, by her desire to find a more contemporary way to explain why a patient's present – even though decades later – might be still infiltrated by the toxicity of her bygone past. The concept of quantum entanglement fitted the bill. Albert Einstein (Isaacson 2008), after struggling for years to understand the laws governing the mysterious nonlocal forces that characterize quantum interactions between entities that are separated in time and space, famously derided this strange phenomenon by dubbing it *spooky action at a distance* – shorthand for capturing the essence of these enigmatic interactions that defy the laws of Newtonian physics.

Indeed, Model 5 confronts head-on the quantum entanglement of the patient's present with the toxicity of her past, that is, the spooky coupling of her present dysfunction with the implicitly held, deeply embedded, disempowering, relational constructs about self, others, and the world that the patient, as a young child, had constructed in a desperate attempt to make sense of things.

The goals in Model 5 are therefore quantum disentanglement from these outdated and dysfunctional misconceptions; the construction of more adaptive, more flexible, more reality-based, more present-focused, and more future-oriented mental models; and, going forward, passionate commitment to intentioned, coherent, and embodied action in conformity with these updated and more empowering narratives – such that, ultimately, more fulfilling realities can be realized.

Model 5 also draws upon the uplifting idea that the quantum universe holds infinite potential, relevant for the patient if she can but extricate herself from the erroneous relational preconceptions that she has about self, others, and the world – false beliefs that have been providing the propulsive fuel for her trauma-related symptoms and dysfunctional behaviors. This concept of quantum superposition, which is related to both the wave–particle duality and the Heisenberg uncertainty principle of quantum theory, speaks to the idea that an entity will exist in all possible states simultaneously until it is observed, measured, or (in the author's words and at the heart of the therapeutic action in Model 5) *intended* – at which point the wave will collapse to a particle and will then be the only reality that is expressed.

In order to operationalize the concept of pluripotent potential, imagine that you are holding a coin in the palm of your open hand. Either the head or the tail will be visible. Now, toss the coin up into the air. As long as it is in motion (and has not yet landed), it will hold the possibility of both head and tail simultaneously. Either the head or the tail will manifest only once the coin lands, that is, only once the wave collapses. By the same token (so to speak), the author will be suggesting that a wave of infinite possibilities will collapse into finite, observable behavioral change only once it interacts with a patient's intentioned commitment to change – akin to the *observer effect* of quantum theory.

The automotive titan Henry Ford is credited with having quipped, "Whether you think you can, or you think you can't – you're right." This aphorism speaks directly to the daunting impact of our intentionality on what is subsequently expressed and is a poignant reminder of our power to create our own destiny.

22.4.6 THE CREATION OF DESTABILIZING AND GALVANIZING INTERNAL TENSION TO PROVOKE CHANGE

Against the backdrop of empathic attunement and authentic engagement, optimally stressful Model 5 quantum disentanglement statements are specifically designed to create destabilizing and galvanizing tension within the patient by juxtaposing verbalization (in the first part) of growth-disrupting narratives constructed in the past with verbalization (in the second part) of growth-promoting visions designed for the future.

Quantum disentanglement statements rely upon mindfulness to promote bottom-up (from body consciousness to brain consciousness) retrieval of old programs and intentionality to promote top-down (from brain consciousness to body consciousness) installation of new programs.

Mindfulness facilitates remembering and reactivating; intentionality facilitates reprocessing and eventual reconsolidation.

The first part of the statement – informed as it is by mindful attention – activates the patient's limbic system as she retrieves, from body consciousness to brain consciousness, the implicitly held, procedurally organized, growth-disrupting emotional learnings and relational expectations that have been festering inside and maintaining her recalcitrant symptoms and maladaptive behaviors. In essence, the first part of the statement involves bringing to mind the internal record of unmastered early relational traumas stored, unprocessed, in her right (emotional) brain and the self-limiting narratives that were constructed as a result.

The second part of the statement – informed as it is by intentioned action – deactivates the limbic system arousal and activates the prefrontal executive functioning of the brain as the patient looks ahead and, from brain consciousness to body consciousness, envisions an alternative, preferred reality, takes growth-promoting ownership of her need to change, and, going forward, commits to action in alignment with that inspired vision. In essence, the second part of the statement involves bringing to bear the analytic wisdom of her left (rational) brain and therefore, a more evolved perspective.

22.4.7 MINDFUL AWARENESS

More specifically, the first part of a quantum disentanglement statement privileges the power of mindfulness and is designed to address one, two, or three of the elements of the growth-disrupting triad of *target symptom*, *formative experience,* and *constructed (derivative) narrative* underlying the patient's refractory inertia.

By way of mindful attention to the present moment and facilitated by closing of the eyes, this first part of the statement promotes mindful retrieval and reactivation of outdated narratives deriving from unmastered early traumatic experiences. It encourages the patient both to visualize elements of the toxic triad and to verbalize everything that gets triggered inside her as she begins to remember what her body cannot forget. The patient is guided to pay especial attention to, and make explicit, the somatic elements, physical sensations, visceral reactivity, and sensorimotor perceptions that are being evoked as she delves ever more deeply into remembering and reactivating old memories.

22.4.8 INTENTIONED ACTION

More specifically, the second part of the statement privileges the power of intentionality and is designed to address one, two, or three of the elements making up the growth-promoting triad of *envisioning of possibility, ownership of need to change,* and *commitment to action in alignment with what truly matters.*

As will soon become apparent, the pivotal experience of jolting mismatch prompting adaptive updating of narrative (which constitutes the therapeutic action in Model 5) will be created by the juxtaposition of the first and second parts of these disentanglement statements. Importantly, this mismatch will be triggered when a learned expectation is repeatedly and decisively placed side by side with either an experience that is real in the present or an experience that is envisioned for the future.

In fact, research studies have demonstrated that setting the intention to experience something positive that disconfirms the learned expectation of something negative can be almost as powerful as the actual experience of something positive that disconfirms the learned expectation of something negative.

More specifically, a growing body of evidence supports the finding that simply visualizing something, even though it occurs entirely in the mind, is almost as effective as actually doing it. According to a study done at the Cleveland Clinic (Ranganathan et al. 2004), participants were able to strengthen muscles simply by visualizing physical movement. This impact simply requires concentrated *mental practice*, namely, "the cognitive rehearsal of a physical activity [without movement]" (Saimpont et al. 2013, p. 1). In fact, a recent study demonstrated that subjects wanting to master a particular skill were able to decrease by 50% the number of actual practice hours if they visualized mastery of it (Miller 2018). Indeed, there is mounting support for the idea that mental practice, in combination with physical practice, can improve performance remarkably (Arora et al. 2011).

22.4.9 CO-CONSTRUCTED MODEL 5 QUANTUM DISENTANGLEMENT "I" STATEMENTS

Unlike the optimally stressful statements in Models 1–4 (which are crafted by the therapist and use the pronoun "you" to signify the patient), Model 5 interventions are statements created collaboratively by both patient and therapist and use the pronoun "I" instead of "you." Indeed, because quantum disentanglement statements require of the patient that she take embodied ownership of her need to change, and that she therefore set the intention to commit to action in alignment with that going forward, it is better both that the patient contribute to the crafting of the statements and that the interventions be "I" statements.

A particularly useful exercise is to have the patient write down a series of such statements so that she can review them periodically.

The following Model 5 statements (co-created by the author and several of her patients) are, of course, out of context. Hopefully, however, they will offer the reader a sense of how powerfully effective they can be in creating jolting and embodied mismatch experiences that will then prompt adaptive updating of old, disempowering, and growth-disrupting narratives and jumpstart intentioned action designed to actualize potential.

Even though I feel damaged and broken inside because of how my brother sexually abused me for all those years, I can envision the possibility of someday feeling better about myself as I take more ownership of the fact that I was not really a victim of his abuse because I really liked the attention he was paying me and certainly could have stopped doing it with him at any point. I got more from him than I was getting from my alcoholic parents. And, although I hate to admit this, it made me sad when it stopped.

I always feel so worried that no one will listen to me. I feel that I do not have a right to speak my truth. I was never allowed to speak up in my family and was always silenced. I was made to feel so invisible – and so irrelevant. I remember how awful it felt to be ignored all the time. My body trembles as I remember – and I feel sick to my stomach. I just hated being pushed to the side and being told that I did not matter. It hurt so much. My chest is feeling so tight. I used to try to make myself really small so that I would not take up too much space. It was awful!

But I can envision the possibility of someday feeling good enough about who I am that I will be able to present myself to the world without apology and without self-consciousness. I will have a voice and will use it to express how I really feel. I know that I will need to start taking risks that, to this point, I have avoided taking because I was so afraid. But I know that I need to speak up and let my voice be heard. I want this so bad. I am so tired of holding myself back and being always in the shadows. I've got this! I can do it!

I shun social contact and hide myself away and carry a gun to try to feel safe in this community where so many men now in power were my "johns" when I was a child. They held me in their power and tormented me. But I can now almost envision expanding the safety I feel in my church to a larger world.

I feel the cold dread of my stepfather's driving me to have sex with strange men. I want to flee and hide away, but I can see there must be another way out toward safety. I just need to commit to making myself take care of myself and to believing that I am no longer that vulnerable child I once was.

I feel dirty and hate myself, but I know I deserve better. I know I deserve to love myself and to feel good about who I am. I am hereby committing to showering and washing my hair daily.

Even though I cannot imagine ever finding work that would enable me both to express myself and to make enough money to support myself because my parents were always undermining how I felt about myself and my ability to make good choices for myself, I can imagine that I might someday be able to give myself permission to go where my heart leads me and to find creative ways to figure out the financial piece – so I hereby commit to exploring, with greater freedom, my range of options going forward.

22.5 CONCLUSION

At the heart of the therapeutic action in Model 5 is the neuroplastic synergy of mindfulness (that is, paying attention to the present moment, always with compassion and never judgment, in order to discover the self-limiting and disempowering beliefs that are fueling the patient's refractory inertia) and intentionality (that is, setting the intention to commit to action in the present that will enable the patient, going forward, to live in more harmony with the vision that she has for her future).

The repetitive and ongoing generation of embodied mismatch experiences is the sine qua non for therapeutic memory reconsolidation, the net result of which will be quantum disentanglement of the past from the present, elimination of the target symptom and its behavioral sequelae, and advancement of the patient from refractory inertia to intentioned action – a result of updating the mental programs that had been maintaining the patient's paralysis and thwarted potential.

Indeed, whereas the psychodynamically informed Models 1–4 involve understanding life backward and appreciating that the patient's history is her destiny, the constructivist Model 5 involves living life forward and appreciating that the patient has within her the power to create her destiny – such that, going forward, she will be able to embrace love, work, and play to her greatest potential.

Ann Landers's (1996) simple but profound advice is very much to the point here: "Nobody gets to live life backward. Look ahead, that is where your future lies."

REFERENCES

Alberini CM. 2005. Mechanisms of memory stabilization: Are consolidation and reconsolidation similar or distinct processes? *Trends Neurosci* Jan;28(1):51–56.

Alberini CM, Milekic MH, Tronel S. 2006. Mechanisms of memory stabilization and de-stabilization. *Cell Mol Life Sci May*;63(9):999–1008.

Armstrong C. 2019. *Rethinking Trauma Treatment*. New York: WW Norton & Company.

Arora S, Aggarwal R, Sirimanna P et al. 2011. Mental practice enhances surgical technical skills: A randomized controlled study. *Obstet Gynecol Surv* 66(6):336–338. doi: 10.1097/OGX.0b013e31822c17e1

Bandler R, Grinder J. 1982. *Reframing: Neuro-Linguistic Programming and the Transformation of Meaning*. Moab: Real People Press.

Braid J. 2019. *Magic, Witchcraft, Animal Magnetism, Hypnotism, and Electro-Biology*. Sydney, Australia: The Wentworth Press.

Cahill L, Prins B, Weber M et al. 1994. Beta-adrenergic activation and memory for emotional events. *Nature* Oct;371:702–704. doi: 10.1038/371702a0

Coughlin P. 2004. *Intensive Short-Term Dynamic Psychotherapy: Theory and Technique*. New York: Routledge / Taylor & Francis Group.

Coughlin P. 2016. *Maximizing Effectiveness in Dynamic Psychotherapy*. New York: Routledge / Taylor & Francis Group.

Craig G. 2011. *The EFT Manual*. Carlsbad: Energy Psychology Press.

Davanloo H (ed.). 1977. *Basic Principles and Techniques in Short-Term Dynamic Psychotherapy*. Northvale: Jason Aronson.

Dispenza J. 2013. *Breaking the Habit of Being Yourself: How to Lose Your Mind and Create a New One*. Carlsbad: Hay House.

Doidge N. 2007. *The Brain That Changes Itself: Stories of Personal Triumph from the Frontiers of Brain Science* (reprint ed.). City of Westminster, London: Penguin Books.

Dudai Y, Karni A, Born J. 2015. The consolidation and transformation of memory. *Neuron* Oct 7;88(1): 20–32. doi: 10.1016/j.neuron.2015.09.004

Ecker B, Ticic R, Hulley L. 2012. *Unlocking the Emotional Brain: Eliminating Symptoms at Their Roots Using Memory Reconsolidation*. New York: Routledge / Taylor & Francis Group.

Ecker B, Ticic R, Hulley L. 2013. A primer on memory reconsolidation and its psychotherapeutic use as a core process of profound change. *The Neuropsychotherapist* 1:82–99. doi: 10.12744/tnpt(1)082-099

Eden D, Feinstein D. 2008. *Energy Medicine: Balancing Your Body's Energies for Optimal Health, Joy, and Vitality*. New York: TarcherPerigee.

Eroglu C, Barres BA. 2010. Regulation of synaptic connectivity by glia. *Nature* Nov 11;468(7321):223–231. doi: 10.1038/nature09612.

Erwin E (ed.). 2003. *The Freud Encyclopedia: Theory, Therapy, and Culture* (1st ed.). New York: Routledge / Taylor & Francis Group.

Ethell IM. 2018. Brain's 'support cells' play active role in memory and learning. *Medical News Today* Jun 20. medicalnewstoday.com/articles/322203.

Feinstein D. 2019. Energy psychology: Efficacy, speed, mechanisms. *Explore* 15(5):340–351.

Fosha D. 2000. *The Transforming Power of Affect: A Model for Accelerated Change*. New York: Basic Books.

Frederickson J. 2013. *Co-Creating Change: Effective Dynamic Therapy Techniques*. Kensington: Seven Leaves Press.

Freud S. 1919. Lines of advance in psycho-analytic therapy. *Standard Edition of the Complete Psychological Works of Sigmund Freud* 17:157–168. London: Hogarth Press.

Freud S. 1937. Analysis terminable and interminable. *Int J Psychoanal* 18:373–405.

Gisquet-Verrier P, Lynch JF, Cutolo P et al. 2015. Integration of new information with active memory accounts for retrograde amnesia: A challenge to the consolidation/reconsolidation hypothesis? *J Neurosci* Aug 19;35(33):11623–11633. doi: 10.1523/JNEUROSCI.1386-15.2015

Gisquet-Verrier P, Riccio DC. 2019. Memory integration as a challenge to the consolidation/reconsolidation hypothesis: Similarities, differences and perspectives. *Front Syst Neurosci* Jan 11;12:1–11. doi: 10.3389/fnsys.2018.00071

Gold PE. 2008. Protein synthesis inhibition and memory: Formation vs amnesia. *Neurobiol Learn Mem* Mar;89(3):201–211.

Hayes SC, Strosahl K, Wilson KG. 2016. *Acceptance and Commitment Therapy: The Process and Practice of Mindful Change*. New York: Guilford Press.

Hebb DO. 2002. *The Organization of Behavior: A Neuropsychological Theory*. East Sussex: Psychology Press.

Howard S. 2009. *Skills in Psychodynamic Counselling and Psychotherapy*. Thousand Oaks: SAGE Publications.

Isaacson W. 2008. *Einstein: His Life and Universe*. New York: Simon & Schuster.

Kauffman C. 2006. Positive psychology: The science at the heart of coaching. In DR Stober & AM Grant (eds.), *Evidence Based Coaching Handbook: Putting Best Practices to Work for Your Clients* (pp. 219–253). Marblehead: John Wiley & Sons Inc.

Kierkegaard S, Hannay A. 1996. *Papers and Journals: A Selection. City of Westminster*. London: Penguin Classics.

Landers A. 1996. *Wake Up and Smell the Coffee!: Advice, Wisdom, and Uncommon Good Sense*. New York: Villard Books.

Lee JL, Nader K, Schiller D. 2017. An update on memory reconsolidation updating. *Trends Cogn Sci* Jul;21(7):531–545. doi: 10.1016/j.tics.2017.04.006

Levine P. 1997. *Waking the Tiger: Healing Trauma*. Berkeley: North Atlantic Books.

Lonergan MH, Olivera-Figueroa LA, Pitman RK et al. 2013. Propranolol's effects on the consolidation and reconsolidation of long-term emotional memory in healthy participants: A meta-analysis. *J Psychiatr Neurosci* Jul;38(4):222–231. doi: 10.1503/jpn.120111.

Martin SJ, Grimwood PD, Morris RG. 2000. Synaptic plasticity and memory: An evaluation of the hypothesis. *Annu Rev Neurosci* 23:649–711.

Miller M. 2018. Envisioning your way to success: The power of mental practice. Blog. doi: 6seconds.org/2018/01/15/envisioning-way-success-incredible-power-mental-practice/

Miller WR, Rollnick S. 1992. *Motivational Interviewing: Preparing People to Change Addictive Behavior*. New York: Guilford Press.

Nader K. 2003. Memory traces unbound. *Trends Neurosci* Feb;26(2):65–72. doi: 10.1016/S0166-2236(02)00042-5

Nader K, Schafe GE, LeDoux JE. 2000. Fear memories require protein synthesis in the amygdala for reconsolidation after retrieval. *Nature* 406,722–726. doi: 10.1038/35021052

Ogden P, Pain C, Minton K. 2006. *Trauma and the Body: A Sensorimotor Approach to Psychotherapy*. New York: WW Norton & Company.

Pesso A. 1969. *Movement in Psychotherapy: Psychomotor Techniques and Training*. London: University of London Press.

Ranganathan VK, Siemionow V, Liu JZ et al. 2004. From mental power to muscle power – gaining strength by using the mind. *Neuropsychologia* 42(7):944–956. doi: 10.1016/j.neuropsychologia.2003.11.018

Rossouw P. 2014. *Neuropsychotherapy: Theoretical Underpinnings and Clinical Applications*. Queensland, Australia: Mediros Pty Ltd.

Rubin RD, Fried R, Franks CM. 1969. New application of ECT. In RD Rubin & CM Franks (eds.), *Advances in Behavior Therapy, 1968* (pp. 37–44). New York: Academic Press.

Saimpont A, Lafleur MF, Malouin F et al. 2013. The comparison between motor imagery and verbal rehearsal on the learning of sequential movements. *Front Hum Neurosci* 7:773. doi: 10.3389/fnhum.2013.00773

Schafer R. 1994. *Retelling a Life: Narration and Dialogue in Psychoanalysis.* New York: Basic Books.

Schiller D, Monfils MH, Raio CM et al. 2010. Preventing the return of fear in humans using reconsolidation update mechanisms. *Nature* Jan 7;463(7277):49–53.

Schlichting ML, Preston AR. 2015. Memory integration: Neural mechanisms and implications for behavior. *Curr Opin Behav Sci* Feb;1:1–8.

Schwartz RC. 1997. *Internal Family Systems Therapy.* New York: Guilford Press.

Shapiro F. 2017. *Eye Movement Desensitization and Reprocessing (EMDR) Therapy: Basic Principles, Protocols, and Procedures.* New York: Guilford Press.

Siegel DJ. 1999. *The Developing Mind: How Relationships and the Brain Interact to Shape Who We Are.* New York: Guilford Press.

Small D. 2015. *The Origins of Unhappiness: A New Understanding of Personal Distress.* New York: Routledge/Taylor & Francis Group.

Stark M. 1999. *Modes of Therapeutic Action: Enhancement of Knowledge, Provision of Experience, and Engagement in Relationship.* Northvale: Jason Aronson.

Stark M. 2015. *The Transformative Power of Optimal Stress: From Cursing the Darkness to Lighting a Candle* (International Psychotherapy Institute eBook). www.FreePsychotherapyBooks.org.

Stark M. 2016. *How Does Psychotherapy Work?* (International Psychotherapy Institute eBook). www.FreePsychotherapyBooks.org.

Stark M. 2017. *Relentless Hope: The Refusal to Grieve* (International Psychotherapy Institute eBook). www.FreePsychotherapyBooks.org.

Verkhratsky A, Butt A. 2007. *Glial Neurobiology.* Marlbehead: John Wiley & Sons Inc.

Vredeveldt A, Hitch GJ, Baddeley AD. 2011. Eyeclosure helps memory by reducing cognitive load and enhancing visualisation. *Mem Cogn* 39:1253–1263. doi: 10.3758/s13421-011-0098-8

Wang SH. 2018. Novelty enhances memory persistence and remediates propranolol-induced deficit via reconsolidation. *Neuropharmacology* Oct;141:42–54.

Wang SH, Ostlund SB, Nader K et al. 2005. Consolidation and reconsolidation of incentive learning in the amygdala. *J Neurosci* Jan 26;25(4):830–835. doi: 10.1523/JNEUROSCI.4716-04.2005

23 Mind, Consciousness and the Design Nature of Sound

John Beaulieu and David Perez Martinez

CONTENTS

23.1 INTRODUCTION

The unique vibratory range that comprises the sound spectrum has organizational and design properties that *largely* structure the physical world and all of our mental activity. The physical world is created by subatomic processes subject to vibrational frequencies and patterns that direct matter and the mind into innumerable configurations, forms and mental processes. The mind is a manifestation of consciousness, the bridge between the physical and the immaterial. When we state that the mind and body are one, we are reaffirming the role that consciousness plays in bridging the mind with the physical world. Sound is a perfect tool for understanding this relationship because it *mimics the vibratory nature of the universe, organizes matter into its many forms and serves as a vehicle for consciousness* in creating a sense of self and reality, social identity, physiological activity and different states of mind. Language, music, art, mathematical theory, physics, neuroscience and anatomy illustrate clearly the relationship that exists between mind, consciousness and the design nature of sound.

We can logically conclude that since we are a part of the universe, then who we are reflects an aspect of the universe. When we describe ourselves, we are also describing an aspect of the universe. Our material bodies reflect the physical nature of the universe and as such, are subject to the same set of dynamics that determine the behavior of all matter. Our minds, awareness and sense of self reflect the conscious nature of the universe as manifested in living organisms. Scientific research into the nature of mind and consciousness is still in its infancy, with little agreement on what it is and how it emerges. Modern cosmology, however, postulates that the early universe was not physical in nature. It was a quantum sphere of light, subatomic particles, vibration and movement stemming from electromagnetism, gravity, spin, charge and other fundamental manifestations. The "reality" of the universe therefore cannot be reduced to its material aspect. We are multidimensional beings existing in a vibratory/informational universe of quanta, patterns and possibilities. Living organisms in general, and perhaps human beings in particular, are *designed and shaped* by these fundamental qualities and processes *and programmed* by consciousness.

23.2 VIBRATION

Modern cosmology postulates that the universe came into existence as a big explosion that set everything in motion. Movement/vibration is arguably therefore the most fundamental aspect of the

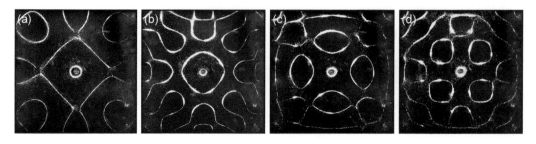

FIGURE 23.1 Chladni sound patterns created on a metal plate by a violin bow dragged across the edge of the plate.

universe; "*everything*" is constantly moving with characteristic frequencies, rhythms and patterns. This is the foundation underlying the first principle of Therapeutic Sound Healing Practices: We are vibrational beings living in a vibrational universe. Movement creates change and establishes new *relationships* that are the engine for the diverse multiplicity observed in the universe. We now know that it is the underlying vibratory field that gives matter its form and shape: This is the second principle of Therapeutic Sound Healing Practices, unwittingly uncovered in 1787 by German physicist Ernst Chladni. He observed that when sand is placed on a metal plate, and a violin bow is dragged across the edge of the plate, the sand on the plate vibrates into different geometric designs based on the frequency of the sound.[1] The changing sand patterns allow us to see invisible frequencies of sound waves that are fundamental to Schrödinger's wave function equation, which shows that all matter has unique wave-like properties[2] (Figure 23.1).

Dr. Hans Jenny, MD, from Basel, Switzerland updated Chladni's work. He called his experiments *cymatics*, which means the study of wave phenomena. He attached an oscillator on a metal plate and used high-speed photography in order to capture the sonic designs created by different frequencies (Figure 23.2).

If you were in Dr. Jenny's laboratory during a cymatics experiment, you would hear the pitch of the sound with your ears, feel the plate vibrating the mechanoreceptors in your skin and see a design

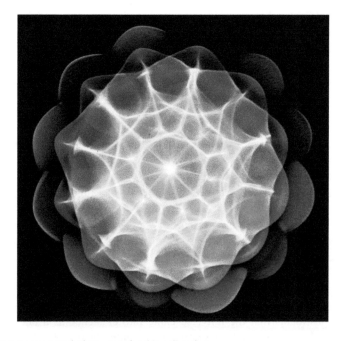

FIGURE 23.2 Water on a metal plate organized by vibration.

form on the plate. Any change in frequency would simultaneously create a change in the geometric design, and the same frequency always produced the same structure. A cymatic sound design may look static as a photograph; however, it is continually vibrating in resonance with its frequency. If you were to attempt to change the design without changing the vibrational frequency, it would immediately return to its original design. And if the vibration were to cease, the design could no longer be sustained.

David Perez Martinez, MD, psychiatrist, expert in the therapeutic use of sound and a self-described "cymatic phenomenologist," has created a unique process of documenting vibrational patterns and cymatic designs in natural and manufactured objects and processes using nothing more than a cellular phone and observation. This process uncovers the principle of Dr. Jenny's work by documenting still and moving images of mundane everyday scenes, objects and events. Water puddles, sidewalks, cloud patterns, flowers and vegetables, rusting garbage dumpsters, fungus growing in rocks, flowing water, pothole covers, trees, architectural structures, etc. are all examples of images documented. Dr. Perez calls them "frozen sound" images that mimic the underlying vibratory field of the physical world and uncover organizational and design patterns that illustrate the vibrational nature of human consciousness. The fact that the same cymatic images observed in nature, from the micro to the "microsphere," are omnipresent in human design across cultures that have had no contact suggests that consciousness is tied somehow to the vibratory fabric of the universe. As an exercise, try to look at these images from a vibrational design perspective without it having to be "something," i.e., sidewalk, mud puddle, broken glass, etc. The "something" of each photo will be listed at the end of the photo section, but while observing, try to perceive the vibrational aspect of the image and what it says to your intuition about the nature of "things" out there, who you are and how you operate.

Since Dr. Perez Martinez's process does not require a laboratory or specialized equipment, anyone with a smartphone can do it. He introduced his process to a group of 50 students in 2019 as part of a class on Sound and Consciousness in Stone Ridge, NY. The students worked in groups of four and were given an hour to work with the following process, take photos and pick three of their favorite sound designs. The group photos were uploaded into a PowerPoint presentation, and each group shared their vibratory experiences, after which the class did their best to guess the object label. Everyone learned to be less involved with labels and more aware of the universal vibratory nature of sonic design in all aspects of life.

The Perez Martinez Process used in class:

1. Make sure you are safe. Safety can be signs warning of danger or/and in general taking photos in a state of mind where you are aware of your surroundings while at the same time prepared to take safe behavior if necessary. This state is like "highway hypnosis," in which your mind is drifting while driving, and if something catches your awareness, you instantly come back to normal driving behaviors.

2. Be mindful, relax your eyes and observe. This is known as having "soft eyes" or listening with your eyes. When something "catches your eye," take a photograph of it with your smartphone. In fact, if you are inspired, take photos from different distances and angles.

3. Look at your photographs and mindfully tune into the vibratory quality of the different designs. After viewing a number of photographs, you will develop an ability to sense vibrational changes.

4. Once you become confident in your experience of vibration and design, the next step is to compare your vibrational experience with the labels and associations you have with the object you have photographed.

5. Share your photos with others without telling them what they are. Allow them to share their experience, and when it is time, let them know what the photo is, i.e., a mud puddle in your backyard, a tree trunk, etc.

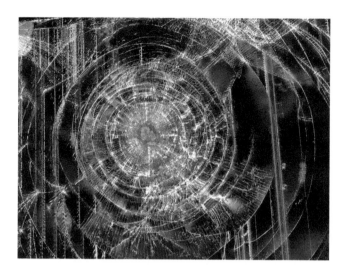

FIGURE 23.3   Photo 1.

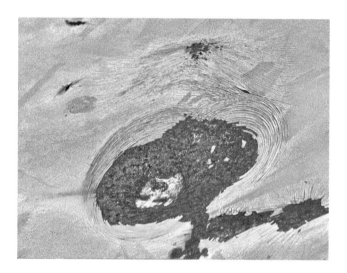

FIGURE 23.4   Photo 2.

Dr. Perez Martinez's work is displayed in the following photos as described in step 3. For steps 4 and 5, see the photographic descriptions in the next section after the last photograph (Figures 23.3–23.10).

23.3   CYMATIC PHENOMENOLOGY DESCRIPTIONS

Photo 1: As I was walking in Chelsea, New York City around April 2019 I noticed that the glass in a commercial light box in a bus stop had been vandalized, producing a classic vibrational pattern of expanding concentric circles. Soon I saw other bus stops with vandalized signs and began photographing them. About a week later the news media reported that the incidents were the work of a vandal that the police was actively looking for and within days he was apprehended. While upset about the vandalism, I was grateful for the images and the teachings extracted from them.

The image illustrates the wave particle duality as represented by the concentric circles (waves) and the linear projections (particles) radiating from the core. It's a visual representation of the vibrational energy released by the Big Bang.

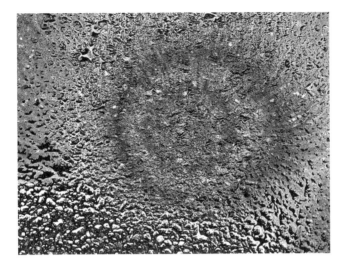

FIGURE 23.5   Photo 3.

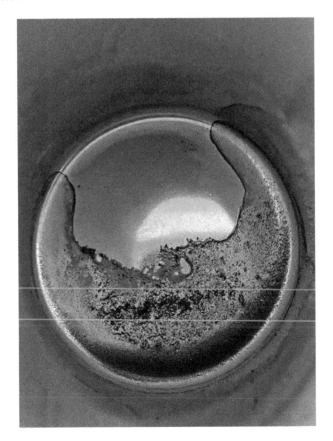

FIGURE 23.6   Photo 4.

Photo 2: Garbage dumpsters in front of construction sites are common in Manhattan and have become one of my favorite places to find cymatic images. The dumpsters are metallic and are typically repainted many times over in different colors to hide the rusting metal. As the paint heats and dries, it cracks and forms stress patterns that visually demonstrate the underlying vibratory forces

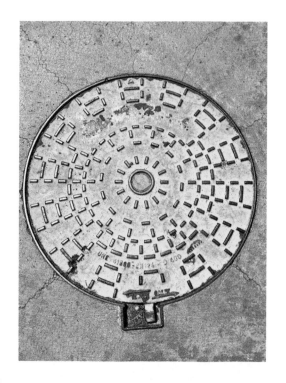

FIGURE 23.7   Photo 5.

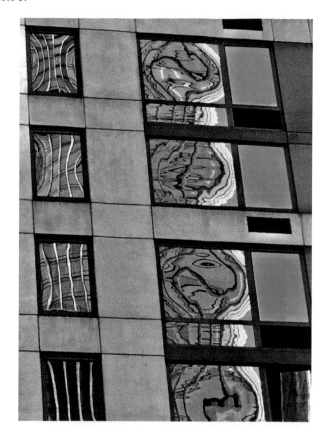

FIGURE 23.8   Photo 6.

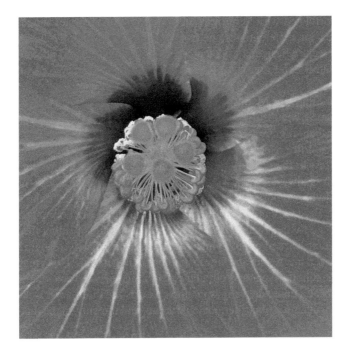

FIGURE 23.9   Photo 7.

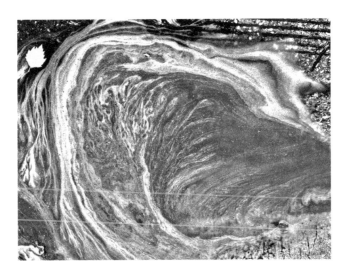

FIGURE 23.10   Photo 8.

creating the phenomenon. The concentric circular patterns around the main structure is a physical consequence and visual manifestation of the energy created and released by the heat/paint/metal complex.

The image reminds me of the energy that comes from within and surrounds the physical body (aura), but also of the consequences when too much energy is accumulated without an outlet when it doesn't flow. As a psychotherapist, I see many individuals with the tendency to hold things in until they explode.

Photo 3: Another classic concentric circle cymatic image formed by gasoline falling on wet pavement. This dirty, toxic pollutant creates a beautiful image that illustrates sonic vibrations (concentric circles) correlated with light frequencies (colors). It illustrates the principle that everything is vibrating and what differentiates one from the other is essentially its unique vibratory rate (color). It shows how we are designed to detect and respond to sonic and photonic frequencies and how consciousness detects and organizes these patterns into the perceptions and sense of reality that we experience.

Photo 4: Image of Sun Over Mountain in blue coffee mug. For years I noticed that my tea and coffee cups often formed beautiful images. Later I realized that they are cymatic in nature and began photographing them regularly. I call them "Coffee Cymatics."

This image of the sun/fire over mountain is the Lu Hexagram in the I Ching: The Wanderer. It instructs us to never rest in the quest for illumination. The wanderer mimics universal vibrational dynamics and as such is always moving, changing, open to new experiences, never holding on to anything, aware that light and darkness, pleasure and pain, are two sides of the same coin and that one leads to the other. Here we cannot tell if the sun is going down or coming up and it doesn't matter. One will always lead to the other and we move, wander through it riding the vibrations.

Photo 5: When I first learned about cymatic images I immediately recognized the patterns in manhole covers all over the world and began photographing them. This image from Mallorca, Spain depicts movement both linear and circular resembling particle wave duality emanating from a central source. It is not a coincidence that manhole covers are circular. It is a culmination of the tendency of certain particles to spin (rotational vibration), and the only shape that prevents the cover from falling into the hole.

Photo 6: Recently I was admiring a new performing arts space in Manhattan's Hudson Yards and wondering when I would see my first performance there. As I turned to leave, I noticed reflections from the performance center in windows across the street and forming moving cymatic images. As I walked, the images and patterns in each window changed as my position did. I started moving and dancing while filming the windows. Alas, my first Hudson Yards performance!

Photo 7: Walking along 7th Ave in Manhattan I spotted a potential gold mine for a cymatic phenomenologist: a white, soapy scummy lump of something moving slowly in the water towards the sewer with all kinds of wave and circular spiral movements internally displaying innumerable forms and structures coming in and out of existence. The image is a snapshot that illustrates many different vibrational currents. It was taken from above but imagined sideways is reminiscent of *The Great Wave of Kanagawa* or a river bed.

Photo 8: This image summarizes for me the vibratory nature of mind and consciousness. It is an image of a living entity in its own aura exposed to vibratory frequencies all around it. The inner core is pentatonic, the primary musical scale of most ancient cultures and civilizations and the basis of the five-pointed star and DaVinci's *Vitruvian Man* representing our concurrent existence in physical and ethereal planes.

I feel a deep spiritual connection to this image and approach it as a source of "good vibes", information and inspiration.

23.4   NEUROANATOMY/HEARING/NEURAL SCIENCE

Life from the very beginning has been structured by its vibratory field and designed to interact with it. All the manifestations of consciousness observed in humans and other "higher" animals can also be observed in the simplest, earliest organisms. Every living organism has structural, functional and behavioral attributes naturally "designed" to resonantly respond to the vibratory patterns in their environment. Early organisms possessed a motoreum and sensorium that allowed them to scan their surroundings, evaluate environmental conditions, and move towards or away from desired versus undesirable conditions.[3, 4] They also had the ability to store information (memory) even before having organized genetic material and used it to make behavioral decisions. Initially, these prokaryotic organisms had a ciliated flagellum used for balance, feeding, locomotion and defense. About half a billion years ago, flagellated cilia evolved into "mechanosensory" hair cells – widely considered to be the precursor of all exteroceptors – and bony fish developed an auditory labyrinth, the precursor of the ear and source of hearing in vertebrates. Amphibians were the first to transform these excitable sensory hair cells in their "bony labyrinth" into a nervous system sensitive to sound and movement. The nervous system and the anatomical structures of the hearing apparatus in vertebrates since then have developed under the influence of and in response to sound and vibration.[5]

The auditory pathway in humans is driven by sound and movement and travels from the external ear to the thalamus, where it is relayed to the auditory cortex. It has tonotopic organization and is lined with neurons designed to fire only at certain frequencies (Hz). Vibrational information carried by the auditory nerve is picked up by the medial geniculate body (MGB) of the thalamus. Whereas early views of the MGB were that it served as a simple one-way gate to the auditory cortex, numerous studies have demonstrated that the MGB, auditory cortex and cerebral cortex are linked together to form a vast network of sensory information network that converges at the MBG.[6] The thalamus via the MGB serves as a central hub that receives and passes on auditory information to every site in the network.

Auditory information is interpreted and abstracted via consciousness in two different ways. Information received by the MGB is a sonic design, as demonstrated by the work of Dr. Jenny, which is relayed to the auditory cortex, where it is interpreted as "something." The practice of mindfulness, i.e., mindful listening or mindful viewing, creates a synchronization between the auditory cortex, its cerebral cortex network sites and the MGB that allows one to phenomenologically experience a resonance between physical reality (something) and sonic design (waves and geometric pattern). Dr. Perez's phenomenological cymatics allows the viewer to tune into sonic designs that manifest in physical reality while at the same time being aware of the many interpretations that may be given to those designs. When the experience of the sonic design and interpretations, i.e., meanings given to different sonic designs, come into sync, a resonant neural coherence is achieved that allows the mind to perceive that which allows the abstraction and interpretation of all information – consciousness.

Nothing illustrates the relationship between mind, consciousness and vibration more clearly than language and the implications for self-exploration and social/communication development. *To the extent that mammals expanded the range of acoustic possibilities, their consciousness expanded.* Mammals were the first vertebrates to develop separate divisions of the auditory nerve into branches for movement (vestibular) and sound (cochlear). They were the first animals to hear above the 16 Hz range and thus, the most acoustically sophisticated. Initially, mammals were very small, vulnerable and dependent at birth, requiring communication and cooperation for survival. They communicated privately around large animals by vastly improving their hearing apparatus and neural circuitry as well as the capacity to emit high-pitched sounds that only they could hear. Eventually, certain sounds were associated with aspects of survival versus safety and wellness, and responses to them were codified, "wired" into the DNA and passed onto future generations, in some cases across different species. Language as we know it began when a particular sound that we are anatomically equipped to hear and produce was associated with a *consensually designated meaning* that was shared with others. Over time, these sounds were associated with visual symbols and codified into a language or code that serves as a tool for self-expression and communication. Over time, hearing capabilities continued to evolve parallel to the evolution and expansion of consciousness as manifested in increased mental activity, social interaction and culture in humans.

23.5 CONSCIOUSNESS

Movement is a change in the vibratory field that yields information. Information is the observance of change created by movement. Observance is an act of consciousness, a poorly understood quality of the universe that allows perception of change, patterns and in humans, awareness of self. It is because of consciousness that we are able to perceive the information created by changes in pressure waves (sound), create a symbol to represent it and designate meaning and value to it. There is no inherent meaning or value to anything in the universe; there is only information, because change is the only thing that can be perceived. The rest is created by consciousness on the basis of experiences. The key to understanding all this lies in the word *create*. We are creators of our self-identity and reality depending on the pattern(s) of change, the vibratory changes that our consciousness can perceive and the state(s) of mind experienced. Our ability to conduct vibrations through our mind and body will ultimately determine our state of mind. The more states of mind we have available to us, the more we will be able to adapt to the infinitely changing currents within a vibrational ocean of possibilities. There are an infinite number of states of mind potentially emerging as responses to patterns in the environment.

The *Nada Bindu Upanishad*, written around 100 BCE, is a sacred Vedic treatise that understood and described this relationship between sound, mind and consciousness. In Sanskrit, *Nada* means sound, *Bindu* refers to consciousness as a point or vortex from which universal energy originates and *Upanishad* means to sit near one's teacher with devotion. The *Nada Bindu Upanishad* is intrinsic knowledge about sound, mind and consciousness. This is learned by listening to sound with devotion. It states that "The mind exists as long as there is sound." And, it goes further into the transcendent and healing aspects experienced in other states of consciousness when it continues:

> [B]ut with the cessation of sound there is a state of being above the mind. Through deep listening the mind becomes absorbed in an everlasting soundless state. The soundless state is the supreme seat. When we become absorbed in the soundless state our attachments to the mind's vibrational patterns are neutralized. There is no doubt about it.[7]

Sound is therefore a vehicle for consciousness to manifest as mind and a meditative tool to help attain states of consciousness beyond the mental.

When we listen deeply to sound, we intuitively experience at a macro level the vibrational behaviors that mimic the quantum behaviors that physicists are observing and measuring at a micro level. *"The mind exists as long as there is sound" is a way of saying that the mind is frequency.* At a micro level, different states of mind can be visualized as frequencies that organize quantum waves/particles into "reality structures." At a quantum level, according to Planck, each energy element (E) is proportional to its frequency (v). Similarly, at a macro level, sound is measured in frequencies that create geometric structures (E), which are expressed as different organized shapes, designs and networks that are proportional to the frequency of the sound. The founders of quantum physics realized that other cultures and traditions had developed a knowledge of the vibrational behaviors they were observing at the quantum level. They wondered how these ancient contemplative traditions could have arrived at an understanding of a vibrational universe without modern mathematics and scientific technology. They discovered that the phenomenological practice of deep listening was the experimental basis for their understanding of mind and consciousness.[8] Erwin Schrödinger, a pioneer of quantum physics, understood that sound has been used for thousands of years to explore the relationship between mind and consciousness. He said: "The unity and continuity of Vedanta are reflected in the unity and continuity of wave mechanics."[9]

The understanding that consciousness derives from vibration is not new. Eastern and Western contemplative and indigenous shamanistic traditions have been listening to and playing sound in different forms as a method of inquiry into the vibrational nature of mind and consciousness for thousands of years. Each tradition has created a unique culture, language and music, and sound practices are found to guide individuals into an inner understanding of themselves as conscious vibrational beings and to communicate better among themselves. The sound practices used in these traditions are based on deep listening and include singing, chanting, drumming and many others. Making and listening to sound in these traditions is more than entertainment and is often misunderstood because it is a subjective phenomenological approach to consciousness, healing and wellness. Following this line of thought is the philosopher David Chalmers, who suggests that the "hard problem" of consciousness is qualia.[10] Qualia is the inner experience of vibration received through sensory perception, i.e., listening to sound. Qualia is a hard problem for researchers because it is subjective and cannot be quantified. As mental health professionals, we have worked with qualia for many years. We listen to our client's inner experiences and allow ourselves to enter into and experience their reality at a vibrational level. Suspending one's rational mind in order to learn from our intuition by having the inner experience of playing and listening to sound is contrary to objectively observing, labeling and quantifying sounds. It is one thing to measure sound and another thing altogether to have the intrinsic experience of what musicians call "being in a sound." When we enter into a vibrational state of consciousness through sound, we are not bound by rational thought processes, and thus, we become open to our intuition.

23.6 CONCLUSION

Movement/vibration is a fundamental aspect of the universe that creates change and yields information. Consciousness manifests itself as an awareness that allows perception of change and processing of information and allows the mind to become a bridge between our bodies, the material world, and the vibratory fields and patterns that define our existence. Like everything else, consciousness is vibratory in origin. The brain is part of the physical substratum that sustains the mind, and it is essentially organized structurally and functionally as a pattern recognizer. The brain is thus structured and organized by responding to information generated by change in the vibratory field and the nature of consciousness. It is the vibratory field and consciousness that direct biology, not the other way around. When a person has a stroke and cannot walk, it is the desire and attempt to walk that recreates the neural circuitry needed to do so; a person does not develop new structures or circuitry without actively trying. Clinical research has demonstrated that neuroplasticity is influenced by emotional and psychological factors and promoted by meditation and music. This is the essence of the relationship between mind, consciousness and the design nature of sound.

REFERENCES

1. Ernest Chladni, (Entdeckungen *über* die *Theorie* des *Klanges [Discoveries in the Theory of Sound]* (Germany: Leipzig, 1787), https://echo.mpiwg-berlin.mpg.de/ECHOdocuView?url=/permanent/library/5M6VYMSC/pageimg&pn=8&mode=imagepath.
2. J. Michael McBride, "Chladni Figures and One-Electron Atoms," *Freshman Organic Chemistry Lecture #9* (Open Yale Courses, Yale University, 2009), https://www.youtube.com/watch?v=5kYLE8GhAuE, 2016-06-05.
3. Gerhard Roth and Ursula Dicke, *Evolution of Nervous Systems and Brains* (Berlin Heidelberg: Springer, Jan. 1, 1970), accessed May 27, 2017, http://link.springer.com/chapter/10.1007/978-3-642-10769-6_2.
4. James E. Peck, *Evolution of Nervous System*, 2nd ed. (Academic Press, Dec. 16, 2016), accessed May 27, 2017, https://www.elsevier.com/books/evolution-of-nervous-systems/kaas/978-0-12-804042-3.
5. Stephen Porges, "The Polyvagal Theory: Phylogenetic Substrates of a Social Nervous System," *International Journal of Psychophysiology* 42 (2001): 123–146.
6. Edward Bartlett, "The Organization and Physiology of the Auditory Thalamus and Its Role in Processing Acoustic Features Important for Speech Perception," *Brain and Language* 126, no. 1 (2013): 29–48.
7. Aiyar K. Narayanasvami, *Thirty Minor Upanishads* (Madras, India: Evinity Publishing Inc., 2009).
8. J.L. Heilbron, *Dilemmas of an Upright Man: Max Planck and the Fortunes of German Science* (Cambridge, MA: Harvard University Press, 2000).
9. Walter Moore, *Schrödinger: Life and Thought* (Cambridge, UK: Cambridge University Press, 1989), 173.
10. David Chalmers, "Facing Up to the Problem of Consciousness," *Journal of Consciousness Studies* 2, no. 3 (1995): 200–219.

24 The Use of Sound and Color in Clinical Application

John Beaulieu, Thea Keats Beaulieu, and Jerry Wintrob

CONTENTS

DOI: 10.1201/b23304-26

24.1   INTRODUCTION

In our chapter, we present an integrated approach to sound and color in the healing arts. We are a group of healing artists coming from different professions, optometry, counseling, naturopathic medicine and creative arts therapy, who recognize that mind–body coherency is necessary to support and enhance the effectiveness of all specific treatments. We also recognize that when a client is coherent, conditions that we may be trained to treat oftentimes resolve as part of a holistic healing process. For this reason, there is an important distinction to be made between specific evidence-based treatments and general holistic practices that have been shown to enhance mind-body coherency. Sound and color, when correctly understood and integrated into a healing arts practice, will induce a relaxation response similar to what we seek when we are in nature. For example, when we sense that we are out of balance, we may naturally go to the ocean and listen to the sound of the waves or view the colors of a sunset in order to seek internal coherence. Afterwards, we feel refreshed, energized and relaxed. Research suggests that the relaxation response lowers our heart rate, normalizes blood pressure and oxygen consumption, as well as alleviating the symptoms associated with a vast array of conditions, including arthritis, insomnia, depression, cancer, anxiety, vision disorders and aging.[1] In other words, our body is self-regulating and will produce all that is necessary in the right amount to achieve balance.

Our focus is on using sound and color practices to create a coherent internal mind–body environment that will prevent the onset of physical and mental conditions as well as support professional treatment for diagnosed conditions. To be sure, sound and color can be used for specific treatment of conditions; however, we have chosen to present three approaches to sound and color practices that can be used by everyone as preventative medicine as well as being suitable to integrate into professional practices to supplement specific treatment goals. The first approach, presented by Dr. Jerry Wintrob, OD, is the successful integration of sound into syntonics, the optometric practice of viewing colors to correct vision disorders. The second approach, presented by Thea Keats Beaulieu, is an intuitive sensory-based model based on feeling tones created by color imagery integrated with sound. Both use sound and color to establish a coherent self-regulating body–mind environment that is able to spontaneously adapt to life changes. We call the third approach Sound and Color Frequency Resonance. This is an experimental method inspired by Dr. Wintrob's work in *Syntonic Phototherapy* and Dr. Beaulieu's work with sound healing designed to phenomenologically explore sensory integration through the use of pure sound and color frequencies.

24.2   HOLISTIC SYNTONIC PHOTOTHERAPY AND SOUND HEALING

Syntonic phototherapy is the viewing of colored light filters by a client in order to rebalance their autonomic nervous system (ANS). Syntonics was first discovered by Harry Spitler, MD, in the 1930s, when he documented the effect that the application of colored light would have on the brain and result in subsequent changes in visual problems.[2] The ANS is comprised of the sympathetic and parasympathetic nervous systems. Syntonics uses color to balance the ANS to reduce stress, improve vision and help clients perform at their peak potential. The five main colors used by syntonic practitioners are given Greek names: Red is alpha, orange is delta, green is mu, blue is upsilon, omega is violet. The colors on the red end of the spectrum stimulate the sympathetic system, and colors on the blue end stimulate the parasympathetic system. Green is the color of balance, and patients view green in a process called *nascentization* in order to enter into a receptive state of balance that enhances treatment with different color combinations (Figure 24.1).

In optometry, syntonics is used to treat vision problems within the modality called vision therapy. Syntonics can also be part of a holistic optometry approach to health and wellbeing. Balancing the sympathetic and parasympathetic nervous systems through color creates a whole-body physiology that improves vision as well as the whole person mentally, emotionally and physically. The

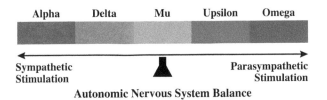

FIGURE 24.1 Autonomic nervous system balance.

holistic effectiveness of colored light therapy cannot be overemphasized. Using the methodology of balancing the ANS with the use of colored light filters for specific visual conditions is quite effective. For example, strabismic patients who exhibit esotropia, a condition where one eye turns in, have an overactive parasympathetic system. As standard, they are treated with colors on the red end of the spectrum, for example alpha delta, a red/orange combination. These patients often present emotional challenges regarding how they relate to their peers. The alpha omega filter combination (red/violet) is a way to balance the patient and treat the emotional component of the visual problem. By using the two ends of the spectrum, we are creating an internal balance that will help to give a patient the emotional support necessary to enable a more holistic form of treatment. Patients must be understood from a multifaceted approach. Treating a patient is necessary from an emotional as well as a visual perspective.

A new analysis of clinical reports and existing research suggests that stress is both consequence and cause of vision loss, which impacts the eye and brain due to ANS dysregulation. Continuous stress and elevated cortisol levels negatively impact the eye and brain due to autonomous nervous system (sympathetic) imbalance and vascular dysregulation; hence, stress may also be one of the major causes of visual system diseases such as glaucoma and optic neuropathy.[3] Stress reduction techniques such as sound healing and music help to create an internal mind–body environment that enhances syntonic treatments as well as possibly preventing or reducing vision loss. Integrating color with sound simply increases the holistic effectiveness of treatments as well as treating specific vision problems.

In the following extract, Dr. Wintrob presents his case experience with color and sound. The names of his patients have been changed, and he is speaking in the first person.

David is a 14-year-old boy. His schooling is very rigorous, and he is in school 12–14 hours per day. If his schedule wasn't challenging enough, his visual findings presented a very difficult case. He has had two strabismus surgeries and now presented as a moderate hyper esotrope, a condition where one eye turns in and up. He was coming for weekly vision therapy sessions. With all my cases, I have them do 20 minutes of daily home syntonic exercises. I believed that his case had a significant emotional component, so his daily syntonic prescription was alpha omega (red/violet) for 10 minutes followed by alpha delta (red/orange) for 10 minutes. He also did an in-office treatment of just alpha omega (red/violet) for 10 minutes. In my experience, patients like David often have poor results from therapy. The strabismus surgery is so invasive that it is very hard to get a good outcome. As an adjunct to David's therapy, I introduced sound healing using Biosonic C and G tuning forks and almost immediately his mood changed. I observed that his anger began to dissipate, and his mother reported seeing a large improvement in his performance at school. I was pleasantly surprised when after 12 sessions of integrating sound and color he began to show fusion, stereo, and an appreciation of depth. There is no question in my mind that the integration of Biosonic tuning forks with color treatments was the deciding factor (Figure 24.2).

24.2.1 Biosonic C and G Tuning Forks

The Biosonic Body Tuner™ tuning forks which sound C and G were developed by Dr. John Beaulieu and are the primary tuning forks used by sound healers in the world today.[4] Biosonic tuning forks are designed to scientific standards using the highest-quality aluminum alloy. They are precisely

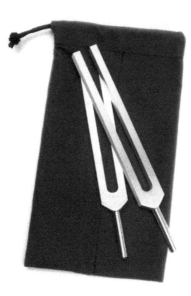

FIGURE 24.2 Biosonic C and G tuning forks.

tuned within 0.5% of the indicated frequency at 20°C. There are two methods that are used to sound the Biosonic C and G tuning forks:

1. Knee Tap or Apple Tap: Hold the tuning fork by the stem with moderate pressure and gently tap the flat side of the prongs on your knee cap. Do not hit or slap your knee cap. If you do not want to tap your knee cap, then tap the tuning fork on an apple or hard rubber surface.
2. Together Tap: Hold the stems of the tuning forks in your left and right hands and gently tap the edges of the prongs together. Play with creating an easy sounding tap versus a banging tap when too much force is used. When you tap them together, move them around off your body. Do not bring the tuning forks directly to your ears.

24.2.2 BIOSONIC TUNING FORK RECORDINGS

A recording of Biosonic tuning forks is included for use with this chapter. The recording includes Biosonic C and G Bodytuners™, a special tuning fork sound color concert called Sound Rainbows, and the individual tones for each color. The Biosonic C and G Bodytuners™ and Sonic Rainbows recordings can be used with all the sound color exercises. The recordings can be listened to with speakers or headphones while viewing a color and can be used with any color visualizations or phenomenological learning exercises in this chapter if Biosonic Body Tuner tuning forks are not available. The recording can also be used with color visualizations if the Biosonic color glasses are not available. The colors in the Color Sensibility and Sound section are the same colors used in the glasses. Mindfully view the color, close your eyes and then visualize the color while listening to the recording of the color.

The Biosonic Tuning Fork Recordings can be accessed via the Supplementary Material section at www.routledge.com/9781032110127.

According to Dr. John Beaulieu, C and G Biosonic tuning forks have been shown to create an immediate relaxation response that is associated with the downregulation of stress via the release of nitric oxide (NO), leading to ANS balance. He and his collaborators published a peer-reviewed article suggesting that NO provides the physiological pathways through which sound and music operate by hypothesizing that sound stimulates the release of anandamide, an endogenous endocannabinoid that in turn stimulates the release of cNO in immune cells, neural tissues and human vascular endothelial cells.[5] In technical terms, nitric oxide is a "gaseous diffusible modulator" that moves through the entire body and central nervous system in waves or puffs of gas. The release of nitric oxide counteracts the negative effects of adrenergic overstimulation. Adrenergic stimulation in the presence of norepinephrine/adrenaline results in a racing heart, high blood pressure, anxiety and greater vulnerability to pain. This in turn triggers a relaxation response to sound by the effects of a wave of nitric oxide gas that signals a reduction in blood pressure, lower heart rate, increased pain tolerance and an overall lowering of metabolism. This positive reaction also appears to inhibit vascular dysregulation and promotes healthy blood flow to the visual system.

In another case, Dr. Wintrob presented Sophie, a 5-year-old girl with refractive amblyopia:

> This is a condition where the two eyes have dramatically different prescriptions. Her left eye has a low farsighted prescription and she easily corrected to 20/20 at both distance and near. Her right eye had a high amount of farsightedness and astigmatism. As a result, in this eye, her best corrected acuity was 20/80 at both distance and near. Her ability to use the two eyes together, i.e., her binocularity was very poor. Testing revealed a significant suppression of the right eye (the brain was ignoring the input from the eye). The reason for this is that she did not wear glasses prior to the age of 3. The right eye did not get the proper stimulation to enable the cells of the macula (the area of the eye used for sharp vision) to develop properly. Normal vision therapy consists of weekly visits for 45 minutes coupled with home syntonics and other vision exercises. In my experience with refractive amblyopia patients, improvement of vision in a patient's eye to 20/40 within a year's time was considered to be exceptional progress. Sophie received the recommended Syntonic Combination of Alpha Delta (red/orange) to stimulate the eye and improve its sight with the addition of the use of Biosonic C and G tuning forks twice a day. After just seven months of therapy, her eye sight improved to 20/20 distance and near, her depth perception improved, and her social skills and general mood were elevated.

In discussing cases, it is difficult to know which intervention caused the shift, or whether it is the combination of interventions that produced the change. David's and Sophie's cases suggest that syntonic color treatments are enhanced when they are complemented with stress reduction practices such as sound healing. We need more clinical studies to confirm the causal role of stress in vision loss and different low-vision diseases in order to evaluate the efficacy of different anti-stress therapies such as sound healing for preventing progression and improving vision recovery in holistic optometry. We are optimistic about the positive effects the integration of sound and color has had in the successful treatment of eye conditions.

24.3 COLOR SENSE ABILITY AND SOUND

People are getting interested in waves, now more than ever. We want to connect to something; we sit at the computer, many hours a day, searching on Google for something to connect to. Light from the sun comes in waves; movement in nature shows us its beauty and its force in waves, as in the rise and fall of the ocean or the delicate flutter of a hummingbird's wing. Light travels in waves. Sound travels in waves. *Color is a sonic wave of light.*

> When you see a rainbow, that vibrant miraculous performance of color, how does it make you feel? When does it happen? Unexpectedly and brilliantly after it rains and the sun peeks through? When we see a rainbow, we see the world through a technicolor lens refracting and bending our thoughts. The rainbow bends the light of the sun into radiant colors in perfect strands, arching across the sky like a magic wand.[6]

The rainbow imagery is designed to activate feeling tones associated with the experience of viewing the colors a rainbow. Emotional information embedded into sound and color frequencies can be positive or negative depending on one's relationship with the embedded memories, thoughts and emotions. From a vibrational perspective, a rainbow is a visual color keyboard sounding a chord that creates a tone. When mental and emotional information is embedded in that tone, it becomes a carrier wave for thoughts and emotions. If the reader were to close their eyes and become mindfully aware of the sensations streaming through their body and less aware of their thoughts and emotions, they would be able to tune into the vibration of the feeling tone. Although feeling tones cannot currently be reduced to mathematical frequencies, they are nevertheless frequency based and have a direct effect on one's mental, emotional and physical state.

The following color sense and sound stories and affirmations show how you can use tuning forks with color images to bring your body to a right environment, where the color goes on a healing journey. The goal is to allow the color and sound feeling tones activated by the stories to stream through your mind and body as pure vibration. It is important to let your intuition be your guide. Tune in, listen and go with the color you feel the most strongly. Tuning into and trusting body sensations in this way is contrary to traditional wisdom, which says it is important to engage in logical deliberative process before making a choice. Research says otherwise. Studies have found that when it comes to making important life choices, such as intuitively choosing sounds and colors for healing, trusting your intuition can lead to better outcomes than logical thinking processes. It is called the "deliberation-without-attention" hypothesis, which has been confirmed in a number of studies.[7]

LET YOUR INTUITION GUIDE YOU IN MAKING YOUR COLOR CHOICES. GO WITH WHAT COLOR COMES TO YOU.

1. Sit in a safe place, close your eyes and mindfully tune into the sound of your breath.
2. Intuitively choose a color that resonates with you.
3. Breathe the color in; as you exhale the color, make a humming sound in resonance with the color.
4. Read the color story, or have someone read the story to you. Tap the tuning forks, close your eyes, and tune into the feeling tones of the story and allow them to stream through your body.

24.3.1 GREEN

I am standing barefoot in the middle of the forest, and I can smell the scent of the pines and feel the cool breeze on my face relaxing. The warm sun feels good, and I raise my arms up toward the sky and open them up to the sides, letting my head fall back and jaw relax. I concentrate on the upper part of my body, taking the color green into every cell in my body and breathing out. I appreciate all that is. I feel more alive than ever before. Holding my hands to my heart, I see myself being calm, finding peaceful solutions to the harmony with Nature.

Tap your Biosonic Body Tuners.

24.3.1.1 Affirmation for Green

I am willing to listen and respect other's points of view without compromising my integrity. Peace and quiet are mine to enjoy now. I have the ability to listen even if I don't agree. Peaceful solutions come my way easily and effortlessly. Anything is possible to bring joy and peace to my world (Figure 24.3).

FIGURE 24.3 Color green.

24.3.2 BLUE

I am standing on a beach, looking out at the horizon, as far as I can see is an endless expanse of blue space. I let my face, my throat and my jaw relax as I take a deep breath in and let it all shake out as I breathe out. I breathe in the color blue to every part of my body, let it go to any area of my body that wants it most. I feel the space opening around my joints and the organs in my body. Each organ of my body knows which one wants more space around it. Breathe blue in and breathe blue out. All I can see is endless infinite space. I feel my jaw and throat relax as I take a deep breath in with the color blue. I can sing. I can dance. I am like a butterfly landing lightly on a flower petal, able to spring off with a happy heart.

Tap the Biosonic C and G tuning forks.

24.3.2.1 Affirmation for Blue

Blue: I express myself and speak the truth with courage. My voice is clear. My thoughts come out as I intend them to. I am understood and appreciated. I stand up for what I believe in (Figure 24.4).

FIGURE 24.4 Color blue.

24.3.3 RED

I am sitting in my favorite room in a house I feel safe in. I sit in my favorite chair, surrounded by pillows. I can adjust them in different ways to find the perfect amount of comfort that is perfect for me. I feel relaxed and comfortable. I get up and walk outside to my beautiful garden. It is a beautiful sunny day, and the smell of the earth is so strong, I kneel down to take a handful in my hand and bring it to my nose to smell. I smell the freshly sprouting herbs I have planted. I see the fruits and the vegetables coming to life after a long winter, I feel my body like a tree, able to bend with the wind. I am flexible and rooted deep in the earth, nourished by water. I can grow in my own way in my own time.

Tap the Biosonic C and G tuning forks.

24.3.3.1 Affirmation for Red

I can warm up any place I go. My presence alone stimulates and inspires all around me (Figure 24.5).

FIGURE 24.5 Color red.

24.3.4 ORANGE

I step slowly into a beautiful pool of clear water on a hot summer day. Easing myself into the water, I let my body relax. I feel the cool sensation on my skin, smell the scent of the sea air, and feel the water slide as I move gracefully swimming around anything that comes my way, I hear the water lap up on the shore in the distance, and see a school of fish underneath me. I am thankful and at peace with myself and others. I can adapt and change to new situations.

Tap the Biosonic C and G tuning forks.

24.3.4.1 Affirmation for Orange

Creative solutions come to any problem coming my way (Figure 24.6).

FIGURE 24.6 Color orange.

24.3.5 YELLOW

Take a moment to visualize or think of something you really want. You don't have to say this out loud since it is only for you. Take the first thing that comes to mind. Don't think too much about it. Now put that image across the room. See it clearly, what is the energy, or element you need to get it. Now sit in a comfortable chair and read the following words out loud to yourself or another.

I am running as fast as I can on a sandy beach with the sun beating down on my back and shoulders. I am strong and capable. I surge forward with determination and feel my purpose with every step. My eyes are focused and I see my path clearly. I jump easily over rocks and sticks and I listen to the sound of the waves lapping up on the shore. Nothing can stop me. As long as I am safe, I will continue forward, honoring my feelings, but not being overwhelmed by them. I go fearlessly towards what I want with purpose and determination, while feeling the warmth of the golden sun.

Tap the Biosonic C and G tuning forks.

24.3.5.1 Affirmation for Yellow

I take action with purpose and enthusiasm (Figure 24.7).

FIGURE 24.7 Color yellow.

24.4 THERAPEUTIC DISCUSSION

Feeling tones are an explanation for sound and color systems that assign different and sometimes contradictory therapeutic qualities to sounds and colors. For example, in one system, the color blue may be associated with being down and out, i.e., "the blues," and in another system, the color blue is associated with peace and tranquility. The color blue, i.e., from light blue to dark blue, is a wave of light consisting of different frequencies. The color blue has no emotion or thought. It does not know right or wrong or sad and happy. It is a frequency perceived as blue that comes and goes just as rainbows refract the light of the sun to appear and disappear. Similarly, music consists of frequencies of sound that become music in the ear of the beholder. A music composition may be uplifting for a listener and depressing for another listener. In the 1950s, rock and roll music was exciting for teens and "the devil's music" for parents. Today, those teens are grandparents who are uplifted by listening to rock and roll tunes.

Thoughts and emotions are embedded into a sound and/or color. They can be positive or negative depending on one's relationship with the event in which they were embedded. For example, a negative experience with rainbows, which is highly unlikely but nevertheless possible, will activate a very different feeling tone response than a positive one. *The colors of the rainbow act as a carrier wave for the feeling tone.* This is the process of mindfully focusing on the felt sense vibration of the feeling tone. In other words, regardless of the "right or wrong," agreements or disagreements, or any emotions that may be associated with the feeling tone, the event cannot be changed. When thoughts and emotions are reduced to a feeling tone, vibration is allowed to pass through the mind–body as a frequency. What we are left with are the colors of the rainbow without an embedded feeling tone. This is the basis of somatic psychotherapy, in which a client is asked to focus on the sensations of a thought and/or emotion rather than the story of a challenging event. The sensations can then be appreciated as pure frequency and allowed to stream through the body as a neutral carrier wave frequency.

By learning about pure sound and color frequencies through direct experience, one can become aware of the feeling tone information that has been unconsciously embedded into these sounds and colors. *Sounds and colors are neutral frequencies of energy waves seeking to move through the body–mind.* They have the ability to become carrier waves for emotions and thoughts that can be positive or negative. When we can consciously differentiate sound and color frequencies from embedded feeling tones, then we have the ability to keep, modify or remove feeling tone information from the carrier wave. We can also choose to consciously add new feeling tone information to any color or sound.

The ability to understand and embed feeling tones is fundamental to music and art as well as indigenous shamanistic practices. Musicians and painters understand that sounds and colors are carrier waves for feeling tones.[8] They learn basic scales and color palettes that are not embedded with thoughts and emotions. During master classes, musicians focus on expressing feelings through sound through tonal color. This is why a listener may prefer one pianist playing the same piece of music over another, e.g., Arthur Rubinstein's Chopin over Vladimir Horowitz's Chopin. The notes are the same, and their playing techniques are masterful, but the feelings embedded in the sound create different colors through the tone. The Sanskrit term *Raga*, which describes the classical music of India, means to use sound to color the mind with emotion.[9] Life is filled with waves of emotion that are expressed through sound and color. This is what Thea Keats Beaulieu calls "Color Love" and perhaps the reason why every progressive artist and composer at the turn of the century was interested in correspondences between music and visual art.[10] Wassily Kandinsky, the painter of sound and vision, said in his journals: "Color acts upon the human body, it is the key touched by man to obtain the appropriate vibration from his creative spirit."[11]

24.5   SOUND AND COLOR FREQUENCY AND RESONANCE

Dr. John Beaulieu and Dr. Jerry Wintrob have developed an experimental sensory integration system using Biosonic tuning forks tuned to special Biosonic color glasses to work with the integration of sound and color frequencies. Sensory integration is the perception of vibrational resonances between the senses. The experience of sensory integration is normal and is an important component of wellness. It is an important component of any natural healing processes that leads to greater mental and physical adaptability in all aspects of life. Because our senses are limited in vibrational range, we see and hear only a small part of the vibrational spectrum. When our senses are organized and working together in a state of neural coherence, we enhance creativity and problem-solving skills.[12] For example, research suggests the importance of integrating sound and vision to enhance an athlete's motor outcomes.[13] The golfing industry has discovered that the sound of a golf shot on impact is very important. Golf club manufacturers work overtime to perfect the sound of their drivers. Scott Mase, a professor of mechanical engineering at California Polytechnic State University says, "it's important to hear that sound, and it's also important from manufacturers' point of view at a point of sale."[14]

Seeking integration between sound and color is not new. Many cultures have developed systems of sensory integration for healing and enhanced wellbeing. In India, China and Japan, sound and color have always been integrated with all the senses and integral to the healing arts and arts. In Ayurveda, the natural healing system of India, the sounds of mantras are associated with different colors, emotions and tastes. For example, the sound of the mantra "Lam" is associated with the color red, sweet tastes and fear. In ancient Greece, the Pythagoreans paired colors with musical notes, which resonated within a system of universal harmony they called "the music of the spheres."[15] Aristotle advocated the existence of a harmony of colors that resonated with the harmony of sounds.[16] In 1590, the Italian painter Guiseppe Arcimboli created a system of colored fabrics to be played by musicians. In 1646, the German artist Athanasius Kircher developed a system of correspondences between musical intervals and colors.[17] The Russian composer Alexander Scriabin believed that the integration of sound and color created a powerful psychological resonance within listeners. His composition *Prometheus, Poem of Fire* is scored with musical notes and colors.[18] In 1704, Sir Isaac Newton proposed in his treatise *Optics* a parallel between colors and notes of the musical scale. Newton mathematically divided the visible light spectrum into seven colors, which, he proposed, resonated with the notes of a musical scale.[19]

We determine sound and color resonance by raising or lowering sound and color frequencies 39 to 41 octaves. An octave is a doubling or a halving of a frequency. Doubling or halving an inaudible sound in octaves in order to hear it is a common practice in modern research. For example, researchers use octaves to transpose the sounds of dolphins, whales and bats from the ultrasonic range into the range of human hearing.[20] Astronomers raise the subsonic sounds of pulsars, planets and black holes into an audible range to better research them.[21]

Frequency Resonance Chart for Biosonic Tuning Forks and Colored Glasses

Tuning (Hz)	Tuning (nm)	Glasses Color
256	533	Green
288	473	Blue
320	426	Indigo
341.3	399	Violet
384	710	Red
426.7	640	Orange
480	568	Yellow

24.6 BIOSONIC COLOR GLASSES

The intention of sound and color frequency and resonance is to allow resonant sound and color frequencies to simultaneously enter the body through visual and auditory channels to promote an enhanced mind–body coherence through sensory integration. To work with sound and color frequency resonance, we use biosonic tuning forks and developed special biosonic colored glasses that are tuned based on peak light transmission through color gels. To ensure accuracy and consistency, each color gel is checked against a scientifically generated set of light transmission parameters. The color gel is then inserted into the color glasses frame (Figures 24.8 and 24.9).

24.6.1 How to Use Biosonic Color Glasses

1. Try on the color glasses. Adjust the temple tips so that the glasses are snug over the back of your ears and the bridge fits comfortably over your nose, allowing effortless viewing. The color glasses can also be adjusted to fit comfortably over your normal glasses.
2. Ideally, go outside to view the sky, but if you are inside, view a neutral wall, preferably while illuminated by full spectrum light. If this is not possible, view a lighted area without focusing on objects or anything distracting. We will call this mindful viewing.
3. Viewing the color glasses over your regular glasses or contact lenses will not have the same effect. These lenses decrease the absorption of light. Do not be concerned about what you are actually seeing, and just try to be with the color.

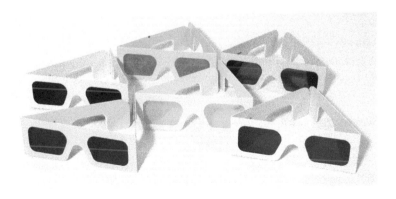

FIGURE 24.8 Biosonic color glasses.

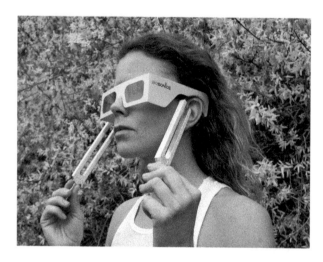

FIGURE 24.9   How to perform phenomenological sensory integration (PSI) exercises.

24.7 PHENOMENOLOGICAL SENSORY INTEGRATION (PSI) EXERCISES

The high quality of the color gels and the tuning forks creates an opportunity for systematic phenomenological exploration that has the potential to generate ideas for more research into sensory integration. Because tuning forks and color glasses have a common tuning baseline, it is possible to systematically record, discuss and correlate experiences with others. When we learn to detach from emotional and intellectual information associated with a sound and/or color, we can then begin to phenomenologically explore the direct effect of any sound and/or color on our mind and body.

All PSI exercises begin with the establishment of coherence through breath and sound. Coherent breathing promotes comfort and relaxation as well as pleasantness, vigor and alertness. This in turn reduces anxiety, depression, anger and confusion. This leads to greater heart rate variability and central nervous system coherence.[22] Find a safe, comfortable place to practice coherent breathing. Close your eyes and focus on your natural breath, and when you are ready, breathe in for 5 seconds and then out for 5 seconds for approximately 1 minute.

24.7.1   PSI Exercise 1: C and G

As explained in the Holistic Syntonic Phototherapy and Sound Healing section, C and G is a sonic interval that can enhance the effect of any color.

1. Choose a color to explore and put on your color glasses.
2. Close your eyes, tap C and G Bodytuner tuning forks, and mindfully listen.
3. Open your eyes and mindfully view the color for a specific length of time.

24.7.2   PSI Exercise 2: Specific Sound and Color Explorations

1. Choose a color and resonant sound to explore and put on your color glasses.
2. Close your eyes and tap the tuning fork that resonates with the color you have chosen.
3. Hum a sound in resonance with the tuning fork.
4. Open your eyes and view the color.
5. Take a deep breath and hum the sound of the color.

24.7.3 PSI Exercise 3: The Purpose of This Exercise Is to Build Trust in Your Sensory Integration Abilities

1. Without tuning forks or color glasses, imagine a color and hum until your humming sound comes into resonance with your visualized color.
2. Color Balloon Breathing: An example of a therapeutic application through a variation of sound and color integration.

Imagine a color filling the space in whatever part or organ of your body needs your attention at this time, maybe a part that hurts you or is giving you pain, If it could give you a color, what color would it give you? Take that color and breathe it into your body, filling up your lungs like two balloons, and then gently exhale a humming sound in resonance with the color. Repeat as often as you like, targeting the area. Imagine your diaphragm filling up like a balloon, let the color freely change if it needs to. Let your intuition be your guide.

24.7.4 PSI Exercise #4: A Result of Working with Tuned Sound and Color Resonances Is the Ability to Develop and Trust Your Sound and Color Sensibility

1. Tune into and view a color in your environment and hum until your humming sound comes into resonance with the color.
2. When a sound attracts you, tune into it. Hum with the sound and simultaneously visualize a color until it comes into resonance with the sound.

24.7.5 PSI Discussion

PSI exercises can be used to tune into and explore colors in many ways to develop and gain confidence in our sensory integration abilities. For example, in 1850, the chemist William Henry Perkins accidentally discovered the first synthetic organic dye in history, which he called the color mauve (Figure 24.10).

24.7.5.1 Mauve

He was looking for a way to obtain affordable quinine to treat malaria when he accidentally discovered a purple-blue residue in the bottom of his test beaker. Although his experiment failed, he soon realized that he had made the first synthetic organic color dye in history. He called the bluish-purple color mauve. Before his discovery, the only way to obtain the color mauve was through the mucus of the predatory sea snail *Bolinus brandaris*. Perkins' discovery of mauve inspired a revolution in medicine and fashion. Mauve is used in medicine to color cells in order to study chromosomes under a microscope and played an essential role in the discovery of the bacillus responsible for

FIGURE 24.10 Color mauve.

tuberculosis and in chemotherapy research. The discovery of mauve led to an explosion in the world of fashion. In 1862, Queen Victoria wore a long mauve gown, and in the next 5 years, 28 dye factories sprang up across Europe to produce all the fashionable garments dyed with the color mauve. Historians referred to this time as "The Mauve Decade," the color that changed the world.[23] In order to phenomenologically explore mauve, we created mauve tuned color glasses with a resonant tuning fork frequency of 341 Hz. One can look at the color, visualize and hum in resonance with the color, and then compare one's humming sound with the sound of the tuning fork.

24.8 OVERVIEW AND CONCLUSION

There is much more that could be written about and researched in the area of sound and color integration. What is most important is that the experience of sensory integration be understood as normal and further researched as an important component of a natural healing process that leads to greater mental and physical adaptability in all aspects of life. The integration of sound and color has been in the past and ideally, going forward into the future a place where science and art meet. Seeing and simultaneously hearing colors as sounds or sounds as colors used to be considered a rare congenital condition called synesthesia, in which sensory stimuli cause unusual experiences that are associated with neurological dysfunction and mental illness.[24] Many people who reported synesthetic experiences risked being labeled as strange or weird or worse, being diagnosed as schizophrenics or drug addicts and consigned to mental hospitals. This resulted in the erroneous belief that the experience of sensory integration might be an indicator that something is physically or mentally out of balance. Whereas previous studies indicated that synesthesia occurred at a rate of 1 in 25,000, newer studies have suggested that synesthesia is a common condition, with a rate of 1 in 23 people who demonstrate over 150 different forms of synesthesia.[25] Today, people are paying for training designed to increase synesthetic experiences in order to enhance cognitive ability and increase neural plasticity, leading to greater creativity and problem-solving skills.[26] In the field of consciousness research, the experience of synesthesia is a gateway into the neural correlates of consciousness.[27, 28] We suggest that the term *synesthesia* gives way to *sensory integration*, a term that allows the freedom for everyone to explore sound and color integration and for researchers to systematically show the many specific healing effects found in sound and color practices.

REFERENCES

1. Herbert Benson, *The Relaxation Response* (New York: William Morrow and Co., 1975).
2. Raymond L. Gottlieb and O.D. Wallace, Syntonic Phototherapy. *Photomedicine and Laser Surgery* 28, (Nov. 2010): 449–452.
3. Bernhard A. Sabel et al., "Mental Stress as Consequence and Cause of Vision Loss: The Dawn of Psychosomatic Ophthalmology for Preventive and Personalized Medicine," *EPMA Journal* 9 (2018): 133–160.
4. John Beaulieu and David Perez-Martinez. *Sound Healing Theory and Practice Nutrition and Integrative Medicine* (New York: CRC Press, 2019), 449–471.
5. John Beaulieu et al., "Sound Therapy Induced Relaxation: Down Regulating Stress Processes and Pathologies," *Medical Science Monitor* (2003).
6. Kathleen Keats-Beaulieu, *Journey Through the Color Worlds* (Stone Ridge: Biosonic Enterprises Press, 2016).
7. Ap Dijksterhuis et al., "On Making the Right Choice: The Deliberation-Without-Attention Effect," *Science* 311 (2006): 1005, https://doi.org/10.1126/science.1121629.
8. David Rudhyar, *The Magic of Tone and the Art of Music* (Boulder: Shambhala, 1982).
9. Tejaswinee Kelkar, *Color Wheel for Music: Tonal Pitch Space and Color Mapping for Ragas Research* (May 2015), https://www.researchgate.net/publication/277308068_colour_wheel_for_music.
10. H. Heyrman, *Art and Synesthesia: In Search of the Synesthetic Experience* (Spain: University of Almería, July 2005), http://www.doctorhugo.org/synaesthesia/art/index.html.
11. Wassily Kandinsky, *Concerning the Spiritual in Art* (New York: Tate Publishing, 2001).

12. Daniel Bor et al., "Adults Can Be Trained to Acquire Synesthetic Experiences," *Scientific Reports* 4 (Nov. 18, 2014).
13. Fabrizo Sors et al., "Audio-Based Interventions in Sport," *The Open Psychology Journal* (Jan. 2015): 212–210, https://www.researchgate.net/publication/288992706_audio-based_interventions_in_sport.
14. Scott Simon, *The Sound of the Golf Swing* (NPR Weekend Edition, Aug. 11, 2018), https:// www.npr.org /2018/08/11/637780597/the-sound-of-the-golf-swing.
15. A. Ione and C. Tyler, "Synesthesia: Is F-Sharp Colored Violet?" *Journal of the History of the Neurosciences* 13 (2004): 58–65.
16. L.E. Marks, "On Colored-Hearing Synesthesia: Cross-Modal Translations of Sensory Dimensions," *Psychological Bulletin* 82 (1975): 303–331.
17. J. Jewanski, "What Is the Color of the Tone?" *Leonardo* 32, no. 3 (1999): 227–228.
18. Cretien van Campen, *The Hidden Sense: Synesthesia in Art and Science* (Cambridge: MIT Press, 2007).
19. Isaac Newton, commentary by Nicholas Humez, *Opticks: A Treatise of The Reflexions, Refractions, Inflexions and Colors of Light* (Palo Alto: Octavo, 1998).
20. Australian Government Department of Agriculture, *Whales, Dolphins, and Sound: Water and the Environment*, https://www.environment.gov.au/marine/marine-species/cetaceans/whale-dolphins -sound.
21. Maggie Masetti, *Can You Hear a Black Hole* (Blueshift, NASA Aeronautics and Space Administration, Oct. 2013), https://asd.gsfc.nasa.gov/blueshift/index.php/2013/10/29/maggies-blog-can-you-hear-a -black-hole/.
22. Andrea Zaccaro et al., "How Breath-Control Can Change Your Life: A Systematic Review on Psycho-Physiological Correlates of Slow Breathing," *Frontiers in Human Neuroscience* (2018), https://www .ncbi.nlm.nih.gov/pmc/articles/PMC6137615/.
23. Simon Garfield, *Mauve: How One Man Invented a Color That Changed the World* (New York: Norton and Co., 2000).
24. J.E. Harrison and S. Baron-Cohen, "Synesthesia: An Introduction," in *Synesthesia: Classic and Contemporary Readings*, eds. S. Baron-Cohen and J. E. Harrison (Blackwell Publishing, 1997), 3–16.
25. J. Simner et al., "Synesthesia: The Prevalence of Atypical Cross-Modal Experiences," *Perception* 35 (2006): 1024–1033.
26. Daniel Bor et al., "Adults Can Be Trained to Acquire Synesthetic Experiences," *Scientific Reports* 4 (Nov. 18, 2014).
27. N. Sagiv and C.D. Frith, "Synesthesia and Consciousness," in *Handbook of Synesthesia* (New York: Oxford University Press, 2013), 924–940.
28. Tessa M. van Leeuwen, Wolf Singer, and Danko Nikolic, "The Merit of Synesthesia for Consciousness Research," *Frontiers in Psychology* (2015), https://www.frontiersin.org/articles/10.3389/fpsyg.2015 .01850/full.

BIBLIOGRAPHY

Babbitt, Edwin D. *Principles of Light and Color* (New York: Babbitt & Co., 1878).
Bartram, Lyn, Abhisekh Patra, and Maureen Stone. "Affective Color in Visualization." In Proceedings of the 2017 CHI Conference on Human Factors in Computing Systems, May 2017. https://doi.org/10.1145 /3025453.3026041.
Beaulieu, John. *Music and Sound in the Healing Arts* (Barrytown: Station Hill Press, 1987).
Beaulieu, John. *Human Tuning* (Stone Ridge: Biosonic Enterprises, Ltd., 2010).
Beaulieu, John, and David Perez–Martinez. "Sound Healing Theory and Practice." In *Nutrition and Integrative Medicine: A Primer for Physicians*, edited by Aruna Bakhru (Boca Raton: CRC Press, 2016).
Benson, Herbert. *The Relaxation Response* (New York: William Morrow and Co., 1975).
Clark, Linda. *The Ancient Art of Color Therapy* (New York: Simon & Schuster, 1975).
Clark, Linda, and Yvonne Martine. *Color Breathing* (New York: Berkley Medallion Books, 1976).
Elliott Salamon, Minsun Kim, Beaulieu, and John, George B. Stefano. "Sound Therapy Induced Relaxation: Down Regulating Stress Processes and Pathologies." *Medical Science Monitor* 9 (5): RA96–RA101.
Groffman, S. "Psychological Aspects of Strabismus and Amblyopia: A Review of the Literature," *Journal of the American Optometric Association* 49 (1978): 995–999.
Kobayashi, Shigenobu. *Color Image Scale* (New York: Kodansha America, 1990).
Kyoiku, O., M. Yamakawa, N. Tanaka, H. Muraakami, and S. Hori. "Influence of Sound and Light on Heart Rate Variability." *Journal of Human Ergology* 34 (2010): 25–34.

LaViolette, Paul A. "Thoughts about Thoughts about Thoughts: The Emotional Perceptive Cycle Theory." *Man-Environment Systems* 9 (Sept. 1979).

Leiberman, J. *Light Medicine of the Future* (Sante Fe: Bear and Co., 1995).

Stefano, G.B., G.L. Fricchione, B.T. Slingsby, and H.Benson. "The Placebo Effect and the Relaxation Response: Neural Processes and Their Coupling to Constitutive Nitric Oxide." *Brain Research Reviews* 35 (2001).

Spitler, Harry Riley. *The Syntonic Principle* (Eugene: Resource Publications, 2011).

25 The Human Body: A Biological Sound Healing Instrument

Shawn Marie Higgins

CONTENTS

DOI: 10.1201/b23304-27

When you think vibrationally and then act on it with discipline, you open the doorway to new possibilities.

John Beaulieu, ND, PhD

25.1 INTRODUCTION

Sound healing practices have been used by humans for thousands of years across many cultures to span all continents. The use of musical instruments and the human voice for healing still remains widespread throughout the world. The following pages present a compelling stance that the human voice is possibly the most powerful sound healing instrument that exists for human beings. For is it not from the human vocal tract that many musical instruments were modeled in the first place? And many wind instruments cannot be operated without the player's breath … breath from which the individual tone and timbre of the player's natural voice adds to the quality of sound produced by the instrument.[1]

Vocal cords and ears are two obvious pieces of proof that we are designed to make, interpret and function in response to *sound*. You will learn in the coming pages that they are by far not the only ones. And, the instinctive development of language amongst every human culture is testament that not only are we designed to make sound, but we are compelled to use it as a source of creative power by means of communication and affirmation. Our vocal tracts are instruments that can be played to create anything we choose – art, healing or destruction.

It is the human voice that has created much chaos in the way of wars. And, it is the human voice that can create peace. It is the human voice that allows us to make change in our *external* lives by transforming our living, working and social situations with conversation, discussion and debates, and by voicing our needs and wants. What we say has impact. It has potential to have both positive and/or negative effects on others, our environment and ourselves. The *intention and emotion* of what we say adds even more power to our words as we experience their effects, steering the course of our lives.

The human voice also allows us to make changes to our *internal* lives, our physical and emotional health and wellbeing. Through vocal healing practices such as mantra and prayer, as well as simply voicing words of love and compassion to others, we open our hearts to self-awareness and intuition. We open doors to our self-guidance systems of knowing what is right for us. The vibration of our own voice even has the power to initiate healing changes on a cellular level within our own bodies.

25.2 WHAT IS SOUND?

What humans call *sound* is the spectrum of *vibrational* frequency that can be sensed by our ears and transmitted to the brain to be interpreted as something we hear. Sound is energy that is conducted as a wave via pressure gradients through any medium, such as air, water, glass or metal. These waves are measured in frequency, which is the speed at which they are vibrating in oscillations or cycles per second (also expressed as Hertz). Since sound is vibration, which is a wave of pressure, then it has physical force. It has the ability to affect all that is in its environment.

In a two-dimensional drawing as shown in Figure 25.1 (bottom), we see a sound wave in air as a sine wave, or a curved line. However, in our three-dimensional world, a sound wave is really a *traveling disturbance* caused by pressure to particles in the air – as shown in Figure 25.1 (top).

25.2.1 WAVE PROPAGATION

Vibration is an oscillation or back and forth movement about a point of equilibrium. When there is a focal disturbance to a medium, the particles (molecules) within it that were exposed to the distur-bance begin to vibrate. Let's again use air as an example. The air around us is made up of molecules.

SOUND WAVES

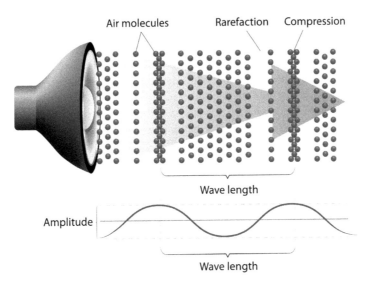

FIGURE 25.1 The top wave depicts a three-dimensional sound wave showing particle disbursement – periods of alternating compression (increased density) and rarefaction (decreased density) of the air particles. The bottom depicts a sound wave as a two-dimensional sine wave.

Air is mostly composed of nitrogen (78%) and oxygen (21%), but also contains trace amounts of other molecules such as carbon dioxide, argon, neon, methane, helium, hydrogen and others.[2] When molecules in the air become disturbed they vibrate and collide with adjacent particles. Then those particles become disturbed and collide with particles next to *them*, and so on, to create a chain of motion, a *wave of pressure*. The particles transmit the waves but do not travel with them. Thus, a wave *transfers energy without transferring matter*.[3]

The movement of air flowing with sound oscillates back and forth with an overall propagation in the direction that the sound wave is traveling. What we get are periods of alternating compression (increased density) and rarefaction (decreased density) of the air particles,[4] as shown in Figure 25.1 (top).

25.3 EVERYTHING IS VIBRATION

Quantum theory tells us that everything in the universe, whether visible or invisible, is vibrating and in a constant state of motion. In physics, the word *quantum* is defined as "the minimum amount of any physical entity involved in an interaction."[5] In simple terms, quantum refers to the smallest possible unit of something. Most (if not all) physics and chemistry books will tell us that all matter, living or nonliving, is made up of cells. All cells are made up of molecules, which are made up of atoms. An atom broken down consists of subatomic particles, which are protons, neutrons and electrons – the smallest possible units of anything.

Consider the Newtonian structure of an atom, the version many of us learned about in chemistry class. It depicts a neatly packaged nucleus of protons and neutrons orbited by spherical electrons on a seemingly preorganized fixed and orderly path. How neatly predictable, right? Well, not so much. As Bruce Lipton, PhD, explains in his revolutionary book *Biology of Belief*, the field of quantum physics (versus Newtonian physics) has determined that atoms are actually made entirely of "vortices of energy that are constantly spinning and vibrating." These tiny vortices are called *quarks*, and each one spins or "wobbles" to its own rhythm. Each quark and each atom has its own unique energy imprint. Thus, each *collection* of atoms also vibrates at its own frequency.[6] Each object, organism, person, *everything* vibrates a unique frequency into the universe. These frequencies can change in response to influencing factors. For example, if a person's physical, mental and/or spiritual life circumstances change, this may affect their overall health (by way of affecting the spin and vibration of the atoms that make up their body) and thus, their net vibrational frequency that is being emitted into the environment.

Dr. Lipton also explains that if viewed under a high-powered microscope, atoms have no structure and are actually invisible. If viewed on *low* power focus, from more of a distance, an atom may appear as a hazy orb. However, the more closely we look with the microscope the more and more invisible the atom becomes until there is no structure at all. It does not appear as a Newtonian atom. There is just invisible energy, which appears as nothing, "a physical void." Thus, everything is energy, it is movement, it is vibration ... and matter does not even really exist.[6]

25.3.1 VIBRATION IS THE UNIVERSAL LANGUAGE

Since everything in the universe is vibration, then it is this level through which everything can communicate with everything else, at which everything is on the same playing field. Vibration is the language that everything speaks and thus, becomes an *interdimensional bridge* for communication between all forms, a meeting place for resolution of all conflict and a transformational platform from which all may expand.

Vibrations exists in many forms. *Sound* is the form of vibration that is most accessible to human beings, which is most evident in the fact that we are designed with highly sophisticated mechanisms with which to make *and* interpret it. The human voice is unique in that it successively recruits energy through various dimensions. It begins in the spiritual realm of thought but then rapidly enters the physical realm as it triggers neurons in the brain to fire the appropriate synapses for the physical body functions necessary for vocal tract expression of sound in the form of *speech*. The original thought vibration is transduced through a series of dimensions until it ends up in audible form within the etheric realm, the air, where it then has the capacity to reach the spiritual thought-space of *others* – because it can then be *heard*. Sound bridges us not only between dimensions but also between each other.

25.4 VOICE

Voice is any type of sound produced within and transferred through the *vocal tract*. The *human voice* originates at the vocal cords. Its primary sound source is vocal fold vibration and includes talking, humming, singing, laughing, crying, screaming, yelling, shouting, etc. There are other sounds emitted through the vocal tract that convey meaning or emotion, such as sighing, huffing, blowing, etc. However, these do not require the involvement of the vocal cords. These sounds are produced by passive air friction and thus, are not referred to as "voice."[7]

The vocal tract refers to the cavity through which sound travels from its source at the vocal cords to its exit from the mouth and/or nose. It includes the larynx, pharynx, oral cavity, nasal cavity and interior aspect of the lips. The entire *vocal system* also includes the lower respiratory tract, since the source of exhaled airflow comes from the lungs.[7, 8]

Larynx: Includes the rami glottis (the opening or space between the vocal cords), the vocal folds, laryngeal muscles that alter the position and tension of the vocal cords, and the sub- and supra-glottal lumens.

Pharynx: Includes muscles that change the quality of sound by adjusting the shape of the pharyngeal lumen. It is also a primary resonating cavity of the human vocal tract.[9]

Oral cavity: Includes the tongue, lips, hard and soft palates and teeth. The tongue, mandible and lips are a few major articulators that shape the vibrating air into distinct words and sounds as it flows through the oral cavity to exit the mouth.[9]

Nasal cavity: Includes the nasal conchae and turbinates. Air is streamed through the nasal cavity when pronouncing nasal consonants and other nasal sounds during speech.[8]

Human voice production is divided into three main parts by current literature: "respiration, vibration and articulation."[8]

1. Pressurized airflow is supplied by the lower respiratory tract in order to produce the force of exhaled air necessary for voice production.
2. Vibrating the air occurs as it passes between vocal cords, thus creating the *source of sound*. Changing the position and tension of the vocal cords alters the frequency of vibration that is imparted onto the out-flowing air. This changes the quality of the sound produced.
3. Shaping the sound source into distinct units of sound, such as phonemes, syllables and words, is the process of *articulation*. As the vibrating air flows through the vocal tract, it is shaped with the very fine-tuned intricate motor capability of the articulator muscles of the larynx, pharynx and oral cavity (most significantly the tongue). It then flows into the atmosphere and is picked up by our ears and interpreted by our brains as speech or song sound.

A*rticulation* is the process of purposefully "shaping" the vocalized sound into meaningful speech[8] or melodious song. It conveys meaningful content in the form of language and artistic content in the form of singing. In the case of singing, even though sounds may be formed that convey no cognitive meaning, voice *quality* such as tone, pitch, prosody (rhythms of accent and intonation in speech) and volume are skillfully manipulated to create a desired sensation in melody and emotion.

25.5   VOICE PRODUCTION REQUIRES THE ENTIRE BODY

By definition, the vocal tract is considered a fairly finite space. However, the process of vocalization does not even begin without the cooperation of nearly the entire body. Before we can even engage the vocal tract we must first access an array of other physiological mechanisms which work in cooperative effort to produce meaningful sound. In some way, almost every part of our physical bodies is touched by the power of the voice.

The respiratory tract: In order to speak or sing we must first take an inhalation. We must delve deep within the body, all the way down to even the tiny alveoli of our lungs, waking up the cellular components of gas exchange at the interface of capillary walls. The change in gas concentrations in our blood and pressure differences between the respiratory tract and the outside environment cause us to exhale. It is the pressurized air from the lungs that creates the force of exhaled air through the vocal tract which becomes our voice.

Through respiration we involve not only the movement and shaping of air through our bodies in the process of vocalization. We also involve the blood and the entire vascular system. As we inhale before speaking we oxygenate our blood which circulates nourishment to all organs and tissues. As we speak or sing we exhale, simultaneously excreting unneeded carbon dioxide and other gases from the body. Here we must also include the bones and marrow, the birth place of blood cells from the start.

I find it interesting that respiration, a most vital, life-sustaining bodily process, is absolutely required for the functioning of the human voice. Our need for oxygen parallels our ability to voice. In order to use our voices, we must oxygenate our blood. The two cannot be separated. *Voice is a form of self-expression that is cast from the body. It is the body function that reaches the furthermost outside of us. The vital exchange of gases during respiration is the most intimate process and is the body function that reaches the centermost within us. Voice (sound) bridges these two extremes of our being – the innermost with the outermost.*

Nervous system: In order to explore the full "reach" of voice, we must meander all the way up into the cerebrum of the brain, where thought premeditates our every spoken word, and where emotion predetermines spontaneous vocalizations of passion or fear. This involves both *cognitive* and *emotional* centers of the brain. Additionally, as we will discuss later, the process of *hearing* is highly linked with speech. Therefore, the entire ear apparatus and auditory centers of the brain are also involved in voice production.

Cerebrospinal fluid: Even more primal than the respiration of air via the lungs is *primary respiration*. This is an inherent involuntary mechanism within the central nervous system (CNS) that involves the entire body and can be palpated by trained practitioners from *anywhere in the body*.[10] Dr. William Garner Sutherland, founder of cranial osteopathy (although he credited the discovery to Dr. A.T. Still, the founder of osteopathy), called it *the breath of life*. It is inherent motion, a rhythmic expansion and contraction of the CNS (the brain and spinal cord) in synchronization with the fluctuation of cerebrospinal fluid (CSF).[11]

Primary respiration is influenced by secondary respiration. Evidence supports that thoracic inhalation significantly promotes CSF fluctuation, whereas holding the breath actually decreases it. CSF that is in direct contact with the thoracic paraspinal epidural venous plexus system senses pressure changes during thoracic respiration. This directly affects the direction and force of CSF flow.[12]

The diaphragm: If we must use the respiratory tract for vocalization, then we must also consider the accessory structures required for its proper functioning and all of the interconnecting fascia in between. The diaphragm is the main muscle for respiration. [13] Its expansion and contraction during respiration greatly affects all other organ systems and musculoskeletal structures via pneumatic pressure differences and fascial interconnections.[13, 14]

The diaphragm forms the floor of the thoracic cavity and the roof of the abdominal cavity. It directly attaches to the xiphoid process and symphysis of the *sternum*, costal cartilage of *ribs 6 through 10* and directly to *ribs 11 and 12*, the *spine* at thoracic vertebra T12 and lumbar vertebra L1-3, the *anterior longitudinal ligament* at those levels, the *medial and lateral arcuate ligaments*, the fascia of *quadratus lumborum* and *psoas major*.[13]

The diaphragm has three major openings through which vital structures pass, thereby affecting these as well. The *esophageal hiatus* contains the esophagus and the posterior and anterior vagal nerves, the *vena cava opening* allows passage of the inferior vena cava and sometimes the phrenic nerve (the diaphragm's own innervation via cervical spinal nerves C3, 4 and 5). The *aortic hiatus* passes directly behind and adjacent to the diaphragm between the left and right crus. This passageway contains the aorta, the azygos vein and the thoracic duct.[13]

The diaphragm plays the largest role in creating pressure differences between the thoracic and abdominal cavities and the atmosphere. Contraction of the diaphragm moves it inferiorly into the abdominal cavity, thereby increasing intrathoracic volume and decreasing intrathoracic pressure. Intrathoracic pressure decreases to lower than atmospheric pressure which encourages air to flow into the lungs. Relaxation of the diaphragm moves it superiorly, reversing the process and allowing passive exhalation.[13, 14]

Through its fascial connections diaphragm movement can affect pretty much the entire body. For example, fascia is continuous from the diaphragm all the way up to the superficial and deep cervical structures, soft tissues and bones. From there it even continues to the cranial bones, through the foramina and all the way up into the dura. It continues downward to the pharynx, larynx, lungs and heart.[14]

The ribs and intercostal muscles also play a major role in inspiration and thus, voice production. Their contraction and relaxation "pumps" the rib cage and sternum, adjusting intrathoracic volume and pressure in harmony with respiration, echoing the effects of the diaphragm.

The spine and *spinal cord* move during respiration. During inhalation all of the spinal curves flatten. The entire cervical, thoracic and lumbar spine moves with every inhalation and exhalation. Additionally, as mentioned earlier, the thoracic and lumbar vertebra are diaphragm attachments and subsequently move with its contraction and relaxation. The cervical spine also contributes to respiration by supplying the innervation of the diaphragm via the phrenic nerve, cervical spinal nerves 3–5.[13] *Spinal cord motion*, especially in the antero-posterior direction, is affected significantly by respiratory influences. The cervico-thoracic and thoraco-lumbar junctions are two areas that have shown the most movement.[15]

Sacrum: During inspiration the sacrum counternutates as the thoracic and pelvic diaphragms descend. During exhalation the sacrum nutates as the thoracic and pelvic diaphragms ascend.

The pelvic diaphragm and pelvic floor muscles change tension and configuration with sacral movement.

The head and neck are involved in sound and speech production. As previously discussed, air flows through from the lower respiratory tract to the trachea, larynx, between the vocal cords and then to the pharynx. It then exits through the oral and nasal cavities. On its way through the vocal tract it is also shaped into distinct sounds or words. The *articulator muscles* are responsible for this. They are located in the larynx, pharynx and mouth as well as all muscles associated with the *jaw, cheeks, teeth, gums, lips, palate and tongue.* The feeling and emotion associated with what we voice involves all of the *muscles of facial expression.* The *cranial sinuses* act as resonators for the sound produced by the vocal cords. These include the frontal, sphenoid, ethmoid and maxillary sinuses.

25.6   OUR BODIES ARE RESONATORS FOR SOUND

Here we must explore the concept of *space.* Just as it is required of the body to supply the nerve impulses, muscles and blood supply for the proper working of the vocal cords, it must also supply the room for them to work – the space. The body responsibly validates its purpose in vocalization by ensuring its fullest expression. We are well equipped with resonating cavities with which to express our words and song to all that is around us. Even the empty space within our bodies is hollowed with purpose, such as to carry and amplify its own voice.

Most musical instruments also contain *resonators* (empty spaces or cavities), which intensify the original sound waves to increase their strength or volume. *Resonance* occurs when the moving sound waves contact the sides of a cavity or chamber, causing *it* to vibrate and amplify the original sound waves. For example, the body of a guitar is an air-filled cavity. It resonates the sound produced from the plucked, vibrating guitar strings.

Our bodies' living resonators are quite remarkable compared with those of the guitar or other instruments, because they are not fixed in shape. They are flexible and dynamic. They can voluntarily change shape, thus having very fine control of the essence (tone, pitch and quality) of sound produced. Voice resonators are responsible for the idiosyncrasies that uniquely identify each one of our voices.

Our natural voice resonators include the "empty space" of the vocal tract itself – the larynx, pharynx, and oral and nasal cavities. The pharynx is a very effective resonator due to its flexibility. Whereas the oral cavity is largely involved in resonance of vowels and the nasal tract for consonants, *all* vocalized sounds have equal resonance through the pharynx. The dynamic nature of the pharynx is due to its interdependence on several surrounding structures, to include the larynx, velum, tongue and mandible.[9]

Other resonators include the frontal, sphenoid, ethmoid and maxillary sinuses. Research support for the function of paranasal sinuses as voice resonators is still underway[16] but personal experience tells us that they are resonators to at least some degree. When our sinuses are irritated or inflamed our voices change significantly. In fact, the sound of a blocked cranial sinus is very distinct and we can tell at once that the speaker has a cold or sinus inflammation.

25.7   THE VOCAL CORDS

The source of vocalized sound begins at the vocal cords. Vocal cords, or *vocal folds,* are tissue folds in the larynx that impart vibration onto the air flowing out of the lungs in order to produce sound. The *rima glottis* is the opening or space between the vocal folds. The geometry of the glottis is highly dynamic in that it changes in response to the position and tension of the laryngeal muscles and thus, the vocal folds.[7] Very detailed control of glottal geometry is necessary for speech and contributes to the individual nuances in each of our voices. It accounts for even subtle changes in intonation that convey great variation in meaning and emotion in language.

During normal breathing, the glottis is open, as air flows passively in and out of the lungs. The vocal cords are not tensed during relaxed breathing. The glottis is wide open, allowing free flow of air and full respiration. Sound produced here is due to passive air friction and not considered "voice."[7] It is the closure of the glottis (adduction of the vocal folds) causing resistance against the airflow that triggers the vocal cords to vibrate. We voluntarily tense the vocal cords when we speak, for example, which decreases the amount of space within (closes) the glottis. This in turn obstructs the airflow, which sets the vocal cords vibrating.

Phonation is the process of producing sound via the *alternating* opening and closing (vibration) of the vocal folds. The vocal folds open in response to high-velocity air pressure from the lungs. The vocal folds close as a result of the *Bernoulli effect*, which is a principle that is defined as "an increase in the speed of a fluid that occurs simultaneously with a decrease in its static pressure or potential energy."[17] What this means for phonation is that right after high air pressure from the lungs opens the vocal folds, the resultant decrease in pressure forces the vocal folds shut again. This action is repeated as air continues to stream through the vocal folds, causing the rhythmic opening and closing action (vibration)[9] (Figure 25.2).

25.7.1 Muscle Anatomy and Functions of Vocal Cords

The intrinsic laryngeal muscles are responsible for the detailed manipulation of glottal geometry (and vocal cord tension) that is needed for phonation (particularly for speech). This fine motor control of vocal fold position and glottal geometry must also instantaneously coordinate with thought, emotion, reasoning and response-related neurological networks in order for communication to occur fluently. Thus, the mind is involved, which takes us out of the physical body altogether. Vocal cords provide the perfect connection, or bridge, between the body and the mind.

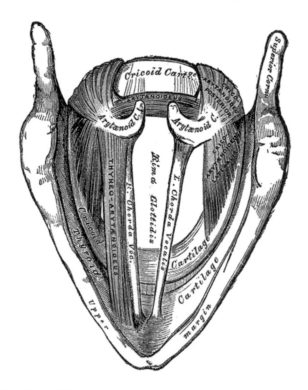

FIGURE 25.2 Superior view of the vocal cords showing the glottis (space between the vocal folds) and the intrinsic laryngeal muscles involved in vocal fold tension and control. (Image by Henry Vandyke Carter, Public domain, via Wikimedia Commons – https://commons.wikimedia.org/wiki/File:Gray960.png)

TABLE 25.1

Actions of the Major Intrinsic Laryngeal Muscles Involved in Vocalization

Muscle	Acton on Vocal Folds	Effect of Glottal Shape
Thyroarytenoid	Adducts	Closes
Transverse Arytenoid	Adducts	Closes
Posterior Cricoarytenoid	Abducts	Opens
Lateral Cricoarytenoid	Adducts	Closes
Vocalis	Tenses	None
Cricothyroid	Tenses	None

The vocal folds are attached to the arytenoid cartilages which articulate with the cricoid cartilage. There are controlled degrees of both rotational and sliding motions around the cricoarytenoid joint. There are motions along both a long and a short axis, very finely controlled.[7] When the intrinsic muscles of the larynx contract, they pull on the arytenoid cartilages, which causes them to pivot. The major muscles involved are the thyroarytenoid, lateral cricoarytenoid, posterior cricoarytenoid, interarytenoid and cricothyroid. All are innervated by the current laryngeal nerve except for the cricothyroid which is innervated by the superior laryngeal nerve. Both nerves are branches of the vagus nerve.[18] Contraction of the posterior cricoarytenoid muscle abducts the vocal cords, contributing to opening the rima glottis. The lateral cricoarytenoid muscle adducts the vocal cords, closing the rima glottis.[7] Table 25.1 outlines the actions of the major intrinsic laryngeal muscles involved in vocalization. Refer to Figure 25.2 for an illustration of them (Table 25.1).

25.7.2 VOCAL FOLD STRUCTURE

Contrary to what one might assume from the simple rope-like structures that we have traditionally seen from a superior view with a laryngoscope, the vocal cords are not just thin horizontally oriented strands. The vocal folds are comprised of an elaborate "three-dimensional" multilayered composite of highly differentiated tissue layers.[7] Each layer has highly specialized function so as to achieve the very fine control of vocal fold tension and position. Precision determines the glottal geometry which is necessary in order to convey the numerous, yet intricate and oftentimes subtle, nuances in vocal sounds, pitch, tone and parody that exist within languages. A very subtle difference in overtone can convey a great difference in meaning.

Figure 25.3 shows these layers. The deep layer is the vocalis muscle. Over that (more superficial) is a tissue layer that varies in thickness vertically (thicker at the top). Moving outward is the external mucosa, the superior portion of which is the vocal fold tip, composed of tissue similar to that of skin. A space exists just beneath the external mucosal layer, Reinke's space, permitting autonomous movement of the external mucosal layer, free from the other tissue layers. The vocal folds are highly elastic. It is this quality plus the freedom of movement of the external mucosal layer that allows them to vibrate at very high frequencies.[8]

25.7.3 WAVE MOTION OF THE VOCAL CORDS

Notice the tissue differentiation both medial-laterally *and* vertically. It is this quality of vertical tissue differentiation plus the ability of the external mucosal layer to move independently that permits a vertical change in air pressure. There is a "vertical phase difference in vocal fold surface motion." This is also called a "mucosal wave" that is happening only at the *surface* layer along the longitudinal (vertical) length of the vocal fold mucosa. During vibration this surface layer moves in and out in

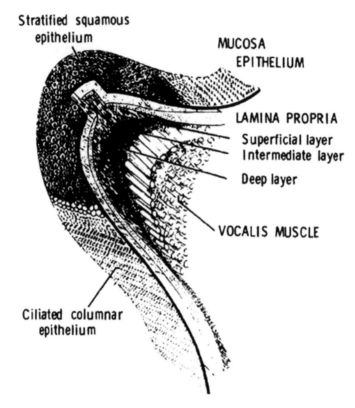

FIGURE 25.3 Schematic depicting the three-dimensional structure of the vocal folds. (Reprinted with kind permission from Henrich, N., *Logopedics Phoniatrics Vocology*, 31, 15–16, 2006.)

a repetitive motion. However, the entire longitudinal length of this layer does not necessarily vibrate as one unit.[7] Motion varies at each level and synchronizes as a wave-like movement.

25.7.4 THE GREAT UNKNOWN

Nerve impulses from the brain control the muscles that alter the *position and tension* of the vocal cords, but they cannot account for the *vibration*. Although it seems apparent that airflow between the vocal folds starts them vibrating, it is still not known what *sustains* the vibrations. Hence, the actual "origin of vocal cord vibration" is still not known. It was postulated by a French speech and language therapist, Raoul Husson, in 1950 that each vocal cord vibration is stimulated by a single impulse from the recurrent laryngeal nerve.[19] But this theory doesn't hold up, because brain-to-vocal cord nerve impulse transmission cannot attain the high speeds at which the vocal cords are capable of vibrating. At high pitches nerve transmission speed simply cannot keep up with the vocal cords. Therefore, it is not purely the work of nerve impulses that causes vocal cord vibration.[8]

The "myoelastic-aerodynamic theory," previously proposed in 1958 by Dutch speech scientist Jan Willem van den Berg, accounts for vocal fold vibrations, but with obvious unknowns. Although it describes an apparent energy transfer between the *vocal folds and the air itself*, which is the basis of "self-sustained" vocal fold vibration, exactly *how* the exchange occurs has still not been found. But it seems clear that energy is transferred from the airflow to the vocal cords due to differences in intraglottal pressure between the opening and closing phases of vocal cord vibration.[7]

Despite the remaining mystery of how vocal cords are able to sustain vibrations at such high frequencies, we can rest assured that whatever the answer, it seems to be at least somewhat governed by the laws of Mother Nature. The human female voice, for example, has a fundamental frequency range of 165–255 Hz[20] which includes that of the average wing beat frequency of honeybees, at about 230 Hz.[21] We will explore in the next section how the articulation, or *shape*, of our voices also aligns with nature … as the expression of speech sound.

25.8   SPEECH SOUND

Speech is a universal means of expression for the human soul.

Rudolf Steiner

Speech is the glue of society. It is the glue within and between all cultures. Although a vast number of species on earth communicate in some way via sound, the human species is the only one that articulates sound into intellectually and emotionally meaningful content. It is quite extraordinary that from the moment of *birth* we are in full use of our vocal cords. Our very first exhalation results in a cry, the first expression of our own unique sound.

However, even before birth, long before we have the ability to *produce* sound, the formative processes of embryogenesis have already prioritized developing the means by which to *hear* it. Humans have the ability to hear *before birth*. We are able to listen to speech originating outside the womb in order to prepare for speaking it at a later time in life.[22]

The first signs of embryological development of the ear are visible to us at about 4 weeks of gestation. They begin as two *otic placodes*, one on each side of the cephalad end of the neural tube. These are essentially metabolic fields of thickened ectoderm created as a result of the compressive forces at play during neural groove development. These metabolic fields serve as "gardens" for further growth and development of the ears.[23]

It has been shown that fetuses can begin to hear sounds originating outside the womb sometime during the second trimester of pregnancy.[24] Studies have reported evidence of fetuses hearing extrauterine sounds as early as 18–19 weeks of gestation.[25] Research outcomes support that the first acoustic stimuli sensed by the developing fetus are its mother's own voice and heartbeat. The fetus actually recognizes its mother's voice by the third trimester and responds to it (versus another voice) autonomically with an increased heart rate.[26]

The fetus has an innate preference for its mother's sounds. It has been shown that prenatal exposure to the maternal voice, versus any other voice, "stimulates language related cortical regions of the brain." Perceiving the mother's heartbeat and voice increases the neuroplasticity of the auditory cortex and stimulates both the language and emotional processing areas of the brain (orbitofrontal cortex and amygdala). What the fetus hears affects memory storage and sets up neural connections for further development of hearing and learning language after birth.[26] The outcomes of these studies reveal to us the close developmental relationship between hearing, speaking and emotional processing.

25.8.1   SPEECH LEARNING IN INFANCY

Let's consider these conclusions along with those of Guenther's research, published in 2006, which describes the mechanism of speech learning after birth. In doing so we can presume that during early fetal development we are already preparing for *speaking after birth*. And this "preparing" begins with hearing.

Generating speech and language requires the coordination of neuronal activity between a multitude of areas located in both the cortical and subcortical brain. These areas include, but are most likely not limited to, the temporal, parietal and frontal lobes of the cerebral cortex for the auditory, somatosensory and motor aspects of speech sounds, respectively. The subcortical structures include the cerebellum, basal ganglia and brain stem, which accommodate the vast number of neuronal interconnections at the rapid speeds required in order to achieve real-time fluency in speech. This degree of intricacy is required in order to generate even very simple speech sounds. Imagine the complexity involved in orchestrating the *additional* synapses necessary for incorporating the thought, intention and emotion required for meaningful, fluent speech.[27]

During infancy the first step in speech production is a "babbling phase," where indiscriminate sounds are vocalized in order to calibrate the neurologic feedback system between sensory and motor functions. When an infant hears a sound, this *perception* results in activation of a small group of neurons which collectively become associated (and activated) with only that sound. This phase of speech learning establishes a neurosensory–motor feedback mapping system with which to later learn *specific* speech sounds and eventually, an entire language.[27]

It's important to note that *hearing* sounds first is important in speech learning and development. When sounds are heardthey initiate synaptic activity to the auditory cortex of the brain. There, "auditory targets" for each sound are developed. They are then stored in memory and will be utilized as a guide for future vocalized attempts at mimicking those sounds. Hearing a sound (sensory) stimulates the same group of neurons that are later involved in speaking (motor) that same sound. In other words, the same group of neurons synapse for both hearing and producing any particular sound. This synaptic connection is the result of *mirror neurons*.[27]

Mirror neurons play a huge role in mirroring another's actions, which is what occurs when infants are learning to speak. Similar to hearing and speech, the same group of mirror neurons fire when an individual *performs* an action as when she/he *observes* another person doing that same action. Evidence also suggests that they help infants understand the empathy and intention behind another's actions. Mirror neurons were first discovered in monkeys and are not exclusive to humans.[28]

As an infant voices garble in its attempts to "hit" an auditory target it becomes more and more accurate with each try. There is an error feedback system that senses any difference between the attempt and what was actually voiced. As volume, tone, pitch and articulator muscle accuracy improves, each attempt gets closer and closer to its target. Once it is "hit," i.e., the word is spoken with enough accuracy, the error feedback system is no longer activated. It no longer picks up a difference between the target and what was voiced. At that point a neurological *feed forward system* is established for that word. Eventually, fluency within the entire language is obtained.[27]

As far as I have discovered, hearing is the only sense, aside from touch, that picks up stimuli across the different dimensions of fluid media on either side of the womb. Touch, however, does not convey the cognitive and emotional information that sound does. Hearing allows us the ability *in utero* to perceive information in preparation for life outside of the womb. Thus, *sound* bridges the abrupt transformation of life from one fluid medium to another – from liquid to air.

25.8.2 THE POWER OF THE WORD

Once we transition to a life in air, we exist in a medium that connects us to everything else within it. Air is freedom and expansion, but at the same time it is exposure and vulnerability. No longer does the liquid compartment of the womb protect us from earth's atmosphere at large, where all other elements are shifted and transformed through the volatile quality of air.

Knowing what it's like to be human, the ego-possessing, opinionated, emotional creatures that we are, it may seem obvious that our bodies would highly prioritize the ability to hear and speak – *to communicate*. Speech, after all, may be the glue of society, but it can also be a repellant between societies, cultures and families. Given the degree of genetic planning in making sure that at the time of hearing development *in utero*, we are already getting the neurologic connections ready for language skills after birth, we cannot assume for one second that the privilege of speech affords us simply the ability to "get our points across to others." Perhaps there is more to the evolutionary privilege of speech with which our species has been blessed.

Perhaps there is more power in our words than most of us realize. Sure, given the array of emotions such as compassion, love, guilt or rage that words can trigger in others, they certainly have the power to stimulate reactions and result in change. However, thanks to the extraordinary work of a few philosophers, teachers and scientists, it is becoming more and more evident that our words have the power to manifest much more change (and much faster) than we have ever realized.

Next, I present the work of a few extraordinary minds that have helped bring to the surface of human awareness the remembrance of our species' true power of being – the power of the word.

25.8.3 VISIBLE SPEECH – AERODYNAMIC SOUND FORMS

It was Rudolph Steiner (1861–1925), an influential Australian philosopher and esotericist, who first theorized in the early 1900s that spoken words are expressed as "visible sound forms." Even without the equipment at that time to scientifically explore laboratory evidence for this, he was able to "see" them forming their own unique shapes in air as they exited the mouth.[8]

Steiner believed that not only does speech express itself as air form, but it also expresses itself through *body* form. Speech can also be expressed both artistically and in a healing capacity through body gestures and movement. This concept became one of the core bases for a healing practice that he developed and named *therapeutic*, or *curative, eurythmy*.[29] Steiner voiced his hope that someday a method would become available to observe the speech air forms. This would help support the core principles of therapeutic eurythmy.[8]

Decades later, in the 1960s, Johanne Zinke (1901 to 1990), a German Waldorf School teacher in Dresden, attempted to find out if Steiner's theories were valid. By using cigarette smoke to illuminate the developing air forms, she was able to visualize, photograph and video record *air shaping into forms* just outside the mouth during speech. She validated Steiner's theory of "visible sound forms!"[8]

But even more astonishing is that these "speech sound figures" proved to be *reproducible*. Each "spoken sound" consistently formed its own *unique flow pattern in air* independent of other factors, such as volume and speaker. Interestingly, the air flow patterns moved in *vortices*. Each sound seemed to be its own process of forming, unfolding and dissolving spirals into the surrounding atmosphere. These "external phonatory turbulences" show that speech is more complex than just any sound. Here, an important distinction must be made between sound and speech sound. Whereas *sound* is vibration, *speech sound* is more than vibration – it is *gesture*.[8]

With great foresight Steiner had actually detailed the exact shape morphology of certain sounds. The more sophisticated laboratory equipment necessary to see and record the air forms was available to Zinke. We now know that he did in fact describe the air form patterns with astounding accuracy. The images in Figures 25.4 and 25.5 show Zinke's photos of the sound forms of two of the five vowels with Steiner's predictions of their shapes 50 years earlier. The images presented here are screen shots taken from a video by speech scientist Serge Maintier, PhD, that accompanies his book *Speech: Invisible Creation in the Air*.[30] Time stamps are included to allow the reader to easily locate the image in the video (Figure 25.4 Figure 25.5).

These images are still shots of Zinke's video of the air form for the vowel "ah" (Figure 25.4) and the vowel "ē" (Figure 25.5) with Steiner's own words describing what he thought the air forms would look like. For the vowel "ah," he described: "As an air gesture, this ah is shaped by a stream of air that flows outward but then becomes bowl shaped as it encounters the density of the air outside." For the vowel "ē," he described: "When we speak ē we basically let it develop right at the front of mouth which gives it a sharply tapering energy. The ē streams out into the density of the external air in form of a sharp arrow-like jet of air, like a sword cleaving the external air."[30]

The revolutionary work of Serge Maintier, PhD, a German speech artist, scientist and Waldorf teacher in Germany, confirmed Zinke's findings with intriguing accuracy. He also expanded upon her work by showing incredibly detailed "morphodynamics" of the air flow patterns and by revealing the phenomenon of "coarticulation in speech."

He used a high-speed camera, laser light and a microphone to simultaneously monitor the sounds' movements as they were being spoken. He used oscilloscope and spectrogram recordings to track the sounds' voltages (vocal cord vibration) and signal strengths ("loudness"), respectively, over time.

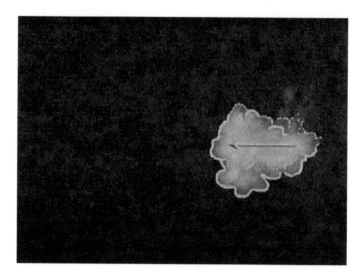

FIGURE 25.4 Time stamp 7:24 from www.youtube.com/watch?v=i6eFtohBEWA 21 (From Maintier, S., Accompanying video to *Speech, invisible creation in the air.*)

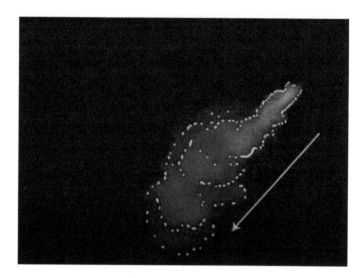

FIGURE 25.5 Time stamp 10:43 from www.youtube.com/watch?v=i6eFtohBEWA 21 (From Maintier, S., Accompanying video to *Speech, invisible creation in the air.*)

He also added audio to the recordings, a missing component in Zinke's experiments. In doing this he was able to capture what these air formations *sounded and looked like* as they were being spoken and heard simultaneously. Analyzing such detailed morphodynamics along with audio allowed him to reveal the "temporal connection" between *vision and sound*.[8] Figure 25.6 shows the beautifully detailed morphology of a voiced vowel "ē."

25.8.4 COARTICULATION IN SPEECH

Maintier also demonstrated the concept of coarticulation in speech. Coarticulation refers to the changes in air flow patterns of sounds that occur with pairing vowels and consonants together. A particular vowel's air shape pattern, for example, changes depending on its preceding or following consonant. Likewise, what comes before or after a consonant may change its flow pattern as well.[30]

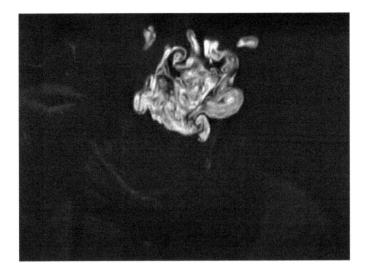

FIGURE 25.6 Time stamp 1:05:40. This is a still shot example of the detail and complexity of the air form patterns that Maintier was able to capture. The vortices are clearly visible. This is the sound of the vowel "ɛ." Image from www.youtube.com/watch?v=i6eFtohBEWA (From Maintier, S., Accompanying video to *Speech, invisible creation in the air.*)

Figure 25.7 shows the variation of air forms of the consonant "k" (which is very sensitive to coarticulation) with various preceding vowels.

In showing the correlation of pronunciation of vowels paired with consonants in relation to the intention of the human being, let's look at two sounds that were examined in Maintier's video: "an" (pronounced "ahn") and "na" (pronounced "nah"). The air forms of the vowel "ah" and the consonant "n" each reveal very different qualities depending on where they are placed in the syllable. [30]

When "an" is voiced, the air form of "a" is soft and "n" is strong. When "na" is voiced, the air form of "n" is soft and "a" is strong. We may be able to hear these differences, but even more interesting is that we can see them in the air forms. Because these air formations were difficult to capture in screen shots, I will refer you to Maintier's video at the *time stamp 21:19* that shows the air forms of both syllables.[30]

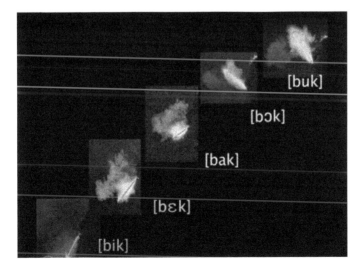

FIGURE 25.7 Time stamp 39:03. This still shot shows coarticulation of the consonant /k/. There is great variation of the air forms with various preceding vowels. Image from https://www.youtube.com/watch?v=i6eFtohBEWA (From Maintier, S., Accompanying video to *Speech, invisible creation in the air.*)

The field of linguistics has previously shown that "vocalization is most active in the vowel core of the syllable." Yet, when voicing "an," the vowel here seems calmed by the following consonant. Rudolf Steiner, decades before, said that the sound "an" causes us to "hold back into ourselves," to "linger within." In order to calm the strength of the vowel we follow it with a consonant that captures it to "go within."[30]

If we reverse the syllable, we see that the forces of each sound are also reversed. When voicing "na," the shape of the "a" here is strong. It's almost as if the consonant is "throwing" the vowel, or setting it free, rather than capturing it as it did with pronouncing "an." Steiner's words 50 or so years prior said that when we say the sound "na," "we merge to the outer world."[30]

25.8.5 THE NASAL CAVITY

With consonants, in some cases, the lips are closed, forcing the exhaled air through the nose. Video reveals that air exhaled through the nasal cavities during vocalization is also spiraled. Voicing the consonant "m," for example, completely closes the lips. All air is forced through both nasal cavities, creating two vortex jets (Figure 25.8). Due to the lack of flexibility and articulator muscles like those contained in the oral cavity, the nasal cavity spirals its airflow with the shape and position of the nasal turbinates.[30]

The effect of nasal turbinates is to increase the contact surface area for air to warm and humidify as it is *inhaled* through the nasal cavity. The concha bones themselves are spiral shaped. This further increases the surface area but also *spins the air flow into vortices*. Vortical flow results in turbulence, allowing more vigorous contact with the mucosal walls, slowing due to the chaotic nature of the flow, and increased time for air mixing and filtering before it enters further *into* the body through the respiratory tract[31] (Figure 25.9).

Let's recall that Zinke and Maintier have demonstrated that *exhaled* air (speech) is spiraled. But why would air need mixing on its way *out* of the body? In answering this question, we refer back to Maintier's work which has shown us the true "gesture like nature of speech sound."

25.8.6 SPEECH IS GESTURE

As the video tracking shows, these "external phonatory disturbances" are continually transforming vortices, forever unfolding, even as they dissolve away into the open atmosphere.[8] Whether speech

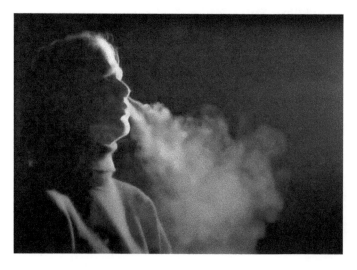

FIGURE 25.8 Two spirals right outside the nostrils with pronunciation of the consonant "mm." Image from https://www.youtube.com/watch?v=i6eFtohBEWA (From Maintier, S., Accompanying video to *Speech, invisible creation in the air.*)

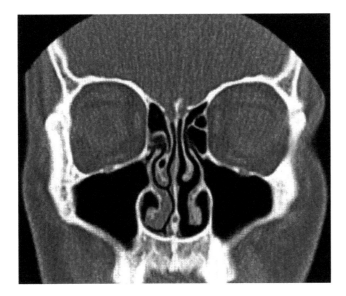

FIGURE 25.9 In a computed tomography front view cross section of a normal nose, notice the spiral shaped conchae. (Image obtained and modified for resolution quality from Wikimedia Commons contributors, "File: NormalNose-CT-Front-cross-section-common-wiki.jpg," *Wikimedia Commons, the free media repository,* https://commons.wikimedia.org/w/index.php?title=File:NormalNose-CT-Front-cross-section-common-wiki .jpg&oldid=487315137 (accessed March 10, 2021).)

exits the mouth or the nares, it is vortexed; it *gestures* as it leaves the body. The boundless realm of ether receives the spiraling speech forms and absorbs them as they fade and then disappear from our visible and audible spectrums. Butthey still exist in the effects they create.

Air is the medium on which the arrow of speech soars. Our ears are the target. When we say something, we have a reason to be heard. We have a target audience, a target purpose. Speech is *gesture*; it is sound *actualizing*. As it enters the atmosphere it begins the actual formative process of creating what we say. *But how?* As we have already discussed, the language of the universe is vibration, motion. The language between human beings is vibration with *gesture*, the *vortex*.

25.9 THE VORTEX – A PHENOMENON OF NATURE

The vortex is a natural phenomenon found in all of nature. It has no mass and consists entirely of energy – it is pure motion. Vortices themselves are invisible, but we can see their *motion* in nature's fluid mediums. In physics, simply put, fluids are defined as substances that cannot stop flowing against an applied external force. Fluids are liquids, gases and plasmas.

Vortices are the result of contrast. They occur when two or more fluid mediums of differing make-up, quality or behavior meet. The purpose of the vortex is to buffer opposing forces until there is harmony amongst the elements. Both "pools of substance" are changed in the mixing, even if only a little bit. And in a world that pretty much *is* contrast, the purpose of the vortex is to *integrate*.[32]

We see vortices in water when a mountain stream flows into a lake of dissimilar composition. We see them in air as winds of varying pressure and temperature collide. We can see vortices in the fluids and particles that they displace, such as the dust and debris of a tornado and the star dust and interstellar gases that reveal the spiraling formation of galaxies.

In my own words, *the vortex is the great integrator of life*. It creates the turbulent chaotic state necessary for allotting sufficient space-time for all mixing parties of various composition to agree, or at least compromise. It is the peacemaker between all that is.

How does this relate to speech? Speech "exists solely in the element of air," which is the element that connects all terrestrial things on earth. Air is a fluid medium and behaves as such, forming vortices as it blends. Likewise, the speech carried on that air follows the same laws of fluid dynamics in nature – it spirals. We see the great integrator at work with the human voice just as it is with everything else. Only this time, we are integrating sound gestures that carry deliberate intent and the power to create.

> *Air is the medium on which the arrow of speech soars.*
> *Speech is the medium on which the arrow of intent soars.*

Speech is the carrier of change. Just as a small body of streaming of water forms a vortex as it meets a larger one, so do our words as they flow into the open atmosphere. Our words fulfill themselves as blooming vortices to alchemize with all that is around them. They blend with the words and intentions of all other humans, to ultimately rest on one collective reality. It is likely that each speaker's words change the collective whole to a small degree and their own personal experience to a larger degree.

The power of the word is buffered in its degree of materialization. What we say will be manifested only to the extent allowed by an intelligence much greater than our own. When we speak meaning and intention that emits a vibration in close proximity to that of nature, the tangible results of our desires seem easier and greater. There is less opposition between the two mixing substances.

Although weather and galaxies can eventually agree, unfortunately, it seems, humans cannot. But we cannot hurt ourselves *too* much … not immediately, anyway. Our words, no matter what their intention, are buffered in their blending before coming to fruition with the current state of perceived reality of the collective human consciousness. Thus, we can thank our lucky stars for this great buffering system that even protects us from ourselves.

Not only that, but the respiration required for voicing anything insists that we oxygenate our blood. Whether in the act of voicing empathy or antipathy, it is required that we vitalize our bodies with oxygen at the same time. Thus, even voicing negative gestures sustains our own lives. Thankfully we will feel the dissonance of these two contradictory events, and the worst harm is done to ourselves.

Voicing anything also contributes to the wellbeing of *other* life forms, as those gestures are carried on the carbon dioxide we exhale as a product of speech. Even negative words offer vital nutrients to other beings on earth with which we are in symbiotic relationship via gas exchange. No matter what we say or do, *we must breathe*. No matter how hard we try we cannot be all bad, because the very fact that we *live* requires that we harmonize with the natural world.

25.10   THE CREATIVE POWER OF SPEECH IN ANCIENT ARTWORK

Support for the notion that spoken words become our reality is seen not only in their formation of vortical gestures but in the great complexity of them. The great work of Zinke and Maintier has shown us that the variations between even just voiced *syllables* show vast, yet uniquely identifying, changes in their aerodynamic behaviors and three-dimensional shape formations. Even a simple syllable knows what it is! And it *becomes* itself as it is voiced. It is added to the collective reality of life experience on earth and perhaps even within the whole universe.

It seems that ancient cultures already knew this. The spiral is seen throughout ancient drawings, sculptures and even enormous works of architecture across the globe. Ancient civilizations on every continent have left evidence of their knowledge of the significance of the vortex. And they took great effort in displaying this wisdom in the form of art and architecture. Was this because, like speech, all artistic expressions have the power to manifest? Or was it because they somehow knew that humanity would turn, would *forget* the power of their own being?

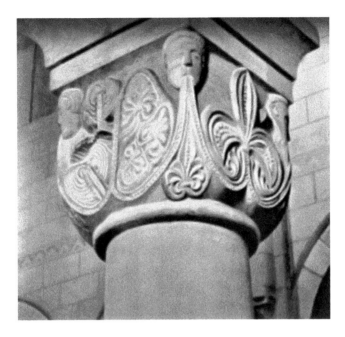

FIGURE 25.10 Time stamp 1:08:45. The "spirits of the four corners of the earth," Romanesque capital in the church of Oberstenfeld. Image from https://www.youtube.com/watch?v=i6eFtohBEWA (From Maintier, S., Accompanying video to *Speech, invisible creation in the air.*)

Figure 25.10 shows the Romanesque capital in the church of Oberstenfeld. It shows the creation of life forms and sustenance with speech. I came across this picture in Theodor Schwenk's book *Sensitive Chaos* and in Serge Maintier's video. I use it again here because it literally shows the manifesting power of speech. The ancients knew this before Rudolf Steiner himself spoke of it and before Zinke and Maintier validated it. This surviving artwork supports their findings, hundreds or even thousands of years later.

Figure 25.11 is an image of the Vézelay Marie-madeleine South Nave capital showing "The Spirits of the Four Winds" using antique bellows to blow creation into being. Wind, the element of air, was used to create and to connect heaven and earth. A further look into the symbolism on one face of the architecture shows one human clothed and the other naked, indicating transformation.[33]

The ancients portrayed the power of speech in their art. There is also an art to speech. Its craft is in its precision. Its precision intensifies power. Just as a laser is condensed light, spoken words are condensed commands. We can *choose* our words, organize them and vary their content to thoughtfully craft the architecture of our own lives. Wouldn't *all* forms of art allow us to do this? Is it possible that the artistic expression of the human being in any form is a means through which we manifest?

Our vocal tracts are instruments that can be played to create anything we choose. If we have the power within us to have such great effects with just syllables, then what about with words? Sentences? Stories? And how does this change with intention and emotion? The power of the word can cultivate unity or it can create war. All wars begin with words. They begin with a simple exchange of words between parties that do not agree. And then further exchange of words can create insults, anger, threats. We can use our words in any way we wish. Human beings have *conscious choice*. We can premeditate what we want and then create it. Even if we don't agree we can create balance. I don't think we're even supposed to agree! We have all heard the well-known philosophy of many ancient sages that the whole purpose of our life experience is to learn how to come together in tolerance and compromise. As in the natural selection and mixing of genetic pools biologically, the greater the variation between the individuals compromising to create one community, the greater its collective intelligence. The greater its potential.

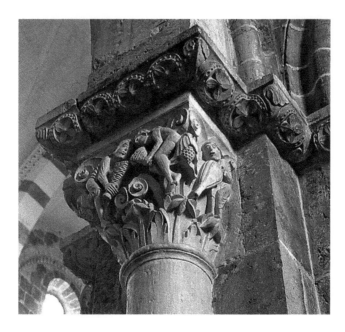

FIGURE 25.11   "The Spirits of the Four Winds" at Vézelay Marie-madeleine South Nave capital. "The Four Cardinal Points" represented gateways between man and the heavens, where the Winds could enter man's world. (Image used with kind permission from https://compostela.co.uk/symbols/vezelay-spirits-four-winds/

25.11   THE SENSORY CYCLE

Earlier in the chapter we discussed human hearing and speech development both in utero and during infancy. In researching this process something quite extraordinary occurred to me. This highly resembles an ancient and very sacred "call and response" type of healing practice known as *kirtan* (which we will discuss later in the chapter). Speech learning in infancy is a form of *kirtan*. It is *the first kirtan*, for which we are preparing to participate even before birth.

To me, this demonstrates a genetically prioritized *sensory cycle* between hearing and speech. Embryogenesis determines that both hearing something and speaking it are controlled by the exact same nerve bundle. More specifically, hearing *our own speech* is the only means by which we can assess its quality. As infants we must *self-assess* our own speech in order to mimic auditory targets to learn language and perfect the accuracy of our speech. As adults we must self-assess our own speech in order to improve not its accuracy but its *content*. It is the content of our speech that reflects its intention, which then reveals our state of mental and emotional health.

25.11.1   THE MIRROR OF THE SOUL

Through voice, our thoughts are manifested into physical waves and spirals that apply force to *all* ear drums within audible range. These vibrations ultimately end up as perceptions in the brain that affect emotions and may even cause *others* to react. *What we say actually vibrates a physical part of someone else's body.* What we say must be self-assessed, as we have such great power to potentially affect all that is around us.

Sensing our own voice allows us to "see" ourselves, moment to moment, through what we say. Once voiced aloud, the impact of our words can become stark, and oftentimes, we regret what we say. Speech has great power in intention, yet it is ethereal and can be instantaneously corrected. In the form of speech, then, sound becomes our truest and most malleable mirror. It becomes the mirror that reflects back to us the image of our own intentions. *Speech is the mirror of the soul.*

Through our speech, we can receive wisdom from higher sources. Have you ever *really* understood or realized something only after you have voiced it to someone else or an audience? The popular notion that teaching something helps us to learn it is true. It is because when we say something aloud, we can "see" it. When lecturing to an audience about a subject that inspires us, we sometimes spontaneously incorporate brand new information right there in the moment. This knowledge is coming from a higher source, channeled to us via the open doors that we create through inspired action. And it's not just speech through which we channel. It can be done through any form of inspired art. But it is the *sound* we produce that allows us to *hear* ourselves. We can then access the most receptive sensory cycle organ, *the ear*, poised perfectly to reflect our innermost state of wellbeing.

25.12 THE EAR

Although not involved in sound *production,* the ear is involved in sound perception and interpretation. Primitively, the ear is one of the most delicate yet crucial sensory organs necessary for human (and land-dwelling vertebrate) survival. This is evident, at least in part, from its highly protected and hidden location. As we voyage through the three main compartments of the ear we retreat further and further away from the outer world towards the center of the cranium, where its most sensitive parts are encased in the hardest bone found in the human body.[34]

Dr. Maintier describes three routes of "dialogue between the ear and larynx," ways in which our own voices come back to us. Our voice travels to our own ears via air directly from mouth to ear and after it has been modified by the surrounding environment on its way to our ears. Vocal vibrations are also conducted from their source at the vocal cords directly through the bones of the skull[8] to the cochlea via the otic capsule (the bony labyrinth) of the inner ear.[35] Figure 25.12 shows a schematic of the outer, middle and inner ear.

25.12.1 THE EXTERNAL EAR

In sensing our own sound, the spiraling air forms of speech are introduced to the ear via another spiral – the inward spiral of the auricle. Again, the mirror – the resting inward spiral – receives its mirror image, the vortexing outward spiral. Stillness receives motion. Even in life experience, quiet perception receives answers.

The auricle of the external ear funnels sound waves into the external auditory canal, where they are oriented to "hit" the ear drum/tympanic membrane (TM) at right angles (so that sounds retain their relative frequencies).[36] This causes the TM to vibrate, thereby starting a chain reaction of transmission through various mediums that carry the sound waves on a "journey through the elements."[32]

Let's now take that journey to discover how the human body converts airborne sound waves into brain perceptions. It does this by first amplifying the wave's force, but only to break it in the cochlea, thereby sending it on a succession of transduction events which end up as nerve impulses to the brain that affect our interpretation and impressions of the environment around us.

25.12.2 THE MIDDLE EAR

Via the TM the pressure waves are passed from air to the bones in the middle ear. Here, we see the conversion of wave energy to mechanical energy. The main goal of the middle ear is to provide "impedance transference"[36] of the sound waves, which matches each sound wave's pressure with the increased force needed to transition it from air to the denser fluid/membrane medium of the inner ear. The vibrations are amplified as they are passed along a chain of ossicles, the malleus, incus and stapes, that act as "mechanical levers" to increase and concentrate the wave energy.[34] There is also an increase in acoustic energy as the pressure waves travel from the large TM to the stapes

The Internal Ear

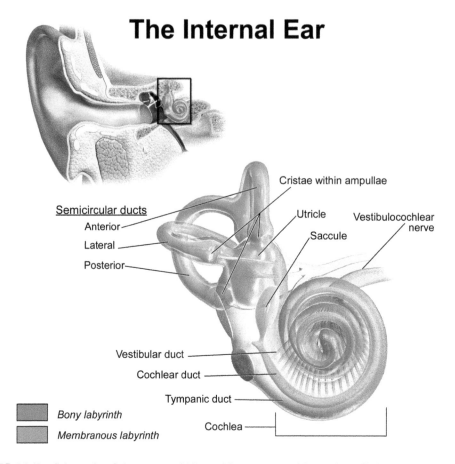

FIGURE 25.12 Schematic of the outer, middle and inner ear; cochlea and vestibular apparatus. (Image modified for resolution optimization from original source: Wikimedia Commons contributors, "File:Blausen 0329 EarAnatomy InternalEar.png," *Wikimedia Commons, the free media repository,* https://commons.wiki-media.org/w/index.php?title=File:Blausen_0329_EarAnatomy_InternalEar.png&oldid=501289841 (accessed March 10, 2021).)

footplate that contacts the small oval window.[36] The decrease in area between the TM and the oval window increases wave pressure, contributing to the increased force needed to match each specific frequency as it passes into the fluid environment of the cochlea.

25.12.3 The Inner Ear

The inner ear is comprised of a bony labyrinth that houses the organs of hearing and balance, the cochlea and vestibular apparatus. Together, they reside in a membranous labyrinth that floats inside the bony one. Just as the brain and spinal cord are protected within the buoyant fluid environment of CSF, so is the endolymph filled *membranous labyrinth* as it floats within the liquid perilymph of the *bony labyrinth*.[37] The perilymph communicates directly[38] and the endolymph indirectly[39] with the CSF. In this way the inner ear brings the soul's reflection of sound deep within the cranium to be gazed upon by the most intimate parts of ourselves – the central nervous system.

The cochlea is a conical fluid-filled cavity within the bony labyrinth that contains the sensory organ for hearing (the organ of Corti). Its job is to convert the altered sound waves delivered by the ear ossicles into electrical energy to be transmitted as nerve impulses via the auditory nerve to the brain. The cochlea consists of three liquid compartments running in parallel, all coiling together,

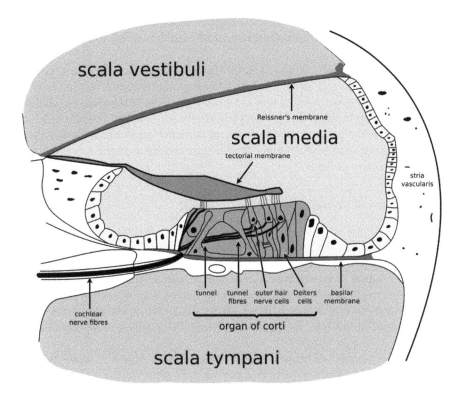

FIGURE 25.13 Cross section of the cochlea, which shows the three fluid compartments and the organ of Corti. (Image modified for resolution quality from Wikimedia Commons contributors, "File:Cochlea-cross-section.svg," *Wikimedia Commons, the free media repository,* https://commons.wikimedia.org/w/index.php ?title=File:Cochlea-crosssection.svg&oldid=510916813 (accessed March 10, 2021).)

forming a spiral of about 2.5 turns (in humans).[34] The two perilymph-filled chambers, the scala vestibuli and scala tympani, are divided by the endolymph-filled scala media flowing between them (see Figure 25.13) The ionic composition of each pool of fluid varies, the endolymph-filled scala media being very high in potassium and the perilymph high in sodium.[40]

The organ of Corti comprises specialized sensory epithelia consisting of outer and inner sensory hair cells situated along the length of the basilar membrane, a dividing barrier between the endolymph and perilymph compartments, as shown in Figure 25.13. Each hair cell has stereocilia embedded at its apex that project into and are bathed in the potassium-rich endolymph of the scala media.[41] The stereocilia project upward and close to, but not touching, the overlying *tectorial membrane.*

Through the oval window, which sits at the base of the cochlea, mechanical vibrations from the middle ear enter the scala vestibuli and propagate as traveling waves along the basilar membrane of the cochlea, from its base toward its apex.[40] Each wave "breaks" at a place along the cochlea that corresponds with its wavelength (frequency). The cochlea is frequency mapped so that high-pitched sounds that have shorter wavelengths break at the base of the cochlea, shortly after they enter the perilymph. Low-pitched sounds with longer wavelengths travel further and break closer to the apex.[37]

The outer sensory cells of the organ of Corti are disturbed at the point at which the wave breaks along the basilar membrane, thereby opening pores and exposing them to the high-potassium environment of the endolymph above them. The potassium-rich endolymph has high positive electrical potential[42] which depolarizes the cells. The outer cells *muscle contract* towards the inner cell hair cells, and due to the wave break elevating them, their stereocilia touch and move the tectorial membrane. Through the endolymph, this force is passed to the inner hair cells, disturbing and depolarizing them as well.[37] This causes the release of neurotransmitters which trigger action potentials in the auditory nerve.[41]

If we glimpse a bird's eye view of this "journey through the elements" we can see the energy transduction from sound waves in air, to mechanical energy via osseous levers in the middle ear, to fluid traveling waves, to muscle contraction and electrical energy in the inner ear, and finally, to nerve action potentials that travel to the brain. As beautifully portrayed by Theodor Schwenk in his book *Sensitive Chaos*, "The passage into the cavity of the inner ear is like a journey through the elements, from air via the solid medium to the liquid, and every form on the way reveals its origin in the archetypal movement of fluids."[32]

25.12.4 THE VESTIBULAR SYSTEM

The vestibular system senses head movement and acceleration via two types of end organs, the cristae and maculae, respectively. The membranous vestibule consists of three fluid-filled semicircular canals, a utricle and a saccule, all housed together with the cochlea within the bony labyrinth of the inner ear. Head rotation in various planes of motion is sensed by the cristae located within the ampulla of the semicircular canals. Acceleration along various axes of motion is detected by the maculae, also known as the otolith organs, which are located in the utricle and saccule. The utricle and saccule are housed in the bony recesses that separate the vestibule from the cochlea.[40] (See Figure 25.12.)

Why are the sensory organs of hearing and movement housed together? Both the cristae and maculae are specialized sensory epithelia that contain hair cells similar to those found in the cochlea.[40] The hair cells of the vestibular system sense *body* motion, whereas the hair cells of the cochlea sense *wave* motion. In my thinking, the common denominator here is *movement*. They develop and evolve together because they are both sensing *motion*. And since everything in the universe is motion (vibration), then this sensory ability is of the utmost importance. The vestibular apparatus senses motion of the head – movement originating *within* the body. The cochlea senses vibrations in the form of sound waves originating *outside* the body.

25.13 VOICE AS A HEALING INSTRUMENT

Now that you see how the expressed air forms of speech sound affect us from without and all that is around us, let us explore how we can harness the power of voice to affect and heal us *within*.

Since ancient times, the power of voice has been utilized for purposes way more expansive than inter-human communication. It is true that voice is the root of language, the glue between cultures. However, the human voice may also be used as a *self-healing musical instrument*.

It is even theorized that early man's first spoken language was sung, and it mimicked the sounds of nature. More evidence can simply be observed in children, who oftentimes instinctively sing their sentences and move their bodies in playful (or agitated) romping rhythms in sync with the melody of their mood.[43] Music is instinctively expressed through our every motion at every turn. As Wallace Stevens writes in his poem "Life Is Motion," our body's movements and actions become our dance with life, our "marriage between air and flesh."[44] Withal, our body's voice becomes our song of life, our marriage between air and self-expression.

Most, if not all, ancient cultures such as Hindu, Tibetan, Chinese, Sumerian, African, Egyptian and others, practiced some form of self-healing with voice. Although not performed as widely among the human race as in ancient times, these practices are still utilized throughout the world today. In addition to speaking with kindness and purpose, ways to heal through voice include practices such as *tonal singing*, *mantra* and *direct vibration through body tissues*. These practices bring dormant or passive forces of healing already present within us to the forefront of our consciousness.

25.13.1 The Chakras and Auras – the Body's Energy Template

The body's physical topography is paralleled by a vibrational (energy) template. This template is structured with seven main energy centers, or *chakras*, positioned adjacent to corresponding endocrine glands and organs.[45–47] Chakras are vortical energy channels that filter energy flow to and from the outside environment, encouraging balance among the body, the earthly environment and the heavens or spirit world.[46] Just like all vortices in nature, chakras serve to integrate. They occur when two substances of varying quality meet. Chakras form in response to the contrast between our bodies and the outside environment, whether earthly or spiritual. They also create balance among the various energy layers of the body's *aura*.[47] Each chakra is the vibrational equivalent of its synonymous physical body parts and functions.[45, 46] Figure 25.14 shows the location and vortical shape of the seven chakras.

The *human aura* is also called the *human energy field* or *subtle energy body*.[45, 47] All living beings have auras that enclose the physical body. They are created by the totality of energy emitted from the whole being. It has also been postulated the other way around, that the physical body is the result of energy condensation of the original spiritual layers of being. In the books *Hands of Light* by Barbara Brennan and *The Book of Chakras* by Ambika Wauters, the human aura is described as consisting of seven layers of various energy bodies. Each body exists within a plane of energy that is encased by the one above it. Each has defining qualities and purpose, and each corresponds to a particular chakra.[46, 47]

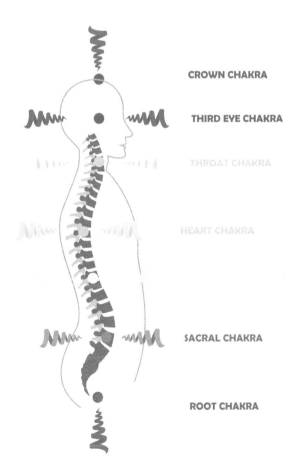

CROWN CHAKRA

THIRD EYE CHAKRA

THROAT CHAKRA

HEART CHAKRA

SACRAL CHAKRA

ROOT CHAKRA

FIGURE 25.14 Chakra anatomy showing the shape and location of the seven main chakras of the human body.

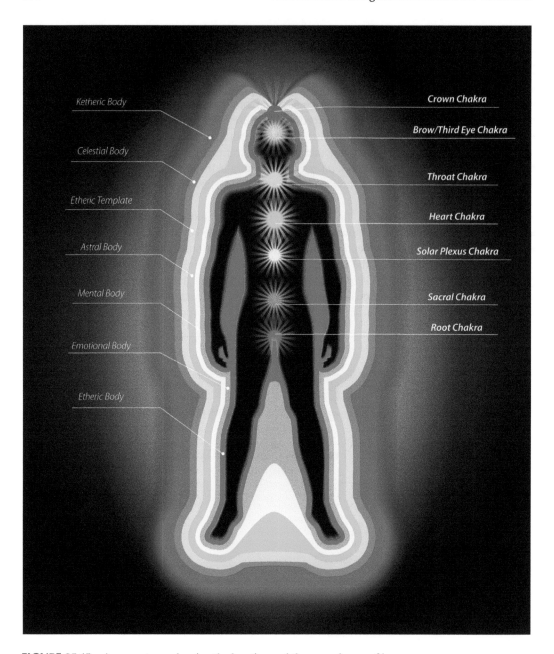

FIGURE 25.15 Aura anatomy showing the location and the seven layers of human auras.

The seven auric layers are depicted in Figure 25.15, although they are named differently according to various sources. Table 25.2 identifies the endocrine glands, emotional aspects and body physiology as they correlate with the seven chakras and auric layers. The state of health and wellbeing of the body is reflected in the quality of the aura and can now be photographed and diagnosed with *Kirlian photography.*[48]

Table 25.2 shows the seven auras and their associated chakras, emotions, endocrine glands, physiology and musical tone.[45–47]

Chakras are of great importance to our physical, emotional, mental and spiritual health. On a physical level, when they are activated, they are capable of triggering hormone release from their corresponding endocrine glands. Endocrine glands are ductless; hence, they secrete hormones

TABLE 25.2
Auras and Chakras

Aura (Brennan)	Chakra	Emotion	Endocrine Gland	Body Systems	Note
Etheric	Root	Trust	Adrenals	Spine, kidneys	C
Emotional	Sacral	Creativity	Gonads	Reproductive system	D
Mental	Solar Plexus	Power Wisdom	Pancreas	Gastrointestinal/CNS	E
Astral	Heart	Love, Healing	Thymus	Cardiac/circulatory, CNS	F
Etheric	Throat	Communication	Thyroid	Vocal/respiratory tract	G
Celestial	Third Eye	Awareness	Pituitary	Ears/nose, left eye, lower brain	A
Ketheric	Crown	Spirituality	Pineal	Right eye, upper brain	B

directly into the bloodstream, thereby affecting our physical and emotional health quite quickly. Chakras also work to affect us spiritually, as the emotional aspects of each connect us with our own karmic lessons and life purpose.

The vibration of each chakra resonates at a frequency that can also be represented by musical tone; therefore, one powerful way to access and awaken chakras is through voice. We can do this by simply singing along to songs we love, by voicing a chakra's specific musical tone and/or its meaning with sacred words. Doing this initiates a *vibrational* force *using* a *physical* body part – the vocal cords. The gesture of voice once again demonstrates itself as a bridge between the physical and energy bodies, allowing them to communicate and harmonize.

25.13.2 Vocal Toning

Vocal toning is voicing or humming in harmony with sacred musical scales, or simply sustaining any note that feels good in the body. The vibration of the vocal cords resonates the power of those vibrational frequencies through your body and activates the corresponding chakras. Vocal toning also physically resonates vibration into the cranium via bone conduction.[49] Direct vibration though the facial bones resonates to all other articulating cranial bones and to their soft tissue attachments, including the dura and brain.

Vocal cords vibrate the nasal bones most strongly, according to recent literature.[49] Vibration is then transferred from the nasal bones to the ethmoid and then to the sphenoid bone, within which the pituitary gland sits. This results in activation of the pituitary gland itself, thus stimulating hormone release that affects growth, metabolism, thyroid function, cardiovascular and sexual health and health during lactation and pregnancy. When voice is used with good intention, such as for kindness to others or self-healing, pituitary function is affected positively, encouraging a healthy balance of all body systems involved.

As resonance continues, the pineal gland is activated, affecting melatonin production and circadian and seasonal body rhythms. It resonates the vibration through the chest, opening up the heart and lungs. It sends vibrations into the spine, aligning posture and straightening our bodies to allow room for proper organ function, blood flow and lymphatic drainage. And when the sacred tones access our spirit, emotional healing parallels that of the physical. Sometimes this comes in the form of sorrow or grief, as the contrast between where we are and where we should be is revealed. But this pain is brief and very much worth the effort.

25.13.3 Mantra

Other types of voice healing include *mantra* and *kirtan*, which involve chanting sacred words. *Mantra* is the utterance of sacred words or groups of words that produce spiritual awakening. *Kirtan* is the act of chanting a mantra that is then repeated or "answered" by another person or group of people. It is a call and response approach, which heightens the collective spiritual awakening of the group.[50]

There are many types of mantra, such as *Bija* (seed), *Saguna* (with form) and *Nirguna* (without form). For example, *Bija Mantra* in particular is the "seed mantra." It consists of "one-syllable seed sounds" that when spoken aloud, with discipline and in repetition, create sound vibrations that resonate through the body and empower various aspects of the soul.[51] The combination of each word's meaning, articulation and tone is divinely matched to create a harmony that awakens certain core *energy centers* in the body. When spoken in certain ordered sequences, they become even more specific and powerful.

Chanting mantras activates the sacred seeds within us, allowing us to express them in whichever way exemplifies our own truth. Although we may all chant the same seed sounds, they blossom differently within each of us, creating infinite flavors of expression of self-awareness and truth.

Here are the *Bija* seed sounds, pronunciations, associated chakras[51] and meanings:

LAM (LUM) for the earth chakra (1) – Red – Root Chakra – *I am.*
VAM (VUM) for the water chakra (2) – Orange – Sacral Chakra – *I feel.*
RAM (RUM) for the fire chakra (3) – Yellow – Solar Plexus Chakra – *I do.*
YAM (YUM) for the heart chakra (4) – Green – Heart Chakra – *I love.*
HAM (HUM) for the throat chakra (5) – Blue – Throat Chakra – *I speak.*
AUM (OM) for the third eye (6) – Indigo – Third Eye Chakra – *I see.*
Silence, AH, OM for the crown chakra (7) – White light/Violet – Crown Chakra – *I heal.*

When matched with the divine tone of its chakra (Table 25.2), the seed sound becomes more precise in its healing. For example, voicing the word "LUM" in a C note aligns vocal cord vibrations with the root chakra in both seed meaning *and* tone. You can voice any tone, but voicing a C with LUM will add more precision to the vibrational effect.

Similarly to when infants learn to speak, we *adults* learn to speak new words when we chant mantra. Mantra includes the added task of voicing the musical tone with the word, which adds another dimension of brain function to the challenge. Both hearing and voicing *svaras* in tones that we have never voiced before triggers the brain to develop new auditory targets. Auditory targets are instinctively and automatically developed during infancy. When the adult brain attempts to establish new auditory targets, brain function that is merely a remnant of our infancy is reawakened and put back to work.

Healing through vocal vibrations is a perfect representation of what my dear mentor and friend, Dr. John Beaulieu, ND, PhD, once told me in conversation. "When you think vibrationally and then act on it with discipline, you open the doorway to new possibilities." This is exactly what is happening here. Our intention is to use voice as the vibrational force to heal and integrate body, mind and soul. Then, we act in discipline by taking the time and effort to sit with intention to harmonize our breathing with the correct sounds, sequences and melodies, in combination with positive intentions, to produce a deliberate healing effect.

25.14 *ALANKAR* – MY PERSONAL EXPERIENCE WITH SOUND HEALING THROUGH VOICE

During my quest for research on the healing power of voice and speech sound, I came across an Indian "voice yoga" teacher, Lakshmi Santra, who teaches a type of the vocal healing called *Alankar.*

Alankar is an ancient Indian practice that, like *Bija* Mantra, voices sacred words with intent and correct tone. *Alankara* literally means "adornment" or "decoration." *Alankar* is the personal creative process of decorating or embellishing a piece of music or musical genre based on ancient

Indian principles and classical music. *Alankars* are composed of a succession of *svaras*, words that designate and hold a particular note on a musical scale.[52]

Like *Bija*, in *Alankar* there are seven words that each hold one of the seven core soul meanings. Although there are few words, the effect of each sound may vary greatly in response to even subtle changes in word order, intention, strength and evenness of the tone, allowing the nuance of each *svara* and *alankar* to change without limit. Although there is slight variation among different regions of India, the words, pronunciations, musical notes and meanings are as follows:[52]

SA – (Sah) – C – self, meditation, it holds the energy of all the notes
RE – (Ray) – D♭ – practice
GA – (Gah) – E♭ – deepness
MA – (Mah) – F – sweetness
PA – (Pah) – G – purity
DHA – (Dha) – A♭ – patience
NI – (Nee) – B♭ – continuation, action

My intention was to immerse myself in the practice of mantra as a form of research for my book. My initial expectation was to learn about the practice and to truly feel the healing power of voice. Through this immersion I would gain the experience needed in order to write about it authentically. Suffice it to say I did gain all of that. But much to my surprise, I gained much more.

When I began training with Lakshmi I just so happened to be going through a very difficult time in my life. We started easy, with only the first three or four *svaras*. But voicing them on pitch with a strong nonwavering voice was more difficult than I had anticipated. At first, I found myself out of breath quite easily. However, as the hour-long session progressed, I was able to harmonize the movement between my diaphragm, breath and vocal cords. I completed the first session with obvious improvement. To my delight, after that session, I had an easier time hitting higher pitches with songs I sing at home, playing my guitar. My breathing expanded; I felt clear and energized.

During my second session, I was tasked with voicing *all* of the *svaras*. Lakshmi progressed quickly up the entire scale, hitting very high notes, some of them in half tones. With repetition, my voice finally responded wonderfully by opening and allowing me to hit the notes on pitch. Everything seemed to be going well.

As I continued to repeat the higher *Alankars*, I suddenly felt a terrible sensation slowly welling up in my left chest, near my heart. It was very stark and localized. It had shape and color. I felt death, terror, panic. It felt inevitable. I had had a short history of panic attacks previously in my life for other reasons, but I had never felt anything so despairing, especially while I was engaged in a beautiful healing practice. But there it was, welling up to the point where I could no longer even take a breath, let alone use my voice. I didn't know how to exist with the feeling, it was so intense. I wanted to run away from it, but I couldn't – it was *within me*. It was the most intense sensation of emotional pain that I had ever experienced in my conscious adult life.

Lakshmi kept chanting, expecting me to repeat her string of sacred singing, but I was suddenly immobilized. My voice, my breath – it just stopped. I began shaking and started to softly cry. Lakshmi stopped too, turned off the music and said in her sweet Indian accent, "ok, you talk to me."

I could barely utter words of explanation, but they somehow spilled out of me in weak, choppy phrases. I didn't need to say much, which was a surprise to me. I didn't need to go on about the dramatic specifics that defined my seemingly awful situation. Somehow, right then, I only needed to utter enough words to form the skeleton of it all – just the bones. The stuff between the bones, the "spaghetti" that filled it all in, was unnecessary.

Lakshmi listened. I had never felt so completely understood with so few words. I discovered something in that moment – something that I never could have learned from any reference book or research paper. In order to allow this healing process to become fully activated within me, *I needed to speak in my own native language (English) only the words that paralleled the sacred Hindu ones that had just opened my soul.* Nothing more.

We don't ever really need to say too much, considering that there are a mere seven sacred core essences that completely define the meaning of all that exists. We need not get wrapped up in details or take things too seriously. There is great healing in simplification.

You could take any complicated scenario in life and boil it all down to one of these seven core principles of existence. When we chant these words in sequences, in repetition, we are calling all of the messed-up circumstances in our lives to simplify to one word, one meaning, that defines its soul lesson, the laser point version of the whole complicated story. We have exposed the problem's true identity and thus, inactivated its power. The key has found its door. The door then swings free of its dead bolt and instantaneously unleashes emotions that cleanse the soul. This was the intense pain I felt during my session with Lakshmi. Chanting the words unlocked areas of energy block in my body that had been holding on to emotional pain for many years. *But, how?*

As mentioned earlier, each word in *Alankar* is paired with a musical tone – it is a *svara*. We must say the word in perfect pitch. Some of these tones are flat notes, or half tones, that are not typically used in spoken language and not typically voiced in song in these particular sequences. At first, my voice had difficulty finding the flat notes. Interestingly, at first, I even had trouble *hearing* them! I had never experienced this, even though I am an amateur musician and a somewhat talented singer.

My first sequence required voicing the flat note of "Re." At first my "Res" were begun with a brief yodeling-like maneuver around the note before my voice could find it. But after many tries, I was hitting it right on pitch in sequence with the other tones. Success! But alas, Lakshmi moved fast up the musical scale to another half tone in a much higher pitch – more difficult. And then another, even higher. These were completely foreign to me.

My vocal cords had rarely, if ever, deliberately intended those vibrational frequencies. I had never consciously efforted towards voicing the half tones. These musical sequences are not intuitive from an artistic perspective like music that we listen to on the radio. It was awkward. It seemed almost *forced.* It required great focus and effort. As an active person who exercises regularly, I surprisingly found my whole body getting fatigued.

When my voice finally hit the pitch of the high half tone, in combination with the specific *svara*, I felt a sensation in my vocal cords. It felt as if they were falling or "fitting" into something, like a puzzle piece that slips down into place as it finds its designated space in the puzzle. My vocal cords "fit" into that flat note. That note "hit" something within me. First, I felt surprise that my voice had found this new vibrational platform on which it could dwell. And now I could go there at will, since I now had the skill to find this note on my own. A new place for hanging out, a new *space.*

Then, I felt something welling up within my chest, behind my sternum. First pressure, then a slow expansion of emotional pain that I described earlier. Slow as it was, its intensity increased to the point of silencing me. I felt the connection between the musical note and the dis-ease within my body and spirit. I cannot name the dis-ease, but I can name the new perspectives of which I am now consciously aware. I remember the old ones and can even compare the two. I now see how certain old perspectives and beliefs were hurting me.

In *Alankar* each word *is* sanctified meaning. Each is the purest expression of its own voiced being. In my experience, when spoken in unison with its paired musical tone, the two become activated as one and work as an interdimensional key for unlocking energy blocks in the person who spoke it. When *svaras* are spoken in sequence, as in *Alankar*, this further adds variety and dimension to the healing potential. It reveals awareness of an aspect of one's true self. This glimpse initiates both the discovery and healing of the defect, simultaneously.

Although there are relatively few core meanings in mantra practices, the number of sequences possible allow much variety and depth to cover the vast array of human dilemmas. For example, you may have heard the well-known concept that the entire array of human emotion stems from only two core emotions – love and fear. Love is truth. That which is not truth does not exist.

Through this practice we are brought to the awareness that we are only ever voicing ourselves. Although we are all voicing the same syllables and notes, no two vocal tracts can produce exactly the same voice. Each voice differs in tone on levels that have never been explained by science. You may even recognize a family member or friend just by hearing their voice. I believe that each vocal tract produces the exact quality in tone that is needed to heal the human it belongs to. We are born with the means to heal *ourselves*. It is the going *within*, the healing of the self, that leads to the enlightenment of one's own gifts, one's own capacity to love, to trust, to tolerate, to forgive.

SOUND HEALING AND VIBRATION TRAINING AND LEARNING OPPORTUNITIES

Osteopathic Wellness, LLC
Raymond, Maine
Go to www.osteopathicwell.com for more information and to contact Dr. Higgins.

REFERENCES

1. Wolfe, Joe, Garnier, Maëva and Smith, John. Vocal tract resonances in speech, singing, and playing musical instruments. *HFSP J.* 2009;3(1):6–23.
2. Sharma, Sandeep, Hashmi, Muhammad F, Rawat, Deepa. *Partial Pressure of Oxygen.* Treasure Island: StatPearls Publishing; 2020 Jan. https://www.ncbi.nlm.nih.gov/books/NBK493219/
3. Russell, Dan, What is a wave? *Acoustics and Vibration Animations*, https://www.acs.psu.edu/drussell/Demos/waves-intro/waves-intro.html, April 2002.
4. Russell, Dan. Longitudinal and transverse wave motion, *Acoustics and Vibration Animations*, https://www.acs.psu.edu/drussell/Demos/waves/wavemotion.html, August 1988.
5. Wikipedia Contributors, *"Quantum," Wikipedia, The Free Encyclopedia*, https://en.wikipedia.org/w/index.php?title=Quantum&oldid=1011197508 (accessed March 10, 2021).
6. Lipton, Bruce H. *The Biology of Belief: Unleashing the Power of Consciousness, Matter & Miracles*, Carlsbad, CA: Hay House, Inc. 2008, p. 70–71.
7. Zhang, Zhaoyan. Mechanics of human voice production and control. *J Acoust Soc Am.* Oct. 2016;140(4):2614–2635.
8. Maintier, Serge. *Speech: Invisible Creation in the Air.* Great Barrington, MA: Steiner Books, Edited by Rainer Patzlaff; 2016.
9. Kummer, Ann W. Disorders of resonance and airflow secondary to Cleft Palate and/or velopharyngeal dysfunction, *Seminars in Speech and Language*, May 2011, 32(2):141–9.
10. Becker, Rollin, *Life in Motion.* Portland: Stillness Press, LLC. Edited by Rachel E. Brooks; 1997, p. 41.
11. Sutherland, William Garner, DO. *Contributions of Thought*, 2nd ed. The Sutherland Cranial Teaching Foundation, Yakima, WA, 1998.
12. Dreha-Kulaczewski, Steffi, Joseph, Arun A., Merboldt, Klaus-Dietmar, Ludwig, Hans-Christoph, Gärtner, Jutta and Frahm, Jens, Inspiration is the major regulator of human CSF flow. *J Neurosci.* 2015;35(6):2485–2491.
13. Shahid Zainab, Burns Bracken. Anatomy, abdomen and pelvis, diaphragm. Treasure Island: StatPearls Publishing; Jan. 2020. https://www.ncbi.nlm.nih.gov/books/NBK470191/
14. Chaitow, Leon, Bradley, Dinah, Gilbert, Christopher, Ley Ronald. *Multidisciplinary Approaches to Breathing Pattern Disorders*; Elsevier Science Ltd., Netherlands, 2002, Ch.1, pp. 1–41.
15. Winklhofer S, Schoth, F, Stolzmann, P, Krings, T, Mull, M, Wiesmann, M, Stracke, C.P., Spinal cord motion: Influence of respiration and cardiac cycle. *Fortschr Röntgenstr* 2014; 186: 1016–1021.
16. Havel M, Ertl L, Bauer D, Schuster M, Stelter K, Sundberg J. Resonator properties of paranasal sinuses: preliminary results of an anatomical study. *Rhinology.* 2014 Jun;52(2):178–82.
17. Wikipedia contributors, *"Bernoulli's Principle," Wikipedia, The Free Encyclopedia*, https://en.wikipedia.org/w/index.php?title=Bernoulli%27s_principle&oldid=1009085357 (accessed March 10, 2021).
18. Sataloff, Robert T., Heman-Ackah, Yolanda D., Hawkshaw, Mary J., Clinical Anatomy and Physiology of the Voice, *Otolaryngol. Clin. N. Am.* 2007; 40:909–929.
19. Froeschels, Emil, The question of the origin of the vibrations of the vocal cords, *AMA Arch Otolaryngol* Nov. 1957; 66:512–516.

20. Titze, Ingo R. *The Principles of Voice Production*. Prentice Hall, Hoboken, New Jersey, 1994, p. 188.

21. Altshuler, Douglas L, Dickson, William B, Vance, Jason T, Roberts, Stephen P, and Dickinson, Michael, Short-amplitude high-frequency wing strokes determine the aerodynamics of honeybee flight. *PNAS* December 13, 2005;102(50):18213–18218.

22. Uchida-Ota, M., Arimitsu, T., Tsuzuki, D., Dan, I., Ikeda, K., Takahashi, T., & Minagawa, Y. (2019). Maternal speech shapes the cerebral frontotemporal network in neonates: A hemodynamic functional connectivity study. *Developmental Cognitive Neuroscience, 39,* Article 100701.

23. Blechschmidt, Erich, *The Ontogenetic Basis of Human Anatomy*. Berkeley: North Atlantic Books. Edited and translated by Brian Freeman, 2004. p. 187–188; 113-118.

24. Querleu, Denis, Renard, Xavier, Versyp, Fabienne, Paris-Delrue, Laurence, Crépen, Gilles. Fetal hearing. *Eur. J. Obstet. Gynecol. Reprod. Biol.* 1988;29;191–212.

25. Hepper, Peter G, Shahidullah, Sara B. Development of fetal hearing. *Arch Dis Childhood* 1994;71:F81–F87

26. Webb, Alexandra R., Heller, Howard T., Benson, Carol B. and Lahav, Amir. Mother's voice and heartbeat sounds elicit auditory plasticity in the human brain before full gestation. *PNAS* 2015;112 (10):3152–3157.

27. Guenther, Frank H. Cortical interactions underlying the production of speech sounds, *J. Commun. Disorders*, 2006;39:350–365.

28. Acharya, Sourya and Shukla. Mirror neurons: Enigma of the metaphysical modular brain, *J Nat Sci Biol Med.* 2012 Jul–Dec; 3(2): 118–124.

29. Steiner, R. *Eurythmy as visible Speech*, audio lec. 1, June 1924, Dornach found at https://wn.rsarchive.org/Lectures/GA279/English/RSP1967/19230826p01.html

30. Maintier, Serge, Accompanying video to *Speech, invisible creation in the air*, found at https://www.youtube.com/watch?v=i6eFtohBEWA 21

31. Petekkaya E, Ulusoy M, Bagheri H, Şanlı Ş, Ceylan MS, Dokur M, Karadağ M. Evaluation of the golden ratio in nasal conchae for surgical anatomy. *Ear Nose Throat J.* 2021 Jan; 100(1):NP57–NP61.

32. Schwenk, Theodor, *Sensitive Chaos – The Creation of Flowing Forms in Water and Air, Sophia Books*, Rudolf Steiner Press, East Sussex, 1962 (revised translation 1996).

33. Meisner, George, Vézelay: The capital of the four wind spirits, Compostela - The joining of Heaven and Earth, https://compostela.co.uk/symbols/vezelay-spirits-four-winds/

34. Brownell, William, E, Ph.D., How the Ear Works – Nature's Solutions for Listening, *Volta Rev.* 1997; 99(5): 9–28. Author manuscript available in PMC 2010 June 21.

35. Ruggero, Mario, A, Cochlear Delays and Traveling Waves: Comments on 'Experimental Look at Cochlear Mechanics,' *Audiology.* 1994; 33(3): 131–142. Author manuscript; available in PMC 2013 February 22.

36. Leurs, Jan Christoffer, and Hüttenbrink, Karl-Bernd, Surgical anatomy and pathology of the middle ear, *J. Anat.* (2016) 228, pp338–353.

37. Husemann, Armin, *Human Hearing and the Reality of Music, Steiner Books*. Anthroposophic Press, Great Barrington, MA, 2013.

38. Binhammer, Robert T., CSF anatomy with emphasis on relations to nasal cavity and labyrinthine fluids, *Ear, Nose Throat J.* n.d.;71(7):292–299.

39. Lo, William W. M., Daniels, David L., Chakeres, Donald W, Linthicum Jr, Fred H., Ulmer, John L., Mark, Leighton P. and Swartz, Joel D., The endolymphatic duct and sac. *Anatomic Moment AJNR* May 1997;18:881–887, 0195-6108/97/1805–0881 © American Society of Neuroradiology.

40. Ekdale, Eric G, Form and function of the mammalian inner ear. *J. Anat.* 2016;228:324–337.

41. Raphael, Yehoash and Altschuler, Richard A., Structure and innervation of the cochlea: Review. *Brain Res Bull.* 60 (2003) 397–422. © 2003 Elsevier Science Inc.

42. Robles, Luis and Ruggero, Mario A, Mechanics of the mammalian Cochlea. *Physiol Rev.* 2001 July;81(3):1305–1352. Author manuscript; available in PMC 2013 March 07.

43. Meymandi Assad, DLFAPA, Music, Medicine, Healing, and the Genome Project, *Psychiatry.* 2009 Sep; 6(9): 43–45.

44. Stevens, Wallace. *Life is Motion*, a poem from the *book Harmonium*, Alfred A. Knopf, Inc. 1919.

45. Ross, Christina, Energy medicine: Current status and future perspectives. *Glob Adv Health Med.* 2019;8:1–10.

46. Wauters, Ambika, *The Book of Chakras*, Quarto Publishing plc, London N7 9BH, 2002, p. 6, 11–2

47. Brennan, Barbara, *Hands of Light*, Bantam Books, New York, 1987, p. 42–43.

48. Priya, Shanmuga B., and Rajesh, R. Understanding abnormal energy levels in aura images, ICGST AIML-11 Conference, Dubai, UAE, 12–14 April 2011, CMS College of Science and Commerce, Coimbatore, India TDC, NeST, Technopark, Thiruvananthapuram, India.

49. Chen, Fei C, Ma, Estella P-M, Yiu, Edwin M-L. Facial bone vibration in resonant voice production. *J Voice*. 2014 Sep;28(5):596–602.

50. Brown, Sarah, *"Every Word Is a Song, Every Step Is a Dance": Participation, Agency, and the Expression of Communal Bliss in Hare Krishna Festival Kirtan*, Florida State University Library.

51. Heather, Simon, How to sound the Bija mantras for the chakras, May 2012, http://www.simonheather.co .uk/pages/articles/how_to_sound_bija_mantras.pdf

52. Lakshmi Santra is a well-known *Alankar* teacher and sound healer in Pondicherry, India. During my sessions with her, we discussed the meaning of the *svaras* and the philosophy of the practice of *Alankar*.

26 Art in Medicine
Tapping into Creativity for Healing the Mind/Body

Susan Imholz and Judy Sachter

CONTENTS

26.1 INTRODUCTION

A notable 2013 study showed that the activity of observing art work considered to be beautiful by the viewer generates the same brain cortical activity as being in love.[1] Neuroscience is now validating the power of engagement with art activities as brain food[2,3,4] in addition to experimental evidence of improved immune functioning, and enhanced physical and psychological health.[5,6,7,8] This probably comes as no surprise; most of us consider a trip to a museum a form of relaxation, recreation, eye candy – it can also be exhilarating and inspiring. These activities also figure prominently in our (the authors') model of mind. We are moving toward a model of mind body holism that is now informed by a finer understanding of biophysiology but at the same time, increasingly honors the mysteries of the power of symbolic thinking. It's clear that evolving models of mind dictate the approach to and language of health and healing. Our selective review of mental models (see Figures 26.1 and 26.2) illustrates that metaphors for mind are cyclical.[9] Periodically, the role of creativity and imagination is elevated in cultural discourse (i.e., Jung 1954, Vygotsky 1970, Gardner 1985).[10,11,12] In our current time, advances in biophysiology dominate academic thinking and language for describing the mind. Choice of theory and language set the parameters of a clinical encounter. Therefore, we begin with a historical overview of our changing model of mind and its relationship to the integration of art and imagination into the healthcare encounter.

The authors' qualifications for writing on the subject of art as elixir include three decades of work experience in cross-disciplinary product development and test-bed technology projects that aimed to integrate higher levels of creativity as a starting place for design. Additionally, we authored a book series on the use of technology in clinical practice, emphasizing the integration of new media research and collaboration across disciplines.[13,14] Both authors are artists and former art teachers – a

DOI: 10.1201/b23304-28

Development of Metaphors of Mind 300A.D. – 20th Century

Century: 400 – 300 B.C. Plato (429-347 B.C.). Main contribution is defining epistemology and philosophy as disciplines. His stance on perceived reality is limited; all we can know empirically is the essence of things, not the ultimate reality of the world.	Century: 300 B.C. Aristotle (384-322 B.C.) A member of Plato's academy, started his own school, the Lyceum (334-323 B.C.). Creates a hierarchy of ranking mental functions, introducing the first classification model which includes morality and aesthetics, logic and science, politics and metaphysics.	Century: (4th Century A.D.) Vasubandhu was a teacher of the Mahayana Buddhist tradition and the no-self doctrine; this conception of mind rejects a permanent manifestation of self to enable access to higher consciousness and enlightenment.
Century: 10th, Avicenna (d. 1037); an Islamic scholar known for contributing subject/object distinctions in logic. Articulated "second intentions", defined as the properties of concepts acquired when attaining knowledge of a particular subject.	Century: 16/17th, Thomas Hobbes (1588-1679); a founding member of the Royal Society of London. Articulated the differences between individual behavior and how people interact as groups. The group mind vs. individual mind	Century: 16/17th, Rene Descartes (1596-1650). Best known for introducing what we call the mind/body split; proposing that there is a disjuncture between these two systems.
Century: 17/18th, John Locke (1632-1704). Locke is cited as the originator of modern conceptions of identity and the self, and first proposed the "tabula rasa" metaphor of mind as blank slate upon which experience writes the man.	Century: 18/19th, Immanuel Kant (1724-1804). Kant is a central figure in modern philosophy and great synthesizer of early metaphysics, epistemology, ethics and philosophy; his ideas bridge the "Enlightenment" and "Romantic" periods.	Century: 19th, Charles Darwin (1802-1882). Darwin is one of the first true empirical scientists— separating himself from the tradition of combining philosophy and religious belief with writings about evolution, and by extension, human development.
Century: 19/20th, Wilhelm Wundt (1832-1920). Known as the father of experimental psychology, Wundt was a laboratory psychologist who studied sensation and perception, he also argued for a non-reductionist account of consciousness.	Century: 19/20th, William James (1842-1910). Noted as the father of American psychology, James claimed to be an empiricist who also believed that "science is nothing but the finding of an analogy" which are fluxational.	Century: 19/20th, G. Stanley Hall (1844-1924). Hall is known as the founder of the child study movement in the US, and for defining the discipline of educational psychology.

FIGURE 26.1   Development of metaphors of mind from 300 AD to the twentieth century.

Development of Metaphors of Mind 19 – 21st Century

Century: 19/20th, Sigmund Freud (1856-1939). Freud's metaphors of mind were drawn from social & political life, mythology, hydraulics, anthropology and the natural world. Ego, ID, and superego are his signature conceptual contributions to the structure of mind.	Century: 19/20th, Emil Kraepelin (1856-1926). Kraepelin formed the first nosology system of mental illness that described and matched physical symptoms and brain functions with categories of mental disorders. This system was widely used in hospitals and health care settings.	Century: 19/20th, Carl Jung (1875-1961). Jung names psychological types (i.e., introvert, extrovert). He differed from psychoanalytic colleagues by incorporating spiritual life and myth into theories of personality. He originates and defines the theory of a collective unconscious.
Century: 19/20th, James B. Watson (1878-1958). Known as the father of human behaviorism, Watson applied Pavlov's classical conditional protocols to infants (Little Albert), and showed that fear could be taught using associative stimulus/response conditioning.	Century: 19/20th, Harry Stack Sullivan (1892-1949). Sullivan laid the groundwork for understanding he individual based on the network of relationships in which he or she is enmeshed in society; a sociometric understanding of personality.	Century: 19/20th, Lev Vygotsky (1896-1934). Vygotsky theorized about the social basis of cognitive development (vs. biological) and contributed new perspectives on the role of social interaction and symbolic mediators in the acquisition of knowledge and culture.
Century: 19/20th, Jean Piaget (1896-1980). Considered the father of genetic epistemology, or a biological basis for cognitive development. He also provided rich descriptive accounts of conceptual change in childhood.	Century: 20th, B.F. Skinner (1904-1990). Skinner is remembered for taking behaviorism (stimulus-response learning--mind as table rasa) to the extreme; he is also known for using his own children in his experiments.	Century: 20/21th, Albert Bandura (1925-) Cited as the father of social cognitive theory; provides a more comprehensive overview of human cognition in the context of social learning and social mediators than previous cognitive theorists.
Century: 20/21st, Marvin Minsky (1927-2016). Society of mind; mind is a product of a vast society of cognitive agents, each with their own purpose, language, methods, and knowledge base. Intelligence comes from the diversity of human experience.	Century: 20/21st, Howard Gardner (1943-). Authored texts on multiple intelligences; social, visual, mathematical, emotional-- elevating the role of creativity and imagination in human development.	Century: 20/21st, Michael Gazzaniga (1939-). Cited as the father of the field of cognitive neuroscience, the study of the neural basis of mind. Studies cerebral lateralization and split-brain research

FIGURE 26.2   Development of metaphors of mind from the nineteenth to the twenty-first century.

foundation that informs our thinking about software development and a design approach. We believe real transformation of professional disciplines is rooted in meaningful interactions between people with diverse expertise working side by side every day. We highly prize interdisciplinary dialogue and exchange, and were fortunate to have the opportunity to attend the MIT Media Lab as graduate students in its early years, where cross-disciplinary collaboration is well established, and where we learned to "see around corners."

Our chapter is written in two parts; in Section 26.2, we examine how *art* and *creativity* have remained consistent features of models of mind over time – yet their importance eludes our full understanding. In Section 26.3, we report on new software and devices that embody our ideal design processes and involve creative participation on the part of the users. While broad in scope, the chapter suggests that *creative design, creative collaboration,* and *creative expression* underlie most worthy human accomplishments and are the driving forces behind both personal and cultural development. If these activities lead us forward in our thinking and doing, then they are also powerful forces for self-healing that can't be ignored. Our chapter content is limited to analysis of Western milestones. We acknowledge that the Indo-Asian traditions provide deep insight into the subjects of health, healing, and creativity, which we don't address. We wanted to provide an informative and engaging narrative, with a wealth of citations for those interested in delving deeper into this subject matter.

26.2   ART AND CREATIVITY IN HISTORICAL PERSPECTIVE

The health centers of antiquity known as Greek asclepieia were ancient healing sanctuaries that embraced the arts, simple nutrition, guided meditation and dream interpretation in practice: A good starting place for citing the importance of creativity in healing.[15,16,17] These activities are also offered in the best spas and recuperative centers across the world today.[18] In other words, these activities have withstood the test of time as essential components of what constitutes a therapeutic healing environment. Our modern-day understanding of why they work is grounded in biophysiology, brain and neuroscience research.[19,20,21,22,23] In ancient times, it was believed that the creative urge of the poet and the painter came from divine inspiration. Today, we have traded metaphors for the animating force behind creativity – without gaining greater clarity on its source.

We are educated to believe there is a firm correlation between the passage of time and what we call progress; however, a more nuanced understanding of where we came from reveals that written and oral history conceal as much as they preserve about our past. In *Metaphors in the History of Psychology*, David Leary (1990)[9] observed that metaphors for mind are more than linguistic conventions of their time – they are more fundamentally a form of thought having basic epistemological functions (p.1), and they play a vital role in shifts in thinking at the frontier of scientific exploration (p.347). As it relates to our subject of creativity for healing, an important anchor to our proceeding discussion is noting when and where linguistic conventions of artists and scientists diverged in significant ways. From the time of Plato until the industrial revolution, analogy and metaphoric language were acceptable in all forms of discourse. In the mid-1600s, the Royal Society of London for Improving Natural Knowledge decreed that scientists were to adopt "plain speaking" in conducting experiments and leave metaphor to poets and novelists (K. Gergen in Leary, p.268).[24] So began the scientific method, or *logical positivism*. This divide marked the beginning of philosophical and linguistic tensions between artists and scientists that still exist today in the form of skepticism about ancient wisdom or old knowledge not born under a microscope or measuring stick. We may also peg the origin of *technical rationality* to these same circumstances, demonstrated by manufacturing and industrial growth in the 1700s. Here, we define technical rationality as a philosophy of instrumental problem solving made rigorous by the application of logical positivism (hereafter, scientific materialism) (Schön 1983, p.21).[25]

In summary, scientific materialism set in motion a competing cultural dialogue between ancient wisdom and philosophical teachings (all religious and esoteric traditions and philosophies preceding the seventeenth century) and disciplines that emerged under its influence. Our ancient traditions are "the keepers of the magic"; creativity, symbolic thinking, semiotics, divergent thinking, intuition and the arts. Going forward, we will refer to this disposition as *humanistic holism*. On the other hand, scientific materialism values efficiency, technocentric thinking, convergent thinking, systems thinking, control systems and data. Going forward, we will be referring to this disposition as *technical rationality*. How these two forces coalesce and blend to form our future is an ongoing process. In turn, they are defining our models of mind and influence how we use creativity in our daily lives or for healing. What follows are several examples of how these two competing narratives have shaped professional activity and our ideas about creativity. We limit our review of models of mind to developments in the field of psychology and psychiatry over the past 150 years. Due to the constraints of writing a single chapter on this topic, we've had to compress our discussion to highlights. The challenge has honed our focus to research milestones and events that seem most relevant to future medical practice.

26.2.1   Turn of the Century (Nineteenth to Twentieth)

At the turn of the nineteenth century, modern American psychologists were in step with the new lingua franca of logical positivism in Europe. In an early American Psychological Association presidential address, Dr. James Cattell (1896)[26] reportedly characterized his peers engaged in laboratory experiments as factory workers and fact gatherers – noting that laboratory work was "scarcely more stimulating than the routine of the factory or the farm" (Leary, p.21).[9] In retrospect, historians did not think this was an inspiring view of psychology, remarking that nothing of significance came of fact finding in America during this period – no lasting theory in particular. However, Cattell's comments reflected a radical new approach to the study of human nature by proxy – through animal studies and experiments. Inherent in this view was a deliberate avoidance of subjective philosophical musings on the formation of human character from previous centuries. Then (and now), this break in the lineage of thought is rationalized by the need to exorcize religion from scientific exploration.

On the subject of art and creativity, there were major contributions from psychologists and psychiatry in the making. For example, Otto Rank's seminal book *Art and Artist* expounds upon the development and change in meaning of art-forms from similar changes in the idea of the soul from pre-history to the twentieth century (p.12).[27] Rank's cross-continental cultural analysis is intertwined with emerging theories of personality, which were the cutting edge of psychology in 1932, when the book was first published. From this point onward, academic research began focusing on the biological basis of creativity as a process situated within human cognitive growth, and in so doing, started down the path of reductionist thinking. There were many interdisciplinary thinkers and outliers to this trend who championed the belief that *the whole is greater than the sum of its parts* and who persisted in reminding us that history harbors a rich legacy on the healing powers of creativity; among them were Carl Jung,[28] Jacob Moreno[29] and Abraham Maslow.[30] These authors remain relevant because of the complexity of their thinking and for our purposes, their unwillingness to quarantine creative thought from human development as a process that is separate from personality growth.

Jung is recognized as one of the most original thinkers in the history of psychology today. In his time, he was admonished by his peers for deriving theory from clinical findings and mythic sources rather than empirical investigation.[31] Jung is credited with devising the use of "active imagination" (inducing a meditative state wherein one calls forth images or fantasies from the unconscious mind for analysis) as a therapeutic technique. Jung's *Red Book* (aka *Liber Novus*), published in 2009[32] (but created in the first decades of the twentieth century), is one of the most stunning examples of the use of mystic symbols and art making in psychoanalysis – *his own*. For Jung, as opposed to Freud, the journey of life became more interesting with maturity, or adulthood. In theory, Freud placed more emphasis upon the early stages of human development in forming character. Jung believed the goal of maturity was to overcome the inadequacies of early life; additionally, he thought mature mental faculties were more suited to "the exercise of imagination" that constituted his analytic process.[33]

Jacob Moreno was the founder of the clinical psychotherapeutic practice of "psychodrama." Moreno thought mankind's ability to generate surplus realities (e.g., fantasy, harnessing imagination in the service of self-reflection, conflict resolution and self-actualization) was our most valuable mental ability. Of all his contemporaries, no one more than Moreno championed the power of creativity and spontaneity as therapeutic energies that could conquer all of life's challenges if properly channeled. He never doubted the necessity of art and believed that artistic drive was a force that underlies all worthy human accomplishments, which was very unusual for a psychiatrist of his era. Moreno received his training as a physician at the University of Vienna, graduating in 1917, and conceived of psychodrama as the natural evolution of psychoanalysis.[34, 35]

Abraham Maslow began his career as an experimental psychologist doing animal behavior studies (circa 1934) but gradually rejected the prevailing scientific methodologies for studying people as being terribly inadequate. Today, he is best known for his "pyramid of needs" schematic, which illustrates his theory of personality structure and priorities. Maslow is credited with establishing three sub-divisions of psychology that now represent creative holism: Humanistic, transpersonal and positive psychology.[36] However, it's more accurate to say Maslow laid the groundwork for positive psychology to flourish at a later date.[37, 38] By the time Maslow became president of the American Psychological Association in 1967, he wanted to expand the scope of psychology as a domain to integrate all religious perspectives, including transcendent or peak experiences, and in 1969, founded the Association for Transpersonal Psychology.

Over the 70-year period (1896–1967) that we've just traversed, Cattell and Maslow showcase the polarities of academic thought within psychology on how to define and accomplish its mission of modeling minds and human development. In our present-day environment, the continuing rivalry between humanistic holism and technical rationality is represented by transpersonal psychology versus trans-humanism. The first disposition retains a curiosity to plumb the depths of who we are and what we are capable of, recognizing what we still don't know about ourselves from a scientific stance, and supports divergent thinking. The second disposition assumes supreme knowledge (the right to determine what *is* definitive science) with the goal of enhancing human capacities to converge with industrial technological needs and serve commercial interests. These are important distinctions that are not fully articulated as differing models of mind in public debate. Why is this important? We believe that choice of a model of mind determines the language and parameters of the clinical encounter. Furthermore, choice of model of mind is a primary driver of any complex software design process in product development, which we will discuss in Section 26.3. All to say, the root assumptions one brings to the design of technology for clinical purposes matter greatly.

26.2.2 Mid-Twentieth Century

At the height of scientific materialism's influence on Western culture in the early and mid-twentieth century, art making, history and culture as contexts for analysis became too big and unwieldy for experimental psychology and other emerging sub-divisions of psychology, with two exceptions: Education and clinical settings. In the field of education, John Dewey[39] and Herbert Read[40] were redefining the childhood curriculum by emphasizing the central place of art making and the apprenticeship model of craft production in schools. The holistic view of creativity in health took root in the expressive therapies (i.e., art therapy, music therapy, journaling, psychodrama and gestalt therapy) within clinical psychology and psychiatry.[41,42,43,44] The discourse in clinical psychology preserved the language and techniques of the shaman, symbolic thinking and semiotic analysis as legitimate methods for assisting in the healing of illness.[45,46] In Europe, social movements like the Anthroposophical Society (founded in 1912 in Cologne and banned from Germany by the National Socialists in 1935) harnessed esoteric traditions to rewrite the narrative of personal development and human evolution anew in response to the emerging technocentric view of man.

The Anthroposophists are well known for elevating creative process in every area of life, including farming (inventing biodynamic farming), medical botany (founding Weleda) and education (founding of Waldorf schools).[47]

In 1950, Dr. John P. Guilford's presidential address to the American Psychological Association directly dealt with the lack of attention that creativity had been receiving from academic researchers in psychology, emphasizing that it merited serious study; consequently, he dedicated the latter part of his career to it. Simonton (2001) credits Guildford's address with spearheading resurgence in critical analysis of creativity as a driving force in human development that would last several decades.[48] As an interesting counterpoint to scientific materialism in the United States, there was unprecedented growth in art education in public schools, and the establishment of new art museums and community art centers across America, in the early and mid-twentieth century.[49,50] These major investments signaled that the United States did value creativity as an expression of cultural sophistication, if not foundational knowledge for personal growth. Alternatively, perhaps, American society was asserting the significance and appreciation of the creative arts as a response to the increasingly fragmented and atomistic models of mind coming from psychology research at its most respected institutions. At Johns Hopkins University, Watson (1925)[51] introduced the idea of behaviorism, the study of behavior divorced from introspection. Skinner (1953)[52] further amplified the notion that behavior and consciousness were mutually exclusive by narrowly defining learning as a system of rewards and punishments (operant conditioning) at Harvard. At Stanford, Bandura (1963)[53] also espoused operant and classical conditioning (Pavlov 1927)[54], emphasizing the role of imitation in learning. The atomistic model of mind represents the ultimate metaphor of mind as machine; mind broken down into component parts that can be reconfigured, re-engineered or re-programmed.

While major discoveries were being made about the micro-world of the brain in microbiology and genetic studies, which explained the underlying basis for cognitive and human development, this discussion was narrowly technical in scope.[55,56,57] In public forums, this information was often simply characterized as the nature versus nurture debate to make it more relevant to the lay person and daily life. Surreptitiously, much of psychology was also beginning to fall under the influence of instrumental reasoning and technical rationality fostered by computer science.[58,59] The machine learning agenda and the race to develop artificial intelligence were now dominating America's best technical colleges and universities, funded by a robust military-industrial complex. Atomistic models of mind were the perfect "fuel" for building and programming smart machines. Meanwhile, art and artists of this period (1940–1980) dove into abstract expressionism, minimalism, pop art and conceptual art, providing a visual analogue of the stripped-down nuts-and-bolts narrative of human nature that was being offered by biological and behavioral research – now devoid of philosophy, spirituality or historical references.[60]

Returning to what was happening in clinical psychology and psychiatry mid-century, much was being written on the "holding environment" that allows healing to take place in a therapeutic relationship.[61,62,63] In psychodynamic theory, this concept was and is often described in terms of discourse analysis between client and healer during a verbal therapy session; in art therapy and the expressive therapies, analysis also extends to the art-making activities and *intermediary objects* (i.e., art, music, dance, staged psychodrama) that are produced in the therapy process. Research in these modalities necessitates both therapeutic aesthetics and empirical frameworks. Shaun McNiff (1998) put it this way:

> What is most intriguing about creative arts therapy research is that it requires the integration of the two elements that have been polarized throughout the past four centuries of debate over what constitutes appropriate scientific methodology. Art-based research comprises both introspective and empirical inquiry. Art is by definition a combination of the two. The artist-researcher initiates a series of expressions as a means of personal introspection, and the process of inquiry generates empirical data which are systematically reviewed.[64]

(p.57)

It's worth noting that while the expressive therapies took root in psychiatric settings, now, you are likely to encounter art therapists on every medical unit of the hospital and in diverse social-work settings. In defining the principles and practices of expressive arts therapy, Knill et al. (2005)[34] introduce the *metaphor* of "food as medicine" to re-orient our perception of art making in psychotherapy. First, Knill invokes the origin of the word diet – *diaita* from Greek – which originally meant a manner of living or lifestyle to maintain health; an idea that extends far beyond the current usage. "Within a psychosomatic understanding, we ... refer to the regulated nourishment of psyche or soul ... [as] diet [which] would also concern corrective regulation of psychic nourishment and metabolism" (p.87). Secondly, Knill applies similar reasoning to the concept of medicine: "[medicine] must be composed in such a way that it can be metabolized by the system ... and ... it must interact in a constructive way with the self-regulating forces in the system" (p.87). With this schema, Knill is now ready to prescribe art activities in tandem with the psychotherapy process: (a) paint daily, go to your easel instead of turning on the tv [diet], (b) read the poem that helped you during your session every time you get stuck on that theme [medicine], (c) make a place for the sculpture you made so that you can see it easily and look at it when you get lost in doubts [medicine] (p.88). Here, we see the essence of using images of the imagination to anchor and enliven the healing process. These same principles are at work in Buddhist culture, where a particular Thangka painting may be prescribed for someone to meditate upon as a healing ritual. While anecdotal evidence exists for how mental focus on symbolic mediators might work to influence our metabolism, we still don't know why empirically. Conversely, scientists have written about artists in history who were forerunners of scientific discoveries; artists who very precisely articulated in prose processes in biology that would later be confirmed under the microscope. Leher (2007) presents a compelling treatise on how science is not the only path to knowledge in his analysis of the lives of artists (e.g., Walt Whitman, August Escoffier, Marcel Proust, Gertrude Stein, Igor Stravinsky, Paul Cezanne) who intuitively grasped cognitive and perceptual architecture that was later defined empirically.[65]

Just as the psychology and psychiatry community was contributing to the reunification of old world knowledge and scientific materialism through the lens of empirical methods in its research, the medical profession in the United States was beginning a parallel pursuit under the banner of "integrative medicine." The establishment of Dr. Herbert Benson's Mind/Body Medical Institute at Harvard in 1975 (along with his research on *the relaxation response* and its benefits for those suffering from chronic stress) is cited as a landmark beginning for integrative practices.[66,67,68] In 1979, Dr. Jon Kabat-Zinn's mindfulness-based stress reduction program at Massachusetts Medical School at Worcester, and the creation of the Center for Mindfulness in Medicine, Health Care, and Society, also solidified the trend of integrating complementary and alternative modes of healing with traditional medicine. Today, we can add to this list several other research initiatives that are all supporting cross-disciplinary and integrative approaches to human health. They include the Mind & Life Institute in Charlottesville, VA; Stanford University's Center for Mind, Brain, Computation and Technology, and the Center for Compassion and Altruism Research; the Mind Science Foundation in San Antonio; Harvard's Mind/Brain/Behavior Initiative, to name a few.

Many of the academic centers mentioned here are gravitating toward the next frontier of mind/brain research – understanding what consciousness is. This area of exploration is playing a vital role in shifting our ideas about what mind is, as well as drawing other science disciplines into the conversation.

26.2.3 LATE TWENTIETH CENTURY TO THE PRESENT

The kaleidoscope of human perception is ever changing. Our model of mind would change again due to an unlikely source: Quantum physics. David Bohm once remarked that science is primarily a perceptual enterprise and not about gaining knowledge.[69] This observation is particularly true when it comes to metaphors for mind. Historical perspective highlights how our collective perceptual focus shifts when a new cultural imperative appears. At the close of the twentieth century, what physicists call "the measurement problem" began to unravel basic assumptions that underlie all natural sciences. The measurement problem is short-hand for the baffling outcome of the repeated double-slit experiments, where photons revealed their double life as both particle and wave under observation.[70,71,72] These experiments are the cornerstones of quantum physics. Karl Pribram (1990) makes the connection to models of mind in this way:

> Heisenberg (1930/1984) pointed out that in microphysics, the observed varies with the instrumentation of the observer. Bohr (1928/1985) enunciated his principle of complementarity on the same grounds … This enfoldment of observation into the observable has led some physicists and philosophers (e.g., Whitehead 1938) into panpsychism in which consciousness is a universal attribute [of all living things] rather than an emergent property of brain organization … Such views have interesting consequences … bringing the concept of consciousness closer to that [of] Eastern mystical tradition and the spiritual religious view of the West.[73]

(p. 97, 1990)

Here, Pribram is acknowledging the shift from scientific materialism toward something else, which consensus science has yet to name. What seems clear is that a research methodology that focuses on the relationship between things, rather than phenomena in isolation, is where we are headed.

Much of the academic history of creativity reads as a subject in search of a meaningful experimental context that encompasses its magnitude. Mid-twentieth-century computers enabled researchers to perform multiple regression analysis, factor analysis and time series studies of creative people, but as in Cattell's fact gathering, nothing significant came from research conducted on the head of a pin. Changing the way we conduct science increases the likelihood that we can come to a fuller understanding of creative powers and their usefulness. The problem may be that academia (due to its current siloed structure) is asking the wrong questions. Recent consciousness studies have conjoined research on creativity with that on psi phenomena. These studies attempt to understand a range of extrasensory perceptions: remote viewing, precognitive perception, and what's come to be known as the "experimenter bias effect" (aka the measurement problem). The outcome of efforts to reproduce the double-slit experiments by removing human participation (by using video cameras, random number generators or computers that give commands to other technical apparatus) in observing the performance of electrons only confounded scientists.[74,75] It was proved that the phenomenon of experimenter bias was robust, as it continued to appear under a variety of controlled conditions.[76] Many of these studies imply that experimenter intention (belief or desired outcome) is what determines the outcome of the experiment.[77,78] In a frequently quoted exchange between the Dalai Lama and Princeton researchers studying mind/matter interactions, his Holiness was asked whether machines (random number generators) can be conscious – to which the Dalai Lama replied, "if you think it is so, it is," implying that humans can impart, confer or perceive consciousness in what we think of as inert matter. The Society for Scientific Exploration has been hosting lively forums and debates on the issues of experimenter bias, the decline effect, precognitive effects and the machine consciousness phenomenon in research.[79] The pursuit of a definition of consciousness is producing a growing number of research studies in college and university settings on psi across disciplines (physics, psychology and engineering). These studies represent the forefront of our understanding of creativity as much as they explain extrasensory perception and consciousness.[80]

On another front, the National Institute for Mental Health (NIMH) identified the 1990s as "the decade of the brain"[81] and the first 10 years of the twenty-first century as "the decade of discovery".[82] Its current strategic-plan priority for brain research is unusually broad; it is to *define the mechanisms of complex behavior*. The stated goal of this research activity is to advance drug treatments.[83] The study of epigenetic mechanisms is included in this mandate. Epigenomic factors in human health (e.g., the effect of environment, personal experience and the microbiome on health) add enormous complexity to research studies on the etiology of mental illness. Understanding the interplay between genomic and epigenomic influencers that define risk for developing illness will be a multi-decadal enterprise. As described by Dr. Bruce Lipton (2006, 2009), Dr. Pelletier (2018) and others, acknowledging the insights epigenetics brings to the study of human development changes everything.[84,85,86,87] It's another paradigm shift of great significance in regard to how we conduct science, and an important milestone in recognizing the value of integrative medicine. Lipton has summarized these changes in our view of health and healing as follows: (1) The epigenetic view of human development supersedes the Newtonian definition of matter (preferring the quantum view of universal connection), making what's invisible just as important as what we can see; (2) if genes are no longer seen as the sole determining factor of human potential or illness, the mind and psychological health become major factors, not minor players in the treatment planning process for all illness. These new ground rules alter our model of mind from one that is primarily linear in development and controlled by biological determinants to a dynamic model where cognitive executive functions are in fact co-creators of our state of health and wellness. The shift from germ theory (Lister & Pasteur 1852)[88] to terrain theory (Béchamp 1912)[89] as the cause of disease (an organism's state of balance is seen as the primary instigator of illness) also supports the notion that self-regulation is paramount. *Now*, the question for clinical practitioners becomes: How do we elevate the role and involvement of the individual in his/her healing process to utilize these newly realized capacities? While this assessment may seem speculative to some, these ideas are spurring change in medical care. A 2010 survey of 714 hospitals noted that 42% were offering *complementary and alternative medicine* (hereafter CAM), up from 37% in 2007 (different respondent pool, *n* not noted).[90] A more recent survey of non-institutionalized patients by the National Center for Complementary and Alternative Medicine showed that 33% of adults used some form of complementary health (both physical fitness – defined as yoga, tai chi, qi gong or chiropractic adjustments – and use of non-vitamin/non-mineral supplements).[91] The surveyed subjects spent $28.3 billion dollars in out-of-pocket expenditures in 2012. Culturally, the populace has clearly gotten the message that diet and exercise are key factors in maintaining health; creativity remains more ineffable in terms of its quantification value.

As our theoretical model of mind has changed, academic and clinical psychology has evolved from asking *what is creativity, and where is it located?* to *what can creativity do?* This turns out to be a much more fruitful approach to understanding creativity and its uses for activating innovative thinking and doing. Our thesis in this section was that models of mind are intimately linked to our approach to health, healing and creativity. Now, we turn our attention to how technology is changing healthcare and amplifying creativity. We have embedded our discussion in a competing framework of philosophies – holistic humanism versus technical rationality – and will continue to use these distinctions in the next section while discussing new technology.

26.3   NEW TOOLS FOR HEALTH AND WELLNESS

There is currently a wave of innovation and venture capital flowing to life sciences software development globally. Medical expertise is migrating to mobile platforms, making it possible to bring expertise anywhere and to enable patients to manage their health in new ways. In the previous century, the creation of therapies and the design of hospitals and places of recovery were driven by theories and ideas we no longer find as useful. In their place, research on the micro-world of mind and body, including biology, genetics, epigenetics and neurophysiology, now provides micro-data streams for diagnosis and analysis. The shift from macro theory to micro data has opened up an entirely new set of parameters for designing health interventions. One's model of mind and understanding of human development and human potential are key drivers of any complex software design process in healthcare product development. They determine the language used in the clinical encounter, the timing of intervention, the parameters of analysis, and how goals and objectives are established. Furthermore, we believe that if your model of mind is robust and values human creativity, then it will enrich the software design process, resulting in more expansive and dynamic design solutions. As mentioned earlier in the chapter, new developments in mind/brain research confirm that activity-based therapies for mental health and optimal functioning play an important role in recovery from illness, remediation of addiction and behavioral imbalances, as well as self-actualization and personal growth.[3–9] Additionally, we noted that the expressive therapies (art, music, movement and psychodrama) have a rich history in the use of *intermediary objects* to facilitate healing in psychotherapy and psychotherapeutic processes, thereby furnishing us with useful information on what constitutes a good holding environment outside the clinical encounter.[42–47] By definition, an intermediary object is any object, work space or medium that continues, advances and expands upon the patient/therapist dialogue and therapeutic relationship outside a clinical appointment.[14]

Together, micro-sensors for assessing physiological or mental states, and understanding the modes of communication or holding environment that supports therapeutic goals beyond clinical meetings, form a new design template for all kinds of medical interventions. The notion of embedding clinical assessments in creative authoring tools or activities that we enjoy (e.g., art making, music making, journaling) is also a recommended starting place for conceptualizing the design of intermediary objects. This approach, in our opinion, is well suited to the CAM and integrative medicine ethos. Mobile apps in medicine are nurturing a focal shift from *talking* with healthcare providers as the medium of the therapeutic encounter, to *doing/making/experimenting* and sharing data with healthcare providers. For example, heart rate variability (hereafter HRV) biofeedback devices like *Inner Balance*, or brain training platforms like *Lumosity*, are experiences which clients/patients self-direct. In this genre of tools, health education becomes a primary goal along with management of illness. Increasingly, the objective of many medical software interventions is to make lifestyle changes to avoid or reverse chronic illness.

Table 26.1 outlines two competing mind sets that are driving design innovation and their main characteristics. Much of future product development across the fields of science and healthcare will be initiated by professionals with deep subject matter expertise who apply their knowledge to the creation of products with no previous object identity – what do we mean by this? That the design of intermediary objects will be first-of-kind, akin to the way in which cell phones with visual screen interfaces changed our understanding of what a phone was or could be.[92,93] What follows is our critique of four software tools that embody a holistic design approach to human health in the use of digital media. In choosing among a variety of new materials and software devices, we use the opportunity to elucidate the differences between creative design and tools that are simply repurposing or adapting current tests and assays to a digital format. Innovation, in our opinion, implies that new contributions are being made to scientific research, new tools are emerging from evolving research, and new ways of engaging patients and educating people about their health result from the previous two conditions.

TABLE 26.1
Characteristics of Holistic versus Technocentric Design

Holistic Design Characteristics	Technocentric Design Characteristics
• Values clients as collaborators, views professional consultation as a reflective conversation; encourages creative input and participation – tech design is rooted in a holistic model of mind	• Values central control and authority as it relates to client interactions, ownership of client data (test results, analysis, lab results); tech design is rooted in economic priorities of greater efficiency and relies on a behaviorist model of mind
• De-mystifies professional knowledge as being the purview of experts	• Fortifies boundaries between experts and clients; evokes parent/child relationship metaphors (e.g., we know best) to characterize alliance
• Incorporates the client's knowledge and learning process, and acknowledges its value in shaping solutions	• Compliance rather than education of clients is valued and monetized

26.3.1   Four Examples of Holistic Design

Here, we present four tools with very different learning objectives:

> *Inner Balance* (a phone app designed to improve well-being and emotional coherence through heart rhythm pattern training).
>
> *OpenBCI* (mobile biosensing wearables that capture EEG/EMG/ECG – reporting real-time brain activity, muscle activity and heart rate, plus emotion detection, using open-source code and components for research and education).
>
> *ChoiceCompass* (a phone app that assesses heart rhythms to assist in decision making).
>
> *Akila AI* (a diabetes prevention solution that uses an AI-powered digital health coach to make lifestyle changes for better health).

These four companies represent innovators and investigators at very different stages of development and design experimentation. *Inner Balance* (made by the Institute for Heart Math) represents over 29 years of research; the tool itself is the result of four product development cycles. Inner Balance uses heart rate variability feedback to assist users in reducing stress and increasing happiness. *OpenBCI* was established in 2013 and has been growing its product line consistently, specializing in low-cost, high-quality hardware to allow greater numbers of researchers, educators, artists and hobbyists to participate in brain/body experimentation. It has fabricated headsets to measure EEG activity (brainwaves), bio-sensors to measure EMG (muscle) and ECG (heart beat) activity and emotional states, and interface boards, along with a variety of other specialized sensors. *ChoiceCompass* was launched in 2015 after a year-long testing period, with research on its algorithms ongoing. This tool allows you to compare two different or opposing choice-scenarios from your smartphone to determine which is producing more heart coherent signals, an indication of best choice. Lastly, *Akila AI* is a tech-driven platform that is currently delivering a diabetes prevention program in clinical trials. The company is in an early development phase. In Table 26.2, we briefly categorize the functionality of each tool.

What is it about these four tools that distinguish them as exceptional creative innovators from our point of view? They employ what we call *reflective research development practices* (Schön 1983).[26] Drawing upon our experiences as technology project/product designers, we'd like to share our "best

TABLE 26.2
Holistic Design Examples and Characteristics

Website	Tech	What Is It?	What Does It Do?
https://heartmath.org (Inner Balance)	Biosensing device (ear or finger clip)	Smartphone app and biofeedback device that tracks heart rhythms for coherence and incoherence	Aims to increase well-being and happiness through raising awareness about physiological processes and their impact on health
https://openbci.com	Multiple tool set, tool maker	EEG/EMG/ECG biosensing tools that interface with open-source and commercial software	Open-source platform for experimentation that also values its community of users as collaborators
https://choicecompass.com	Biosensing tool that works with your phone's camera	Smartphone app that taps into heart activity patterns related to intuition	Aids in decision making by allowing users to query their own physiological data
https://akila.ai	Virtual coach focusing on the mind/body environment	Tech-driven diabetes prevention program aimed at changing diet and exercise behaviors	Using Fitbit and cell phone technology, the learning platform supports behavioral change and facilitates greater awareness of eating habits

practice principles" in design, knowing that physicians are increasingly applying their expertise to tech-tool making both for research and for their patients in private practice. First, we will give a brief overview of our guiding principles. Then, we will use these concepts to evaluate and comment on our chosen four companies. The principles that we recommend relate to the project planning cycle and early product development cycles. They include: (a) *frame analysis*, (b) *repertoire-building research*, (c) *fundamental methods of inquiry and theory*, and (d) *process reflection-in-action practices* (Schön 1983, pp.309–323).

Frame analysis, as Schön conceived it, is the first step in project modeling. Simply stated, it is the lens through which you define a project or product. When practitioners are unaware of their "frames" for roles or problems, they do not experience the need to choose among them. When a practitioner becomes aware of frames, the possibility of alternative ways of framing reality enters the conversation. A role frame is super-ordinate to, and longer lasting than, the setting of the problem context. We recommend model of mind as a foundational frame. A new framing of a research issue is often the impetus for a new product, as illustrated by ChoiceCompass.

Repertoire-building research serves the function of accumulating and describing outlying exemplars or problems in ways that expand the boundary of thinking and drive the evolution of inquiry. When practice situations and problem contexts do not fit available theories, models of phenomenon or techniques of control, they may nevertheless be inappropriately assigned to pre-existing memes/theories. The cutting edge of medical research is engaged in repertoire-building research, defining new areas of study that have no precursors. Later, we discuss Inner Balance and the Institute for HeartMath as an example of how repertoire-building research was transformed into product development.

Research on fundamental methods of inquiry and theory naturally follow from frame setting and determining the body of research that one uses to begin product development. A practitioner's fundamental methods are closely connected to both frames and repertoire of exemplars. One way of facilitating this dialogue is through the use of process-flow modeling and action research methods, whereby an overarching theory and a generic method of inquiry are used to restructure a situation so that one can validly say that the theory fits the problem-situation. Our example of Akila AI showcases how adapting a well-studied and widely used pre-diabetes education program to an AI technology platform altered the goals of the program and resulted in altering inquiry methods.

Process Reflection in Action: In the reflective research principles we are recommending, researchers and practitioners enter into modes of collaboration very different from the forms of exchange usually implemented in applied science. The practitioner does not function as a mere user of the developer/researcher's product or data. She reveals the ways of thinking she brings to professional practice and draws on reflective research as an aid to personal development. These characteristics are commonly found in the open-source coding community. We offer OpenBCI as an exemplar of best practices in process reflection in action.

Next, we elaborate on best practices principles as they've been embodied by our chosen four companies.

26.3.2   Frame Analysis – ChoiceCompass as Example

The science behind algorithms that capture heart rate patterns is still quite young. The ingenuity of ChoiceCompass is that it allows users to query their own physiological data and invites them to learn about their psychophysiology through problem-solving queries. The phone app user defines a question with two solutions and employs the app to render a decision about which scenario produces a more coherent physiological response in terms of heart rhythms. By thinking about one solution and then the other (each for a period of 50 seconds) while holding a finger over a smartphone camera, the Mossbridge algorithm deciphers changes in heart beats based on the variations in blood color and the interval between heart beats to give feedback. ChoiceCompass is an exemplar of frame analysis because it "broke the mold" in terms of how HRV data had been used in the past, resulting in a novel learning tool. Drawing upon her deep understanding of human psychology, intuition and physiology, culminating in a novel model of mind, Mossbridge expanded upon previous heart variability uni-modal training tools (with different algorithms) by taking advantage of the breadth of variation in the phenomenon – meaning heart rate variance is highly individualistic. Mossbridge is seeing a more complex picture of heart rate variance (including gender differences) and can collate that data with client queries; moreover, ChoiceCompass stimulates reflective and creative thinking in the user.[94]

26.3.3 Repertoire-Building Research – Inner Balance as Example

The HeartMath Institute is our exemplar of an organization that adopted repertoire-building research activity to fill a void in the scientific literature. HeartMath's scientific studies on the psychophysiology of stress, resilience, and the interactions between the heart and the brain over 29 years have made a significant contribution to our understanding of how the autonomic and parasympathetic nervous systems work together. HeartMath used their research to design biofeedback tools that help people regulate and repattern learned behaviors that are beneath awareness (i.e., automatic responses to stress and frustration) and bring them into conscious awareness. Their studies demonstrate that patterns of heart activity have distinct effects on cognitive and emotional functions. During times of stress and negative emotions, the heart rhythm pattern is erratic and disordered. The corresponding pattern of disturbed neural signals traveling from the heart to the brain inhibits higher cognitive functions. Thinking clearly, remembering and learning are disrupted as a result. Conversely, more ordered, stable and coherent heart pattern input to the brain during positive emotional states has the opposite effect.[95] The Inner Balance mobile tool guides people into their coherence zone, providing graphical visual displays of heart rhythms to enhance the learning process. The tool is being used in both clinical and educational settings for all ages. The Institute of HeartMath is a shining example of an organization that employs repertoire-building research.

26.3.4 Research on Fundamental Methods of Inquiry and Theory – Akila AI as Example

When used to enhance human experience, AI technology or platforms that "remember" and make recommendations based on user-inputs can provide "just in time" learning experiences for patients, which occur on their own time, based on their own needs. This level of customization is important in making lifestyle changes. In adapting a face-to-face pre-diabetes program to an AI platform, Akila AI designers made use of a body of knowledge on learning theory and cognitive-behavior change not usually applicable to classroom education settings. The AI enhanced support platform engages the client in a two-way dialogue (through cognitive-behavioral-therapy prompts and user-generated voice inquiries). This interface allows more frequent interactions than face-to-face educational programs or asynchronous learning portals. AI prompts might be reminders to get up and walk for at least 5–10 minutes during the day or suggestions for lunch just before lunch time. Through the use of process-flow modeling and action research methods in clinical trials, the company is improving personalized health coaching.

26.3.5 Research on Process Reflection in Action – OpenBCI as Example

OpenBCI is an open-source platform that makes tools for human experimentation – including mobile EEG (brainwave sensors), ECG (heart beat sensors) and EMG (muscle activity sensors) gear, helmets and sensor interface boards (4, 8 and 16 channels). The company name denotes its kinship with open-source software (hereafter OSS) values, and the acronym BCI stands for brain–computer interface. The early OpenBCI model of product development involved creating an extensible, collaborative studio where the company's designers requested feedback from the researchers who use their products, thereby enhancing OpenBCI's iterative product development cycle. Additionally, the company provided space for researchers to showcase their studies on its website, and it continues to log and link to research that has been conducted using OpenBCI hardware. A hallmark of the OSS philosophy is the explicitness with which the relationship between designer/coder and user is spelled out with the goal of creating equal partnerships. Data ownership is clearly stated, sharing code (allowing for customization and enhancement) is what makes it all work as a communal enterprise, standards regarding financial remuneration are clearly stated, and tracking of information for any purpose (i.e., marketing) is optional or restrained. Exchanges between users and code writers are welcomed. To a large extent, the OSS community has already assimilated all four of Schön's principles of practice (i.e., frame analysis, repertoire-building research, research on fundamental methods of inquiry and theory, process reflection in action). Many would argue that the open-source community has manifested higher levels of creativity as a result. In this paradigm, divergent thinking and exploration are rewarded. OpenBCI exemplifies the fullest expression of *process reflection in action*.

In summary, today's technology-rich milieu offers unique opportunities for medical professionals to extend their expertise using and creating software design tools. Becoming a designer has its challenges. It's not necessary to acquire an engineering degree to tinker; there are many ways to collaborate. The most important decisions you make as a designer, surprisingly, are those that are least discussed by both the professional engineering and design communities. We have repeatedly emphasized model of mind as a fundamental frame for designing as starting place, knowing that it is understated in the design literature. Inherent in your model of mind and the depth to which it is articulated clearly in the design process are the values and user capacities that will guide you in decision making about tool design, the quality of the software environment you are designing, the quality of care your clients/patients receive through the use of the tool, and the quality and form of collaboration manifest in tool design.

Many medical practitioners are endowed with the resources (both as individual practitioners as and institutional affiliates) to conduct their own research and development process. In our books on *Psychology's New Design Science*,[14, 15] we encourage the adoption of the design literature and implementation of design studios in clinical training programs, citing the huge expense of engaging software engineers in the open market place. We think that clinical training programs can play an important role in challenging technocentric design by injecting alternative value systems into the software economy, based on real human needs. The debut of design studios within clinical training programs is underway in psychology and psychiatry,[96] and they are increasingly apparent in medical schools across the country. Design thinking and design reasoning underlie the evolution of all professions. Clinical graduate training programs not only represent the places where deep knowledge resides about medicine; they are also the places that have continuously interfaced with hospitals, clinics and healthcare facilities over time. Medical technology that grows in these contexts is much more likely to embody holistic design sensibilities (with a healthy respect for scientific method), because they are rooted in the reality of human/patient interactions and the standards of care applied in these settings. Practically speaking, introducing design studios into medical graduate training can be achieved through collaboration with engineering, art and psychology departments in university settings without tremendous investments.

26.4 CONCLUSION

Creativity is a verb. Like Jacob Moreno, we believe that our ability to create surplus realities is one of our most valuable mental abilities. Creativity is something that can be accessed from within in service to self-reflection, conflict resolution, problem solving, healing and self-actualization. The arts provide foundational experiences in bringing ideas to life, from concept to rendering, enabling belief in ourselves as capable doers and sparking innovation. Human facility for greater aliveness and joy, greater harmony and greater awareness may well be related to the wealth of creative outlets in our living environment in all phases of life.

In Section 26.2, we anchored our discussion to models of mind, noting that creativity has been a topic of concern academically for over 150 years but receives only intermittent focus from psychology and psychiatry. We are currently in a period of resurgent interest in creativity, supported by other disciplines, including physics, engineering and design. This confluence of interest is a promise of greater understanding of what creativity is and how we can harness it to develop human potential.

In Section 26.3, we featured four products that embody best practices in holistic design principles, which support and advance creative thinking. In elaborating upon the design process, we again emphasized what model of mind one chooses for designing, citing its importance to the quality and outcome of project/product development. Additionally, we provided best practice guidelines for beginning designers contemplating the use of new media to extend their expertise.

The extent to which the medical engineering community values creativity, human health and wellbeing is the extent to which it can overcome what we call the technical rationality ethos of tool making and product development. Technocentric design is driven by economic efficiencies, which in turn, are *framed* by the singular priority of commercial return on investment. The 5G cell phone infrastructure technology, for instance, is our exemplar of worst practices in technocentric design. The 5G design process has ushered in the era of building utilities for machines (as the identified consumer), now a business-to-business enterprise. As a result, human health and environmental health were altogether ignored in the build-out. The global backlash under way was swift and furious. Using our best practices principles as a comparative guide in this case, we can re-frame the issues in terms of the design process: (1) Accountability for decision making was insular, meaning that community stakeholders were not identified and brought into the process of design; (2) no articulated model of mind and human development was employed *as a foundational frame*, ostensibly removing human beings from *process-flow modeling* in the planning process; (3) new research to support its implementation was conducted but without testing the exposure toxicity of the 5G WiFi signals on people and the environment.[97,98,99,100] While outside the realm of medicine, the 5G build-out highlights how important design decisions are. This is both an ethical problem and a regulation problem.

As it relates to medicine, a recent article in the *LA Times* warned of the dangers of mixing tech corporate design practices (heavily biased toward technocentric design) with developing medical technology.[101] With the subtitle "Artificial intelligence has come to medicine … Are patients being put at risk?", the author cited tech's mantra of "fail fast and fix it later" as the culprit. The article documented doctors' and consumer advocates' concerns that regulators are not doing enough to keep consumers safe from flawed technology. It also suggested that design practices for invasive medical technology should be subject to the same testing requirements imposed on drug manufacturers, including rigorous scientific review and human trials – but they aren't. The author interviewed doctors actively engaged in life science venture capital firms, who noted that "most [medical] AI products have little evidence to support them." The reason given was that software developers find the Food and Drug Administration (FDA) process too onerous and too expensive. Here, we clearly see how our competing paradigms – humanistic holism and technical rationality – are playing out in the marketplace. It's very likely that we will continue to see more reports in the news similar to the *LA Times* article. The business marketing approach is to overwhelm public news media channels with upbeat stories of AI's wondrous accomplishments and the inevitability of its dominating economic progress. Time and again, critical analysis of acclaimed new tech products or services shows that what is at stake are competing value systems: efficiency (convergent thinking, systems thinking, control systems) versus personal involvement and the ability to exercise personal preferences (creativity, symbolic thinking, divergent thinking, intuition).[102,103] Technocentric thinking will always favor and be driven by economic efficiencies. Humanistic holism will predominantly favor enhancing the quality of human experience as a driver of innovation. Preserving the balance between these forces is necessary for a brighter future – this will be a true challenge for all future designers and medical practitioners.

We have woven together many strands of discussion on creativity, which shows that art in medicine is a much broader topic than imagined; creativity in medicine lies at the core of innovation and how therapeutic interactions are conceived and take shape. We hope that our perspective on these topics will help others to formulate their own ideas and criteria for thinking about project/product design and for evaluating new technologies.

REFERENCES

1. Ishizu T., Zeki S. (2013). The brain's specialized system for aesthetic and perceptual judgment. *Eur. J. Neurosci.* 108. https://10.1111/ejn.12135
2. Heilman K.M., Acosta L.M. (2013). Visual artistic creativity and the brain. *Prog. Brain Res.* 204, 19–43. https://10.1016/b978-0-444-63287-6.00002-6
3. Vartanian O., Bristol A.S., Kaufman A.B. (eds.) (2013). *Neuroscience of Creativity*. Cambridge, MA: MIT Press.
4. Chatterjee A. (2006). The neuropsychology of visual art: Conferring capacity. *Int. Rev. Neurobio.* 74, 39–49. https://10.1016/s0074-7742(06)74003-x
5. Richards R. (2010). Everyday creativity: Process and way of life – four key issues. In J.C. Kaufman, R.J. Sternberg (eds.), *The Cambridge Handbook of Creativity*. Cambridge, UK: Cambridge University Press.
6. Richards, R. (2007). *Everyday Creativity and New Views of Human Nature: Psychological, Social, and Spiritual Perspectives*. Washington, DC: American Psychological Association.
7. Runco M., Pritzker S.R. (eds.) (1999). *Encyclopedia of Creativity* (1–2). San Diego: Academic Press.
8. Staricoff R., Loppert S. (2003). Integrating the arts into healthcare: Can we affect clinical outcomes? In D. Kirklin, R. Richardson (eds.), *The Healing Environment Without and Within*. London, UK: Royal College of Physicians; 2003:63–80.
9. Leary D. (ed.) (1990). *Metaphors in the History of Psychology*. New York: Cambridge University Press.
10. Jung C. (1954). *The Development of Personality*. New York: Princeton University Press.
11. Vygotsky L. (1970). *Thought and Language*. Cambridge, MA: MIT Press.
12. Gardner H. (1985). *The Mind's New Science*. New York: Basic Books.
13. Imholz S., Sachter J. (eds.) (2017). *Psychology's New Design Science and the Reflective Practitioner*. River Bend: Libra Lab Press.
14. Imholz S., Sachter J. (eds.) (2014). *Psychology's New Design Science: Theory and Research*. Champaign: Common Ground.
15. Castiglioni A. (1947). *A History of Medicine*. London, UK: Routledge. https://doi.org/10.4324/9780429019883; ebook ISBN 9780429019883 published in 2019.
16. Marketos S., Fronimopoulos J.N., Laskaratos J. (1989). The treatment of eye diseases in the asclepieia. In H.E. Henkes, C.L. Zrenner (eds.), *History of Ophthalmology* (ACOI vol 2) Switzerland: Springer Nature. https://doi.org/10.1007/978-94-009-2387-4_5
17. Oberhelman S.M. (2013). *Dreams, Healing, and Medicine in Greece: From Antiquity to the Present*. Surrey, UK: Ashgate Publishing.
18. To name a few: The Golden Door in Escondido CA, Mii Amo in Sedona AZ, Sunrise Springs Spa in Sante Fe NM, Art of Living Center in Boone NC, Preidlhof in South Tyrol Italy, Hotel Palacio in Lisbon Portugal. Many of these spas are surrounded by hundreds of acres of pristine natural beauty. They feature the use of native plants in their treatments, and they all promote organic unprocessed food. Note the variety of activities: Yoga, kickboxing, trail trekking, mineral baths, sweat lodges, forest bathing, bird watching, fishing, sea sports, in addition to art classes, meditation, poetry and journaling classes, dance as ritual and other healing activities.
19. Zaidel D.W. (2013). Biological and neuronal underpinnings of creativity in the arts. In O. Vartanian, S. Bristol, J.C. Kaufman (eds.), *Neuroscience of Creativity*. Cambridge, MA: MIT Press.
20. Sawyer K. (2011). The cognitive neuroscience of creativity: A critical review. *Creativ. Res. Jrl.* 23, 137–154. https://doi.org/10.1080/10400419.2011.571191
21. Finger S., Zaidel D.W., Boller F., Bogousslavsky J. (eds.) (2013). *The Fine Arts, Neurology and Neuroscience: History and Modern Perspectives*. Oxford, UK: Elsevier.
22. Dietrich A., Kanso R. (2010). A review of EEG, ERP and neuroimaging studies of creativity and insight. *Psych. Bull.* 136, 822–848. https://doi.org/10.1037/a0019749

23. Krout R.E. (2007). Music listening to facilitate relaxation and promote wellness: Integrated aspects of our neuro-physiological response to music. *J. Arts Psychother.* 34(2), 134–141.

24. Gergen K. (1990). Metaphor, meta-theory, and the social world. In D. Leary (ed.), *Metaphors in the History of Psychology.* New York: Cambridge University Press.

25. Schön D. (1983). *The Reflective Practitioner: How Professionals Think in Action.* New York: Basic Books.

26. Cattell J. (1896). Address of the president before the American Psychological Association, 1895. *Psychol. Rev.* 3, 135–48.

27. Rank O. (1975). *Art and Artist.* New York: Agathon Press.

28. Jung C., von Franz M-L., Henderson J., Jacobi J., Jaffé A. (1964). *Man and His Symbols.* Garden City: Doubleday.

29. Moreno J.L. (1993). *Who Shall Survive?* McLean, VA: American Society of Group Psychotherapy & Psychodrama.

30. Maslow A. (1968). *Toward a Psychology of Being.* New York: Van Nostrand Reinhold.

31. Hall C., Lindzey G. (1970). *Theories of Personality.* New York: John Wiley & Sons.

32. Jung C.G. with Shamdasani S. (ed.) (2009). *Red Book (Liber Novus).* New York: Philemon Series/W.W. Norton.

33. Knill P., Levine E.G., Levine S.K. (2005). *Principles and Practice of Expressive Arts Therapy.* London, UK: Jessica Kingsley.

34. Blatner A. (1988). *Foundations of Psychodrama: History, Theory and Practice.* New York: Springer.

35. Fox J. (ed.) (1987). *The Essential Moreno: Writings on Psychodrama, Group Method, and Spontaneity by J.L. Moreno.* New York: Springer.

36. Seligman M., Csikszentmihalyi M. (2014). Positive psychology: An introduction. In M. Csikszentmihalyi (ed.), *Flow and the Foundations of Positive Psychology.* Dordrecht: Springer. 279–298.

37. Hoffman E. (2008). Abraham Maslow: A biographers reflections. *J. Human. Psychol.* 48(4), 439–443.

38. Goud N. (2008). Abraham Maslow: A personal statement. *J. Human. Psychol.* 48(4),448–451.

39. Dewey J. (1915). *The School and Society.* Chicago: University of Chicago Press.

40. Read H. (1945). *Education Through Art.* New York: Pantheon.

41. McNiff S. (1992). *Art as Medicine: Creating a Therapy of the Imagination.* Boston: Shambhala.

42. Peters J. (2000). *Music Therapy: An Introduction.* Springfield: Charles C. Thomas.

43. Pennebaker J. (ed.) (1995). *Emotion, Disclosure, and Health.* Washington, DC: American Psychological Association.

44. Zausner T. (2007). *When Walls Become Doorways: Creativity and the Transforming Illness.* New York: Harmony/Random House.

45. Eliade M. (1964). *Shamanism: Archaic Techniques of Ecstasy.* New York: Pantheon.

46. Hillman J. (1977). *Re-visioning Psychology.* New York: Harper and Row.

47. Prokofieff S. (2015). *The Esoteric Nature of the Anthroposophical Society.* West Midlands: Wynstones Press.

48. Simonton D. (2001). *The Psychology of Creativity: A Historical Perspective.* See: https://simonton.faculty.ucdavis.edu/wp-content/uploads/sites/243/2015/08/HistoryCreativity.pdf

49. Stocking G.W. (1985). *Objects and Others: Essays on Museums and Material Culture.* Madison: University of Wisconsin Press.

50. Hudson K. (1975). *A Social History of Museums.* New York/London: MacMillan Press.

51. Watson J.B. (1925). *Behaviorism.* New York: Norton.

52. Skinner B.F. (1953). *Science and Human Behavior.* New York: McMillan.

53. Bandura A., Walters R.H. (1963). *Social Learning and Personality Development.* New York: Holt Rinehart and Winston.

54. Pavlov I.P. (1927). Translated by Anrep G.V. Conditioned reflexes: An investigation of the physiological activity of the cerebral cortex. *Nature* 121 (3052), 662–664. https://doi.org/10.1038/121662a0

55. Dobzhansky T. (1937). *Genetics and the Origin of the Species.* New York: Columbia University Press.

56. Hebb D. (1949). *The Organization of Behavior: A Neuropsychological Theory.* New York: John Wiley & Sons.

57. Piaget J. (1971). *Genetic Epistemology.* New York: W.W. Norton.

58. Wiener N. (1954). *Human Use of Human Beings: Cybernetics and Society.* Boston: Da Capo Press.

59. Newell A., Simon H.A. (1972). *Human Problem Solving.* Upper Saddle River: Prentice Hall.

60. Drucker J. (2005). *Sweet Dreams: Contemporary Art and Complicity.* Chicago/London: University of Chicago Press.

61. Winnicot D.W. (1964). *The Maturational Process and the Facilitating Environment*. New York: International Universities Press.

62. Kohut H. (1997). *The Restoration of the Self*. New York: International Universities Press.

63. Kohut H. (1984). *How Does Analysis Cure?* Chicago: University of Chicago Press.

64. McNiff S. (1998). *Art-based Research*. London/New York: Jessica Kingsley.

65. Leher J. (2007). *Proust was a Neuroscientist*. New York: Houghton Mifflin.

66. Benson H., Greenwood M., Klemchuk A.B. (1975). The relaxation response: Psychophysiologic aspects and clinical applications. *Int. J. Psychiatr. Med.* 6(1–2), 87–98.

67. Benson H., Klipper M.Z. (1975). *The Relaxation Response*. New York: Avon.

68. Benson H., Dusek J.A., Sherwood J.B., Lam P., Bethea C.F., Carpenter W., Levitsky S., Hill P., Clem D.W., Janoj K.J., Drumel D., Kopecky S., Mueller P., Marek D., Rollins S., Hibberd P.L. (2006). Study of the therapeutic effects of intercessory prayer (STEP) in cardiac bypass patients: A multicenter randomized trial of uncertainly and certainty of receiving intercessory prayer. *Am. Heart J.* 151(4), 934–942.

69. David Bohm on perception: from: https://transitionconsciousness.wordpress/2011/09/03/david-bohm-on-perception/, accessed December 12, 2019

70. Frabboni S., Gazzai G.C., Pozzi G. (2007). Young's double-slit interference experiment with electrons. *Am. J. Phys.* 75(1053), 5.

71. Davisson C.J., Germer G. (1927). The diffraction of electrons by a crystal of nickel. *Bell System Tech. J.* 7, 90–105. https://10.1002/j.1538-7305.1928.tb00342.x

72. Bach R., Pope D., Liou S-H, Batelaan H. (2013). Controlled double-slit electron diffraction. *New J. Phys.* 15 033018. https://10.1008/1367-2630/15/3/033018

73. Pribram K.H. (1990). From metaphors to models: The use of analogy in neuropsychology. In D. Leary (ed.), *Metaphors in the History of Psychology*. New York: Cambridge University Press.

74. May E., Utts J.M., Spottiswoode J.P. (1995). Decision augmentation theory: Toward a model for anomalous mental phenomena. *J. Parapsychol.* 59, 195–220.

75. Schmidt H. (1970). PK test with electronic equipment. *J. Parapsychol.* 34(3), 7.

76. May E., Paulinyi T., Vassy Z. (2005). Anomalous anticipatory skin conductance response to acoustic stimuli: Experimental results and speculation upon a mechanism. *J. Altern. Complement. Med.* 11(4), 695–702.

77. Radin D., Nelson R., Dobyns Y., Houtkooper J. (2006). Assessing the evidence for mind-matter interaction effects. *J. Sci. Explor.* 20(3), 361–374.

78. May E., Spottiswoode J.P. (2011). The global consciousness project: Identifying the source of psi. *J. Scie. Explor.* 25(4), 663–682.

79. See https://www.scientificexploration.org, accessed December 12, 2019.

80. Smith P.H., Moddel G. (2015). Applied psi. In J. Palmer, D Marcusson-Claverty (eds.), *Parapsychology: A Handbook for the 21st Century*. Jefferson: McFarland & Co.

81. National Institute of Health Website, accessed December 5, 2019: https://www.nih.gov/about-nih/what-we-do/nih-almanac/national-institute-mental-health-nimh

82. National Institute of Health Library, accessed December 5, 2019: https://www.ncbi.nlm.nih.gov/pmc/articles/PMC1936236

83. National Institute of Health Website, accessed December 5, 2019: https://www.nimh.nih.gov/about/strategic-planning-reports/strategic-objective-1.shtmlu

84. Lipton B. (2006). *The Wisdom of Your Cells: How Your Beliefs Control Your Biology*. Louisville, CO: Audio Book: Sounds True Publishers. ISBN: 1591795222

85. Lipton B., Bhaerman S. (2009). *Spontaneous Evolution: Our Positive Future and How to Get There from Here*. Carlsbad, CA: Hay House Press.

86. Francis R.C. (2001). *Epigenetics: How Environment Shapes Our Genes*. New York: Norton & Company.

87. Pelletier K. (2018). *Change Your Genes, Change Your Life: Creating Optimal Health with the New Science of Epigenetics*. San Rafael, CA: Orion Press.

88. Lister J., Pasteur L. (1852). *Germ Theory and its Applications to Medicine on the Antiseptic Principle of the Practice of Surgery*. Amherst, MA.

89. Béchamp A (1912). *The Blood and Its Third Anatomical Element*. M.R Leverson & translator (eds.). London, UK: John Ouseley Limited.

90. See https://www.hhnmag.com/articles/5496-more-hospitals-offering-cam, accessed December 27, 2019.

91. See https://nccih.nih.gov/about/strategic-plans/2016/use-complementary-integrative-health-approaches-2012, accessed December 27, 2019.

92. LeMasson P., Hatchuel A., Weil B. (2011). The interplay between creativity issues and design theories: A new perspective for design management? *Creativity and Innovation Management*, 20(4), 217–238.

93. LeMasson P., Weil B., Hatchuel A. (2010). *Strategic Management of Innovation and Design*. Cambridge, UK: Cambridge University Press.

94. See https://www.ChoiceCompass.com, accessed January 3, 2020.

95. See https://www.ChoiceCompass.com, accessed Jan 3, 2020.

96. See Sofia University's, Transformative Technology Lab, and Stanford University's Innovation Lab within the Department of Psychiatry.

97. NGO response to 5G health issues: https://ehtrust.org/wp-content/uploads/Scientist-5G-appeal-2017 .pdf, https://ehtrust.org/epa-recommendations-and-reports-on-cell-phones-radiofrequency-and-electro-magnetic-fields/

98. Industry promotion of 5G masquerading as research: https://spectrum.ieee.org/news-from-around-ieee /the-institute/ieee-member-news/will-5g-be-bad-for-our-health, https://www.sdxcentral.com/5g/defini-tions/importance-5g-research

99. US Senate committee meeting with industry leaders admitting no research has been done on human effects: https://www.blumenthal.senate.gov/newsroom/press/release/at-senate-commerce-hearing-blu-menthal-raises-concerns-on-5G-wireless-technologys-potential-health-risks

100. See peer reviewed studies on wifi: https://ehtrust.org/science/peer-reviewed-research-studies-on-wi-fi/

101. Szabo L. (2020). Can medical artificial intelligence live up to the hype? *Los Angeles Times*, January 3, 2020.

102. Wood P. (2015). *Technocracy Rising: The Trojan Horse of Global Transformation*. Mesa: Coherent Publishing.

103. Zuboff S. (2019). *The Age of Surveillance Capitalism*. New York: Public Affairs/Hachette Book Group.

27 Information Medicine for the 21st Century
Physicks and Physics

Nisha J. Manek

CONTENTS

27.1 INTRODUCTION

Books about integrative medicine have become commonplace, but the approach taken here is not at all common. This chapter is about the human organism and how its energetic and informational systems function. It builds on fundamental principles of the laws of nature, of physics, which underpin all processes in the universe. The premise is that human healing and vibrant wellbeing can be elegant, simple and far less convoluted than current medical science wisdom purports it to be. The chapter aims to elucidate these laws from the basics of physics and build a solid ground of the best of translational medicine.

Medical science has gone on the premise that by looking for fundamental building blocks of the physical body, we can reverse engineer and understand the mechanisms of health. The language "building blocks" reinforces the abstraction we see. The main purpose of science is to understand the cell, enzymes and biochemical machinery and then to fix it. What is the problem with this kind of scientific thinking? Compartmentalization, physical separation and discrete objects in space and time. The properties of the whole cannot be analyzed by way of the parts. The human being cannot be divided.

So, how does science handle that? We don't. We ignore the problems of treating separate parts. It's generally felt not to be necessary. The body is seen as separate parts, and one hopes that someone else pays attention to another area. The separation is treated as real. Medicine has adopted the scheme of separating systems, which is a useful approximation when dealing with seemingly inanimate objects but not when dealing with living systems and especially conscious, self-motivated humans.

The great meltdown of 2020–2021 has exposed how the lockdown, that soul-crushing exercise in economic suicide, isn't working. If there's a silver lining here, it is that people are getting a closer look at the true, self-interested character of today's medical system. We can't survey the circumstances without feeling a call to action. We must respond with an exercise designed to redraw the boundaries of our free thought. The cost of moving slowly is increasingly clear. We cannot blame a virus for the destruction of large parts of society. Fear has eroded reason and curiosity and replaced

DOI: 10.1201/b23304-29

these virtues with whatever is most expedient. Developing further biochemicals for human diseases as the best way to defeat illnesses is now being fundamentally challenged. It is also the incompetence of a broken system. We need a broader strategic framework to understand the deeper patterns of how health may be achieved. The problem, simply put, is this: We dispense medical care to heal a body with a disease, but we now know that this is grossly inaccurate. We should do away with the separate systems sooner rather than later and replace them with something more holistic. What is common? Undivided wholeness. Keeping wholeness front and center gives a course correction, empowering people to prevent illness and absolve themselves from the prevailing narrative.

Empowering people summons a key inquiry. Can intention be therapeutic? A powerful question indeed. This chapter will examine the data of the power of humans to change the properties of materials under controlled conditions. At least as it's understood in the broader context of integrative medicine, the idea of intention has startling implications. Intention-based healing is information medicine.

The technical description to follow will be challenging for some readers. How was I to proceed? I have attempted to make the content user-friendly by keeping mathematical equations to a minimum. Any mathematical notation is explained in the most elementary terms. For many of you, try to keep a sense of where we are going with this. We are entering an exciting new territory of science beyond today's accepted physics.

27.2 BIOLOGY RUNS ON LOW ENTROPY

Much of this chapter was written in California, where the warm sunshine provides a never-ending reminder of the overarching influence of solar energy flux for sustaining life. At school, I was told that it is energy that makes the world go round. Energy activates plant growth, powers our machinery and engines, and spurs us to wake every morning full of vitality. We need to get energy – for example, from the sun, from fossil fuels or nuclear power. When unifying concepts for life are sought, they reside in the distribution of energy in the universe. If thermal inequalities were eliminated, no intelligent life would be possible. The flow of energy through a system acts to organize that system.[1] Biology is a manifestation of energy movement.

The study of energy and its transformations is thermodynamics. The foundations of thermodynamics are contained in the First and Second Laws of Thermodynamics.[2] The First Law says that energy is conserved. Any conservation law states that something doesn't change, and any use of the Law involves accounting. There is a fixed amount of energy, and we need to find and add up the various pieces to account for the total. The remarkable thing about this accounting scheme is its generality. It applies equally to living matter and to inanimate stuff. It plain works!

The Second Law says that within the conservation framework, we can't have it any which way we like.[2] Things are not going to be perfect. The Second Law invokes a quantity called *entropy*, something that is not familiar in the medical sciences. I will come back to entropy. The general, condensed version of the Second Law is:

$$G = PV + E - TS$$

The "G" stands for "Gibbs free energy" and energy to do *useful work*. Differences in free energy functions drive all processes in nature. The "PV" term or pressure times volume ($P \times V$) on the right side of the equation underpins the 19th-century age of the power of steam engines. Gibbs free energy can also result from changes in internal energy (ΔE), temperature (ΔT) and entropy (ΔS). In classical physics, quantities such as pressure, volume and temperature can easily be related to daily experience. Other parameters, such as work, heat and energy, are harder to conceptualize but make contact with familiar ideas. Finally, we have quantities such as entropy that are almost entirely dependent on abstractions.

Taking the example of the steam engine, the overall motive power can be understood and calculated as the kinetic energy of water molecules bouncing around in myriad ways. We don't need to know what each water molecule is doing to get the whole system's behavior. In other words, we don't require information on the great number of microscopic states that make up the engine's interior. Ludwig Boltzmann, an Austrian physicist, described this in some detail in the late 1800s.[3] Boltzmann showed that entropy exists because we cannot distinguish particular atoms/molecules and cannot, for example, assign a specific number to each one. He demonstrated that entropy is precisely the quantity that counts the great number of the different molecular/atomic configurations that we cannot distinguish between. This does not mean that our inability to differentiate between microstates is a mental construct; it depends on actual, existing physical interactions. Entropy is not an arbitrary quantity. It is a relative one, like speed. Heat and entropy are statistical descriptions of nature.

The famous Boltzmann equation is:

$$S = k \log(W)$$

This equation tells us that we do not need to know what every molecule in the engine is doing. The Boltzmann constant, k, is a conversion factor relating energy to its temperature at the individual molecule level. Boltzmann's constant is a tiny number to balance out the giant W, a bridge between microscopic and macroscopic worlds. The "S" term is the thermodynamic entropy, and W represents the number of ways the individual tiny molecules (such as water molecules) can arrange themselves and is a vast number. If we know some of the factors affecting W, such as the number of molecules or the volume change, we can calculate the system's entropy. The number of molecules could be a dozen or a standard mole (6.022×10^{23} molecules). The logarithm function allows more straightforward calculations for huge numbers. Boltzmann ushered in "statistical physics," and its triumph has been understanding the probabilistic nature of heat and temperature.

Boltzmann's probabilistic theory explained why heat flows from hot to cold, why swirls of ink disappear into the water to a uniform pale blue, and why smoke from a cigarette vanishes into the air. We understand the direction of each process and its irreversibility. Energy transformation – be it chemical, mechanical, electrical, and so on – loses some energy, and there is no free way of getting it back to reuse. In this transformation, the energy is conserved, but entropy increases. It is entropy that cannot be turned back. The Second Law specifies this. Succinctly written, the Second Law is:

$$\Delta S \geq 0$$

What makes the world go round is not sources of energy but sources of low entropy.[4] Without low entropy, energy would dilute into uniform heat, and the world would power down in a state of thermal equilibrium – no processes would occur. The sun is nature's supply of low-entropy energy, which allows all biological life to grow. Behind the seemingly simple equation of entropy constantly increasing, an entire world awaits discovery.

27.3 INFORMATION, THE IRREDUCIBLE FACTOR IN NATURE

The universe is made of energy, matter and information, but information makes the universe interesting.[5] Without information, the universe would be a featureless, amorphous soup. It would lack the structures and shapes, the aperiodic ordering and fractal arrangements that give the universe its elegance and complexity. Information, like matter and energy, is a fundamental principle of nature. It gets even more interesting. Through its relationship with thermodynamics, information can *drive* processes that we see in nature. How is information a source of Gibbs free energy? Secondly, where does the information come from?

In 1948, Claude E. Shannon published a paper titled "A Mathematical Theory of Communication."[6] Communication theory, or information theory as it is nowadays called, was one of the most important scientific advances of the last half-century, and it revolutionized the basis of modern communications systems. Because of information theory, we can talk to a loved one via the telephone, view television entertainment and download photos on our devices. Specifying or selecting the choice between two equally probable alternatives, which might be messages or numbers to be transmitted, involves one bit of information. By quantifying the number of bits – yes (1) or no (0) – we need to encode messages, the bit is a universal measure of the amount of information in terms of choice or uncertainty. Next, if we want to compress and squeeze a string of characters, the probabilities become key. Shannon bumped into the same principle as Boltzmann: *Probability.* Boltzmann described all the countless probable arrangements of gas molecules of a system so we can "see" how the whole behaves; that is, entropy refers to an average of physical states (such as temperature). In the analogous information function, Shannon described all the countless probable arrangements of the letters of the English alphabet to understand how they transmit communication. In Shannon's formula, information refers to a particular physical state (such as the specific sentence "Dinner is ready.").[6]

The fact that Boltzmann and Shannon both derived the same equation points to the deeply physical nature of information. Yet despite the differences in interpretation that mire down the reconciliation of Shannon's and Boltzmann's ideas, we can still conclude that not only are messages made of information, but most things are. Shannon's theory is more general than Boltzmann's because it applies to any aggregates or physical order. Think of virologists talking about the information contained in virus RNA, or the information in an aria, a video of your child playing on your phone, or the word sequence in this section. Information refers to the presence of order. Shannon's theory applies to any linear array of order in symbols. His theory remains eternally valid.

In his 1962 book *Science and Information Theory*, French physicist Léon Brillouin showed that every experiment conducted on the system yields specific information about the system.[7] Consider this as a type of informational order in an otherwise chaotic system of gas molecules; it has been labeled as the creation of negentropy (less entropy). The crux of this scientific argument is that there is a type of equivalence between negentropy and information. An information increase in a physical event represents a decrease of equal magnitude in the system's entropy.

Coming back to the second question: Where does information come from? We can now consider the nature of consciousness. This brings up many philosophical points about what consciousness is. But, let's go further and ask what consciousness *does*. We see that it creates and manipulates information in symbols such as language, numbers and mathematics, creativity such as art and music, and more. We can appreciate the broad meaning and importance of information in our lives. We share information, knowledge, stories, concepts, opinions, ideas, experiences, wishes, emotions, feelings and moods. Human beings are creative beings. Human consciousness creates information by intention.[8] Just as heat and motion can be communicated, so can strength and weakness and disease. The prevailing struggle in the universe is the war between order and disorder, between entropy and information.

The first question: How is information a source of Gibbs free energy? To get to the answer, we need to go to the basement in Stanford University's Department of Materials Science and Engineering.

27.4 TARGET EXPERIMENTS SHOWING THE POWER OF HUMAN INTENTION TO ALTER MATERIAL PROPERTIES

In the late 1990s, Professor William A. Tiller at Stanford University conducted a series of "target experiments" to test if human intention could impact materials.[9] For each target experiment, Tiller chose a novel two-stage procedure. He took water as his test material. Water is familiar to us. It's critical to biological life. The body's acid/alkaline balance is exquisitely controlled at a pH of 7.4. Any deviation of half a pH unit up or down can mean disruption of cellular function and even death. Tiller chose to change purified water's pH by one whole unit, a significant change and beyond random noise. His protocol centered on the idea of creating information – with intention – and holding the intention in meditation to "imprint" into a simple circuit device. The intention for water was as follows: To activate the indwelling consciousness of the system so that the intention host device (IHD) decreases (or increases) the pH of the experimental water by one pH unit, that is, the hydrogen ion (H+) content by a factor of ten compared with the control.

In the first stage, Tiller, with three of his Stanford graduate students, settled around a table in the physics laboratory, with the electric device in the center. They went into a meditative state – like a communion. Tiller's reading out the intention broke the silence. Then, silence for more than 30 minutes as they held the core intention in mind. The "host" device was thereby imprinted with the information.[10] The imprinted device was "meta-stable," excited above the thermodynamic equilibrium state with subtle energy information. The IHD was protected with aluminum foil to reduce ambient electromagnetic field effects and leakage of the information.

In the second stage, the imprinted IHD was shipped to Minnesota, where the actual experiments were conducted. The receiving laboratory was blinded to the primary intention imprinted in any IHD. Controls, unimprinted devices or UEDs, were also tested for their capacity to change the target material, purified water. The IHD was switched on precisely 6 inches from a water vessel with an electronic pH meter continuously measuring the pH with an accuracy of ± 0.001 pH units. The initial experiments on water pH took about 2 months, and the data were resounding. The water pH would change in line with the information imprinted into the IHD. The UED controls had no effect.[11] No chemical or electrical energy was applied to the water sample.

Tiller went on to use his two-stage protocol to significantly increase (25% at $p < 0.001$) the *in vitro* chemical activity of the liver enzyme alkaline phosphatase[12, 13] and to significantly increase the *in vivo* ratio of adenosine-5'-triphosphate to adenosine diphosphate in the cells of the fruit fly *Drosophila melanogaster* larvae so that they would have a significantly reduced (25% at $p < 0.001$) larval developmental time to the adult fly stage.[14]

Astonishingly, all of these experiments were successful. There is a very low probability for consciousness to affect a physical experiment in today's scientific worldview. Furthermore, to imbed an intention in a host device, which can then be transported to another laboratory site and generate such effects, would be considered impossible. These results are nothing short of dramatic. Other independent investigators have replicated the water pH target experiments in their own laboratories.[15] A device could be imprinted by highly conscious humans, and that device was stable for enough time to affect a target material. This science has revolutionary implications. It tells us that focused human intention has coherent energy to impact physical materials in a specific direction.

27.5   DUAL REALITIES AND FIELD EFFECTS

The target intention experimental data is compelling and has been replicated by Tiller's laboratory. Although other independent laboratories have successfully reproduced the protocol of changing water pH with an IHD, it is primarily a single-laboratory experience. The target experimental data demands a new scientific framework whereby the results are lawful and understandable.

With repeated target experiments, Tiller and colleagues discovered a remarkable phenomenon. Using an IHD in the laboratory testing space over extended periods – 3 to 4 months – the conditions of the laboratory space shifted.[9] Observations of the ambient air temperature, water pH and water temperature showed each to oscillate precisely. For example, an examination of air temperature oscillations showed large 3°C fluctuations in a rhythmic pattern. The air temperature fluctuated at the target experiment setup location and various positions around the room and into the hallway. The instrument accuracy of 0.001°C allowed detailed examinations of these huge temperature waves. They were not associated with air-conditioning or with diurnal cycles of day and night-time. Taking the real-time air temperature waves, Tiller used Fourier analysis to convert them to an amplitude spectrum. The Fourier mathematics revealed unusual behavior. Different spatial locations and the respective frequency at each location nested into each other like harmonics. In other words, all the spectral frequencies of the air temperature "nested" into each other from the different probe locations. Typically, no nesting harmonics would be expected for the air temperature; this is anomalous behavior.

Similarly, the water pH and water temperature also had precisely oscillating wave shapes. Fourier mathematics for both sets of waves "nested" in harmonics. All these oscillations were present over long periods – more than 4½ years – demonstrating something unusual about the physical space wherein the target experiments were conducted. In Tiller's description, it was as if the whole lab space was coherently pumping![9]

Tiller took a further step and checked whether the air temperature oscillations were due to a convection pattern known as Bénard convection. Bénard convection describes air density inversion and rotating currents that bring about oscillating temperature readings. Setting up forced convection with a fan, one would expect the temperature oscillations to disappear instantly if they were due to air currents. With two fans, each with enough force to blow sheets of paper across the room, Tiller recorded the nature of the oscillations. Such a forced convection arrangement *didn't obliterate* the oscillating behavior. This could mean only one thing: The air temperature oscillations *were not due to air molecules*.

It was clear from the data that the space itself is critical to the robustness of the target experiments. The space itself became transformed in fundamental ways. Tiller calls the changed lab space "conditioned." Applying physics terminology, the experimental space altered from a normal state, termed the U(1) EM (electromagnetic) gauge symmetry, to the next higher one, termed the SU(2) EM gauge symmetry state.[16] The higher SU(2) EM gauge symmetry state is also a higher thermodynamic free energy per unit volume state from physics theory. Tiller named the two unique realities Direct space (D-space) to signify U(1) EM gauge and Reciprocal space (R-space) to signify SU(2) EM gauge.

A pivotal "signature" of conditioned space is the magnetic polarity effect. This was done to tease out the evidence for a dual nature: one electrical and particle-like (D-space) and the other magnetic wave information (R-space). Magnets are dipolar. No magnetic monopoles have been discovered to exist in nature. In normal D-space, Tiller repeated the water pH experiment. The water pH with the North pole facing into the water vessel and then the South pole facing into the water would have identical results in terms of H⁺ content. The pH results for either magnetic pole would be predicted by established thermodynamic standards and be equal to zero. In an IHD-conditioned space – R-space – the same setup with a dipolar magnet had very striking results on water pH. The North pole of the magnet *decreased* the water pH, and the South pole *increased* the water pH. Somehow, an IHD-conditioned space allows measuring instruments to access magnetic monopoles.[17]

An important consequence of a conditioned space (R-space) is non-local connectivity between locations separated by huge physical distances over thousands of miles. The connectivity has been termed macroscopic information entanglement.[18] Table 27.1 summarizes some of the general features of D-space and R-space.

Tiller's intention experimental findings answer: How is information a source of Gibb's free energy? The answer is tied to space. The physical space is also called "physical vacuum" and was originally termed "empty space" by the British physicist Paul Dirac.[19] The physical vacuum is critical to understanding the laws of physics and provides a framework in which the world is embedded. Dirac's equations predicted magnetic monopoles.[20] Today, more than 80 years later, science hadn't discovered magnetic monopoles until Tiller's intention experiments. In Reciprocal space, magnetic monopole effects become possible.

The R-space has a higher thermodynamic free energy per unit volume than the usual electric atom/molecule level of reality (D-space). The conditioned space "pumps" energy to do useful work, that is, alter the water's hydrogen ion content in the direction specified by human intention! Energy flows from a higher energy potential to lower potential until equilibrium status is reached.

The entanglement effects of R-space over huge distances provide the backdrop for healing intention broadcast (sent) over large distances to specific physical locations. Remember, R-space isn't electromagnetic. Its magic is a magnetoelectric wave information substance.

TABLE 27.1
Characteristics of Direct Space and Higher Gauge Reciprocal-Space[a]

	Direct Space (U(1)) Gauge	**Reciprocal Space (SU(2)) Gauge**
Medical model	Conventional medicine	Integrative (complementary) medicine
Constituent elements	Electric atom-molecule Electromagnetic (EM) waves	Magnetoelectric information waves (analogue in vacuum level)
Coordinates	Space and time dependent	Reciprocal domain with *frequency* coordinates
Mathematical properties[b]	Scalar and vector quantities	Vector and tensor quantities
Signature of the physical space	Electric monopoles accessed	Magnetic monopoles accessed
Entanglement between parts of a system	Present very locally	Non-local entanglement over extensive (thousands of miles) distances
Information as a source of thermodynamic free energy potential[c]	Information has negligible effects using the Boltzmann's constant	Information effects of significant magnitude as Boltzmann's constant analogue of higher order and change in entropy

[a] Physical measurements quantitatively consist of two parts, one from D-space and one from R-space, when there is space conditioning. Space conditioning may be present from human biofields or from imprinting with an intention host device.

[b] Scalar quantities can be specified by one number, such as temperature and pH values. Vector quantities have magnitude, direction and phase angle to properly define the property. Tensor quantities have geometric mapping associated with any measurement at any point in space.

[c] Boltzmann's constant: 1.380650×10^{-23} joules per Kelvin ($J\ K^{-1}$)

27.6 FROM BENCH TO REAL-WORLD APPLICATION OF INFORMATION MEDICINE

We can move to the human biofields and subtle energies.[21] The understanding of unique levels of the physical space and the signature of the R-space to differentiate magnetic monopoles applies to the human body. Generally, chiropractors and naturopathic physicians are more familiar with the use of magnets to identify imbalances in the body. Generally, holding a magnet close to the body, the South pole strengthens whereas the North pole weakens the muscle groups. Since muscle proprioceptors are intimately connected to the acupuncture meridians, this is evidence that the human body already has *a higher gauge state system* within it.

The acupuncture-meridian/chakra system is the subtle energy "pump" energizing all processes in the body: The body's digestive juices, the brain cells coming alive as I type this sentence, the myocardium's tempo for sending forth blood and nourishment to all parts of the system, and much more. Underneath the hood is the higher thermodynamic power of the acupuncture system. The benefit of priming the acupuncture and energetic systems cannot be over-emphasized.[22] The physical body's acupuncture-meridian system is aligned powerfully in the higher gauge state, which in turn, influences the chemistry and cellular function to a restorative milieu. Tai chi, Qigong, yoga are powerful, subtle energy practices. Adding intentionality to the energy medicine "coheres" the practice and brings coherence. Tiller has studied Qigong masters. A master healer's intentionality in a healing session charges the subtle energy systems of his body. A coupling between the subtle energy system and the physical body creates a pulse of the magnetic vector potential, which is the "bridge" between the subtle, unobservable energies and physically observable electric fields outside the physical body.[23] The primary dipole origin is in the lower abdominal region, traditionally known as the *Hara*.

The higher gauge meridian system is magnetoelectric and distinct from electromagnetism. For processes involving subtle energy systems, we must add the magneto-electrochemical potential: The product of a magnetic charge and magnetic potential. This addition is an expansion of the familiar electrochemical potential that drives cellular functions. I submit theoretical implications of the science thus far to medicine using the "chemical medicine" system. Is it possible that in a higher symmetry state space, pharmaceuticals can begin to demonstrate different, more powerful and less harmful potentials? Essentially, focused human intention can set up a conditioned R-space. Hence, a whole new reality opens and becomes one in which the mind and emotion domains can perform physical and higher-dimensional work.

In medical sciences, we are on the quest for personalized medicine. Tiller's work demonstrates that human intention (information) can change the properties of materials and whole living systems (such as the fruit fly) in a *specific* and *particular* direction. By using human intention, an *individual* human body and human health can be impacted positively. Tiller uses the term "information medicine" in this application as distinct from energy medicine. There is an exchange of energy and information at multiple levels in a human, and information has a higher potential in terms of free energy to drive a process. Tiller used information medicine for a gentleman who suffered from ankylosing spondylitis, a diagnosis of chronic inflammatory arthritis.

This man had waxing and waning arthritis of his knees and elbow joints treated with conventional anti-inflammatory drugs for more than 17 years.[24] His condition worsened to the point of requiring a state-of-the-art class of medicines called biologics to control his pain and get him back to work. With multiple specialists – rheumatology, neurology, pain management, orthopedics, physical medicine and rehabilitation, to name a few – as well as frequent radiographic monitoring and blood tests, his condition was on a downward spiral. Energy therapy with a Qigong master helped, but only transiently for 1 day.

Excellence in chemical medicine and energy healing failed to alleviate his misery. Tiller proposed that his imbalance did not lie in the cellular chemistry or the subtle energy acupuncture systems; instead, it likely lay with informational order. To craft an intention statement, Tiller and I used the man's "wish list," that is, what was meaningful to him for health and living a full life.[8] Getting key points required careful review and revisions until everyone was satisfied with the intention. Tiller and his team imprinted an IHD for him, which was shipped to his home in Minnesota. He plugged the IHD in his home for around-the-clock information broadcast into the space of his bedroom. The IHD was re-imprinted every 3 months to keep it meta-stable and away from equilibrium. The patient submitted regular validated outcome measures. His background conventional medical care was left up to his physicians. When the patient started information medicine, he was not on biologics any longer.

The first aspect to shift in the information medicine program was the gentleman's emotional status to a more hopeful and optimistic state. It was an "inside-out" healing. The physical pain took longer to ease. Unlike conventional medicine with a linear dose–response scheme of chemical interventions, information medicine is non-linear in that the multiple levels in his being were impacted. The active information medicine program was 24 months. His follow-up continued beyond that 2-year time point. Three years after the start of the personalized information medicine program, his joint pain suddenly "disappeared over a few days." By this time, he had stopped seeing multiple medical specialists and his rheumatologist. His improvement has been sustained for more than 4 years. This patient has rejoined society and reactivated his gym membership, is skiing again and is running a successful philanthropy.

Could this successful information medicine outcome be a coincidence? Miracles in medicine are not uncommon. However, as a rheumatologist with 20 years of clinical experience, I have not encountered a case of sudden resolution of refractory ankylosing spondylitis. A noteworthy difference from conventional chemical medicine is the direction of information exchange; there's an active response to the patient's questions and desires. It diverts from a fix-it attitude to something more profound, which has more meaning for the client. The information exchange initiative addresses the underlying problems head-on and helps to lighten the footprint of unnecessary prescriptions and subscriptions. None of this is to deny the need for traditional medicine. There are serious diagnoses and real threats to life that require applying the familiar tools of medical treatment.

Information medicine deals with creating beneficial changes in the participant at higher-dimensional and subtle energy levels of integration (emotional, mental and spiritual). It also impacts the cellular, neurological and pharmacological aspects of the atom/molecule aspect of the physical body with zero intentional use of pharmaceuticals. If we think of how the actual structural changes might occur at the various levels of the person, first, a thermodynamic free energy driving force for a change must build up in the system. Next comes a partial deconstruction of the original structure, followed by a rearrangement of the primary structural elements into a new configuration amenable to lowering the existing thermodynamic free energy driving force. This transforming process is repeated until all the excess thermodynamic free energy driving force (created by the IHD) has been used up.

The second example of information medicine takes advantage of field effects. A key aspect of R-space is entanglement and connectivity between parts of a system separated over any physical distance. Recall R-space isn't electromagnetic. Its magic is a magnetoelectric wave information substance. Fields are continuous without gaps. The preceding provided Tiller with the confidence to "broadcast" intention information from his laboratory in Arizona, United States, to children diagnosed with autism spectrum disorders. The 44 children lived in the United States and all around the globe, as far away as Australia. Tiller had never physically met with any of the participants.

In the year-long information medicine program, the objective was to broadcast specific intentions to the children (recipients). The primary outcomes were scores in the validated Autism Treatment Evaluation Checklist (ATEC).[25] The ATEC Questionnaire is a one-page parent-report questionnaire designed to evaluate change in autistic behaviors in children. It consists of 4 subtests: I. Speech/Language Communication (14 items); II. Sociability (20 items); III. Sensory/Cognitive Awareness (18 items); and IV. Health/Physical/Behavior (25 items). Tiller concentrated on some aspects of the ATEC scoring, such as sociability. His main thrust was to support the integration of these children to function and integrate more readily.[26]

One crucial piece in the design of this information medicine program was that Tiller made a controversial but definitive decision: "There will not be any controls. When we do something from the heart, it doesn't make sense to have controls." Once the IHD was switched on in Arizona, within 24 hours, the first feedback arrived. A mother from Australia called: "My three-year-old! She said: 'I love you, Mama.'"[27] The most this child had spoken in the past was nonsensical utterances and single words not necessarily appropriate for the situation. Moreover, the little girl said about 20 different words that day in perfect context. The mother exclaimed: "We couldn't believe what we were hearing. Just amazing!"

During the information medicine broadcast, kids as old as 15 who had never spoken began to form words. This is nothing short of amazing to an expert in the field. The kids improved from 48% who could use four or more words to more than 60% 4 months into the broadcast. The IHD was re-imprinted every 3 months to ensure that it remained meta-stable away from equilibrium.

There are many questions. What happens to the space of the child's home itself? We don't know. How does the intention information "know" which home to reach? How does information reach a precise home address in Australia? Remember, there is no direct sensory input from Tiller and these families, some of them thousands of miles away from Arizona. The families signed a consent form. They are part of the system and connected by field effects. In Tiller's physics, the IHD initially "conditioned" his lab space in Arizona. This space was strongly entangled to transmit information via R-space fields from Tiller's location to each specific address. In simpler terms, intention information reaches each home via R-space information entanglement.

This preliminary data on with-intention broadcast is exciting. Here, we see an act of love by a physicist, his way to support children for whom medicine has few answers. The scientific community has an opportunity to take this early work and propose steps to bring information medicine into broader know-how.

27.7 GOD'S UNIVERSE AND CONCLUSIONS

We have just seen how human consciousness, in the form of intention, can raise the symmetry level of space to a higher or conditioned state. That conditioned space affects the physical properties of matter. Crucially, information is the bridge between energy and consciousness. We can expand the well-accepted relationship of matter and energy, $E = mc^2$, that Einstein derived to include information as follows:

$$Mass \Leftrightarrow Energy \Leftrightarrow Information \Leftrightarrow Consciousness$$

Looking at the Second Law of thermodynamics, which drives all natural processes, the master equation to account for information and entropy is the following:

$$\Delta G = PV + E - T(S_0 + \Sigma \Delta Ij)$$
$$j$$

Therefore, all terms contributing to changes of Gibbs free energy, ΔG, include pressure (ΔP), volume (ΔV), internal energy (ΔE), temperature (ΔT), entropy, a measure of disorder (ΔS), and information, denoted "I." Information is related to entropy; information change can be regarded as negative entropy change (negentropy). The term in the brackets, S_0, is the original entropy, plus the sum, over all the different types (denoted: j), of information change (ΔIj) active in the process. Consciousness via intention manipulates information of all kinds: Numbers, letters, pictures, symbols, etc. A process producing an increase of information, ΔI, leads to a decrease of thermodynamic entropy, ΔS, by the same amount.

Intention is the creative potential that all humans have. For this potential to be realized, meditation is a prerequisite to clarify and quiet the thinking mind. Then, it is the invisible chain of events needed to transfer information in the very fabric of nature itself. It is a question of creating a path that connects all the chain links and then designing and testing a protocol that would allow credible scientists and imprinters to supply the information to the medical armamentarium. People with mastery of stilling the conscious mind and holding an intention to imprint an IHD summon the scriptural teaching from Matthew 18:20: For where two or three are gathered together in my name, there am I in the midst of them. Tiller often said: It's the Unseen colleagues doing the heavy lifting (in the imprinting), signifying man's connection to divinity in the scientific protocol.

Properly understood, consciousness via intention is powerful. It's a source of energy, and information is the link. It is a catalyst for our awakening. Tiller's science shows us that as we become inner-self managed to a high degree, and focus our intentions, remarkable changes are possible in ourselves and in nature. The development of information in various layers of the human infrastructure can be a positive thermodynamic driving force. It invites us to investigate mechanisms of spiritual reality embodied in the human experience and bring it to a pragmatic and practical use.

Tiller's physics opens an exciting new era. People can receive healing information 24 hours a day in their homes, potentially reducing the cost of medical care significantly. It's not too hard to imagine. The science protocol is before us to take it and make something of it. Numbers tell the story. We need numbers on the ground, and comparable numbers in comparable physical locations not receiving the informational directive. Controls are difficult to do in subtle energy research, but we must not let that fact deter the experiment. The challenge before us is to explain this process to those workers and leaders who hold power in making decisions. We must allow bold medical dreams.

Integrative and conventional medical practitioners must be aware of the similarities and significantly different science foundations involved in their medical considerations. Tiller's body of work is vital to all integrative medicine practitioners because it carries them beyond chemical medicine and even electromagnetic medicine. It allows them to seriously enter the domain of information medicine. Whether we use the biomedical model, the energy medicine model or even the information model will depend on us. For while no one is looking, it is the forgotten people, the suffering, who inherited the surface of the earth, and they will forever favor whoever helps them use their legacy to create a better life rather than destroy it.

REFERENCES

1. Morowitz, H.J., *Energy Flow in Biology*. 1979, Woodbridge: Ox Bow.
2. Van Ness, H.C., *Understanding Thermodynamics*. Kindle ed. 1969, New York: Dover Publications, Inc.
3. Broda, E., *Ludwig Boltzmann: Man, Physicist, Philosopher*. 1983, Woodbridge: Ox Bow Press.
4. Morowitz, H.J., *Entropy for Biologists: An Introduction to Thermodynamics*. 1973, New York: Acad. Pr.
5. Hidalgo, C., *Why Information Grows: The Evolution of Order, from Atoms to Economies*. Kindle ed. 2016, New York: Basic Books.
6. Shannon, C.E., A mathematical theory of communication. *Bell System Technical Journal*, 1948. **27**(3): p. 379–423.
7. Brillouin, L., *Science and Information Theory*. 1962, Mneola, New York: Dover Publications.
8. Manek, N.J., *Bridging Science and Spirit: The Genius of William A. Tiller's Physics and the Promise of Information Medicine*. 2019, Yorba Linda: Conscious Creation LLC.
9. Tiller, W.A., W.E. Dibble, and M.J. Kohane, *Conscious Acts of Creation: The Emergence of a New Physics*. 2001, Walnut Creek: Pavior.
10. Tiller, W.A., M.J. Kohane, and W.E. Dibble, Can an aspect of consciousness be imprinted into an electronic device? *Integrative Psychological and Behavioral Science*, 2000. **35**(2): p. 142–62; discussion 163.
11. Dibble, W. and W.A. Tiller, Electronic device-mediated pH changes in water. *Journal of Scientific Exploration*, 1999. **13**(2): p. 155–176.
12. Kohane, M.J. and W.A. Tiller, Anomalous environmental influences on in vitro enzyme studies part 1: Some Faraday cage & multiple vessel effects. *Subtle Energies & Energy Medicine Journal Archives*, 2000. **11**(1): p. 75 –97.
13. Kohane, M.J. and W.A. Tiller, Anomalous environmental influences on in vitro enzyme studies Part 2: Some electronic device effects. *Subtle Energies & Energy Medicine Journal Archives*, 2000. **11**(2): p. 99 –122.
14. Kohane, M.J. and W.A. Tiller, On enhancing nicotinamide adenine dinucleotide (NAD) activity in living systems. *Subtle Energies & Energy Medicine Journal Archives*, 2001. **12**(3): p. 157–181.
15. Pajunen, G.A., et al., Altering the acid/alkaline balance of water via the use of an intention-host device. *Journal of Alternative and Complementary Medicine*, 2009. **15**(9): p. 963–8.
16. 't Hooft, G., Gauge theories of the forces between elementary particles. *Scientific American*, 1980. **242**(6): p. 104–141.
17. Tiller, W.A. and J.W.E. Dibble, New experimental data revealing an unexpected dimension to materials science and engineering. *Material Research Innovations*, 2001. **5**(1): p. 21–34.
18. Tiller, W.A., et al., Toward general experimentation and discovery in conditioned laboratory spaces: part IV. Macroscopic information entanglement between sites approximately 6000 miles apart. *Journal of Alternative and Complementary Medicine*, 2005. **11**(6): p. 973–6.
19. Dirac, P.A.M., A theory of electrons and protons. *Proceedings of the Royal Society London A*, 1930. **126**(801): p. 360–365.
20. Dirac, P.A.M., The theory of magnetic poles. *Physical Review* 1948. **74**(7).
21. Tiller, W.A., What are subtle energies? *Journal of Scientific Exploration*, 1993. **7**(3): p. 293–304.
22. Manek, N.L., Chunyi, Qigong, in *Textbook of Complementary and Alternative Medicine, Second Edition* E.J.B. Chun-Su Yuan, Brent A Bauer, Editor. 2007, Informa Healthcare, Taylor & Francis Group LLC: Boca Raton, FL. p. 199–210.
23. Tiller, W.A., et al. Towards explaining anomalously large body voltage surges on exceptional subjects part I: The electrostatic approximation. *Journal of Scientific Exploration*. 1995.
24. Manek, N.J.T. and A. William, Information medicine as delievered by intention host devices: A case report, in International Research Congress on Integrative Medicine and Health. 2014, IRCIMH: Miami, FL.
25. *Autism Research Institute (ARI)*. 2021 [cited 2021 7/1/2021]; Educational and information for Autism]. Available from: http://www.autism.com/index.php/ind_atec.
26. Miller, S.R.C., F Tang, N.J. Manek, W.A. Tiller, Impact of broadcast intention on autism spectrum behaviors, in International Research Congress on Integrative Medicine and Health (IRCIMH). 2014: Miami, FL.
27. Tiller, W.M., R.C. Suzy, and J. Yotopoulos, *White Paper XXX. The Globally Broadcast Autism Intention Experiment: Part I, at the Four-Month Stage of a Twelve-Month Program*. 2013, William A. Tiller Institute: Payson, Arizona. p. 86.

28 Birthing the Light, Making Childbirth a Positive Experience

Payal Chaudhary and Manju Puri

CONTENTS

"Kim Jyotis tava bhanumaan ahani me. Ratrau pradeepadikam.
Syaad evam ravi deepa darshana vidhau kim jyothiraakhyahi me.
Chakshuh tasya nimeelanaadi samaya kim dheeh dheeyo darshana kim
Tatra aham athah bhavan paramakam jyothih tadasmi prabho"

Sri Sadhguru Adi Sankaracharya's Eka Sloka Prakaram

TRANSLATION

"What is your light?" "For me sun in the day and lamp in the night."
"Let it be." "By what light do you see sun and lamp?" "Eyes."
"When you close your eyes, what is the light?" "Intellect."
"What light helps to see intellect?" "Me (self)."
"So, you are the ultimate light (self-luminous Self)." "Yes, that's so, my lord."

DOI: 10.1201/b23304-30

28.1 INTRODUCTION

In Spanish, childbirth is *Dar la luz*, which means birthing the light. In the Indian context, it is light that comes in and powers the body, giving us life. By welcoming the new-born that enters this world through the mother's womb, we are welcoming this light by the many rituals in different cultures, for instance, bathing the baby. For example, see this beautiful video on you tube: https://youtu.be/PpvbfuF0ENo

Other rituals include massaging the baby, singing to the baby., etc. In many cultures, the entire village is involved in welcoming the new-born and the mother, helping at every turn. This is a cultural aspect, for each family and mother should be respected, and the creative power should be honored while a mother births her baby. Making childbirth a joyful and natural experience for the mother, the baby and the whole family is therefore a duty of everyone who is involved in assisting in the process of childbirth. This includes birth companions like spouse, partner, family member or doula and healthcare providers like midwives, nurses or doctors, all of whom need to work towards the common goal of making the childbirth a positive experience for the mother as well as the baby.

To give birth to a life is a gift that is the prerogative of a female body, which is why many cultures honor her as the divine or the sacred feminine. It is the energy of creation in its most ethereal form. This force is powerful and highly intuitive. But in this process, women are not just a means to an end. To accomplish this, they need to be in harmony within themselves, with nature and with the rest of creation. Sadly, most of the times in our current paradigm when a woman brings forth life into this world, this may not be the case.

Childbirth should be a wonderful time for a woman and her baby and not something to dread and be fearful of. However, at the present time, outcomes have taken more importance than the process itself. We need to align and realign ourselves with nature's powerful design, which translates into a positive childbirth experience for a woman, and empower her in more ways than one to enjoy motherhood, to bond with her baby, and to nurture him or her to his or her full potential.

In a survey spanning over 140 countries around the world based on a questionnaire, the "positive experience index" and "negative experience index" were measured. "Positive experience index" was assessed by respondents' experiencing wellbeing on the day before the survey in terms of feeling well rested, being treated with respect all day, smiling or laughing a lot, learning or doing something interesting, and experiencing enjoyment.[1] Positive experiences can help us thrive, flourish and be creative and optimistic about life in general.

To give birth to a healthy baby in a clinically and psychologically safe environment with continuity of physical and emotional support from a birth companion and kind and technically competent staff is what defines a positive childbirth experience.[2] This stems from the fact that women do want a physiologic labor that is safe but also wish to be involved in the decision-making process for any intervention when the need arises.

It seems that with the aim of reducing maternal and perinatal morbidity and mortality during childbirth, the natural process of human birth, which unfolds itself automatically and is orchestrated by the fine interplay of various hormones like oxytocin, endorphins, catecholamines and prolactin, is forgotten. These hormones are released in a manner that makes the whole birthing experience ecstatic, creates a special bond between the mother and the baby, and smooths the transition of the new-born into the world. The mother–baby duo get to develop the bond of a lifetime, and for the mother, it is like a new birth into a far greater and more powerful role. All this happens when birth is undisturbed and allowed to progress naturally; however, at the present time, this has become a rarity due to the high rates of medical intervention. Cesarean section is perceived as an easier and safer mode of delivery as compared with vaginal birth by pregnant women and obstetricians. There is an urgent need to move slowly but steadily from a totally medicalized birth to an "Undisturbed Birth."[3]

28.2 HISTORICAL PERSPECTIVE OF CHILDBIRTH

Since time immemorial, childbirth has remained a highly private affair, which was practiced behind closed doors. Female relatives and midwives helped during childbirth. Midwives passed on the knowledge and skills from generation to generation. Some of them were highly skilled at easing the process, rotating the malpositioned baby and much more.

In ancient India, certain Vedic practices (1500 BC) were started 3 months prior to conception, were followed throughout pregnancy, and continued after the birth of the baby. These were described in the *Garbhopanishad* from the *Krishna-Yajur-Veda*.[4, 5]

They included certain basic ingredients like healthy, home-cooked, nutritious, vegetarian food, a focus on good thoughts and spirituality, music, a peaceful environment and doing certain breathing exercises (called *Garbh Sanskar*).[6] The practices were started 3 months prior to conception, which meant that they could potentially influence the quality of human eggs. This was meant to provide a healthy environment for the growing fetus so that it could attain its maximum physical and intellectual potential and was also claimed to nurture the best genetic pool for the baby. Virtue in the baby seems to emanate from the mother and her experience during pregnancy via the neurotransmitters released in the mother's brain. Also highlighted were practices like perineal massage to prevent tears during birthing, and rubbing the breasts with a paste of sandalwood and lotus stem for suppleness to help in breast feeding.[7]

All these practices ensured that the "mother to be" was taken care of and also, was guided about the process of childbirth and new-born care by the elders in the family. But, the unavailability of formal medical care at that time meant wide disparities in the quality of care and high maternal and infant mortality.

Between the 18th and the beginning of the 20th century, obstetric practices saw a sea change, especially in European nations. Male midwives or surgeon practitioners came forth and started attending deliveries, using forceps and handling abnormal labors, but the maternal mortality rate did not see any change. It was not until 1936 that maternal mortality rates began to fall. The major contributing factor was the introduction of antibiotics (sulfonamides).[8] Times changed, and the last 100 years or so saw a huge escalation in the practice of modern medicine, the availability of anesthesia and safe surgical practices.

As per Centers for Disease Control (CDC) data,[9] maternal and infant mortality fell drastically from the early 1900s to 1999 in the United States. In the early 1900s, 6–9 mothers per 1000 live births in the United States died of pregnancy-related complications, and approximately 100 infants out of 1000 live births died before their first birthday. Maternal mortality declined by almost 99% and was reported at 0.1 of 1000 live births in 1997, and the infant mortality rate also declined by 90% to 7.2 per 1000 live births. Major advances in medicine and improvements in healthcare were major contributors to this decline in numbers.

Medicalization of childbirth, although it brought about a change in morbidity and mortality, also meant that the control of a birthing woman's body and the profound and natural process it was meant to go through was taken over by healthcare providers.

In an article written in *Journal of Perinatal Education* in 2003,[10] the author talks about the childbirth journey of three generations of her family: her grandmother, her mother and herself. The narrative highlights how childbirth has changed over these three eras and how women need to reclaim their childbirth and their families. Her grandmother, in 1936, had a childbirth controlled by a male obstetrician, a nurse periodically woke her out of a drugged stupor to admonish her for her inconsiderate behavior, and she had a forceps delivery; plus, she never could breastfeed her daughter. Her own mother just remembered being unconscious and going through a Cesarean section. For her own birth, she had a birth plan and labored with her husband and midwives with medical backup incorporated, just in case. She also went on to breastfeed her daughter for 3 years. The ecstasy of her own childbirth was something that brought her confidence and a sense of purpose (Figure 28.1).

28.3 THE JOURNEY BEGINS: UNDERSTANDING CONCEPTION AND THE ZINC FLASH

The activation of an egg to form an embryo has been seen to be marked by a distinct event called the "zinc spark." So, why do sparks literally fly at the moment of conception? Back in 2011, the

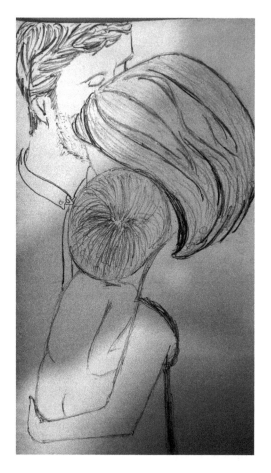

FIGURE 28.1   Reclamation of the family.

Northwestern University team discovered that sparks of zinc exploded at the point of conception in mice. It took them a few years to figure out how to image this event, but by 2014, they'd managed to film the event for the first time ever, and watched as billions of zinc atoms were released at the exact moment when a mammal's egg was pierced by a sperm cell. Using a new fluorescent sensor that was able to track the movements of zinc in live cells, the team caught a glimpse of an egg's zinc-storage capabilities and found some 8000 zinc compartments, each one containing around 1 million zinc atoms, just ripe for exploding. The tiny "firework" that resulted was found to last for about 2 hours after fertilization.

Now, the same team has managed to film this event occurring in a human egg at the point of conception. In this landmark study published in 2016,[1111] it was seen that there was a meiotic maturation–dependent acquisition of the ability of the gamete to mount a zinc spark, with cells arrested at prophase I having on an average a smaller zinc spark compared with those arrested at metaphase II. These results suggest that the machinery that elicits the zinc spark is likely not fully established until just prior to fertilization, which may be an important mechanism to prevent premature egg activation. This information is really powerful in more ways than one. Not only does it pave the way for future selection of good-quality eggs, thus increasing the success rates in ART (assisted reproductive technology) cycles, but it also reinforces that the conception of a new being in nature is marked by the release of energy (zinc flash). On a more spiritual level, this also implies that the origin of a new living being in nature is an event marked by release of energy at a subatomic level, highlighting the importance of interchangeability of matter and energy in living systems.

Matter has been converted into energy, such as burning firewood creating light and heat. However, has energy been demonstrated by science to be converted into matter?

Scientists studying particle collisions at the Relativistic Heavy Ion Collider at the US Department of Energy's Brookhaven National Laboratory found that particles of matter and antimatter could be created by colliding very energetic photons (quantum packets of light), essentially converting light energy into matter in a single step. This is called "The Breit–Wheeler process" and is related, of course, to Einstein's equation, $E = mc^2$. Matter has been converted into energy before, for instance by nuclear reactors, but this is the first time that scientists have converted electrons and positrons, i.e., light, into matter.[12]

28.4 MODELS OF CARE – TECHNOCRATIC TO QUANTUM

Bringing a new life to this earth is the quintessential most powerful force of nature and drives everything at its most basic level. It is the start of a new relationship between a mother and her baby. Soul-level connections are created and nurtured, and the right nurturing could mean the creation of a whole generation of human beings who are mentally and physically strong and capable of making this world a better place to live.

An overview of the Primal Health Research data bank founded by Michel Odent demonstrates how health is shaped during the primal period (from conception until the first birthday). The research also suggests that the way we are born has long-term consequences for sociability, aggressiveness and our capacity to love.[3]

Simon et al.[13] studied how natural birth in mice led to triggering of UCP2 (mitochondrial uncoupling protein 2) expression in hippocampal neurons of mice. UCP2 is induced by cellular stress and is involved in regulation of fuel utilization, mitochondrial bioenergetics, cell proliferation, neuroprotection and synaptogenesis in the adult brain, and inhibition of UCP2 led to reduction in the number and size of neurons, their dendritic growth and certain complex behaviors in adults. This study implied that UCP2 expression leads to development of hippocampal neurons, and as expression of this protein is seen to be triggered by the stress of labor, this means that physiologic labor stress has a crucial role to play in the development of hippocampal neurons and their circuits. This means that more research is needed to understand whether absence of labor stress, as in elective Cesarean section or non-natural births, means no upregulation of UCP2 protein and hence, long-term effects on the functioning of the brain.

For the longest time, health agendas and policies all over the world have been focusing on survival for both the mother and baby during childbirth. In this "technocratic model,"[14] women are not seen as individuals with their own fears and beliefs. They were meant to follow a system of health management that ensured physical safety during childbirth, but this also meant that their individual choices were either ignored or not given precedence. Fear of litigation of the healthcare staff and the unpredictability of childbirth also meant that Cesarean sections appeared to be a safer option.

It is about time that our actions should now aim at "transformational healthcare," as envisioned by the Global Strategy for Women's, Children's and Adolescent Health.[15] This could mean adopting a "quantum model" of care, which implies that what each woman goes through, and what she believes in, matters. There is evidence that each woman has her own attitude and beliefs regarding pregnancy and childbirth based on the information she receives from her family, peers and care providers.[16] Three clusters of women are described as self-determiners, take it as it comes, and fearful women. Self-determiners believe in pregnancy and childbirth as a normal physiological event and have no fear of birth, compared with fearful women, who are afraid of birth and have an increased likelihood of a negative birth experience and poor emotional health. Take it as it comes women are not afraid of birth but are likely to agree to interventions easily.[17]

Each pregnant woman needs to be treated at an individual level, and her thoughts and fears must be taken into consideration. This works to create a holistic and positive childbirth experience for every woman.

28.5   HORMONES AS MESSENGERS – REPRODUCTIVE AND BIRTHING HORMONES

Four major hormones[18] orchestrate the start of labor and the journey of childbirth. They are oxytocin, beta endorphins, prolactin and the epinephrine-norepinephrine system. Figure 28.2 shows how the hormonal interplay leads to effective labor progression, analgesia and a positive childbirth experience.

A mother's body readies for labor by increasing estrogen levels. An increase in uterine oxytocin receptors towards the end of pregnancy plays a vital role in uterine responsiveness to oxytocin, thus leading to effective uterine contractions and helping to prevent postpartum hemorrhage after childbirth. An increase in central receptors for beta endorphins leads to natural analgesia and helps in producing a trance-like state for mother, thus helping her in coping with the stress of labor. Simultaneously, an increase in mammary and central oxytocin and prolactin receptors plays key roles in mother–child bonding post birth and in initiating breastfeeding. Not only does the mother's body undergo these changes; the fetus has its own flow of hormones for optimization of survival after birth. Cortisol release in the fetus in the prelabor phase has a role in initiation of labor. It also causes the maturation of lungs and other organ systems. There is an increase in epinephrine-norepinephrine receptors, which ensures protection from labor-induced hypoxia (caused by late labor catecholamine surge) and neuroprotection and promotes effective energy metabolism after birth.

As per the integrative neuro-psychosocial model of childbirth, which integrates neuroendocrinological, physiological and psychosocial aspects of what a woman goes through during a physiologic

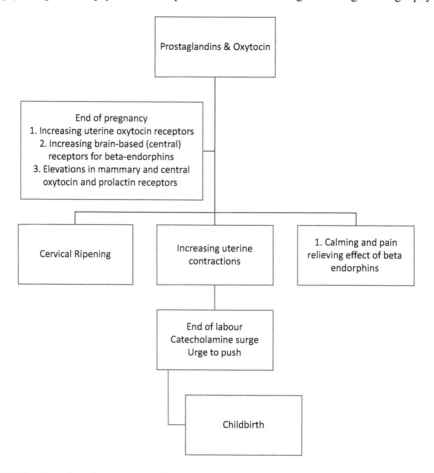

FIGURE 28.2   Flow chart for interplay of maternal hormones during childbirth.

birth,[19] oxytocin not only stimulates uterine contractions during labor but also influences the mother's experiences, behaviors and physiology to facilitate birth.

This is a more holistic way of visualizing childbirth, which is not just a physiological event but has psychological experiences and neuroendocrine events occurring to not only facilitate birth but also act as a transformative experience for the woman and prepare her transition into motherhood. This model of childbirth has been derived after integrating the findings from two previous systematic reviews, one on maternal plasma levels of oxytocin during physiological childbirth[20] and one meta-synthesis of women's subjective experiences of physiological childbirth.[21]

Over the last few decades, the place of birth shifted from home to hospital, which did mean better monitoring during labor and effective handling of complications, but also meant more intervention than was needed and pregnancy being seen as a medical disease, whereby fear of complications became the main driving force for interventions and Cesarean sections. Induction of labor is planned for various indications, like post-dated pregnancy, hyperglycemia in pregnancy, hypertensive disorder of pregnancy or fetal growth restriction. Sometimes, the labor may not go as planned, such as in conditions when babies are not positioned right in the pelvis, for example occipitoposterior position, a big baby or a small pelvis, better referred to as cephalopelvic disproportion, requiring interventions in the form of either an instrumental delivery or a Cesarean section. This may disrupt the hormonal interplay as described earlier for natural childbirth. There is an increased chance of ineffective contractions leading to failed inductions, instrumental births and postpartum hemorrhage. In the baby, it increases the chances for immature development of protective mechanisms like the catecholamine surge, leading to fetal distress and poor adaptation post birth in the form of breathing difficulties, hypothermia and hypoglycemia. There is also a probability of long-term adverse impact on epigenetic programming in babies due to faulty release of hormones and their effects, as shown in some animal studies.[22] This is an area that requires more research to find conclusive evidence on whether there are epigenetic oxytocin-mediated effects on the mother and infant during childbirth[23] (Figure 28.2).

28.6   MICROBIOME – THE KEY TO HUMAN HEALTH

The role of mode of delivery and exposure of an infant to the vaginal microbiome of the mother and its effect on gut health and indirect effect on priming of the immune system is increasingly becoming clear. It has a role to play in the appearance of certain diseases later in life, such as allergies, obesity and inflammatory disorders.[24–26]. It has been argued that the impact of Cesarean birth on the microbiome is also influenced by intrapartum antibiotics and diminished success of breastfeeding after Cesarean section. In a recent study,[27] it was proved that there was a modest difference in the incidence of respiratory illnesses in early life and need for antibiotics depending on the mode of delivery, with Cesarean-born children showing a higher tendency. This difference has been linked to difference in abundance of several biomarker bacteria, like Bifidobacterium species, which are seen in vaginally delivered children, and the abundance of potential pathogens from the genera Klebsiella and Enterococcus in children born by Cesarean section. This difference is independent of peripartum antibiotic usage or breastfeeding pattern.

28.7   HIGHLIGHTING THE CURRENT PERSPECTIVE

28.7.1   Patient's Point of View

To formulate the World Health Organization (WHO)'s intrapartum guidelines, a systematic review done by methodically including 35 studies that had moderate- to high-quality data, certain pertinent findings were derived for what women actually want during childbirth.[28]

These studies were from the time period of 1997 onwards, so taking into consideration the current perspective of women. They represented the views of more than 1800 women, from a wide range of ethnic backgrounds, ages (14–49) and socio-demographic groups. The quality was mostly moderate to high (B or above).

It was concluded that women all over the world want to have a positive childbirth experience, which entails being in a supportive environment during childbirth with a companion of their choice. Beliefs about what matters to women do vary based on local cultural beliefs and practices, but most women want to go with the flow in the presence of technically competent staff, be involved in the decision making, and use their inherent capabilities to give birth to a healthy baby in a clinically, culturally and psychologically safe environment.

For a long time, the medical management–central approach to childbirth has determined how clinicians have looked at childbirth. In recent times, the focus has now shifted to understanding how women view childbirth and their beliefs and attitudes regarding the same, as this determines the long-term psychosocial health of the women and also the outcome and mode of delivery in most cases. This "women-centered approach" means shifting the focus from a risk-centered approach to individualized care wherein what each woman thinks or believes is taken into consideration and acted upon.

A major factor that determines what matters the most to women during childbirth is their inherent attitude towards childbirth. In a Swedish Australian study[17] with prospective longitudinal cohort design with self-report questionnaires, women's attitudes toward childbirth were divided into three clusters: "Self-determiners" (clear attitudes about birth, including seeing it as a natural process and no childbirth fear), "Take it as it comes" (no fear of birth and low levels of agreement with any of the attitude statements) and "Fearful" (afraid of birth, with high safety concerns and not agreeing to see labor as a natural process). Attitudes have been conceptualized using a three-component model: Affective, cognitive and behavioral.[19] The affective component consists of positive or negative feelings toward the attitude object; the cognitive part refers to thoughts or beliefs; and the behavioral element represents the actions or intentions to act upon the object.

At 18–20 weeks' gestation, it was concluded that when compared with the 'Self-determiners," women in the "Fearful" cluster were more likely to prefer a Cesarean (odds ratio [OR] = 3.3, confidence interval (CI): 1.6–6.8), to have less positive feelings about being pregnant (OR = 3.6, CI: 1.4–9.0) and about approaching birth (OR = 7.2, CI: 4.4–12.0), and less than positive feelings about the first weeks with a new-born (OR = 2.0, CI: 1.2–3.6). At 2 months postpartum, it was seen that "Self-determiners" were least likely to have a Cesarean section, whereas the "Fearful" cluster had the highest chance of having an elective Cesarean (OR = 5.4, CI: 2.1–14.2) or epidural placement if they labored (OR = 1.9, CI: 1.1–3.2) and to experience their labor pains as more intense than women in the other clusters. The "Fearful" cluster were more likely to report a negative experience of birth (OR = 1.7, CI: 1.02–2.9). The "Take it as it comes" cluster had a higher likelihood of an elective Cesarean section (OR 3.0, CI: 1.1–8.0). This should serve as a powerful piece of information, because if midwives or doctors delve into what an individual woman thinks and know her beliefs and attitudes towards childbirth, they can work constructively by addressing the various concerns.

28.8 FACTORS INFLUENCING BIRTH PREFERENCES

28.8.1 Childbirth Classes

As humans, fear of the unknown is deeply embedded in our intellect. This drives every creature to its safe domain. Fear of the unknown also has a huge role to play in how women perceive childbirth, especially in the case of primigravidae who have never experienced labor. Fear of pain, and also self-doubt about their own ability to handle pain, is what compounds the fear of childbirth in a woman. Thus, empowering women by knowledge can logically lead to a reduction in this fear.

In a study done on 204 primiparous pregnant women attending health centers in Tabriz, Iran,[30] women were divided into three groups: Not attending, irregularly attending (attending one to three sessions of classes) and regularly attending (attending four to eight sessions of classes). Childbirth fear, pregnancy-related anxiety and depression questionnaires were filled through interviews and were assessed by a general linear model. It was concluded that the scores for fear of childbirth ($p < 0.001$), anxiety ($p < 0.001$) and depression ($p = 0.006$) were significantly lower in the group of pregnant women regularly attending the classes compared with the non-attending group of women. No significant differences were observed between the regularly attending and irregularly attending groups in terms of fear of childbirth ($p = 0.066$), anxiety ($p = 0.078$) and depression ($p = 0.128$).

28.8.2 OWNING ONE'S CHILDBIRTH

Despite there being no operational definition for fear of childbirth, the term itself is self-explanatory. It is normal to be afraid of the unknown as humans. It is normal to feel some anxiety due to the unpredictability of childbirth, and first-time mothers may have certain preconceived notions about childbirth based on what they may have heard from their peer and elders or incomplete information they may have garnered from social media or certain singular experiences of near and dear ones. An important factor that may amplify this fear in times to come is the increase in the number of Cesarean sections all over the world. There is a whole generation of mothers who have had a Cesarean birth and have not experienced natural childbirth. These mothers become promoters of Cesarean sections as a mode of delivery

The prevalence of fear of childbirth in pregnant women worldwide was 14%, and in a subgroup analysis according to parity it was 16% in nulliparous women versus 12% in multiparous women, according to a systematic review and meta-analysis.[31] The fear in women is not the only factor that dictates the childbirth choices; it is also determined by how the father to be or the partner feels about childbirth, and in predominantly patriarchal societies, this can play a huge role in the choice of birth preferences. A recent meta-synthesis on women's experiences of interventions for fear of childbirth highlights a very important narrative, which underlies a basic human mental tackling mechanism, that is, "owning one's childbirth."[32] If a woman is made aware of an all-pervasive truth, that nature has inherently bestowed upon her this inner knowledge and strength to go through childbirth, she can handle it and come out stronger by taking charge of her own mind and body during her birthing journey. An important first step in handling anxiety around childbirth is first to acknowledge and identify the individual fears of each woman. Once women identify their individual fears, they can be empowered to self-manage with adequate support from partners and staff.

28.8.3 ROLE OF PHYSICAL AND MENTAL STRENGTH BUILDING IN PROSPECTIVE MOTHERS

The process of birthing a baby requires hard work on the part of laboring women. In older times, working in fields or even while doing household work, moving around and squatting multiple times during the day was a part of life. This led to improvement in muscle strength and stamina, which eased the process of labor. With advancement in technology, machines do a whole lot of day-to-day work for us. Thus in present times, the majority of women lead a sedentary lifestyle.

Also, fatigue in pregnancy is a common symptom, and its association has been seen to predict an increase in the rate of Cesarean births and depression.[33] In a study by Ward-Ritacco et al., women between 23 and 25 weeks of pregnancy with back pain or history of back pain were assessed for positive psychological changes after acute bouts of resistance exercise.[34] It was seen that the majority of these generally healthy pregnant women (i.e., $\geq 77\%$), when they performed low- to moderate-intensity exercises twice a week for 12 weeks, reported increased feelings of energy and reduced feelings of fatigue after a single bout of low- to moderate-intensity muscle strengthening exercise.

Various studies have shown that yoga and meditation during pregnancy reduce stress and build stamina. In a systematic review of randomized controlled trials, yoga was seen to improve pain and reduce perceived stress levels, anxiety levels and depression and also improved quality of life for pregnant women as compared with the control group in four of these studies.[35] Two studies on depressed pregnant women were included, and one such study reported an improvement in anxiety, depression, anger, and leg and back pain, though the second study did not find any difference from the control group. In one study, which included women with high-risk factors like obesity or advanced age, yoga during pregnancy seemed to reduce their risk of pregnancy complications like hypertension, diabetes or fetal growth restriction. In one study, yoga significantly reduced pelvic pain compared with the control group.

28.8.4   Role of Birth Companion in Labor

A birth or labor companion may be the woman's partner, family member, trained supporter (doula) or nurse/midwife. Informal labor companions have been present during labor since time immemorial, especially when home births were the norm. In the present-day setting of childbirth in a healthcare environment, Labor companions, though usually present in high-income settings, are not allowed in the labor room in low-income or middle-income countries, especially in heavy-load public health facilities. In low- and middle-income countries, neglectful, abusive and disrespectful treatment of women during childbirth in health facilities is a known phenomenon. This has been known to occur in high-income countries as well, although not as overtly but in a covert fashion. This mistreatment can occur at the level of an interaction between the woman and healthcare provider and also due to systemic failures at the healthcare facilities.[36] For a birthing woman to have a birth companion could mean having someone who can look after her rights along with providing physical and psychological support.

According to a recent Cochrane database review of 51 studies that mainly highlighted women's perspectives regarding the presence of a birth companion in high-income settings,[37] labor companions supported women in various ways, which included physical support, helping the women to move around and providing massage or hand holding wherever needed. They also help in providing non-pharmacologic pain relief. In the case of a trained doula, it also means providing information about childbirth, thus bridging the communication gap and acting as an advocate of women's rights. Emotional support is also an important component, as reassurance and well-meant praise and hand holding can make a woman feel confident and in control.

28.8.5   Role of Healthcare Providers

Midwives create a calm birthing environment without architectural design but ensuring that the rooms offer the elements of women-centered care, offering privacy and calmness, facilitating oxytocin.[38] Protecting the space of the mother to be reduces unnecessary traffic into the birthing room and keeps her safe, which will enable the release of natural endorphins, facilitating physiological and healthy labor and birth.[39]

Evidence shows that skilled, knowledgeable and compassionate midwifery care reduces maternal and new-born mortality and stillbirths, keeping mothers and babies safe, and promoting health and well-being.[40] When educated to international standards, midwives can cater to 87% of the needed essential care for women and new-born babies. The State of the World's Midwifery Report, 2014 (SWMR, 2021),[41] launched in May 2021, summarized an analysis of 88 countries that account for most of the world's maternal and neonatal deaths and stillbirths. The report showed that a substantial increase in coverage of midwife-delivered interventions (25% increase every 5 years to 2035) could prevent 40% of maternal and new-born deaths and 26% of stillbirths. Even a modest increase (10% every 5 years) in coverage of midwife-delivered interventions could prevent 23% of maternal and neonatal deaths and 14% of stillbirths. Overall, universal coverage of midwifery would prevent 65% of maternal and neonatal deaths and stillbirths.

Midwives view childbirth as a normal physiological process and have been trained to view childbirth as a non-pathogenic event. Equally, they are trained to identify any changes in the normal physiological process and escalate appropriately to obstetricians. Research has suggested that midwifery-led care offers high-quality services with reduced interventions and Cesarean sections, high rates of maternal satisfaction, and maternal bonding with successful breastfeeding.[42] Midwife-led continuity of care with women also has a profound impact on care, experiences and outcomes, for example 15% less likely to have epidural analgesia, 24% less likely to have a premature birth, and 16% less likely to have an episiotomy. Midwives contribute to the transition of birth by reducing unnecessary interventions such as Cesarean sections, where babies are birthed out of the abdomen and not through the vagina, reducing the natural microbiomes, which have been shown to offer natural immunity for the start of life. This will also reduce unnecessary anesthetic procedures. The individual support a midwife offers to support and facilitate and breastfeeding, keeping mother and baby together, helps remove harmful practices.[43]

The ability to see birth and support birth as a normal phenomenon brings childbirth to a level of placing the mother in the center of holistic care. Midwives practice evidence-based care and respect women and their individual choice, which places the women in an empowering position to have the knowledge of birth and make decisions about their birth. Healthcare professionals can make or break experiences, and we know that women who have had a previous traumatic birth may not access care due to fear. Midwives can bridge and provide high-quality respectful care, reducing abuse, discrimination and non-consented practices. Midwives work in unison with multi-disciplinary healthcare professionals to provide women and their families with the holistic care they deserve to have a safe and positive birth.

Midwives offer women their choice of birthing in positions of their individual preference and support mothers to birth in calm environments and using hydrotherapy and water births as an option. Research into offering hydrotherapy and water births has shown that it can reduce the need for epidural analgesia and offer birth satisfaction. Midwives offer water births, normalizing births for women and their new-borns.

28.9 CLOSING THE LOOP OR COMING FULL CIRCLE

28.9.1 THE BIRTH ATLAS: UNDERSTANDING THE UTERUS, CERVIX, AND DILATION AND EFFACEMENT

When viewed from a medical perspective, labor is a physiologic process during which the fetus, membranes, umbilical cord and placenta are expelled from the uterus. Labor is traditionally divided into three stages that are defined as definite milestones in a continuous process. The first stage of labor begins with regular uterine contractions and ends with complete cervical dilatation at 10 cm. The first part of this stage is the latent phase, when contractions are mild and irregular. These help in priming the cervix by causing softening and effacement of the cervix. The cervix gradually becomes soft and short till it merges with the uterus. This phase smoothly transitions into the active phase of the first stage (cervical dilatation could be anywhere between 3 and 6 cm) when contractions are progressively more rhythmic and stronger, and cervical dilatation and descent of the head are relatively more rapid, and ends at full dilatation (10 cm) of the cervix. The second stage of labor begins with complete dilatation of the cervix and ends with delivery of the baby. In nulliparous women, the second stage is considered prolonged if it exceeds 3 hours if regional anesthesia is administered or 2 hours in the absence of regional anesthesia. In multiparous women, the second stage is considered prolonged if it exceeds 2 hours with regional anesthesia or 1 hour without it.[44] The period between the delivery of the fetus and the delivery of the placenta and fetal membranes is defined as the third stage, which may take 10–30 minutes. Active management of this stage often involves prophylactic administration of oxytocin or other uterotonics (prostaglandins or ergot alkaloids), cord clamping/cutting and controlled traction of the umbilical cord.

28.9.2 CARDINAL MOVEMENTS OF LABOR: HOW THE BABY NAVIGATES THE PELVIS

The mechanisms of labor, also known as the cardinal movements, involve changes in the position of the head of the fetus during its passage through the maternal pelvis. Although labor and delivery occur in a continuous fashion, the cardinal movements are described as the following seven discrete sequences:[45] engagement, descent, flexion, internal rotation, extension, restitution and external rotation, and lastly, expulsion.

When viewed in medical terms, labor and delivery seem to involve certain set standards, which need to be adhered to for it to be called a normal physiologic process, and any deviation from this defined normal is likely to require intervention. This also requires an intravaginal examination at certain intervals by the healthcare provider supervising the labor.

28.9.3 The Holistic Stages of Labor: A New Language for a New Paradigm

Holistic stages of labor is a birth philosophy that envisions labor as an instinctive process that a pregnant woman goes through when it is time to bring the baby out into the world. Whapio Diane Bartlett, a midwife working in the field of natural birthing for the last 40 years with the Matrona foundation,[46] feels the need to train midwives in birthing that envisions childbirth as a natural event in most circumstances and not something that should be thought of as a high-risk event with decision making incorporated into it if the pattern deviates from anything that is considered normal, thus medicalizing the childbirth completely. It views holistic stages of labor as a continuum, which includes embarking on the journey of labor (latent phase), entering the veil (active phase, beyond 4–5 cm of dilatation), on the mountain (active first stage), the summoning (end of first stage, transition), quietude (the resting phase), the breakers (second part of second stage – pushing) and emergence (birth of the baby) into the world in a position of her choice. It highlights the second stage of labor in two distinctive phases, the first, in which there is no natural urge to push, and the second phase, when there is an involuntary urge to push when the head is at the perineum.

It is when a mother is not allowed to behave instinctively and is directed by her caregiver that the control of her own self and the empowerment it brings for her is lost, and the experience may become agonizing and unbearable, prompting her to ask for intervention, which she may come to regret later.

In the middle of the 20th century, Grantley Dick Read described "physiologic labor," which is a labor undisturbed by mechanical, physical or psychological means.[47]. He talks further of a woman following the lead of her uterus during the second stage of labor and not to initiate pushing on the instructions of the healthcare provider.

Constance Beynon (1957) described her observations, which emphasized that women should engage in what she termed "the spontaneous second stage."[48] Included in these observations was the fact that most women required less voluntary straining than was practiced at the time; that as the fetal head neared the pelvic floor, the straining efforts became involuntary and irresistible; that the patient's involuntary straining did not begin until well after the contraction had been established; and that the amount of straining and exertion by the woman varied significantly with each contraction.

28.10 CONCLUSION

Each childbirth is precious. It is a signal of bringing forth light and hope into this world. Medical advances have been a boon for mankind in more ways than one. They have led to huge reductions in maternal and fetal morbidity and mortality. The overarching theme that emerges with evolving times is that we must evolve as well in our perceptions and attitudes towards childbirth. This requires us to see childbirth not as a medical event but rather, a physiologic one, which requires a woman to be comfortable in her own skin, to allow her to choose a partner while birthing and to let her choose the pace at which she wishes to move forward. But before doing this, it also requires her to fully understand and "own" her body and her childbirth journey. While doing so, the role of medical intervention when truly needed should not be undermined.

ACKNOWLEDGEMENTS

Indie Kaur, Professional Midwife, Director of Midwifery Fernandez Foundation, Telangana, India, for her perspective on role of midwives in birthing.

Dr Nikita Sobti, Obstetrician and Gynecologist, for sharing her views on the role of yoga meditation and parental counselling in reducing Cesarean section rates.

REFERENCES

1. OECD. Positive and negative experiences, in *Society at a Glance 2011: OECD Social Indicators*. Paris: OECD Publishing; 2011. https://doi.org/10.1787/soc_glance-2011-23-en.
2. *WHO Recommendations: Intrapartum Care for a Positive Childbirth Experience*. Geneva: World Health Organization; 2018. Licence: CC BY-NC-SA 3.0 IGO.
3. Undisturbed birth. *AIMS J*. 2011;23(4). https://www.aims.org.uk/journal/item/undisturbed-birth.
4. *Garbha Upanishad गर्भ उपनिषद् - LSU*. n.d. Retrieved March 10, 2022, from https://www.ece.lsu.edu/kak/GarbhaUpanishad.pdf
5. *Thirumantiram and Garbha Upanishad: An Overview*. n.d. Retrieved March 10, 2022, from https://www.researchgate.net/profile/Leelavathy-Nanjappa/publication/331199149_Thirumantiram_and_garbha_upanishad-an_overview/links/5c6bd5574585156b5706e748/Thirumantiram-and-garbha-upanishad-an-overview.pdf
6. Sarkar S. Pregnancy, birthing, breastfeeding and mothering: Hindu perspectives from scriptures and practices. *Open Theol*. 2020;6:104–116.
7. Sharma P. Caraka Samhita *Vol.I*, Chapter 2. Varanasi: Chaukhamba Orientalia; 2018.
8. Loudon I. Deaths in childbed from the eighteenth century to 1935. *Med Hist*. 1986 Jan;30(1):1–41.
9. *Achievements in Public Health, 1900–1999: Healthier Mothers and Babies*. Morbidity and Mortality Weekly Report, Centers for Disease Control and Prevention. https://www.cdc.gov/mmwr/preview/mmwrhtml/mm4838a2.htm
10. Behrmann BL. A reclamation of childbirth. *J Perinat Educ*. 2003;12(3):vi–x.
11. Duncan F E, Que E L, Zhang N, Feinberg E C, O'Halloran T V, Woodruff T K. The zinc spark is an inorganic signature of human egg activation. *Sci Rep*. 2016 Apr;6:24737.
12. Adam J, Adamczyk L, Adams J R, Adkins J K, Agakishiev G, Aggarwal M M, et al. Measurement of e $^{+}$ e^{-} momentum and angular distributions from linearly polarized photon collisions. *Phys Rev Lett*. 2021 Jul;127(5):052302.
13. Simon-Areces J, Dietrich MO, Hermes G, Garcia-Segura LM, Arevalo M-A, Horvath TL. UCP2 induced by natural birth regulates neuronal differentiation of the hippocampus and related adult behavior. *PLoS One*. 2012;7(8):e42911.
14. Davis-Floyd R. Culture and birth: The technocratic imperative. *Birth Gaz*. 1994;11(1):24–25.
15. *Global Strategy for Women's, Children's and Adolescents' Health (2016–2030)*. New York: Every Woman Every Child; 2015. Available from http://globalstrategy.everywomaneverychild.org/
16. Potts S, Shields SG. *The Experience of Normal Pregnancy: An Overview. Women-Centered Care in Pregnancy and Childbirth*. Edited by Shields SG, Candib LM. Oxford: Radcliffe Publishing; 2010.
17. Haines H M, Rubertsson C, Pallant J F, Hildingsson I. The influence of women's fear, attitudes and beliefs of childbirth on mode and experience of birth. *BMC Pregnancy Childbirth*. 2012 Jun;12:55.
18. Buckley SJ. Executive summary of hormonal physiology of childbearing: Evidence and implications for women, babies, and maternity care. *J Perinat Educ*. 2015;24(3):145–53.
19. Olza I, Uvnas-Moberg K, Ekström- Bergström A, Leahy-Warren P, Karlsdottir SI, Nieuwenhuijze M, et al. Birth as a neuro- psycho-social event: An integrative model of maternal experiences and their relation to neurohormonal events during childbirth. *PLoS One*. 2020 Jul;15(7): e0230992.
20. Uvnas-Moberg K, Ekstro̊ m A, Berg M, Buclkey S, Pajalic Z, Hadjigeorgiou E, et al. Maternal plasma levels of oxytocin during physiological childbirth—a systematic review with implications for uterine contractions and central actions of oxytocin. *BMC Pregnancy Childbirth*. 2019 Aug;19(1):285.
21. Olza I, Leahy-Warren P, Benyamini Y, Kazmierczak M, Karlsdottir SI, Spyridou A, et al. Women's psychological experiences of physiological childbirth: A meta-synthesis. *BMJ Open*. 2018 Oct;8(10):e020347.
22. Kenkel WM, Perkeybile A-M, Yee JR, Pournajafi-Nazarloo H, Lillard TS, Ferguson EF, et al. Behavioral and epigenetic consequences of oxytocin treatment at birth. *Sci Adv*. 2019 May;5(5): eaav2244.

23. Uvnäs-Moberg K, Gross M M, Agius A, Downe S, Calleja-Agius J. Are there epigenetic oxytocin-mediated effects on the mother and infant during physiological childbirth? *Int J Mo. Sci.* 2020 Dec 14;21(24): 9503.

24. Dominguez-Bello M G, Costello E K, Contreras M, Magris M, Hidalgo G, Fierer N et al. Delivery mode shapes the acquisition and structure of the initial microbiota across multiple body habitats in newborns. *Proc Natl Acad Sci USA.* 2010 Jun;107(26): 11971–5.

25. Sevelsted A, Stokholm J, Bønnelykke K, Bisgaard H. Cesarean section and chronic immune disorders. *Pediatrics.* 2015 Jan;135(1): e92–8.

26. Mueller, N. T, Whyatt R, Hoepner L, Oberfield S, Dominguez-Bello M G, Widen E M et al. Prenatal exposure to antibiotics, cesarean section and risk of childhood obesity. *Int J Obes.* 2015 Apr;39(4): 665–670.

27. Reyman M, van Houten MA, van Baarle D, Bosch AATM, Man WH, Chu MLJN, et al. Impact of delivery mode-associated gut microbiota dynamics on health in the first year of life. *Nat Commun.* 2019 Nov;10(1): 4997.

28. Downe S, Finlayson K, Oladapo O, Bonet M, Gülmezoglu AM. What matters to women during childbirth: A systematic qualitative review. *PLoS One.* 2018 Apr;13(4): e0194906.

29. Rosenberg MJ, Hovland CI. Cognitive, affective, and behavioural components of attitudes. *Attitude Organisation and Change: An Analysis of Consistency Among Attitude Components.* New Haven: Yale University Press; 1960:1–14.

30. Hassanzadeh R, Abbas-Alizadeh F, Meedya S, Mohammad-Alizadeh-Charandabi S, Mirghafourvand M. Fear of childbirth, anxiety and depression in three groups of primiparous pregnant women not attending, irregularly attending and regularly attending childbirth preparation classes. *BMC Womens Health.* 2020 Aug;20(1): 180.

31. O'Connell MA, Leahy-Warren P, Khashan AS, Kenny LC, O'Neill SM. Worldwide prevalence of tocophobia in pregnant women: Systematic review and meta-analysis. *Acta Obstet. Gynecol. Scand.* 2017 Aug;96(8): 907–920.

32. O'Connell MA, Khashan AS, Leahy-Warren P. Women's experiences of interventions for fear of childbirth in the perinatal period: A meta-synthesis of qualitative research evidence. *Women Birth.* 2021 May;34(3): e309–e321.

33. Chien L, Ko Y. Fatigue during pregnancy predicts caesarean deliveries. *J Adv Nurs.* 2004 Mar;45(5):487–94.

34. Ward-Ritacco C, Poudevigne MS, O'Connor PJ. Muscle strengthening exercises during pregnancy are associated with increased energy and reduced fatigue. *J Psychosom Obstet Gynecol.* 2016; 37(2): 68–72.

35. Kawanishi Y, Hanley SJB, Tabata K, Nakagin Y, Ito T, Yoshioka E, et al. Effects of prenatal yoga: A systematic review of randomized controlled trials. *Nihon Koshu Eisei Zasshi.* 2015;62(5):221–31.

36. Bohren MA, Vogel JP, Hunter EC, Lutsiv O, Makh SK, Souza JP, et al. The mistreatment of women during childbirth in health facilities globally: A mixed-methods systematic review. *PLoS Med.* 2015 Jun 30;12(6):e1001847.

37. Bohren MA, Berger BO, Munthe-Kaas H, Tunçalp Ö. Perceptions and experiences of labor companionship: A qualitative evidence synthesis. *Cochrane Database Syst Rev* 2019 Mar;3(3): CD012449.

38. Macuhova J, Tancin V, Kraetzl W-D, Meyer HHD, Bruckmaier RM. Inhibition of oxytocin release during repeated milking in unfamiliar surroundings: The importance of opioids and adrenal cortex sensitivity. *J Dairy Res.* 2002 Feb;69(1): 63–73.

39. Uvnäs-Moberg K. *Oxytocin: The Biological Guide to Motherhood.* 14th ed. Amarillo, TX: Praeclarus Press; 2016.

40. Freedman LP, Kruk ME. Disrespect and abuse of women in childbirth: Challenging the global quality and accountability agendas. *Lancet.* 2014 Sep;384(9948): e42–4.

41. The state of the World's Midwifery 2021. https://www.unfpa.org/sites/default/files/pub-pdf/21-038-UNFPA-SoWMy2021-Report-ENv4302_0.pdf

42. Sandall J, Soltani H, Gates S, Shennan A, Devane D. Midwife-led continuity models versus other models of care for childbearing women. *Cochrane Database Syst Rev.* 2016 Apr;4(4): CD004667.

43. Homer CSE, Friberg IK, Dias MAB, Ten Hoope-Bender P, Sandall J, Speciale AM, et al. The projected effect of scaling up midwifery. *Lancet.* 2014 Sep;384(9948): 1146–57.

44. ACOG. American College of Obstetricians and Gynecologists Practice Bulletin. *Dystocia and Augmentation of Labor. Clinical Management Guidelines for Obstetricians-Gynecologists.* No 49. Washington, DC: American College of Obstetricians and Gynecologists; December 2003.

45. Norwitz ER, Robinson JN, Repke JT. Labor and delivery. Gabbe SG, Niebyl JR, Simpson JL, eds. *Obstetrics: Normal and Problem Pregnancies.* 3rd ed. New York: Churchill Livingstone; 2003.

46. The Holistic stages of birth. https://thematrona.com/the-holistic-stages-of-birth/
47. Ellis H. Grantly Dick-Read (1890–1959): Advocate of "natural" childbirth. *Br J Hosp Med.* 2009 Jun;70(6):355.
48. Beynon CL. The normal second stage of labour; a plea for reform in its conduct. *J Obstet Gynaecol Br Emp.* 1957 Dec;64(6): 815–20.

29 An Introduction to Hidden Societal Enigmas That Have Significant Impact on Mental, Physical and Spiritual Health

Dona Biswas

CONTENTS

29.1 INTRODUCTION

The art and science of healing is one as old as mankind itself. Ever since the first hunter-gatherers formed primitive human society, healing has been a part of all human traditions in all parts of the world. Healers, or shamans, have existed since the Paleolithic and Upper Paleolithic era, and they played a pivotal role in cognitive and social evolution through visual symbolism, group bonding rituals and analogical thought processes (Winkelman, 2004).

Since the scientific renaissance and separation of religion and science, dualistic thinking has replaced holistic thinking in Western society. As a consequence, Western health practice has become extrospective, relying on conquering and manipulating the environment rather than introspective and diving within our own unconscious. Yet increasingly, Western medical practitioners are realizing the limitations of current health treatments, especially in defining and enhancing our rich social, cultural and spiritual internal lives, which refuse to be boxed into neat categories of illness.

DOI: 10.1201/b23304-31

In this chapter, we will explore some hidden but universal societal enigmas that have existed since the beginning of civilization and are in fact wired into our very biology, and that have a huge impact on our physical, mental and spiritual health.

29.2 SHAMANS AS HUMANITY'S FIRST HEALERS

Ever since human beings gathered into primitive societies, belief in our connection with the rest of the universe has been a universal feature of all cultures. Spiritual traditions like shamanism and mysticism have been healing humanity for centuries, even before the concept of modern science or medicine existed.

The word "Shaman" is derived from the Siberian Tungus word "saman," literally meaning "someone who can see in the dark" (Beery, 2017). Shamanism is not a religion but a belief system that cuts across all faith and creed, reaching deep levels of ancestral memory (Matthews, 2001). There are as many forms of shamanism as there are cultures. Some notable examples are the Eskimo (Inuit) shaman, the Tamang of Nepal, the Laotian Hmong, North American Indians, the Salish of Pacific Northwest and the Kwakiutl of the Pacific Northwest Coast. It is believed that the worldwide distribution of shamanism in different societies is not the consequence of diffusion but is rather, based on human psychobiology (Winkelman, 2013). We are in fact wired for peak spiritual experiences, and shamanism emerged from the human need to connect to the universe and peak experiences of ecstasy.

A shaman is not seen as a magician but rather, as a healer, a communicator with the divine or with the spirit world, and/or a religious figure. They are understood to have the power to invoke blessings and protection, and the negative ones can cause harm to the subject. They can also have traditional herbal knowledge and wisdom of rites and rituals. They can act as priests or religious figures.

Since the 17th century and the emerging dualistic thinking in Western society, shamanism began to be perceived as contrary to rational thought, and shamans were regarded as little more than theatrical performers (Winkelman, 2013). However, some anthropologists played a vital role in the renewed interest in shamanism in post-modern times. Eliade, in *Shamanism: Archaic Techniques of Ecstasy*, said that the core aspect of all shamanistic practices is ecstasy and altered states of consciousness (Eliade, 1972). Shamanism is based on the concept of animism, a belief that all the universe is imbued with an innate intelligence and communicates with us. A shaman is an expert in accessing non-ordinary states of consciousness in which he believes his soul leaves his body and enters the spirit world, allowing him to access powers like divination, clairvoyance, communicating with spirits and recovering lost soul fragments (Krippner, 2000).

In 1980, Michael Harner, an anthropologist who had studied shamanism in the Amazon since 1950, published *The Way of The Shaman*, where he expanded the term and concept of shamanism (Harner, 1990). Another notable figure in the revival of shamanism was Carlos Castaneda, an anthropologist and shaman.

Winkleman identifies several common characteristics of shamans across all cultures, including a dominant social role, use of chanting, singing and drumming to access altered states of consciousness (ASC), including visionary experiences, and abilities of divination, diagnosis and prophecy. The shaman also specializes in healing processes focused on soul loss and recovery and views animal relations as a source of power (Winkelman, 2013).

Soul loss is a concept in shamanism considered to be a fragmentation or dissociation, generally because of trauma or burnout, either mental, emotional or spiritual. Signs and symptoms of soul loss can be depression and self-neglect, unhealthy coping mechanisms, fatigue and loss of purpose; neglecting work and household tasks, self-care such as showering, cleanliness and dressing appropriately, etc.

29.3 PSYCHOBIOLOGY OF SHAMANIC STATES OF CONSCIOUSNESS

Fundamental to all shamanic practices is the ability to access ASC. The shaman achieves these non-ordinary states of consciousness through drumming, singing, chanting, dancing or using psychoactive substances (Bourguignon, 1972). Preliminary preparation before entering into such states of consciousness includes fasting, water or sleep deprivation, as well as the use of extremes of temperature and exercise (Winkelman, 2017).

Bourguignon (1974) conducted a survey of 488 societies, discovered that 89% of them had some form of ASC and concluded that the ability to experience such states was a physiological capacity of all human beings (Bourguignon, 1974). The extensive sympathetic activation associated with the preliminary rituals leads to a collapse and consequent parasympathetic dominant state with theta discharges in the range of 3–6 cycles per second from the limbic and lower brain structures, which synchronize the frontal cortex (Winkelman, 2004). This state is associated with selectively focused attention, heightened suggestibility, various degrees of analgesia and behaviors that are experienced as not under voluntary control. Along with these changes, there is also activation of the serotonergic nervous system and release of endogenous opioids. This psychobiologic state is very similar to a state of meditation and forms the basis for experiences like enlightenment and universal connection. These psychobiologic changes are the foundation of ecstatic states, a need for which is wired into our very biology. It is for this reason that many anthropologists like Winkleman consider shamanism as the original neurotherapy. Current psychotherapeutic approaches focus on the conscious mind and only approach the unconscious through indirect processes. The shaman, on the other hand, invites people to access non-ordinary and expanded states of awareness, which enables them to heal at a deeper level. It is thus no wonder that there has been a revival of the core concepts of shamanism in Western cultures in recent decades.

29.4 NEOSHAMANISM

In today's world, it is not always possible for individuals to travel to indigenous cultures and train under such shamans. Post-modern shamanism or neoshamanism aims to redeem a shamanistic past but with significant changes from the original concept. Michael Harner, who formed the Foundation of Shamanic Studies (FSS), can be regarded as one of the founders of neoshamanism. Neoshamanism retains some of the core elements of shamanism, like accessing ASC, use of spirit guides and power animals, and journeying for soul retrieval. However, notable absences are the use of shamanic powers to kill and for sorcery, hunting magic and war parties (vonStuckrad, 2002). Although some anthropologists consider neoshamanism as a watered-down version of true shamanism, it is gaining immense popularity, especially in the United States and Canada, where it is estimated that there are about 100,000 neoshamanic practitioners.

29.5 THE SHAMANIC VERSUS WESTERN MODEL OF MENTAL ILLNESS

Our current model of mental illness is Eurocentric and does not do justice to the diverse cultures of the world (Krippner, 2007). Although cultural competency is becoming a buzzword nowadays, it is more of a lip service and does little to explore the meaning of mental illnesses in different communities. For example, in many native cultures, it is acceptable to hear messages from the earth and talk to nature, yet such people are often labelled as psychotic according to the Western classificatory system. It is thus common for mediums and channels to practice their art in anonymity for fear of being branded mentally ill (Krippner, 2007).

Our current "scientific" approach considers all unusual mental symptoms to be manifestations of imbalances in brain chemistry. On the other hand, shamanistic traditions view such episodes as a spiritual crisis imbued with personal meaning for the individual and believe that traversing this crisis, rather than suppressing it, leads to the resolution of symptoms. The Western medical model treats the "patient" in isolation, increasing stigma, whereas the shamanistic approach attempts to integrate the person within society and considers him a valued member of the community (Nishimura, 1987). In fact, many individuals who experience a spiritual crisis in traditional societies later go on to become shamans themselves, thus embodying the archetype of the "wounded healer." It thus comes as little surprise that the integrative model of neoshamanism is on the rise in modern society.

29.6   SHAMANISM, PLATONIC AND JUNGIAN PSYCHOLOGY

Carl Jung's psychology has several striking similarities to the shamanic worldview, so much so that many regard Jung as a shaman himself. Jung emphasized the importance of the sacred in healing processes and in fact, considered psychologists to be doctors of the soul, similar to shamans.

Jungian psychology proposes animism and the collective unconscious as central to human existence. The unconscious constantly produces animistic motifs, and the archetype is an expression of such a motif; these can be defined as autonomous energetic blueprints that are common to all human beings (Bright, 2009).

Jung himself was influenced by the Platonic worldview, which has animistic roots, focusing on spiritual nature, that is, the "inner meaning" of beings, which they try to fulfil during their existence on earth. Jung's archetypes have their roots in animism, the difference being that animism represents a metaphysical view of reality, while archetypes belong to the unconscious and behave autonomously.

Both shamanism and Jungian psychology seek to treat soul loss by retrieving and reintegrating the vital essence that is missing in a person's life. In many ways, Jung could be regarded as the modern shaman of psychology. The modern scientific paradigm, on the other hand, originates in the thinking of Aristotle, with his emphasis on empiricism and the observable. Jung mourned the loss of shamanistic perspective in modern society, and he identified our increasing analytic thinking as devastating to our wellbeing (Bright, 2009).

29.7   PARALLELS BETWEEN SHAMANISM AND EASTERN PHILOSOPHY

Many shamanic practices around the world include knowledge of *chakras* and *kundalini* (Raiguel, 2010). For example, the Sami system from Northern Scandinavia, the Buryat tradition from Siberia and the Q'uaro of Peru all mention the existence of chakras along the central axis of the body. In fact, Eliade says that yoga itself developed out of shamanism and is an internalized version of a much older shamanic technique (Elaide, 1972). Many shamanic traditions work with a cosmic force rising through the chakras, leading to illumination and enlightenment. This cosmic force, better known as *kundalini (*in Sanskrit), is represented as a coiled serpent or spiral within the base of the spine. The spiral is an archetypal representation of spiritual development in many spiritual traditions. In cultures like the Australian Aborigines, it is represented as a serpent eating its own tail (Villoldo, 2000).

Interestingly, the universal symbol of medicine, the Caduceus of Hermes, depicts two serpents coiled around a staff. This symbol is found both in shamanism and in kundalini yoga. It is believed to represent the central column of the spinal cord (or *Sushumna Nadi* in Sanskrit), around which the masculine and feminine energies (also called *Ida* and *Pingala* in Sanskrit) are wrapped. The recognition of masculine and feminine energies is also seen in Chinese medicine, where the yin and yang are depicted as being coiled around each other in an eternal dance. Although modern medicine may not recognize it, even its symbolic roots are based in shamanism and Eastern philosophy.

29.8   NADIS, MERIDIANS AND THE PRIMOVASCULAR SYSTEM:

The concept of "vital energy" is shared by many ethnomedical healing and shamanic traditions. Chinese medicine calls this vital energy *chi*, while traditional Indian medicine knows it as *prana*. Shamans have long recognized that a vital energy flows between the shaman and all living things. Energy flows are explicitly described in some shamanistic works, and some techniques, like cupping and needling, are very similar to Chinese acupuncture and utilize the concept of meridians, or channels through which vital energy is thought to flow.

Till recently, it was believed that the meridian system lacked an anatomical basis. However, researchers have now validated the existence of a new body system called the primovascular system

(PVS), which corresponds to the meridians described in Chinese medicine. The system was initially described in the 1960s by Bong-Han Kim of North Korea but did not gain attention till 2002, when its existence was confirmed by researchers in South Korea (Stefanov et al., 2013).

The primovascular system pervades the subcutaneous tissues, organs, fascia, etc. and consists of thread-like structures that contain primo fluid, which is rich in extranuclear DNA, RNA, mononucleotides and amino acids. Primo vessels show electrical activity and are believed to act as optic channels of biophoton emissions, while the DNA in the fluid may act as a photon store. These biophotons are believed to play a key role in cell development and differentiation (Rahnama et al., 2011). The discovery of the PVS is able to explain how vital energy, in the form of biophotons, travels through the body and can be extensively manipulated by therapies like acupuncture to encourage healing. While the PVS is still to be charted in its entirety, the map so far is very similar to the map of the *meridians* in Chinese medicine and the *nadis* in Indian medicine.

29.9   CHAKRA ANATOMY AND THE LUMINOUS ENERGY FIELD

Many shamanic cultures recognize chakras as a part of the anatomy of the luminous energy field, or the biofield, as it is now called. The Maya, the Hopi, the Inka and other native groups described nine gates a person passes through to become a sage. These correspond to the chakras. For the shaman, chakras extend luminous threads or *huascas* that reach beyond the body, connecting us to the trees, rivers and forests (Villoldo, 2000).

The question is: Are chakras simply a metaphysical concept shared by different cultures of the world, or are they a part of the energetic anatomy of humans? Modern medicine only recognizes physical anatomy, and hence, most treatments are based in physicality. Fortunately, over the last few decades, innovative technological development has allowed us to gather evidence of the energetic anatomy of humans. One such technique is gas discharge visualization (GDV), developed by Dr Konstantin Korotkov into the Biowell GDV camera, which uses electrical fields to stimulate photon emission from the skin, which is then captured by the camera and mapped to different organs and energy meridians of the body (Korotkov, 2004).

Candace Pert, a neuroscientist, has demonstrated that the chakras are associated with glands and nerve plexuses that are rich in neuropeptides, or "molecules of emotions" as she calls them. Chakras are rich in neuropeptides and thus like "mini brains" (Pert, 1997). Chakras can also be considered to be energy transducers that convert physical energy to subtle energy and vice versa.

It is widely recognized across cultures that chakras also represent developmental stages that an individual needs to traverse on the path to self-actualization. Interestingly, these chakra stages correspond fairly accurately to the psychosocial stages of human development proposed by psychologist Eric Ericson (Erikson, 1959). The chakras and their role in spiritual development across the life cycle has long been recognized in shamanic practice as well (Wright, 2007).

29.9.1   ROOT CHAKRA: TRUST VERSUS MISTRUST

From birth to 18 months of age, infants are completely dependent on their caregivers and learn to trust the world if the care is consistent and predictable. This corresponds to the development of the root chakra, which forms the basis of our sense of security about the world.

29.9.2   SACRAL CHAKRA: AUTONOMY VERSUS SHAME

Between the ages of 1 and 3 years, toddlers begin to explore the world and themselves and establish their independence. They start exploring their sexual and excretory organs and gain control over them. This corresponds to the development of the sacral chakra, which gives us a sense of well-being and comfort in our own bodies.

29.9.3 Solar Plexus Chakra: Initiative versus Guilt, Industry versus Inferiority, Identity versus Role Confusion

Children between the ages of 3 and 6 learn to assert themselves in their environment and interactions, corresponding to the stage of initiative versus guilt. From the age of 6 to 12 years, they begin to compare themselves with their peers and either develop a sense of pride in themselves and their achievements or feel inferior because they don't measure up. This is the stage of industry versus inferiority. In adolescence, between the ages of 12 and 18 years, individuals start questioning their role in the world or purpose in life in relation to others. This stage is referred to as the stage of identity versus role confusion, where individuals start to form a clearer sense of identity. Successful navigation of these stages results in a confident individual and corresponds to the development of the solar plexus, the seat of our power and self-esteem.

29.9.4 Heart Chakra: Intimacy versus Isolation

During early to mid-adulthood (20–40 years), individuals learn to give and receive love and develop intimate, long-term relationships. Successful negotiation of this stage results in the formation of intimate relationships, and failure to do so results in feeling isolated. This stage corresponds to the development of the heart chakra, when we start to focus away from self to friends, partner, family, community, country and ultimately, the world. Ancient traditions consider the heart chakra as the integrator that merges the lower and higher chakras into a more wholesome human experience. It represents the inner marriage of the divine masculine and feminine, the yin and yang, and a more balanced personality.

29.9.5 Throat Chakra: Generativity versus Stagnation

During mid-adulthood (40 to 60 years), the focus often shifts from individual achievements to contributing to the world and others. This corresponds to the development of the throat chakra, successful negotiation of which results in the satisfaction of expressing our truth and contributing to society. In shamanism, *shapeshifting* is a tool to become that which you have previously wished to become, and it helps navigate the conflict of the throat chakra. According to shamanic traditions, shapeshifting can happen on three different levels: The cellular level, changing the physical form to heal illness; the personal level, healing addictions, relationships and behavioral patterns; and institutional, changing organizations on a larger level.

29.9.6 Third Eye Chakra: Integrity versus Despair

From their mid-sixties to the end of life, individuals reflect on their lives and feel either a sense of integrity or a sense of regret or despair. This corresponds to the development of the third eye, a realization of the bigger picture, something beyond "doing": simply "being."

29.9.7 Crown Chakra: Mastery versus Distraction

Although Ericson's stages end with integrity versus despair, ancient traditions recognized a further stage of development, with the opening of the crown chakra and channeling universal love. This is the stage of mastery versus distraction. The individual with an open crown chakra becomes a master, adept at channeling universal love and subtle energy.

It is important to understand that this is only an indicative and not an absolute model. While psychospiritual development usually follows these stages, the challenges are unique for each individual, and while some people might be highly spiritual at an early age and be able to access their higher chakras, others might only be able to negotiate the first few chakras in their lifetime. Although each person's journey is very individual, there are shamanistic tools that are useful to negotiate each developmental stage.

29.10 THE INTEGRATIVE PSYCHOLOGY OF THE FUTURE

Two decades of working as a psychiatrist has convinced me that talk therapy is often not enough to achieve healing. Modern psychology believes that once you become cognizant of unconscious complexes and drives, you can be free of their influence. However, shamans believe that intellectual cognizance is not enough for healing. Healing has both a developmental and a subtle energetic component. Talk therapy works on a mental level and is unable to erase the imprint of trauma on the energetic field (Villoldo, 2000). This is a fact that is only recently being recognized by psychologists and psychiatrists.

Spiritual traditions like shamanism and Eastern philosophy have been healing humans for centuries, and to ignore the richness of these traditions can only be to the detriment of our future (McKernan, 2007). Science is just one aspect of the world we live in and fails to do justice to the fact that we are rich multidimensional beings and are biologically wired to seek spirituality, transcendental experiences and magic in our lives.

More recently, our relationship with both science and spirituality is changing. On the one hand, we are moving away from rigid and artificial religious structures to explore what intuitively appeals to us and connects us to the universe. On the other hand, the narrow dualistic Newtonian science is giving way to a greater awareness of the intricacies of quantum physics and the role of consciousness in navigating our reality. It suddenly appears as if we have come a full circle – we are now using a new paradigm in science to validate what ancient traditions recognized intuitively. The divide between science and spirituality is gradually being healed to enable us to honor and experience ourselves and our environments as multidimensional beings.

REFERENCES

Beery, I. 2017. *Shamanic Healing: Traditional Medicine for the Modern World*. Destiny Books: Simon and Schuster.

Bourguignon, E. 1972. "Dreams and Altered States of Consciousness in Anthropological Research." In *Psychological Anthropology*, edited by Francis L K Hsu, 403–34. Cambridge: Schenkman Publishing Company.

———. 1974. *Culture and the Varieties of Consciousness. Vol. 47. Addison-Wesley Module in Anthropology*. Boston: Addison-Wesley.

Bright, B. 2009. *The Shamanic Perspective: Where Jungian Thought and Archetypal Shamanism Converge. Written Works of Bonnie Bright*. Depth Insights.

Elaide, M. 1972. *Shamanism: Archaic Technique of Ecstasy*. Princeton: Princeton University Press.

Erikson, E. H. 1959. *Identity and the Life Cycle: Selected Papers*. New York: International Universities Press.

Harner, M. J. 1990. *The Way of the Shaman*. San Francisco: Harper & Row.

Korotkov, K. 2004. *Measuring Energy Field: State-of-the-Science*. Fair Lawn: Backbone; Lancaster Gazelle.

Krippner, S. 2000. "The Epistemology and Technologies of Shamanic States of Consciousness." *Journal of Consciousness Studies* 7 (11–12): 93–118.

Krippner, S. 2007. "Humanity's First Healers: Psychological and Psychiatric Stances on Shamans and Shamanism." *Revista de Psiquiatria Clínica* 34 (1): 16–22.

Matthews, J. 2001. *The Celtic Shaman: A Practical Guide*. London: Ebury Publishing.

McKernan, M. 2007. "Exploring the Spiritual Dimension of Social Work." In *Spirituality and Social Work: Select Canadian Readings*, edited by J. R. Graham, J. Coates, B. Swantzenbribier, B. Quelette. Canadian Scholar's Press Inc.

Nishimura, K. 1987. "Shamanism and Medical Cures." *Current Anthropology* 28 (4): 59–64.

Pert, C. B. 1997. *Molecules of Emotion: Why You Feel the Way You Feel*. London: Simon & Schuster.

Raiguel, J. 2010. "Chakra Rebuilding: A Shamanic Healing Tool." *The International Journal of Healing and Caring* 10 (3). https://irp-cdn.multiscreensite.com/891f98f6/files/uploaded/Raiguel-10-3F.pdf.

Rahnama, M., Tuszynski, J., Bokkon, I., Cifra, M., Sardar, P., Salari, V. 2011. "Emission of Mitochondrial Biophotons and Their Effect on Electrical Activity of Membrane Via Microtubules." *Journal of Integrative Neuroscience* 10 (1): 65–88.

Stefanov, M., Potroz, M., Kim, J., Lim, J., Cha, R., Nam, M. "The Primovascular System as a New Anatomical System." *Journal of Acupuncture and Meridian Studies* 6 (6): 331–338.

Villoldo, A. 2000. *Shaman, Healer, Sage: How to Heal Yourself and Others with The Energy Medicine of the Americas*. New York: Harmony Books.

von Stuckrad, K. 2002. "Re-enchanting Nature: Modern Western Shamanism and Nineteenth Century Thought." *Journal of the American Academy of Religion* 70 (4): 771–799.

Winkelman, M. 2004. "Shamanism as the Original Neurotheology." *Zygon* 39 (1): 193–217.

———. 2013. "Shamanism in Cross-cultural Perspective." *International Journal of Transpersonal Studies* 31 (2): 47–62.

———. 2017. "Shamanism and the Brain." In *Religion: Mental Religion*, edited by N. K. Clements, 355–372. McMillan Handbooks.

Wright, S. 2007. *The Chakras in Shamanic Practice: Eight Stages of Healing and Transformation*. Destiny Books.

Index

Milton Keynes UK
Ingram Content Group UK Ltd.
UKHW052025141024
449569UK00016B/706

9 781032 110127